Therapeutic Monoclonal Antibodies and Antibody Products, Their Optimization and Drug Design in Cancers

Therapeutic Monoclonal Antibodies and Antibody Products, Their Optimization and Drug Design in Cancers

Editor

Veysel Kayser

MDPI • Basel • Beijing • Wuhan • Barcelona • Belgrade • Manchester • Tokyo • Cluj • Tianjin

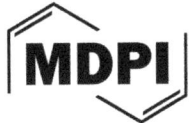

Editor
Veysel Kayser
Sydney School of Pharmacy
The University of Sydney
Sydney
Australia

Editorial Office
MDPI
St. Alban-Anlage 66
4052 Basel, Switzerland

This is a reprint of articles from the Special Issue published online in the open access journal *Cancers* (ISSN 2072-6694) (available at: www.mdpi.com/journal/cancers/special_issues/Antibody_Cancers).

For citation purposes, cite each article independently as indicated on the article page online and as indicated below:

LastName, A.A.; LastName, B.B.; LastName, C.C. Article Title. *Journal Name* **Year**, *Volume Number*, Page Range.

ISBN 978-3-0365-2687-4 (Hbk)
ISBN 978-3-0365-2686-7 (PDF)

© 2022 by the authors. Articles in this book are Open Access and distributed under the Creative Commons Attribution (CC BY) license, which allows users to download, copy and build upon published articles, as long as the author and publisher are properly credited, which ensures maximum dissemination and a wider impact of our publications.

The book as a whole is distributed by MDPI under the terms and conditions of the Creative Commons license CC BY-NC-ND.

Contents

About the Editor vii

Preface to "Therapeutic Monoclonal Antibodies and Antibody Products, Their Optimization
and Drug Design in Cancers" ix

Esteban Cruz and Veysel Kayser
Synthesis and Enhanced Cellular Uptake In Vitro of Anti-HER2 Multifunctional Gold
Nanoparticles
Reprinted from: *Cancers* 2019, 11, 870, doi:10.3390/cancers11060870 1

Haozhong Ding, Mohamed Altai, Sara S. Rinne, Anzhelika Vorobyeva, Vladimir Tolmachev,
Torbjörn Gräslund and Anna Orlova
Incorporation of a Hydrophilic Spacer Reduces Hepatic Uptake of HER2-Targeting
Affibody–DM1 Drug Conjugates
Reprinted from: *Cancers* 2019, 11, 1168, doi:10.3390/cancers11081168 23

Dennis Kirchhoff, Beatrix Stelte-Ludwig, Hans-Georg Lerchen, Antje Margret Wengner,
Oliver von Ahsen, Pascale Buchmann, Stephan Märsch, Christoph Mahlert, Simone Greven,
Lisa Dietz, Michael Erkelenz, Ruprecht Zierz, Sandra Johanssen, Dominik Mumberg and
Anette Sommer
IL3RA-Targeting Antibody–Drug Conjugate BAY-943 with a Kinesin Spindle Protein Inhibitor
Payload Shows Efficacy in Preclinical Models of Hematologic Malignancies
Reprinted from: *Cancers* 2020, 12, 3464, doi:10.3390/cancers12113464 43

Marta Lisowska, Magdalena Milczarek, Jarosław Ciekot, Justyna Kutkowska, Wojciech
Hildebrand, Andrzej Rapak and Arkadiusz Miazek
An Antibody Specific for the Dog Leukocyte Antigen DR (DLA-DR) and Its Novel Methotrexate
Conjugate Inhibit the Growth of Canine B Cell Lymphoma
Reprinted from: *Cancers* 2019, 11, 1438, doi:10.3390/cancers11101438 61

Koichi Saruwatari, Ryo Sato, Shunya Nakane, Shinya Sakata, Koutaro Takamatsu, Takayuki
Jodai, Remi Mito, Yuko Horio, Sho Saeki, Yusuke Tomita and Takuro Sakagami
The Risks and Benefits of Immune Checkpoint Blockade in Anti-AChR Antibody-Seropositive
Non-Small Cell Lung Cancer Patients
Reprinted from: *Cancers* 2019, 11, 140, doi:10.3390/cancers11020140 75

Sarah L. Picardo, Jeffrey Doi and Aaron R. Hansen
Structure and Optimization of Checkpoint Inhibitors
Reprinted from: *Cancers* 2019, 12, 38, doi:10.3390/cancers12010038 89

Katsiaryna Marhelava, Zofia Pilch, Malgorzata Bajor, Agnieszka Graczyk-Jarzynka and
Radoslaw Zagozdzon
Targeting Negative and Positive Immune Checkpoints with Monoclonal Antibodies in Therapy
of Cancer
Reprinted from: *Cancers* 2019, 11, 1756, doi:10.3390/cancers11111756 105

Maria Silvia Cona, Mara Lecchi, Sara Cresta, Silvia Damian, Michele Del Vecchio, Andrea Necchi, Marta Maria Poggi, Daniele Raggi, Giovanni Randon, Raffaele Ratta, Diego Signorelli, Claudio Vernieri, Filippo de Braud, Paolo Verderio and Massimo Di Nicola
Combination of Baseline LDH, Performance Status and Age as Integrated Algorithm to Identify Solid Tumor Patients with Higher Probability of Response to Anti PD-1 and PD-L1 Monoclonal Antibodies
Reprinted from: *Cancers* **2019**, *11*, 223, doi:10.3390/cancers11020223 127

Bastian J. Schmied, Fabian Riegg, Latifa Zekri, Ludger Grosse-Hovest, Hans-Jörg Bühring, Gundram Jung and Helmut R. Salih
An Fc-Optimized CD133 Antibody for Induction of Natural Killer Cell Reactivity Against Colorectal Cancer
Reprinted from: *Cancers* **2019**, *11*, 789, doi:10.3390/cancers11060789 139

Gergely Solecki, Matthias Osswald, Daniel Weber, Malte Glock, Miriam Ratliff, Hans-Joachim Müller, Oliver Krieter, Yvonne Kienast, Wolfgang Wick and Frank Winkler
Differential Effects of Ang-2/VEGF-A Inhibiting Antibodies in Combination with Radio- or Chemotherapy in Glioma
Reprinted from: *Cancers* **2019**, *11*, 314, doi:10.3390/cancers11030314 153

Jessica Cusato, Carlo Genova, Cristina Tomasello, Paolo Carrega, Selene Ottonello, Gabriella Pietra, Maria Cristina Mingari, Irene Cossu, Erika Rijavec, Anna Leggieri, Giovanni Di Perri, Maria Giovanna Dal Bello, Simona Coco, Simona Boccardo, Guido Ferlazzo, Francesco Grossi and Antonio D'Avolio
Influence of Vitamin D in Advanced Non-Small Cell Lung Cancer Patients Treated with Nivolumab
Reprinted from: *Cancers* **2019**, *11*, 125, doi:10.3390/cancers11010125 169

Yuki Katayama, Junji Uchino, Yusuke Chihara, Nobuyo Tamiya, Yoshiko Kaneko, Tadaaki Yamada and Koichi Takayama
Tumor Neovascularization and Developments in Therapeutics
Reprinted from: *Cancers* **2019**, *11*, 316, doi:10.3390/cancers11030316 181

Francesca Bonello, Roberto Mina, Mario Boccadoro and Francesca Gay
Therapeutic Monoclonal Antibodies and Antibody Products: Current Practices and Development in Multiple Myeloma
Reprinted from: *Cancers* **2019**, *12*, 15, doi:10.3390/cancers12010015 197

Mathilde Bonnet, Aurélie Maisonial-Besset, Yingying Zhu, Tiffany Witkowski, Gwenaëlle Roche, Claude Boucheix, Céline Greco and Françoise Degoul
Targeting the Tetraspanins with Monoclonal Antibodies in Oncology: Focus on Tspan8/Co-029
Reprinted from: *Cancers* **2019**, *11*, 179, doi:10.3390/cancers11020179 221

Aena Patel, Nisha Unni and Yan Peng
The Changing Paradigm for the Treatment of HER2-Positive Breast Cancer
Reprinted from: *Cancers* **2020**, *12*, 2081, doi:10.3390/cancers12082081 235

Malgorzata Bobrowicz, Radoslaw Zagozdzon, Joanna Domagala, Roberta Vasconcelos-Berg, Emmanuella Guenova and Magdalena Winiarska
Monoclonal Antibodies in Dermatooncology—State of the Art and Future Perspectives
Reprinted from: *Cancers* **2019**, *11*, 1420, doi:10.3390/cancers11101420 253

About the Editor

Veysel Kayser

Veysel Kayser is an Associate Professor at The University of Sydney (USyd). He completed his B.Sc. degree in Chemistry at Hacettepe University (Turkey) and his Ph.D. in Physical Chemistry at the University of Leeds (UK) in 2004. Subsequently, he undertook post-doctoral fellowships at the Max-Planck Institute of Biochemistry (Germany) and in the Department of Chemical Engineering at MIT (US), and then he worked at MIT for several years as a senior staff scientist. In mid-2013, he took up his current position at USyd. For periods, he was also the Associate Dean for Research and the HDR coordinator at the Faculty of Pharmacy and served in the Multidisciplinary Advisory Board of the Marie Bashir Institute for Infectious Diseases and Biosecurity at USyd (now Sydney Institute for Infectious Diseases).

His research interests are in biologics and vaccines (influenza, rabies, COVID-19, etc.), the development of biosimilars and biobetters, mainly therapeutic monoclonal antibodies (mAbs), antibody–drug conjugates, nanoparticle–antibody complexes, protein engineering, novel formulations of biologics and vaccines, and the mechanisms of protein unfolding and aggregation.

He has obtained five patents, with several more pending, has published over fifty peer-reviewed research publications, has given over 100 talks on biologics and vaccines, and also serves as an editor or member of the editorial board of various journals. He has consulted for and received research funding from industry. He has received numerous awards and fellowships.

Preface to "Therapeutic Monoclonal Antibodies and Antibody Products, Their Optimization and Drug Design in Cancers"

Various forms of antibody products, particularly full-size monoclonal antibodies (mAbs), have been dominating the biologics market due to their specificity and selectivity. They are also the mainstay for the development of next-generation biologics and biobetters for a number of disorders, including cancer. Currently, there are more than 100 approved antibody therapeutics on the market, but thousands are in clinical trials at various stages. It is perhaps not surprising that a considerable number of these medications have been developed for the treatment of different types of cancers.

Biosimilars of some of the top-selling biologics including mAbs are now on the market due to the expirations of patent protections and changes in the regulatory framework around the world; nevertheless, we are yet to see a major global impact of biosimilars. Notwithstanding biosimilar development, a great deal of effort is being made to develop the next-generation mAbs. These include different forms of antibody products including but not limited to bispecific or multispecific mAbs, hyperglycosylated mAbs, antibody–drug conjugates (ADC), single-domain antibodies (nanobodies), and antibody-based nanoparticles. Most of these new developments have been made to address the concerns of the structural stability of antibodies, commonly observed formulation issues, protein degradation, especially due to aggregation, and efficacy and specificity.

Trail-and-error methods still dominate the overall drug development and are commonly applied in different phases of the development of biologics too, including antibody therapeutics. Rational drug development is only possible through the development of novel experimental and computational methods and by elucidating interactions at the molecular level. Most of the drug candidates comprising the next-generation biologics and antibody products would benefit from additional optimization. With the advance of experimental and computational methods, we can now further optimize antibodies as never before.

In this Special Issue of *Cancers*, we have collated sixteen manuscripts, contributed by leading scientists in the field, showcasing the current state of play as well as recent developments in mAb therapeutics and other antibody products used in cancer, their optimization using experimental and/or computational approaches, new developments in immune checkpoint inhibitors, bi-/multispecifics, ADC, nanobodies and antibody-based nanoparticles.

Cellular uptake is an important issue for many drugs and particularly important in several types of cancers and it may be one of the major roadblocks / hurdles when delivering drugs. Several methods have been utilised by Cruz and Kayser to overcome this roadblock, including using a cell-penetrating peptide, where enhanced uptake is achieved when nanoparticles are complexed with such a peptide.

The conjugation of antibodies or antibody products such as fragments to other molecules or nanoparticles has been a subject of study due to its importance when preparing ADCs, bispecifics and antibody–nanoparticle complexes. Conjugation requires introducing a spacer or linker, which may present its own challenges, as Ding et al. demonstrated, where a hydrophilic spacer reduced the uptake of a HER2-targeting affibody–drug conjugate. Kirchhof et al. reported an ADC in hematologic malignancies and Lisowska et al. reported a conjugate for canine B cell lymphoma.

The discovery of immune checkpoint inhibitors has generated excitement around the globe and earned Nobel Prizes in 2018, due to unmatched patient outcomes with regard to several types of cancer. However, blocking the function of immune checkpoint may also be detrimental to the patient due to the triggering of myasthenia gravis. Saruwatari et al. conducted a risk-benefit analysis of immune checkpoint blockage for some non-small cell lung cancer patients. Picardo et al. investigated the structure and discussed the optimization issues of checkpoint inhibitors. Marhelava et al. investigated the targeting of checkpoints with antibodies in cancer therapy. Predicting the response of a patient to a particular therapy is still an onerous task and nearly impossible in many scenarios due to the lack of appropriate factors. Cona et al. attempted to identify parameters that are important as a predictive biomarker response.

Immunotherapy comprises the induction of killer cells against cancer. The Fc domain of antibodies plays a crucial role in inducing this process and many studies have been conducted to enhance this function. Schmied et al. optimized the Fc of the CD133 antibody to induce killer cell reactivity against colorectal cancer.

In some cases, a combination therapy is better than a single approach. Solecki et al. demonstrated that a combination therapy with radio- or chemotherapy with anti-Ang2/VEGF-A displayed better antitumor activity than standard therapies.

Cusato et al. also studied non-small cell lung cancer patients who were treated with Nivolumab and researched the influence of vitamin D.

Katayama et al. reviewed tumor neovascularization and Bonnet et al. targeted tetraspanins with mAbs. Neovascularization is an important process in tumor proliferation and is immature in tumors and affects many aspects of the tumor microenvironment, while tetraspinins play a crucial role in the fixation of antibodies; the functions of Tspan8/Co-029 are summarised in this review.

Bonello et al. reviewed used antibodies and those in development for multiple myeloma. Investigating HER2+ breast cancer, Patel et al. reviewed the new developments for the treatment of HER2+ breast cancer and evaluated new mAbs. Bobrowicz et al. reviewed mAbs in dermatooncology.

I would like to express my gratitude to the *Cancers* editorial office and many colleagues for their help behind the scenes. They worked tirelessly to ensure all submissions were processed smoothly and peer reviews were conducted in a reasonable time and subsequent revisions were completed to the highest standards. I also would like to thank them for allowing me to oversee this Special Issue; it's been an enjoyable journey and I look forward to working together again in the future.

I also would like to extend my appreciation to all the authors for providing quality and informative manuscripts and taking reviewers' and editorial comments seriously and addressing them promptly for timely publications.

Lastly, I would like to thank the reader for supporting us by reading these manuscripts which are the fruits of authors' hard labour and efforts.

Veysel Kayser
Editor

Synthesis and Enhanced Cellular Uptake In Vitro of Anti-HER2 Multifunctional Gold Nanoparticles

Esteban Cruz and Veysel Kayser *

School of Pharmacy, The University of Sydney, Sydney 2006, NSW, Australia; esteban.cruzgonzalez@sydney.edu.au
* Correspondence: veysel.kayser@sydney.edu.au; Tel.: +61-2-9351-3391

Received: 25 April 2019; Accepted: 17 June 2019; Published: 21 June 2019

Abstract: Nanoparticle carriers offer the possibility of enhanced delivery of therapeutic payloads in tumor tissues due to tumor-selective accumulation through the enhanced permeability and retention effect (EPR). Gold nanoparticles (AuNP), in particular, possess highly appealing features for development as nanomedicines, such as biocompatibility, tunable optical properties and a remarkable ease of surface functionalization. Taking advantage of the latter, several strategies have been designed to increase treatment specificity of gold nanocarriers by attaching monoclonal antibodies on the surface, as a way to promote selective interactions with the targeted cells—an approach referred to as active-targeting. Here, we describe the synthesis of spherical gold nanoparticles surface-functionalized with an anti-HER2 antibody-drug conjugate (ADC) as an active targeting agent that carries a cytotoxic payload. In addition, we enhanced the intracellular delivery properties of the carrier by attaching a cell penetrating peptide to the active-targeted nanoparticles. We demonstrate that the antibody retains high receptor-affinity after the structural modifications performed for drug-conjugation and nanoparticle attachment. Furthermore, we show that antibody attachment increases cellular uptake in HER2 amplified cell lines selectively, and incorporation of the cell penetrating peptide leads to a further increase in cellular internalization. Nanoparticle-bound antibody-drug conjugates retain high antimitotic potency, which could contribute to a higher therapeutic index in high EPR tumors.

Keywords: gold nanoparticles; antibody-drug conjugates; cell penetrating peptide; HIV-1 TAT; active-targeting; targeted delivery; trastuzumab; MMAE; valine-citrulline

1. Introduction

Most solid malignancies display a tumor microenvironment with increased interstitial fluid pressures (IFP) that significantly impairs tumor penetration of conventional anticancer agents following systemic delivery. This effect hinders movement of the therapeutic agent from the vascular lumen to the tumor tissue, requiring higher doses to achieve therapeutic efficacy [1,2]. Consequently, the therapeutic index is reduced, and off-target side-effects compromise clinical outcomes. Moreover, inefficient localization in the target tissue can lead to tumor regions exposed to subtherapeutic doses of the drug, whereby cancer cells can undergo phenotypic alterations that render them resistant to the agent administered [3].

In this context, nanoparticles (NPs) have emerged as drug delivery vehicles that can harness the preferential accumulation of nanosized materials in the tumor due to the well-described enhanced permeability and retention (EPR) effect [4]. Several liposome-encapsulated cytotoxic drugs have received regulatory approval on the basis of superior therapeutic indices relative to the free drug [5]. A further attractive feature of nanoparticles is their functional versatility, as their design can be tailored to confer diverse physiological and physicochemical properties to broaden treatment modalities. Myriad distinct NP formats are undergoing preclinical development for various therapeutic and diagnostic applications, e.g., gene delivery, thermal ablation therapy, magnetic resonance imaging (MRI), photoacoustic imaging [6–9].

Among the diverse range of inorganic NPs, gold nanoparticles (AuNP) have been widely appraised as attractive systems for therapeutic applications, e.g., drug delivery, photothermal therapy and radiosensitization [9,10]. AuNPs are easy to synthesize with tunable shapes and sizes, and the strong gold-sulfur (Au-S) interaction allows for the modification of the nanoparticle surface with sulfhydryl containing linkers, through which functional groups can be incorporated to confer biological properties for therapeutic purposes [11]. An analysis of nanoparticle tumor delivery efficiency in in vivo models derived from published data from the year 2005 to 2015 showed that AuNPs had the highest median delivery efficiency among the analyzed inorganic nanoparticle types (including iron oxide, silica, quantum dots and others) [12]. Moreover, a PEGylated AuNP format coated with TNF-α has already shown a promising safety profile and enhanced accumulation in various solid tumors in a phase I dose escalation trial, setting a clinical precedent for gold nanoparticles [13,14].

Adding to the inherent passive accumulation of NPs in solid tumors, the targeting capacity of a nanoparticle carrier can potentially be enhanced by the incorporation of an active targeting agent on the NP surface. Active targeting moieties—e.g., antibodies, peptides, aptamers, affimers—can engage in high-affinity specific interactions with biomolecules overexpressed in cancer subtypes to increase treatment specificity [15]. Within this concept, systemic delivery of the nanocarrier results in passive accumulation in the tumor microenvironment, where the subsequent interaction of the affixed targeting agent with cancer cells can induce receptor crosslinking, receptor-mediated endocytosis and intracellular cargo delivery [16].

In this work, we employed an anti-HER2 antibody, Trastuzumab (Tmab), as an active targeting agent on spherical gold nanoparticles. Tmab is a therapeutic monoclonal antibody that binds to the human epidermal growth factor receptor 2 (HER2) and is approved for the treatment of HER2-positive breast cancer and metastatic gastric cancer [17,18]. Moreover, HER2 overexpression has been documented in esophageal [19], ovarian [20] and endometrial cancer [21] and has been identified as a negative prognostic factor in several of these malignancies [22–24]. Trastuzumab exerts its anticancer activity by binding to the extracellular domain of HER2 to prevent dimerization with other ErbB receptors, thereby inhibiting its key function in cell proliferation and migration. In addition, immune effector components can be engaged through the Fc region of the antibody to destroy cancer cells via antibody-dependent cellular cytotoxicity (ADCC), antibody-dependent cellular phagocytosis (ADCP) and complement-dependent cytotoxicity (CDC) [25,26].

Monoclonal antibodies (mAbs) have become a cornerstone of cancer care since the first therapeutic mAb market approval in 1997 (Rituximab) by virtue of their enhanced treatment specificity. As of early 2019, more than 20 distinct mAbs are indicated for a wide array of solid malignancies, predominantly administered through systemic routes [27]. This notwithstanding, poor tumor penetration and distribution are prominent obstacles that compromise the therapeutic index of mAbs [28,29]. To this end, enhancing drug accumulation in the tumor through the employment of enhanced delivery systems could provide major improvements in therapeutic safety and efficacy.

Conventional designs of active-targeted nanoparticles for drug delivery typically consist of nanoparticles carrying a surface-incorporated targeting agent and a cytotoxic payload either encapsulated within the NP core or loaded onto the surface. In this work, we sought to employ a novel strategy, wherein a cytotoxic drug is conjugated to the antibody initially, and the resulting antibody-drug conjugate (ADC) is employed as a targeting agent-drug carrier on the nanoparticles, thereby broadening the functionality of the active-targeting agent. Herein, we describe the synthesis and physicochemical characterization of ADC-targeted spherical gold nanoparticles. The ADC was produced by chemical attachment of monomethyl auristatin E (MMAE) to Tmab through a cathepsin-cleavable valine-citrulline linker; and further reacted with a sulfhydryl-containing linker for surface conjugation to the gold nanoparticles. We demonstrate that Trastuzumab can be chemically modified in this fashion while retaining high affinity towards its cognate receptor. Since the valine-citrulline linker must be internalized for payload release, we analyzed the intracellular uptake of active-targeted AuNPs on various cancer cell lines. Furthermore, we evaluated the effect of surface incorporation of a cell penetrating peptide to the active-targeted nanoparticle on intracellular uptake.

2. Results

2.1. Nanoparticle Design

Figure 1 displays an outline of the nanoparticle design and conjugation strategy. Attachment of the bioactive moieties—anti-HER2 mAb and HIV-TAT cell penetrating peptide (CPP)—to the gold surface was achieved through the covalent thiol-gold interaction using a bifunctional 5 kDa poly ethylene glycol (PEG) linker with a thiol (SH) and an N-hydroxysuccinimide (NHS) ester end groups (NHS-PEG-SH). The NHS group reacts with ε-amines in lysine residues (and with α-amines present at the N-terminals to a lesser extent) under slightly alkaline conditions to produce stable amide bonds with the protein or peptide [30]. The 5 kDa PEG linker was employed to increase exposure of the functional groups and prevent non-specific interactions between the bioactive groups and the gold surface. Furthermore, PEGylation of gold nanoparticles has proven to be highly beneficial in increasing circulation half-life by preventing adhesion of serum proteins that facilitate uptake by the reticuloendothelial system (RES)—an effect that drastically decreases the amount of nanoparticles that can eventually reach the tumor site [31].

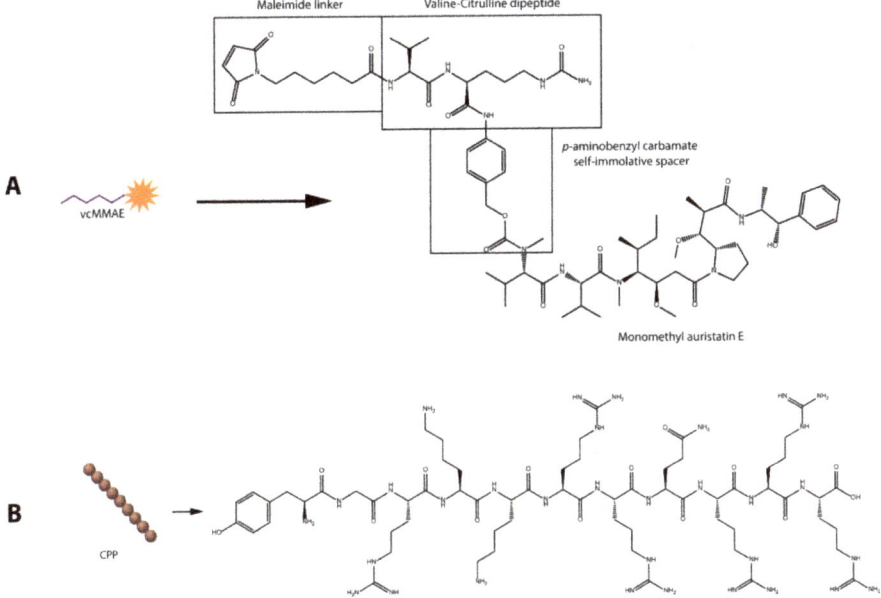

Figure 1. Molecular structures of the bioactive agents utilized for gold nanoparticle (AuNP) surface functionalization. (**A**) Valine-citrulline momomethyl auristatin E (vcMMAE) linker for antibody-drug conjugate (ADC) construction. (**B**) Human immunodeficiency virus twin-arginine translocation (HIV-1 TAT 47–57) protein.

Trastuzumab (anti-HER2 mAb) was employed as an active targeting agent to confer specificity towards HER2 overexpressing cancer cell lines. To enhance the anticancer potency of the antibody, MMAE was attached to Trastuzumab (Tmab) through a valine-citrulline dipeptide cleavable linker (vcMMAE) to produce Tmab-vcMMAE (Figure 1). The valine-citrulline moiety is cleaved by the lysosomal protease cathepsin B; thus, MMAE release occurs primarily following endocytosis and subsequent localization into endosomes or lysosomes. The HIV-TAT cell penetrating peptide was further added onto the surface via the same NHS-PEG-SH linker to increase cellular uptake for intracellular release of the drug cargo (Figure 2B,C).

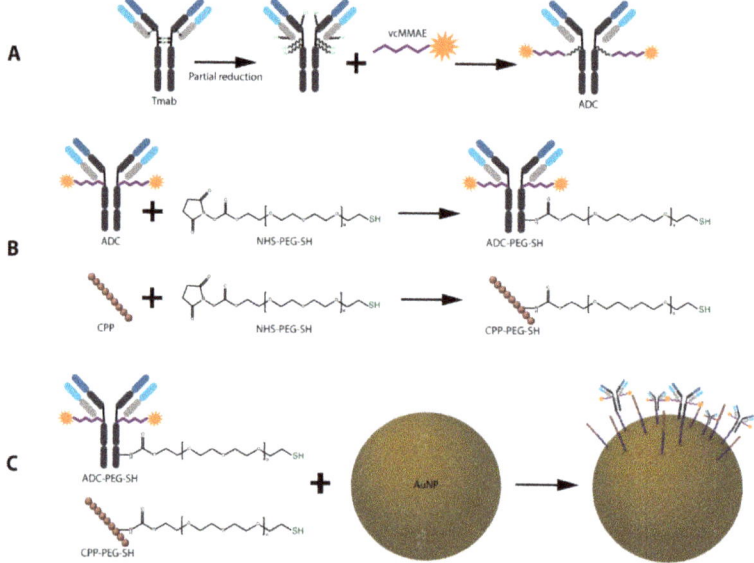

Figure 2. Schematic outline of the design and synthesis of ADC-coated gold nanoparticles with enhanced cell penetrating properties. (**A**) ADC synthesis. (**B**) Trastuzumab and CPP PEGylation for AuNP attachment. (**C**) Conjugation of bioactive agents onto the surface of AuNPs.

2.2. Antibody-Drug Conjugate (Tmab-vcMMAE) Synthesis

MMAE was conjugated to free sulfhydryl groups in Trastuzumab via reaction with the maleimide group in the vcMMAE linker (Figure 2A). To enable protein attachment, Trastuzumab was partially reduced by incubation with dithiothreitol (DTT) at 37 °C in a 3:1 DTT:Tmab molar ratio. Partial reduction produces cleavage of the inter-heavy chain disulfide bonds while preserving non-covalent inter-heavy chain (HC) and heavy-light chain (LC) interactions to conserve full IgG structure.

A colorimetric reaction with 5,5′-Dithiobis(2-nitrobenzoic acid) (DTNB) was performed to confirm the presence of free SH groups following partial reduction. DTNB reacts with SH in a 1:1 molar ratio to produce 2-nitro-5-thiobenzoic acid (TNB^{2-}). Absorption at 412 nm (λ max of TNB^{2-}) can be utilized to calculate the amount of free SH groups per antibody monomer (Figure S1A).

After confirmation and quantification of the presence of free SH groups, the intact structure (no chain dissociation) was confirmed through size exclusion–high performance liquid chromatography (SE-HPLC), whereby the elution time of the reduced antibody shifted by 0.0128 min but did not display peaks at longer elution times indicative of chain dissociation (Figure S1B).

The drug-linker (vcMMAE) was then attached to free SH groups in the partially reduced Tmab as described in the methods section. Successful attachment of vcMMAE was confirmed through intact protein mass spectrometry analysis (Figure 3). The deconvoluted mass spectrum of the ADC displayed up to 3 vcMMAE attachments per antibody heavy chain in the G0F or G1F glycoforms (Figure 3A). Light chain analysis (Figure 3B) showcased a single attachment per LC monomer, consistent with a single free SH in LC obtained from partial reduction of the interchain disulfide bonds.

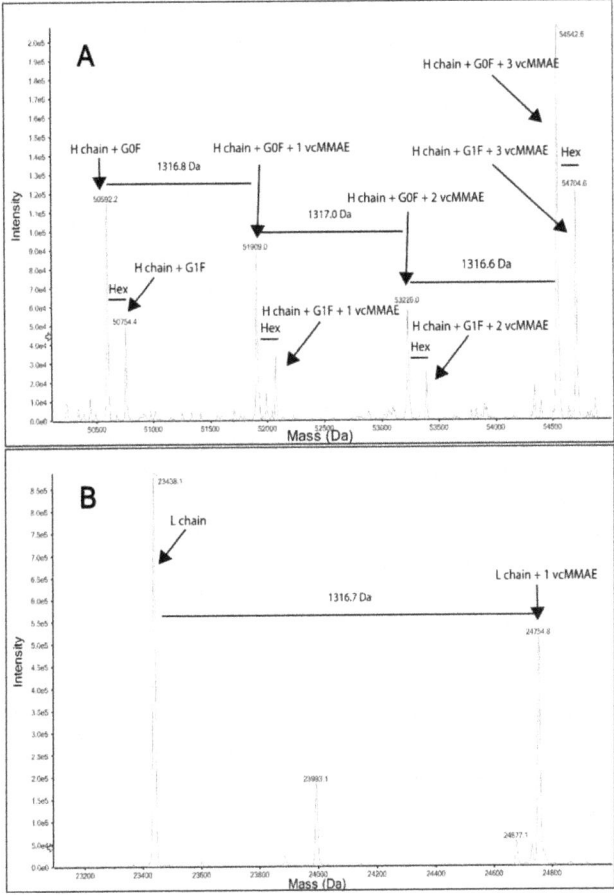

Figure 3. Protein intact mass analysis of Tmab-vcMMAE. (**A**) Deconvoluted spectrum of Tmab-vcMMAE heavy chain. (**B**) Deconvoluted spectrum of Tmab-vcMMAE light chain.

An average drug-to-antibody ratio (DAR) of 2.91 was obtained from analysis of the UV-Vis spectrum of the ADC as described in the methods section (Figure 4).

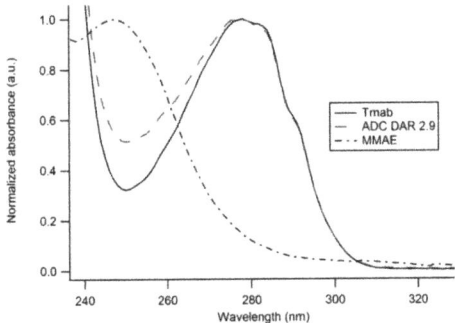

Figure 4. UV-Vis spectra of unmodified Trastuzumab, Tmab-vcMMAE (ADC) and MMAE. The contribution of MMAE to the absorption spectrum of the antibody-drug conjugate enables an estimation of the DAR based on the distinct A_{280}/A_{248} ratios obtained with the unmodified antibody and the ADC.

2.3. Antibody and CPP PEGylation

2.3.1. Structural Characterization

Trastuzumab and HIV-TAT were PEGylated via lysine conjugation chemistry (Figure 1). Antibody PEGylation was confirmed through SE-HPLC (Figure 5). The SE-HPLC chromatograms of the PEGylated Trastuzumab show an increasing shift towards earlier elution times as the PEG-linker/tmab ratio increases (Figure 5). Resolving the exact number of PEG polymers attached per antibody molecule through SE-HPLC separation and other standard protein characterization techniques is challenging, given that the expected molecular weight (MW) increment per individual attachment corresponds to less than 4% of the MW of unmodified Trastuzumab, namely 5 kDa increments to the ~148 kDa expected MW of the antibody. Moreover, PEG molecules display heterogeneity in the number of ethylene glycol units—albeit with only small differences in MW—adding to the ensuing heterogeneity. Nonetheless, detailed characterization and homogeneity are not crucial for subsequent use as targeting agents, as long as the bulk of the protein monomers have been modified and functionality is conserved. A single Trastuzumab monomer possesses 88 lysine residues and 4 amino-terminal groups available for reaction with the NHS group. Hence, reaction with a large number of linkers can potentially impair receptor binding. Consequently, conservation of the functionality of the PEGylated derivative was assessed prior to subsequent surface functionalization of the nanoparticles.

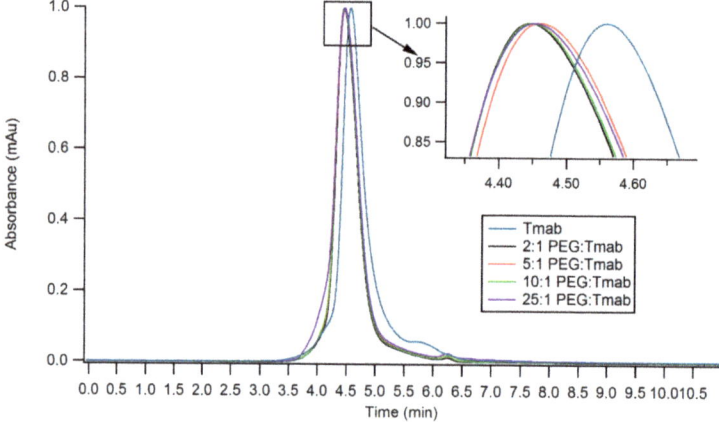

Figure 5. SE-HPLC chromatograms of PEGylated Trastuzumab variants obtained by employing varying ratios of PEG:Tmab ratios. Inset shows the zoomed region displaying small shifts in elution time.

2.3.2. Binding Kinetics of Functionalized Trastuzumab

The chemically modified Trastuzumab variants (Tmab-PEG-SH, ADC and ADC-PEG-SH) were tested for their capacity to retain the binding affinity and binding kinetics to a recombinant HER2 protein after functionalization through surface plasmon resonance (SPR) single cycle kinetic analysis Figure S5).

The binding kinetics to the HER2 receptor were not significantly altered under the assay conditions. The affinity constant (K_D) of the PEGylated antibodies, ranging from 5.46–6.91 pM, showed only minor differences compared to the mean K_D of unmodified Trastuzumab—6.07 pM (Table 1). Kinetic constants for the antibody drug conjugate were also highly similar to the unmodified Trastuzumab. The PEGylated ADC, on the other hand, recorded a slight increase in binding rate constant (K_a) accompanied by a 32-fold increase in the dissociation rate constant (K_d), for a net 14-fold decrease K_D.

The varying molar ratios of PEG-linker utilized for derivatization were deemed appropriate for subsequent attachment to the surface of gold nanoparticles, as the modified antibody did not display significant alterations in binding affinity to the cognate receptor. Henceforth, the highest molar excess (25:1 PEG-mAb ratio) for reaction was employed in order to maximize Trastuzumab attachment to AuNPs. PEGylation of Tmab-vcMMAE caused a significant decrease in K_D; however, the affinity constant remains in the picomolar range, thus it is still expected to exert active targeting capacity.

Table 1. Kinetics and affinity analysis of functionalized Trastuzumab variants.

Trastuzumab Variant	K_a ($\times 10^6$) $M^{-1} \cdot s^{-1}$	K_d ($\times 10^5$) s^{-1}	K_D (pM)
Tmab	3.24 ± 0.15	1.98 ± 0.50	6.07 ± 1.27
Tmab-PEG-SH 2×	3.53 ± 0.15	2.47 ± 0.24	6.83 ± 0.68
Tmab-PEG-SH 5×	2.86 ± 0.03	1.97 ± 0.20	6.91 ± 0.78
Tmab-PEG-SH 10×	2.87 ± 0.11	1.98 ± 0.14	6.89 ± 0.21
Tmab-PEG-SH 25×	2.05 ± 0.03	1.12 ± 0.11	5.46 ± 0.44
ADC	2.25 ± 0.01	1.58 ± 0.09	7.05 ± 0.41
ADC-PEG-SH	7.45 ± 0.07	61.80 ± 0.05	85.01 ± 10.92

2.4. Gold Nanoparticle Surface Functionalization

The surface of 50 nm citrate-capped gold nanoparticles (Cit-AuNP) was functionalized with OH-PEG-SH (OH-PEG-AuNP), Tmab-PEG-SH (Tmab-PEG-AuNP), CPP-PEG-SH (CPP-PEG-AuNP), or a combination of CPP-PEG-SH and Tmab-PEG-SH (CPP+Tmab-PEG-AuNP) through a sequential addition of the bioactive agents.

Transmission electron micrograph (TEM) analysis of the synthesized Cit-AuNPs displayed a mean diameter of 48.29 ± 5.58 nm showing a narrow size distribution and uniform spherical morphology (Table 2). The mean hydrodynamic diameter obtained by DLS was 60.62 ± 0.19 nm (Z-average) with a polydispersity index (PDI) of 0.29. The SPR absorption band of the AuNPs had an absorption maximum (λ max) at 530.5 nm, consistent with the expected λ max for ~50 nm gold nanoparticles according to previously reported determinations of SPR bands of spherical AuNPs [32]. Upon surface functionalization, the λ max shifted towards longer wavelengths (red-shift)—a well-described spectral shift caused by an increase in the local refractive index on the NP surface. In increasing order, the λ max shifts were +1.9 nm for OH-PEG-AuNPs, +2.7 nm for CPP-PEG-AuNP, +3.3 nm for CPP+Tmab-PEG-AuNPs and +3.7 for Tmab-PEG-AuNPs.

Table 2. Size (Z-average), zeta potential (ζ) and absorption maximum (λ max) of surface-functionalized gold nanoparticles.

NP	Z-ave (nm)	PDI	ζ (mV)	λ max (nm)	TEM (nm)
Cit-AuNP	60.62 ± 0.19	0.29	−34.60 ± 0.91	530.5	48.29 ± 5.58
OH-PEG-AuNP	86.61 ± 0.12	0.17	−14.37 ± 0.12	532.4	
Tmab-PEG-AuNP	87.35 ± 0.41	0.17	−1.10 ± 0.46	534.2	
CPP+Tmab-PEG-AuNP	83.42 ± 2.14	0.20	1.5 ± 0.46	533.8	
CPP-PEG-AuNP	81.22 ± 0.39	0.17	6.17 ± 0.71	533.2	
ADC-PEG-AuNP	85.45 ± 1.34	0.19	−2.3 ± 0.37	534.1	

NP: nanoparticle format, PDI: polydispersity index, TEM: transmission electron microscope.

The change in SPR absorption maximum was accompanied by an increase in hydrodynamic diameter (Table 2), where Tmab-PEG functionalization showed the highest increment (87.35 ± 0.41 nm). The PDIs of all surface-functionalized samples decreased relative to Cit-AuNP, indicative of enhanced colloidal stability and a consequent reduction of nanoparticle aggregation. Surface functionalization caused marked alterations in the zeta potential (ζ) of the colloidal dispersions (Table 2). Citrate-capped AuNPs displayed a mean ζ of -34.60 ± 0.91 mV, consistent with a negatively charged surface due to the negatively charged OH^- groups of the citrate moiety. Conjugation with the PEGylated-CPP yielded a mean ζ of +6.17 ± 071 mV, causing a charge reversal attributable to the abundant positively charged arginine residues in HIV-TAT. The combination of cell penetrating peptide and Tmab on the AuNP surface (CPP+Tmab-PEG-AuNP) also had a slightly positively charged zeta potential (+1.5 ± 0.46 mV).

2.5. Cellular Uptake in Various Breast Cancer Cell Lines

2.5.1. Active Targeting in HER2-Positive SBKR-3 Cells

To evaluate the active targeting capacity of Trastuzumab-conjugated gold nanoparticles (Tmab-PEG-AuNPs), SKBR-3 cells (HER-2 positive) were incubated with 20 nm and 50 nm AuNPs coated with Tmab-PEG-SH or OH-PEG-SH. All reported values for gold uptake were obtained from ICP-MS quantification, as described in the methods section. Mean gold nanoparticle uptake per cell was significantly higher for 20 nm Tmab-PEG-AuNP ($t(10) = 6.61$, $p > 0.001$) and 50 nm Tmab-PEG-AuNPs ($t(10) = 6.96$, $p > 0.001$) compared to the OH-PEG functionalized AuNPs counterparts (Figure 6A). Qualitative assessment of cellular internalization through TEM microscopy showed localization into vesicular structures for both nanoparticles formats (Figure 6B,C).

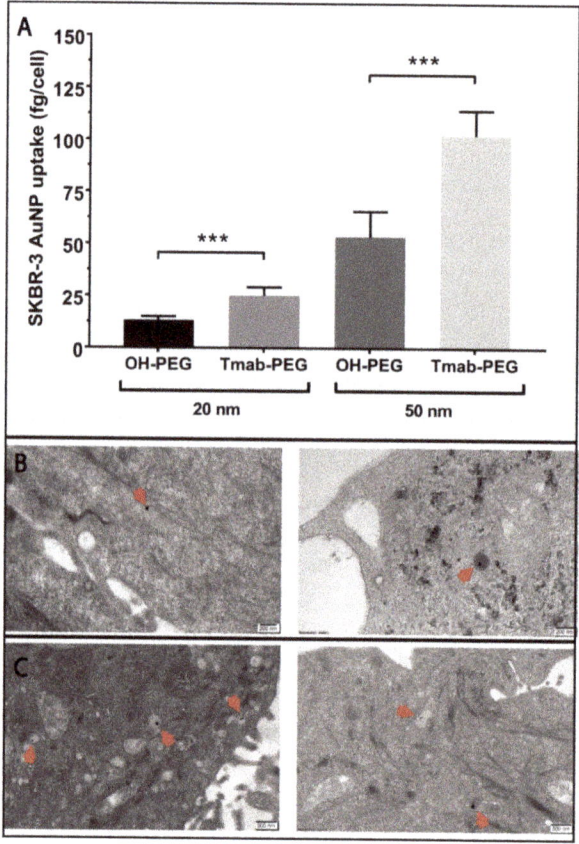

Figure 6. Evaluation of the active targeting capacity of Trastuzumab-functionalized gold nanoparticles. (**A**) ICP-MS quantification of OH-PEG-AuNP and Tmab-PEG-AuNP uptake into SKBR-3 cells after 24 h incubation. Uptake data are reported as means ± SD. *** $p < 0.001$ (Student's t-test). (**B**) TEM micrographs of OH-PEG-AuNPs internalized into SKBR-3 cells. Scale bar 200 nm (**C**) TEM micrographs of Tmab-PEG-AuNPs internalized into SKBR-3 cells. Scale bar: 500 nm.

Trastuzumab coated AuNPs did not display enhanced uptake in two other breast cancer cell lines (MCF-7 and MDA-MB-231) that are not reported to upregulate HER-2 expression (Figure 7) [33]. Uptake into DLD-1 cells (colorectal cancer HER-2 negative cell lines) showed a small increase in mean uptake per cell with no statistical significance. ADC conjugated gold nanoparticles were not employed for cellular uptake assays as the high potency of the drug can cause significant cell death at the concentrations used; thus, evaluation of cellular uptake is not comparable to the other formats.

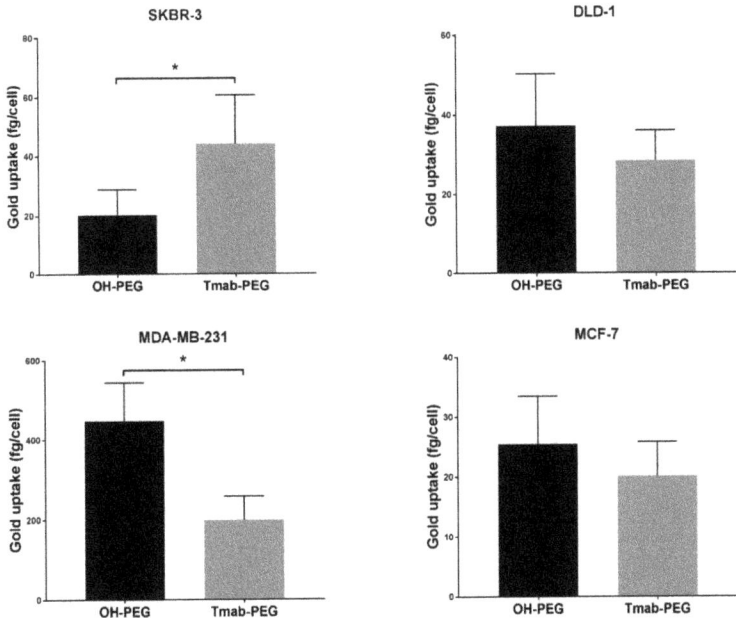

Figure 7. Active targeting of Trastuzumab functionalized gold nanoparticles in various cancer cell lines. Uptake data are reported as means ± SD. * $p < 0.05$ (Student's t-test).

2.5.2. CPP-Driven Enhanced Internalization

To assess the effect on cell internalization using the HIV-TAT cell penetrating peptide as a coating functional group on the surface of the nanoparticles, 4 different cancer cell lines (SKBR-3, DLD-1, MDA-MB-231 and MCF-7) were treated with 25 µg/mL 50 nm gold nanoparticles functionalized with OH-PEG-SH, Tmab-PEG-SH, CPP-PEG-SH, or a combination of Tmab-PEG-SH and CPP-PEG-SH (CPP+Tmab-PEG-AuNP).

A significant increase in uptake, relative to OH-PEG-AuNP, obtained by attachment of the anti-HER2 antibody (Tmab-PEG-AuNP) was recorded for the SKBR-3 cell line (t (4) = 2.22, $p > 0.05$) only (Figure 7). In the same SKBR-3 cell line, AuNP functionalized with the cell penetrating peptide (CPP-PEG-AuNPs) showed approximately 1000-fold increase compared to the Tmab-PEG-AuNP (Figure 8). Similarly, CPP-PEG-AuNPs displayed a high increase in cell uptake relative to OH-PEG-Tmab in all cell lines tested (Figure 8). CPP+Tmab-PEG-AuNP also recorded markedly higher uptake across all cell lines compared to OH-PEG-AuNP. CPP-PEG-AuNP displayed significantly higher internalization than the combination of CPP+Tmab-PEG-AuNP in SKBR-3 and MCF-7 cells, and no statistical difference was observed between these two formats in the DLD-1 and MDA-MB-231 cell lines.

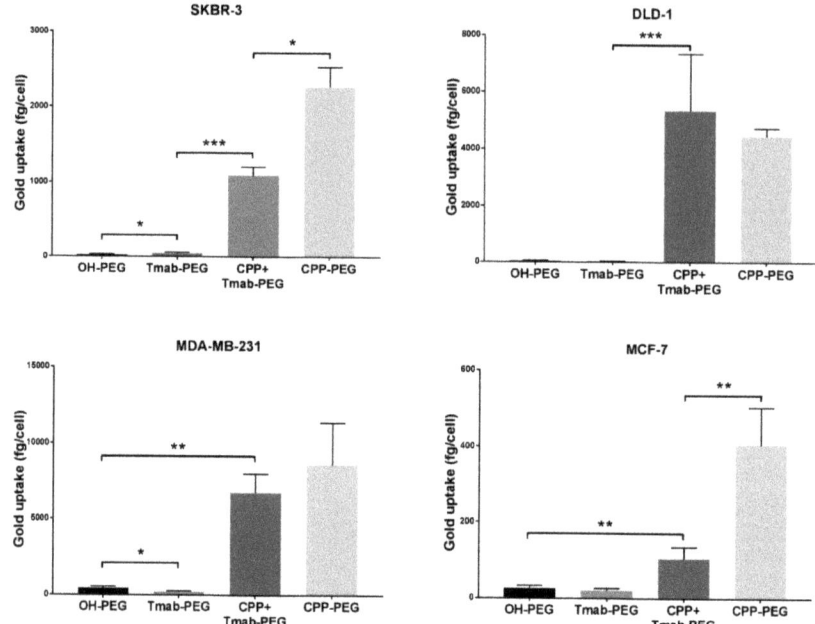

Figure 8. Cellular uptake of cell penetrating peptide (CPP) functionalized gold nanoparticles into various cancer cell lines. Uptake data are reported as means ± SD. * $p < 0.05$, ** $p < 0.01$, *** $p < 0.001$ (Student's t-test).

2.6. In Vitro Cytotoxicity of ADC-PEG-AuNP in HER2 Overexpressing Cancer Cell Lines

To assess the capacity for intracellular release of the drug payload, the in vitro cytotoxic activity of the antibody-drug conjugate bound to the nanoparticles (ADC-PEG-AuNP) was evaluated in two HER2 amplified cell lines: (1) SKBR-3 and (2) SKOV-3 (ovarian adenocarcinoma). Growth rate inhibition (GR) metrics derived from cell growth curves were determined to compare the GR_{50} value of free MMAE, Tmab-vcMMAE, ADC-PEG-AuNP and Trastuzumab (Figure 9 and Figure S6). Growth rate calculations are specified in the methods section. GR_{50} corresponds to the concentration at which $GR(c) = 0.5$. ADC and ADC-PEG-AuNP concentrations reported in Figure 9 correspond to MMAE concentrations based on DAR and antibody per AuNP estimations.

The in vitro cytotoxic activity of free MMAE was higher in both cell lines relative to ADC and ADC-PEG-AuNP (Table 3). MMAE GR_{50} values were subnanomolar for both cell lines. SKOV-3 displayed slightly higher sensitivity to MMAE (GR50 = 0.14 nM) compared to SKBR-3 cells ($GR_{50} = 0.33$ nM). ADC and ADC-PEG-AuNP displayed similar GR_{50} values for both cell lines. Trastuzumab showed a dramatically decreased potency relative to MMAE containing formats, particularly in SKOV-3. Hence, the GR_{50} value was not determined for this cell line due to the high concentration of antibody required to obtain an appropriate dose-response curve. The effect on growth rate inhibition was also determined for OH-PEG-AuNP as a control. The stabilized gold nanoparticles only caused small reductions in growth rate at high nanoparticle concentrations (Figure 9).

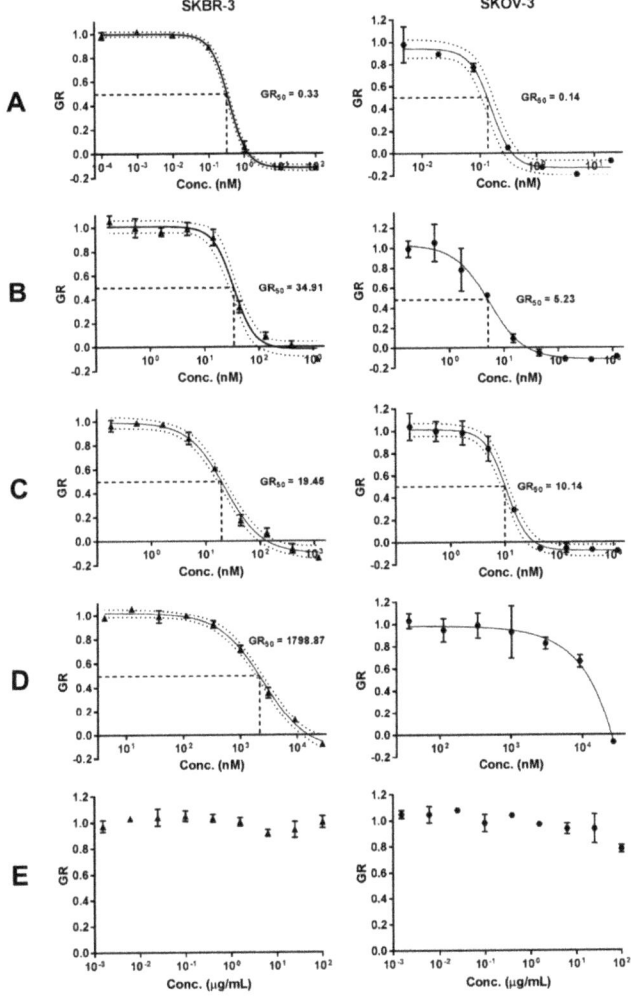

Figure 9. Growth rate (GR) inhibition of (**A**) free MMAE, (**B**) ADC, (**C**) ADC-PEG-AuNP, (**D**) Trastuzumab and (**E**) OH-PEG-AuNP in SKBR-3 and SKOV-3 cell lines. Data are reported as means ± SD. 95% confidence bands are displayed as dotted lines. Concentration of ADC and ADC-PEG-PEG are reported as molar concentrations of MMAE according to the estimated DAR and number of ADC per AuNP, respectively.

Table 3. GR_{50} values with confidence intervals (CI) obtained from dose-response curves in Figure 9.

Sample	SKBR-3			SKOV-3		
Agent	GR_{50} (nM)	GR_{50} 95% CI	R^2	SKOV-3	GR_{50} 95% CI	R^2
Free MMAE	0.33	(0.28–0.37)	0.9986	0.14	(0.11–0.17)	0.9851
ADC	34.91	(29.04–41.02)	0.9847	4.81	(3.56–6.32)	0.9636
ADC-PEG-AuNP	19.45	(16.52–22.80)	0.9913	10.14	(8.55–11.83)	0.9878
Tmab	2118.36	(1849.27–2426.61)	0.9931	N.D.	N.D.	N.D.

N.D.: not defined, CI: confidence intervals, GR_{50}: concentration required to achieve a growth rate inhibition of 0.5.

3. Discussion

The lack of clinical precedent for inorganic nanoparticles has hindered their implementation in cancer therapy. However, the results of the Phase I clinical trial (NCT00356980) of CYT-6091 (PEGylated colloidal gold-rhTNF) published in 2009 were highly promising with regards to safety profile and the capacity to accumulate effectively in a wide range of solid tumors [34]. Considering the remarkable therapeutic potential of gold nanoparticles and the validation of the EPR effect for colloidal gold in human patients, we were prompted to assess three strategies; or a combination thereof, to further enhance the potential of AuNPs for clinical implementation: (1) surface attachment of PEGylated Trastuzumab for targeted treatment of HER2-positive tumors (active targeting), (2) employment of an antibody-drug conjugate as targeting agent to increase the anticancer potency of the system, and (2) surface coating with the cationic HIV-TAT cell penetrating peptide to enhance intracellular delivery.

3.1. Trastuzumab and HIV-TAT PEGylation

Attachment of poly ethylene glycol has become a conventional strategy to increase circulation times and distribution of nanosized structures. PEGylation prevents opsonization and uptake by the RES system—a biological mechanism that severely impedes tumor localization by premature clearance [35,36]. Herein, our results support that Trastuzumab PEGylation for subsequent gold surface attachment can be readily achieved without significant modifications in HER-2 affinity or binding kinetics as was reflected by SPR binding measurements to a recombinant HER2 protein. The same NHS-linker was used for HIV-TAT PEGylation, taking advantage of the two lysine residues in its amino acid composition (Figure 1).

3.2. ADC Construction

MMAE is a cytotoxic payload with exceptionally high potency that has frequently been employed in the construction of antibody drug conjugates. Under our experimental conditions, we obtained an average drug-to-antibody ratio of 2.91, as per UV-Vis spectroscopy analysis, consistent with DARs reported for similar ADC synthesis methods [37,38]. For further structural characterization and confirmation of vcMMAE attachment, the ADC was analyzed through intact protein mass spectrometry analysis. The ADC was buffer exchanged to MeCN 10% v/v to induce inter-heavy and heavy-light chain dissociation, in order to analyze the number of drugs attached to each polypeptide chain. Chain dissociation in MeCN 10% v/v was confirmed by SE-HPLC chromatograms showing the appearance of two peaks at longer elution times (Figure S2). The deconvoluted mass spectra confirmed that vcMMAE can attach to all possible free sulfhydryl groups formed upon partial reduction, i.e., a maximum of three attachments on the heavy chain and one attachment on the light chain.

Herein, our results report on the feasibility of combining two common bioconjugation techniques (lysine and cysteine attachment) to PEGylate Tmab-vcMMAE for nanoparticle attachment. Furthermore, our data show that HER-2 binding affinity decreases by an order or magnitude with ADC PEGylation; yet, the binding affinity remains within the picomolar range. Several studies have combined targeting agents and cytotoxic drugs on nanoparticles; however, the added complexity of the systems also complicates appropriate characterization for implementation, especially in regard to dosage determination as the amount of each individual component requires quantification. To this end, the use of antibody-drug conjugates as targeting agents carrying the payload could simplify this—provided that the DAR is determined, quantification of protein content would be sufficient to estimate drug dosage per nanoparticle.

3.3. Gold Nanoparticle Surface Functionalization

Adding to improved biodistribution and tumor targeting, PEGylation also increases the colloidal stability of gold nanoparticles—a key requirement for long-term storage. Attachment of the bioactive groups was achieved through the thiol moiety of the PEG linker, which, at high pH, can form covalent gold-sulfur (Au-S) bonds, providing stable conjugation to the surface [11]. Indeed, surface functionalization had a pronounced enhancement in nanoparticle stability upon addition of 1% NaCl and cell culture media (Figure S3). Attachment was confirmed by an increase in hydrodynamic size (DLS) and SPR absorption maxima, and most importantly by alterations in the zeta potential that allow to discriminate the presence of the bioactive groups. For instance, the positively charged HIV-TAT caused a charge reversal in zeta potential (+6.17 ± 0.71 mV) for a +40.77 mV shift compared to the citrate-capped gold nanoparticles (−34.60 mV). In contrast, coating with the neutral OH-PEG caused a smaller +20.23 mV shift. Zeta potential values closer to the isoelectric point are generally detrimental to colloidal stability; however, the hydrophilic PEG polymer on the surface impedes nanoparticle aggregation by steric hindrance to prevent surface interactions between AuNPs. The large exclusion volume of the hydration cloud of the PEG linkers is known to prevent interactions between nanoparticle surfaces that lead to aggregation [35].

Quantification of the average number of antibodies that coat individual nanoparticles is challenging, insofar as common colorimetric methods for protein quantitation are difficult to perform due to the much stronger absorption coefficients of gold nanoparticles throughout the wavelength ranges used for protein concentration measurements. Instead, we quantified the amount of antibody by accounting for the ensuing decrease in antibody concentration following attachment, after removal of the functionalized nanoparticles through centrifugation. According to these measurements, an average of 156 antibodies covered the surface of 50 nm AuNPs and 40 antibodies on 20 nm AuNPs (Figure S4).

3.4. Active Targeting and Cellular Uptake

The multivalent presentation of Trastuzumab on gold nanoparticles has been shown previously to promote HER2 receptor crosslinking, leading to enhanced cellular internalization in HER2 overexpressing cell lines [39]. In our experimental setup, Trastuzumab-coated gold nanoparticles were compared to the AuNPs coated with the SH-linker without antibody derivatization, to maximize the similarity in physicochemical properties, excluding the presence of protein. Indeed, the mean hydrodynamic diameter of both formats differed by less than 1 nm according to DLS measurements (Table 2). Electrophoretic mobility determinations, on the other hand, recorded negative zeta potential values for OH-PEG-AuNPs and close to neutral values for Tmab-PEG-AuNP. The drift towards more neutral values—relative to citrate-capped nanoparticles—is consistent with antibody attachment, as Trastuzumab (isoelectric point (pI) 8.7) possesses a net positive charge when dissolved in PBS. A small net positive charge is also expected when suspended in cell culture media (pH 7.4). The effect of nanoparticle surface charge on cellular uptake is well-documented, whereby positively charged nanoparticles have consistently displayed higher uptake rates in nonphagocytic cells [40]. The increase in internalization with positively charged surfaces has generally been ascribed to favorable electrostatic nanoparticle/cell interactions due to the net negative charge of the plasma membrane [40]. In view of the foregoing, it is difficult to rule out a contribution of the more neutral zeta potential of Tmab-PEG-AuNP in enhancing cellular uptake. This notwithstanding, the observation that internalization enhancement was only recorded in a HER2 overexpressing cell line (SKBR-3)—and not in the HER2 basal counterparts (DLD-1, MDA-MB-231 and MCF-7)—supports cellular uptake increase through Trastuzumab-mediated HER2 receptor crosslinking. Interestingly, TEM micrographs of SKBR-3 cells did not show clear distinction between both formats in subcellular localization—i.e., both AuNP designs were primarily localized within vesicular structures, presumably coated preendosomal and carrier vesicles (early endosomes and lysosomes). Alternatively, it is possible that some of these structures are autophagosomes, as gold nanoparticles have been shown to induce autophagosome accumulation [41]. This observation warrants further elucidation of the effect of surface functionalization on uptake mechanism and localization.

3.5. Cellular Uptake Enhancement with HIV-TAT

Due to the relatively low loading capacity of spherical gold nanoparticles, it is essential to ensure maximum cellular internalization when developed as drug delivery vehicles. Having improved selective uptake into HER2 overexpressing cell lines through active targeting, we sought to evaluate the effect of combining a cell penetrating peptide with the antibody targeting agent. HIV-TAT internalization mechanism remains a topic of debate; however, evidence of uptake saturability and energy dependency suggest an endosomal pathway [42]. Endosomal and subsequent lysosomal localization is required for effective drug release of cathepsin B-cleavable linkers, such as those containing the valine-citrulline dipeptide. Enhancing uptake is thus paramount in HER2-targeted conjugates for intracellular release, considering that most ErbB receptors have shown impaired ligand-induced receptor trafficking [43]. To this end, functionalization with the cell penetrating peptide caused a dramatic increase in cellular uptake across all cell lines tested. This enhancement was considerably more significant than that obtained by antibody functionalization only. Conversely, our results did not show improvement in uptake upon combination of both bioactive agents compared to CPP-PEG-AuNP. In fact, uptake was significantly higher with CPP functionalization in SKBR-3 and MCF-7 cells. We presume that this observation stems from the more positive zeta potential of CPP-PEG-AuNPs, in which case engagement through cell membrane/nanoparticle electrostatic interactions is a stronger determinant of uptake rate than antibody-mediated receptor cross-linking.

These findings warrant further investigation into the effect of the highlighted physicochemical and physiological attributes in a more physiological setting. While higher uptake may be desirable in delivery applications, internalization must be specific to the targeted tumor cells. Previous studies have reported that uptake, rather than diffusion, could be the primary mechanism for nanoparticle tumor delivery. Consequently, surface charge has been proposed as a major determinant in tumor distribution upon systemic administration [44]. If indeed transcellular transport has a crucial impact in tumor penetration, then enhancing cellular internalization through strategies such as the attachment of a cell penetrating peptide might provide improved tumor tissue distribution, thus enhancing efficacy and therapeutic index.

3.6. In Vitro Cytotoxicity of ADC-PEG-AuNP in HER2 Overexpressing Cancer Cell Lines

Growth rate inhibition sensitivity in SKOV-3 and SKBR-3 cell lines was markedly higher for free MMAE than for the antibody-drug conjugate and for ADC-carrying gold nanoparticles (Figure 8). It is plausible that the requirement of linker cleavage and self-immolation of the p-aminobenzyl carbamate group in the antibody-drug conjugate hinders conjugated vcMMAE activity compared to the free drug. Additionally, although HER2 binding and cross-linking can induce receptor-mediated endocytosis, free MMAE likely penetrates more readily into the intracellular compartment. Nonetheless, the structural characteristics that presumably hinder conjugated vcMMAE cytotoxicity in isolated carcinoma cells are expected to provide selectivity advantages in more physiological settings.

Comparison of the cytotoxic activity of free ADC and nanoparticle-conjugated ADC displayed similar GR_{50} for both SKBR-3 and SKOV-3 cells (Table 3). GR_{50} values for ADC-PEG-AuNP were lower for SKBR-3 cells and higher for SKOV-3 cells relative to free ADC; however, due to the degree of uncertainty in the estimation of antibodies per nanoparticle it is difficult to establish a significant improvement in MMAE intracellular release and antimitotic activity for either one of the formats. Still, concentrations of ADC-PEG-AuNP required to achieve a 50% growth rate inhibition were extremely low in both HER2 amplified cell lines. As expected, the antimitotic activity of MMAE-containing formats is dramatically higher than that of the unmodified Trastuzumab and PEG-stabilized gold nanoparticles. OH-PEG-AuNPs only caused small reductions in growth rate at high gold concentrations (100 µg/mL) in SKOV-3, which is higher than the equivalent gold concentrations required to achieve a 50% growth rate inhibition in ADC-PEG-AuNPs (> 20 µg/mL). These results confirm that MMAE antibody-drug conjugate retain a highly potent cytotoxic activity when bound to the surface of gold nanoparticles.

These findings warrant further investigation in animal models, as increased accumulation in high EPR tumors could confer potency and safety advantages over the free ADC.

4. Materials and Methods

4.1. Materials

Herceptin® (Trastuzumab) was a generous donation from Genentech (San Francisco, CA, USA). Thiol PEG NHS (NHS-PEG-SH) (5 kDa) linker (Cat. No. PG2-NSTH-5k) was purchased from Nanocs (Boston, MA, USA). The MC-Val-Cit-PAB-MMAE (vcMMAE) linker (Cat. No. BP23969) was obtained from Broadpharm (San Diego, CA, USA). The HIV-1 TAT protein (47-57) (HIV-TAT or CPP) (Cat. No. H0292) was purchased from Sigma-Aldrich (Castle Hill, NSW, Australia). The Series S Sensor Chip CM5 (Cat. No. 29-1049-88), the amine coupling kit (Cat. No. BR-1000-50) and the anti-HIS capture kit (Cat. No. 28-9950-56) employed in the Biacore SPR instrument were purchased from GE Healthcare (Parramatta, NSW, Australia). The recombinant HIS-tagged soluble HER2 (Cat. No. SRP6405) was obtained from Sigma-Aldrich (Australia). Phosphate buffered saline (PBS) was purchased from Astral Scientific (Gymea, NSW, Australia). Amicon 3 kDa (Cat. No. Z740168) and 50 kDa (Cat. No. Z740177) cutoff centrifugal filter units were acquired from Sigma-Aldrich (Australia). Millex-GV syringe filters (0.22 µm, PVDF, Cat. No. SLGV033RS) were purchased from purchased from Sigma-Aldrich (Castle Hill, NSW, Australia). RPMI 1640 and DMEM (high glucose) media were obtained from Life Technologies (Mulgrave, VIC, Australia). All other chemicals and reagents were purchased from Sigma Aldrich (Australia).

4.2. Synthesis of Spherical Citrate-Capped Gold Nanoparticles

Spherical gold nanoparticles were synthesized by citrate reduction of gold chloride in aqueous solution as described by Turkevich [45], and revised by Frens [46]. All glassware employed in this procedure was soaked in aqua regia (3:1 HCl/HNO$_3$ molar ratio) for 3 h prior to the reaction and rinsed with double distilled H$_2$O. Briefly, 100 mL of a 254 µM HAuCl$_4$ solution in double distilled H$_2$O was heated to boiling under stirring. Once boiling, 2 mL or 1 mL of a 1% w/v (34 µM) sodium citrate solution was added to prepare 20 nm and 50 nm, respectively. Following citrate addition, the solution was boiled for 15 min, then cooled to room temperature under stirring for 2 h. Unreacted citrate was removed by decanting after centrifugation at 10,000 g or 3500 g for 30 min to pellet the 20 nm and 50 nm nanoparticles. The synthesized gold nanoparticles were resuspended in double distilled water. Nanoparticle size, size distribution and morphology were assessed through transmission DLS (hydrodynamic size) electron microscopy (size, size distribution and morphology) and shifts in the surface plasmon resonance (SPR) absorption band.

4.3. Tmab PEGylation (Tmab-PEG-SH)

Trastuzumab 21 mg/mL in formulation buffer (L-histidine 4.64 mM, α,α-Trehalose 52.86 mM, polysorbate 20 concentration 73.31 µM, HCl 2.58 mM) was buffer exchanged to sodium bicarbonate (NaHCO$_3$) 0.1 M pH 8.0 using 50 kDa cutoff centrifugal filters to a final antibody concentration of 10 mg/mL (6.87 × 10^{-5} M). The extinction coefficient ε_{280} = 2.25 × 10^5 M^{-1} cm^{-1} was used for all antibody concentration determinations. Buffer exchange was carried out thoroughly to reduce to a minimum the concentration of L-histidine in the formulation buffer, as the primary amine in L-histidine will react readily with the NHS group in the linker. A 5 mg/mL (1 mM) NHS-PEG-SH (5 kDa) linker stock solution was prepared in NaHCO$_3$ 0.1 M pH 8.0 and immediately added to Trastuzumab in 2:1, 5:1, 10:1, 20:1 and 25:1 NHS-linker/Tmab ratios and incubated at 4 °C overnight under stirring. The NHS-linker stock solution in NaHCO$_3$ pH 8.0 was prepared immediately before adding to the Trastuzumab sample, since the NHS ester can undergo rapid hydrolysis at basic pH. Following PEGylation, unreacted NHS-PEG-SH linker was removed by centrifugation through 50 kDa cutoff filters and the PEGylated Trastuzumab (Tmab-PEG-SH) was buffer exchanged to phosphate buffered saline (PBS) 0.01 M pH 7.4 with 1 mM EDTA to a final antibody concentration of 5 mg/mL. EDTA 1 mM was added to inhibit disulfide bond formation between the free SH groups in the linker [47,48].

4.4. HIV-TAT Cell Penetrating Peptide (CPP) PEGylation (CPP-PEG-SH)

HIV-TAT (47–57) peptide was dissolved in NaHCO$_3$ 0.1 M pH 8.0 to a 1 mg/mL (641 µM) concentration. A 10 mg/mL (2 mM) NHS-PEG-SH (5 kDa) solution in NaHCO$_3$ 0.1 M pH 8.0 was added to the HIV-TAT peptide in a 4:1 NHS-linker/CPP molar ratio and incubated overnight at 4 °C under stirring. Unreacted CPP was removed by centrifugation through 3 kDa cutoff filters and the PEGylated CPP (CPP-PEG-SH) was buffer exchanged to phosphate buffered saline 0.01 M pH 7.4 with 1 mM EDTA.

4.5. Tmab-vcMMAE Conjugate Synthesis

4.5.1. Antibody Partial Reduction

Trastuzumab in formulation buffer was buffer exchanged to PBS 0.01 M with 10 mM EDTA in a final concentration of 5 mg/mL (34 uM). A freshly prepared 10 mM stock solution of dithiothreitol (DTT) in PBS 0.01 M EDTA 1 mM was added to the antibody in a 3:1 DTT/Tmab ratio and the reaction was incubated at 37 °C for 90 min under stirring. DTT was then removed by buffer exchanging the partially reduced Tmab with 50 kDa cutoff centrifugal filters to PBS 0.01 M containing 10 mM EDTA to a 10 mg/mL (34 µM) concentration. After partial reduction, the integrity of the full-size IgG molecule was confirmed by SE-HPLC. In addition, free sulfhydryl (SH) groups per antibody were quantified by reaction with DTNB (5,5'-dithiobis(2-nitrobenzoic acid)) and determination of the absorbance at 412 nm for free SH concentration. The final flowthrough of the buffer exchange prior to the DTNB reaction was used as a blank to subtract the potential contribution of residual DTT in the solution. The extinction coefficient $\varepsilon_{412} = 1.42 \times 10^5$ M^{-1} cm^{-1} for the TNB^{2-} reaction product was employed for sulfhydryl quantification.

4.5.2. Conjugate Synthesis

vcMMAE was dissolved in DMSO at a 1.26 mM concentration and added to a chilled 10 mg/mL partially reduced Tmab solution in a 4.6:1 vcMMAE/Tmab ratio. The reaction mixture was incubated at 4 °C with stirring for 1 h. A 20-fold molar excess of cysteine—relative to maleimide—was added to quench the reaction. Unreacted vcMMAE and cysteine were removed by centrifugation through 50 kDa cutoff centrifugal filters and buffer exchanged to PBS 0.01 M pH 7.4 for storage, or NaHCO$_3$ 0.1 M pH 8.0 for subsequent PEGylation. The average drug-antibody ratio (DAR) was calculated based on absorbance values at 248 nm and 280 nm as has been described previously [49]. The following formula was employed:

$$DAR = \frac{\varepsilon_{248}^{Tmab} - F\varepsilon_{280}^{Tmab}}{F\varepsilon_{280}^{MMAE} - \varepsilon_{248}^{MMAE}}$$

F=A248/A280 and the extinction coefficients utilized are listed in Table 4.

Table 4. Extinction coefficients of Trastuzumab and monomethyl auristatin E (MMAE) employed for the calculation of drug-to-antibody ratio (DAR) based on UV-Vis spectroscopy.

Sample	248 nm	280 nm
Trastuzumab	7.75×10^4	2.25×10^5
MMAE	1.59×10^4	1.50×10^3

PEGylation of Tmab-vcMMAE (ADC-PEG-SH) was achieved following the same procedure as for the unconjugated antibody.

4.5.3. Intact Mass Analysis

Trastuzumab and Tmab-vcMMAE were concentrated using 50 kDa cutoff centrifugal filters and buffer exchanged to 10% acetonitrile with 0.1% formic acid. The antibody samples were analyzed through direct injection into a Triple TOF 6600 mass spectrometer (Sciex, Framingham, MA, USA). Infusion was performed at 50 µL/min. The mass range for detection was 100–5000 m/z. Deconvolution of the raw data was achieved using SCIEX Peakview 2.2 (Concord, ON, Canada) and Bruker BioTools software packages (Billerica, MA, USA).

4.6. Binding Kinetics to Recombinant HER2 through Surface Plasmon Resonance

The binding kinetics of derivatized Trastuzumab (Tmab-PEG-SH, Tmab-vcMMAE and ADC-PEG-SH) were tested against a recombinant HER-2 protein using surface plasmon resonance (SPR) in a Biacore T200 instrument (GE Healthcare, Parramatta, NSW, Australia). Briefly, an anti-HIS antibody was bound to a CM5 sensor chip through amine coupling chemistry. Subsequently, a recombinant HIS-tagged HER-2 (4 nM) was bound to the anti-HIS antibody on the sensor chip at a 5 µL/min flow rate for 5 min. 2-fold serial dilutions of the Trastuzumab variants ranging from 8–0.5 nM in HBS-T running buffer (10 mM HEPES, 150 mM NaCl, 0.05% (v/v) Tween 20, pH 7.4) were assayed at 25 °C as single cycle kinetic titrations. The analytes were applied to the sensor surface at 20 µL/min for 2 min, followed by 60 min dissociation times. Analyses of the sensorgrams were performed by fitting a Langmuir 1:1 binding model to derive the association constant (K_a), the dissociation constant (K_d) and the binding affinity (K_D—calculated as K_a/K_d). The analytes were run in duplicate to calculate average values and standard deviation. A goodness of fit (χ^2) value within 5% of the maximum response level (Rmax) was used as acceptance criteria.

4.7. Gold Nanoparticle Surface Functionalization

Trastuzumab-coated (Tmab-PEG-AuNP), OH-PEG coated (OH-PEG-AuNP) and CPP-coated (CPP-PEG-AuNP) gold nanoparticles were produced by incubating citrate-capped gold nanoparticles (OD = 1) with a 1×10^5 molar excess of SH-PEG-Tmab, SH-PEG-OH or SH-PEG-CPP in NaHCO$_3$ 0.01 M pH for 2 h at room temperature while stirring. The unconjugated reagents were removed by pelleting the nanoparticles at 3500 g for 30 min and removing the supernatant. The conjugated nanoparticles were centrifuged four times and resuspended in PBS 0.01 M pH 7.4 for storage at 4 °C. ADC-PEG-AuNP were produced by incubating the nanoparticles with ADC-PEG-SH following the same procedure. CPP+Tmab-PEG-AuNP were obtained by incubation with a 1×10^5 molar excess of CPP-PEG-SH for 5 min followed by the addition of a 1×10^5 molar excess of Tmab-PEG-SH, and further incubation under stirring for 2 h.

4.8. UV-Vis Spectroscopy

UV-Vis absorption spectra were obtained over a wavelength range of 800–200 nm for gold nanoparticles or 400–200 nm for protein samples, using a Shimadzu 2600 UV-Vis spectrophotometer (Shimadzu, Japan). AuNP samples in RPMI media were corrected by blank subtraction of the RPMI.

4.9. Size-Exclusion High-Performance Liquid Chromatography (SE-HPLC)

Size-exclusion chromatograms were obtained with a Zorbax GF-250 column connected to an Agilent 1200 Liquid Chromatography system (Agilent Technologies, Santa Clara, CA, USA), running potassium phosphate buffer 150 mM pH 6.5 as a mobile phase at a 0.5 mL/min flow rate. Peak absorption was detected at 280 nm with an in-line UV signal detector (Agilent Technologies, Santa Clara, CA, USA).

4.10. DLS and Zeta Potential Measurements

DLS and zeta potential measurements of the functionalized gold nanoparticles were conducted with a Malvern Zetasizer Nano ZS (Malvern Instruments, Worcestershire, UK) with a 633 nm Helium

Neon Laser and an avalanche photo diode (APD) detector. The measurements were conducted in triplicate and the values are reported as mean Z-average ± standard deviation. For zeta potential measurements, the functionalized nanoparticles suspended in PBS 1× (phosphate buffer 0.01 M, NaCl 0.137 M, KCl 0.0027 M, pH 7.4) were diluted 1:10 in deionized water. Cit-AuNPs were directly resuspended in PBS 0.1X. The zeta potential was derived from the Henry equation using an $f(Ka)$ of 1.5.

4.11. Cellular Uptake Quantification through Inductively Coupled Plasma Mass Spectrometry (ICP-MS)

The SKBR-3 cell line was provided by Dr. Thomas Grewal. The DLD-1 cell line was purchased from the American Type Culture Collection (ATCC). The MDA-MB-231 and MCF-7 cell lines were obtained from Dr. Fanfan Zhou. SKOV-3 cells were provided by Dr. Pegah Varamini.

To compare the cellular uptake of gold nanoparticles coated with OH-PEG and Tmab-PEG, SKBR-3 cells were seeded at density of 1×10^5 cells/well in 24-well plates in RPMI media containing 10% FBS. Following incubation at 37 °C for 48 h, the cell media was removed, the cells were washed twice with PBS, and fresh RPMI media (10% FBS) containing 50 µg/mL 20 nm and 50 nm gold nanoparticles (coated with OH-PEG or Tmab-PEG) was added, using 6 wells per AuNP sample. The cells were further incubated for 24 h. The AuNP containing media was removed and the cell monolayer washed 4 times with PBS. The cells were detached from the plate using 0.05% trypsin and collected in 1.5 mL centrifuge tubes. Trypsin was removed by pelleting the cells at 300 g for 5 min and the cells were washed twice more with PBS. The cell pellet was digested with 200 µL concentrated HNO_3 (15.9 M) overnight at room temperature. 800 µL concentrated HCl (12.1 M) was then added to dissolve the gold nanoparticles. A 1:4 dilution in Milli-Q water was performed for quantification of gold content through ICP-MS. ICP-MS measurements were carried out with a Perkin Elmer Nexion 300× ICP-MS instrument (Perkin-Elmer, Waltham, MA, USA), calibrated with 5, 10 and 20 parts per billion (ppb) gold standard solutions.

To compare cellular uptake in SKBR-3, DLD-1, MDA-MB-231 and MCF-7 cells, the uptake assays were carried out following the same procedure as described above albeit with the following modifications: (1) 25 µg/mL AuNP concentrations were used, (2) DLD-1, MDA-MB-231 and MCF-7 cells were seeded at 3×10^4 cells/well, (3) MDA-MB-231 and MCF-7 cell lines were cultured in DMEM media containing 10% FBS, (4) each nanoparticle sample was run in triplicate.

The concentration of the gold nanoparticles was determined based on their absorbance at 450 nm using $\varepsilon_{450} = 5.41 \times 10^8$ M^{-1} cm^{-1} and $\varepsilon_{450} = 9.92 \times 10^9$ M^{-1} cm^{-1} for 20 nm and 50 nm, respectively, according to previous determinations [32]. ICP-MS quantification of gold content in the AuNP suspensions was utilized to corroborate that the extinction coefficients used in this method provide appropriate estimations of gold concentrations. The nanoparticles in cell culture medium were filter sterilized through 0.22 µM filters prior to addition to the cells.

4.12. Cellular Uptake Evaluation by Transmission Electron Microscopy (TEM)

SKBR-3 cells were seeded at a density of 1×10^5 cells/well on collagen-coated Thermanox plastic coverslips placed inside each well (24-well plates) and incubated at 37 °C for 48 h in RPMI media containing 10% FBS. Fresh RPMI containing 50 ug/mL 50 nm OH-PEG-AuNP or Tmab-PEG-AuNP was added to the wells and further incubated at 37 °C for 24 h. The wells were washed thrice with PBS. The cells were fixed with 2.5% glutaraldehyde in 0.1 M phosphate buffer pH 7.4. The cell monolayers were subsequently fixed with osmium tetroxide 1% (w/v) in phosphate buffer 0.1 M pH 7.4, then embedded into an epon resin. The monolayers were microtomed into 70 nm sections and stained with uranyl acetate 2% and Reynold's lead citrate. TEM images were obtained with a JEOL JEM-1400 (Tokyo, Japan) microscope with an accelerating voltage of 120 kV.

4.13. Cell Cytotoxicity Evaluation

SKBR-3 and SKOV-3 cells were seeded at 5×10^3 and 3×10^3 cells/well on 96-well plates and incubated at 37 °C for 24 h in RPMI media containing 10% FBS. Fresh RPMI media containing free

MMAE, ADC, ADC-PEG-AuNP, Trastuzumab or OH-PEG-AuNP were added to the wells at the corresponding concentrations in triplicates. RPMI media was replenished for negative control samples. Images (10× magnification) of four different regions per well were acquired at 2-h intervals for 72 h after addition of the antimitotic or control sample using an Incucyte® ZOOM Live-cell Analysis System (Essen BioScience, Ann Arbor, MI, USA). Cell confluence was analyzed with the Incucyte® ZOOM integrated analysis software (v2016A) to generate cell growth curves over time. Growth rate inhibition metrics were employed to assess the antimitotic effect of the samples. Growth rate inhibition metrics have been developed recently to provide more robust and biologically relevant drug response parameters [50]. GR values were calculated as:

$$GR(d) = 2^{log_2(\frac{x(d)_f}{x(d)_0})/log_2(\frac{x(c)_f}{x(c)_0})} - 1$$

where $x(d)_0$ and $x(d)_f$ are the confluence values of cells treated with a cytotoxic agent at time t = 0 h and t = 72 h, respectively. $x(c)_0$ and $x(c)_f$ are confluence values of control wells at t = 0 h and t = 72 h.

GR values were plotted against treatment concentration and the data was fitted to a four-parameter dose-response curve. GR_{50} was obtained by interpolating the treatment concentration at which GR = 0.5.

4.14. Statistical Analysis

Gold uptake quantification was analyzed with a two-tailed, unpaired Student *t*-test. Values are denoted as mean ± standard deviation, and $p < 0.05$ was established as statistical significance.

5. Conclusions

The results presented herein report on the feasibility of utilizing multiple bioactive agents to construct gold nanoparticles with broader therapeutic capabilities. The construction of a thiol-functionalized PEGylated antibody drug-conjugate (PEGylated Trastuzumab-vcMMAE) proved to yield ADCs with conserved high affinity towards the HER2 receptor; thereby enabling coupling to gold nanoparticles to function as targeting agents carrying a cytotoxic payload. ADCs attached to the surface of gold nanoparticles demonstrated to retain similar in vitro cytotoxic potency against HER2 overexpressing cancer cell lines relative to the free ADC. Notwithstanding, enhanced accumulation in high EPR tumors could results in wider therapeutic indices.

Cellular uptake of AuNPs in a HER2 amplified cell line was significantly improved upon covalent attachment of the Trastuzumab targeting agent through the PEGylated-SH linker. Internalization into different cancer cell lines was further enhanced by employing the HIV-1 TAT protein (47–57) as a cell penetrating peptide. Yet, the combination of the antibody targeting agent and the penetrating peptide did not provide improvements in uptake—relative to the penetrating peptide only—in the conditions tested. Our results support previous observations with different nanoparticle formats with regards to the prominent role of surface charge on determining uptake rate into cells, insofar as the charge reversal obtained by incorporating the cell penetrating peptide had a more pronounced impact than the addition of the antibody targeting agent. Efficient cleavage of the valine-citrulline moiety for drug release requires cellular internalization for exposure to cathepsin B in lysosomes or endosomes; therefore, incorporation of the CPP might provide improved intracellular delivery of the MMAE payload in this format.

Supplementary Materials: The following are available online at http://www.mdpi.com/2072-6694/11/6/870/s1, Figure S1: Analysis of the presence of sulfhydryl groups and conservation of intact structure of Trastuzumab after partial reduction with DTT, Figure S2: SE-HPLC chromatograms of partially reduced Trastuzumab in 1 mM EDTA, Tmab-vcMMAE in H2O and Tmab-vcMMAE in acetonitrile 10% with formic acid 1%, Figure S3: AuNP stability upon surface functionalization with Tmab-PEG-SH. Addition of 1% NaCl to citrate capped AuNPs caused aggregation as evidenced by a broad absorption band in the 700–800 nm range, Figure S4: Representative tryptophan fluorescence emission spectra for the estimation of Trastuzumab:AuNP ratio for 20 nm AuNPs, Figure S5: Representative sensorgrams of (A) Trastuzumab, (B) Tmab-PEG-SH 25× and (C) Tmab-vcMMAE binding to recombinant HER2 receptor, Figure S6: Representative SKBR-3 cell growth curves employed to analyze growth rate inhibition activity of MMAE-containing agents at equivalent MMAE concentrations.

Author Contributions: E.C. and V.K. conceived the design. E.C. designed the study, performed all experimental work and data analysis and wrote the manuscript. V.K. supervised the development of the study, contributed to data interpretation and manuscript evaluation and editing.

Funding: This research received no external funding.

Acknowledgments: The authors would like to thank Genentech for their kind donation of Herceptin®. The authors would like to acknowledge the School of Pharmacy of The University of Sydney for financial support. E.C. would like to acknowledge the Ministry of Science, Technology and Telecommunications of the Republic of Costa Rica for postgraduate scholarship.

Conflicts of Interest: The authors declare no conflict of interest

References

1. Heldin, C.H.; Rubin, K.; Pietras, K.; Ostman, A. High interstitial fluid pressure-an obstacle in cancer therapy. *Nat. Rev. Cancer* **2004**, *4*, 806–813. [CrossRef] [PubMed]
2. Netti, P.A.; Baxter, L.T.; Boucher, Y.; Skalak, R.; Jain, R.K. Time-dependent behavior of interstitial fluid pressure in solid tumors: Implications for drug delivery. *Cancer Res.* **1995**, *55*, 5451–5458. [PubMed]
3. Tredan, O.; Galmarini, C.M.; Patel, K.; Tannock, I.F. Drug resistance and the solid tumor microenvironment. *J. Natl. Cancer Inst.* **2007**, *99*, 1441–1454. [CrossRef] [PubMed]
4. Matsumura, Y.; Maeda, H. A new concept for macromolecular therapeutics in cancer chemotherapy: Mechanism of tumoritropic accumulation of proteins and the antitumor agent smancs. *Cancer Res.* **1986**, *46*, 6387–6392. [PubMed]
5. Tran, S.; DeGiovanni, P.-J.; Piel, B.; Rai, P. Cancer nanomedicine: A review of recent success in drug delivery. *Clin. Transl. Med.* **2017**, *6*, 44. [CrossRef]
6. Jin, S.; Leach, J.C.; Ye, K. Nanoparticle-mediated gene delivery. *Methods Mol. Biol.* **2009**, *544*, 547–557. [CrossRef] [PubMed]
7. Manthe, R.L.; Foy, S.P.; Krishnamurthy, N.; Sharma, B.; Labhasetwar, V. Tumor ablation and nanotechnology. *Mol. Pharm.* **2010**, *7*, 1880–1898. [CrossRef]
8. Will, O.; Purkayastha, S.; Chan, C.; Athanasiou, T.; Darzi, A.W.; Gedroyc, W.; Tekkis, P.P. Diagnostic precision of nanoparticle-enhanced MRI for lymph-node metastases: A meta-analysis. *Lancet Oncol.* **2006**, *7*, 52–60. [CrossRef]
9. Lukianova-Hleb, E.Y.; Ren, X.; Sawant, R.R.; Wu, X.; Torchilin, V.P.; Lapotko, D.O. On-demand intracellular amplification of chemoradiation with cancer-specific plasmonic nanobubbles. *Nat. Med.* **2014**, *20*, 778. [CrossRef]
10. Kyriazi, M.-E.; Giust, D.; El-Sagheer, A.H.; Lackie, P.M.; Muskens, O.L.; Brown, T.; Kanaras, A.G. Multiplexed mRNA Sensing and Combinatorial-Targeted Drug Delivery Using DNA-Gold Nanoparticle Dimers. *ACS Nano* **2018**, *12*, 3333–3340. [CrossRef]
11. Xue, Y.; Li, X.; Li, H.; Zhang, W. Quantifying thiol–gold interactions towards the efficient strength control. *Nat. Commu.* **2014**, *5*, 4348. [CrossRef] [PubMed]
12. Wilhelm, S.; Tavares, A.J.; Dai, Q.; Ohta, S.; Audet, J.; Dvorak, H.F.; Chan, W.C.W. Analysis of nanoparticle delivery to tumours. *Nat. Rev. Mater.* **2016**, *1*, 16014. [CrossRef]
13. Alkilany, A.M.; Murphy, C.J. Toxicity and cellular uptake of gold nanoparticles: What we have learned so far? *J. Nanopart. Res. Interdiscip. Forum Nanoscale Sci. Technol.* **2010**, *12*, 2313–2333. [CrossRef] [PubMed]
14. Goel, R.; Shah, N.; Visaria, R.; Paciotti, G.F.; Bischof, J.C. Biodistribution of TNF-alpha-coated gold nanoparticles in an in vivo model system. *Nanomedicine* **2009**, *4*, 401–410. [CrossRef] [PubMed]
15. Byrne, J.D.; Betancourt, T.; Brannon-Peppas, L. Active targeting schemes for nanoparticle systems in cancer therapeutics. *Adv. Drug Deliv. Rev.* **2008**, *60*, 1615–1626. [CrossRef] [PubMed]
16. Rosenblum, D.; Joshi, N.; Tao, W.; Karp, J.M.; Peer, D. Progress and challenges towards targeted delivery of cancer therapeutics. *Nat. Commu.* **2018**, *9*, 1410. [CrossRef]
17. Slamon, D.J.; Leyland-Jones, B.; Shak, S.; Fuchs, H.; Paton, V.; Bajamonde, A.; Fleming, T.; Eiermann, W.; Wolter, J.; Pegram, M.; et al. Use of Chemotherapy plus a Monoclonal Antibody against HER2 for Metastatic Breast Cancer That Overexpresses HER2. *N. Engl. J. Med.* **2001**, *344*, 783–792. [CrossRef]

18. Bang, Y.J.; Van Cutsem, E.; Feyereislova, A.; Chung, H.C.; Shen, L.; Sawaki, A.; Lordick, F.; Ohtsu, A.; Omuro, Y.; Satoh, T.; et al. Trastuzumab in combination with chemotherapy versus chemotherapy alone for treatment of HER2-positive advanced gastric or gastro-oesophageal junction cancer (ToGA): A phase 3, open-label, randomised controlled trial. *Lancet* **2010**, *376*, 687–697. [CrossRef]
19. Fléjou, J.F.; Paraf, F.; Muzeau, F.; Fékété, F.; Hénin, D.; Jothy, S.; Potet, F. Expression of c-erbB-2 oncogene product in Barrett's adenocarcinoma: Pathological and prognostic correlations. *J. Clin. Pathol.* **1994**, *47*, 23. [CrossRef]
20. Berchuck, A.; Kamel, A.; Whitaker, R.; Kerns, B.; Olt, G.; Kinney, R.; Soper, J.T.; Dodge, R.; Clarke-Pearson, D.L.; Marks, P.; et al. Overexpression of HER-2/neu Is Associated with Poor Survival in Advanced Epithelial Ovarian Cancer. *Cancer Res.* **1990**, *50*, 4087.
21. Rolitsky, C.D.; Theil, K.S.; McGaughy, V.R.; Copeland, L.J.; Niemann, T.H. HER-2/neu amplification and overexpression in endometrial carcinoma. *Int. J. Gynecol. Pathol.* **1999**, *18*, 138–143. [CrossRef] [PubMed]
22. Nakajima, M.; Sawada, H.; Yamada, Y.; Watanabe, A.; Tatsumi, M.; Yamashita, J.; Matsuda, M.; Sakaguchi, T.; Hirao, T.; Nakano, H. The prognostic significance of amplification and overexpression of c-met and c-erb B-2 in human gastric carcinomas. *Cancer* **1999**, *85*, 1894–1902. [CrossRef]
23. Santin, A.D.; Bellone, S.; Van Stedum, S.; Bushen, W.; Palmieri, M.; Siegel, E.R.; De Las Casas, L.E.; Roman, J.J.; Burnett, A.; Pecorelli, S. Amplification of c-erbB2 oncogene. *Cancer* **2005**, *104*, 1391–1397. [CrossRef] [PubMed]
24. Yonemura, Y.; Ninomiya, I.; Yamaguchi, A.; Fushida, S.; Kimura, H.; Ohoyama, S.; Miyazaki, I.; Endou, Y.; Tanaka, M.; Sasaki, T. Evaluation of Immunoreactivity for erbB-2 Protein as a Marker of Poor Short Term Prognosis in Gastric Cancer. *Cancer Res.* **1991**, *51*, 1034. [PubMed]
25. Hudis, C.A. Trastuzumab—mechanism of action and use in clinical practice. *N. Engl. J. Med.* **2007**, *357*, 39–51. [CrossRef] [PubMed]
26. Liu, M.; Yang, Y.J.; Zheng, H.; Zhong, X.R.; Wang, Y.; Wang, Z.; Wang, Y.G.; Wang, Y.P. Membrane-bound complement regulatory proteins are prognostic factors of operable breast cancer treated with adjuvant trastuzumab: A retrospective study. *Oncol. Rep.* **2014**, *32*, 2619–2627. [CrossRef]
27. Elgundi, Z.; Reslan, M.; Cruz, E.; Sifniotis, V.; Kayser, V. The state-of-play and future of antibody therapeutics. *Adv. Drug Deliv. Rev.* **2017**, *122*, 2–19. [CrossRef]
28. Thurber, G.M.; Schmidt, M.M.; Wittrup, K.D. Antibody tumor penetration: Transport opposed by systemic and antigen-mediated clearance. *Adv. Drug Deliv. Rev.* **2008**, *60*, 1421–1434. [CrossRef]
29. Lee, C.M.; Tannock, I.F. The distribution of the therapeutic monoclonal antibodies cetuximab and trastuzumab within solid tumors. *BMC Cancer* **2010**, *10*, 255. [CrossRef]
30. Hermanson, G.T. Chapter 18-PEGylation and Synthetic Polymer Modification. In *Bioconjugate Techniques*, 3rd ed.; Hermanson, G.T., Ed.; Academic Press: Boston, MA, USA, 2013; 2p.
31. Gustafson, H.H.; Holt-Casper, D.; Grainger, D.W.; Ghandehari, H. Nanoparticle Uptake: The Phagocyte Problem. *Nano Today* **2015**, *10*, 487–510. [CrossRef]
32. Haiss, W.; Thanh, N.T.K.; Aveyard, J.; Fernig, D.G. Determination of Size and Concentration of Gold Nanoparticles from UV–Vis Spectra. *Anal. Chem.* **2007**, *79*, 4215–4221. [CrossRef] [PubMed]
33. Holliday, D.L.; Speirs, V. Choosing the right cell line for breast cancer research. *Breast Cancer Res.* **2011**, *13*, 215. [CrossRef]
34. Libutti, S.K.; Paciotti, G.F.; Byrnes, A.A.; Alexander, H.R., Jr.; Gannon, W.E.; Walker, M.; Seidel, G.D.; Yuldasheva, N.; Tamarkin, L. Phase I and pharmacokinetic studies of CYT-6091, a novel PEGylated colloidal gold-rhTNF nanomedicine. *Clin. Cancer Res.* **2010**, *16*, 6139–6149. [CrossRef] [PubMed]
35. Suk, J.S.; Xu, Q.; Kim, N.; Hanes, J.; Ensign, L.M. PEGylation as a strategy for improving nanoparticle-based drug and gene delivery. *Adv. Drug Deliv. Rev.* **2016**, *99*, 28–51. [CrossRef] [PubMed]
36. Gref, R.; Minamitake, Y.; Peracchia, M.T.; Trubetskoy, V.; Torchilin, V.; Langer, R. Biodegradable long-circulating polymeric nanospheres. *Science* **1994**, *263*, 1600–1603. [CrossRef]
37. Adem, Y.T.; Schwarz, K.A.; Duenas, E.; Patapoff, T.W.; Galush, W.J.; Esue, O. Auristatin Antibody Drug Conjugate Physical Instability and the Role of Drug Payload. *Bioconj. Chem.* **2014**, *25*, 656–664. [CrossRef] [PubMed]

38. Li, F.; Emmerton, K.K.; Jonas, M.; Zhang, X.; Miyamoto, J.B.; Setter, J.R.; Nicholas, N.D.; Okeley, N.M.; Lyon, R.P.; Benjamin, D.R.; et al. Intracellular Released Payload Influences Potency and Bystander-Killing Effects of Antibody-Drug Conjugates in Preclinical Models. *Cancer Res.* **2016**, *76*, 2710–2719. [CrossRef] [PubMed]
39. Jiang, W.; Kim, B.Y.S.; Rutka, J.T.; Chan, W.C.W. Nanoparticle-mediated cellular response is size-dependent. *Nat. Nanotechnol.* **2008**, *3*, 145. [CrossRef]
40. Cho, E.C.; Xie, J.; Wurm, P.A.; Xia, Y. Understanding the Role of Surface Charges in Cellular Adsorption versus Internalization by Selectively Removing Gold Nanoparticles on the Cell Surface with a I2/KI Etchant. *Nano Lett.* **2009**, *9*, 1080–1084. [CrossRef]
41. Ma, X.; Wu, Y.; Jin, S.; Tian, Y.; Zhang, X.; Zhao, Y.; Yu, L.; Liang, X.-J. Gold Nanoparticles Induce Autophagosome Accumulation through Size-Dependent Nanoparticle Uptake and Lysosome Impairment. *ACS Nano* **2011**, *5*, 8629–8639. [CrossRef]
42. Tkachenko, A.G.; Xie, H.; Liu, Y.; Coleman, D.; Ryan, J.; Glomm, W.R.; Shipton, M.K.; Franzen, S.; Feldheim, D.L. Cellular Trajectories of Peptide-Modified Gold Particle Complexes: Comparison of Nuclear Localization Signals and Peptide Transduction Domains. *Bioconj. Chem.* **2004**, *15*, 482–490. [CrossRef] [PubMed]
43. Baulida, J.; Kraus, M.H.; Alimandi, M.; Di Fiore, P.P.; Carpenter, G. All ErbB receptors other than the epidermal growth factor receptor are endocytosis impaired. *J. Biol. Chem.* **1996**, *271*, 5251–5257. [PubMed]
44. Kim, B.; Han, G.; Toley, B.J.; Kim, C.-k.; Rotello, V.M.; Forbes, N.S. Tuning payload delivery in tumour cylindroids using gold nanoparticles. *Nat. Nanotechnol.* **2010**, *5*, 465. [CrossRef] [PubMed]
45. Turkevich, J.; Stevenson, P.C.; Hillier, J. The Formation of Colloidal Gold. *J. Phys. Chem.* **1953**, *57*, 670–673. [CrossRef]
46. Frens, G. Controlled Nucleation for the Regulation of the Particle Size in Monodisperse Gold Suspensions. *Nat. Phys. Sci.* **1973**, *241*, 20. [CrossRef]
47. Kelly, S.T.; Zydney, A.L. Effects of intermolecular thiol–disulfide interchange reactions on bsa fouling during microfiltration. *Biotechnol. Bioeng.* **1994**, *44*, 972–982. [CrossRef] [PubMed]
48. Trivedi, M.V.; Laurence, J.S.; Siahaan, T.J. The role of thiols and disulfides on protein stability. *Curr. Protein Pept. Sci.* **2009**, *10*, 614–625. [CrossRef]
49. Hamblett, K.J.; Senter, P.D.; Chace, D.F.; Sun, M.M.; Lenox, J.; Cerveny, C.G.; Kissler, K.M.; Bernhardt, S.X.; Kopcha, A.K.; Zabinski, R.F.; et al. Effects of drug loading on the antitumor activity of a monoclonal antibody drug conjugate. *Clin. Cancer Res.* **2004**, *10*, 7063–7070. [CrossRef]
50. Hafner, M.; Niepel, M.; Chung, M.; Sorger, P.K. Growth rate inhibition metrics correct for confounders in measuring sensitivity to cancer drugs. *Nat. Methods* **2016**, *13*, 521–527. [CrossRef]

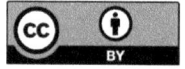

© 2019 by the authors. Licensee MDPI, Basel, Switzerland. This article is an open access article distributed under the terms and conditions of the Creative Commons Attribution (CC BY) license (http://creativecommons.org/licenses/by/4.0/).

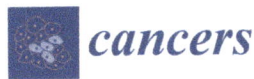

Article

Incorporation of a Hydrophilic Spacer Reduces Hepatic Uptake of HER2-Targeting Affibody–DM1 Drug Conjugates

Haozhong Ding [1,†], Mohamed Altai [2,†], Sara S. Rinne [3], Anzhelika Vorobyeva [2], Vladimir Tolmachev [2], Torbjörn Gräslund [1] and Anna Orlova [3,4,*]

1. Department of Protein Science, KTH Royal Institute of Technology, Roslagstullsbacken 21, 114 17 Stockholm, Sweden
2. Department of Immunology, Genetics and Pathology, Uppsala University, 751 85 Uppsala, Sweden
3. Department of Medicinal Chemistry, Uppsala University, 751 23 Uppsala, Sweden
4. Science for Life Laboratory, Uppsala University, 751 23 Uppsala, Sweden
* Correspondence: Anna.orlova@ilk.uu.se; Tel.: +46-18-471-3414
† These authors contributed equally to this work.

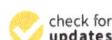

Received: 17 July 2019; Accepted: 12 August 2019; Published: 14 August 2019

Abstract: Affibody molecules are small affinity-engineered scaffold proteins which can be engineered to bind to desired targets. The therapeutic potential of using an affibody molecule targeting HER2, fused to an albumin-binding domain (ABD) and conjugated with the cytotoxic maytansine derivate MC-DM1 (AffiDC), has been validated. Biodistribution studies in mice revealed an elevated hepatic uptake of the AffiDC, but histopathological examination of livers showed no major signs of toxicity. However, previous clinical experience with antibody drug conjugates have revealed a moderate- to high-grade hepatotoxicity in treated patients, which merits efforts to also minimize hepatic uptake of the AffiDCs. In this study, the aim was to reduce the hepatic uptake of AffiDCs and optimize their in vivo targeting properties. We have investigated if incorporation of hydrophilic glutamate-based spacers adjacent to MC-DM1 in the AffiDC, $(Z_{HER2:2891})_2$–ABD–MC-DM1, would counteract the hydrophobic nature of MC-DM1 and, hence, reduce hepatic uptake. Two new AffiDCs including either a triglutamate–spacer–, $(Z_{HER2:2891})_2$–ABD–E_3–MC-DM1, or a hexaglutamate–spacer–, $(Z_{HER2:2891})_2$–ABD–E_6–MC-DM1 next to the site of MC-DM1 conjugation were designed. We radiolabeled the hydrophilized AffiDCs and compared them, both in vitro and in vivo, with the previously investigated $(Z_{HER2:2891})_2$–ABD–MC-DM1 drug conjugate containing no glutamate spacer. All three AffiDCs demonstrated specific binding to HER2 and comparable in vitro cytotoxicity. A comparative biodistribution study of the three radiolabeled AffiDCs showed that the addition of glutamates reduced drug accumulation in the liver while preserving the tumor uptake. These results confirmed the relation between DM1 hydrophobicity and liver accumulation. We believe that the drug development approach described here may also be useful for other affinity protein-based drug conjugates to further improve their in vivo properties and facilitate their clinical translatability.

Keywords: affibody; drug conjugates; hepatic uptake; DM1

1. Introduction

Drug conjugates (DCs) are an emerging class of potent biopharmaceuticals developed to overcome resistance to conventional targeted therapy and reduce off-target toxicity [1–3]. DCs are composed of a targeting agent, specifically interacting with a particular antigen, attached to a biologically active drug or cytotoxic compound via a linker. Antibody drug conjugates (ADCs) constitute the most studied class of DCs [3]. Two common types of drug molecules utilized in many ADCs are the auristatins/maytansines that inhibit microtubule polymerization and the calicheamicins which target the minor groove of DNA to induce double-stranded cuts, leading to cell death in both cases. Today, five ADCs have received market approval by the US Food and Drug Administration (FDA); gemtuzumab ozogamicin (Mylotarg®), brentuximab vedotin (Adcetris®), ado-trastuzumab emtansine (Kadcyla®), inotuzumab ozogamicin (Besponsa®), polatuzumab vedotin-piiq (Polivy®), and many others are still under development or in clinical trials [4,5].

Despite the current success, ADCs still face many limitations [6]. Many conjugation strategies rely on unspecific drug attachment to abundant lysine or cysteine residues in the monoclonal antibodies (MAbs). Even though many strategies for site-specific attachment have been developed [7], many ADCs still have a variable drug-to-antibody ratio (DAR) and variable sites of drug attachment, thus forming a nonhomogeneous final product [3,8]. The lack of homogeneity may lead to suboptimal stability, pharmacokinetics, and activity [9]. A random distribution of payloads may potentially interfere with critical residues on the antigen binding regions of MAbs. Moreover, the rather large ADCs may suffer from limited localization and penetration into solid tumors, thus restricting their antitumor efficacy.

In recent years, alternatives to MAbs have started to emerge. Engineered scaffold proteins (ESPs) are considered the next-generation non-immunoglobulin-based therapeutics [10]. They are derived from small, robust non-immunoglobulin proteins, which are used as "scaffolds" for supporting a surface with the ability to specifically interact with the desired target antigens with high affinity, such as receptors overexpressed on cancer cells. Affibody molecules (6–7 kDa) are one of the most studied classes of ESPs and they are more than 20-fold smaller than MAbs [11,12]. Affibody molecules are based on a 58 aa cysteine-free three-helix scaffold which is derived from one of the IgG binding domains in protein A expressed by Staphylococcus aureus. Affibody molecules have commonly been created by randomization of 13 surface-localized amino acids on helices 1 and 2, followed by phage display selection of binders to different biological targets. Currently, affibody molecules binding with high affinity to several cancer-associated molecular targets, such as human epidermal growth factor receptor 2 (HER2), epidermal growth factor receptor (EGFR), human epidermal growth factor receptor 3 (HER3), insulin-like growth factor 1 receptor (IGF-1R), platelet-derived growth factor receptor beta (PDGFRβ), and carbonic anhydrase 9 (CAIX), have been developed. The cysteine-free structure of affibody molecules permits site-specific conjugation of payloads by introduction of one or more cysteine amino acids at desired position(s) in the scaffold onto which the drug (or any other prosthetic/functional group) can be site-specifically attached. This results in generation of well-defined and homogenous products. The use of affibody molecules as an alternative to MAbs for targeted drug delivery offers several advantages, including efficient production in simple prokaryotic hosts such as *Escherichia coli* [13], efficient and specific drug attachment [14] as well as a relatively smaller size compared to MAbs, which may lead to more efficient penetration and better distribution in solid tumors [15]. However, an important issue for payload delivery using small proteins like affibody molecules is rapid renal excretion. Short in vivo half-life may decrease potency and worsen patient compliance by requiring more frequent administrations. An albumin-binding domain (ABD) was used to prolong the in vivo residence time of affibody molecules by noncovalent interaction with serum albumin [16,17]. We have recently reported on the feasibility of using an anti-HER2 affibody drug conjugate for treatment of HER2-overexpressing tumors in a preclinical murine model [14]. In that study, a HER2-specific affibody molecule, $Z_{HER2:2891}$, was site-specifically conjugated to the antimitotic maytansine derivate (MC-DM1) using maleimide–thiol chemistry. Mice bearing HER2-expressing ovarian cancer xenografts SKOV-3, treated with the tripartite AffiDC, ($Z_{HER2:2891}$)$_2$-ABD-MC-DM1, showed significantly longer survival—twice as long compared to mice in control groups. ($Z_{HER2:2891}$)$_2$–ABD–MC-DM1 was well-tolerated, and no signs of tissue injury or morphological changes were observed after six cycles of treatment [14]. An interesting finding of that study was the relatively high hepatic uptake of the AffiDC compared to the parental non-MC-DM1-containing HER2-targeting affibody construct. Although no histopathological changes were observed in liver sections of the treated mice, earlier reports indicate that hepatotoxicity may be a serious adverse event associated with several FDA-approved ADCs. For example, it has been observed in several clinical studies involving ado-trastuzumab emtansine (T-DM1) that treatment was associated with elevation of hepatic transaminases and hepatic toxicity [18–20]. The mechanism underlying this observed hepatotoxicity remains elusive [20]. A recent report by Yan et al. tried to link hepatic expression of the HER2 receptor to the observed T-DM1-induced hepatotoxicity in a murine model [21]. This study demonstrated that HER2-mediated uptake of T-DM1 by hepatocytes followed by release of DM1 in the cytosol induced several changes, including disorganization of microtubules, nuclear fragmentation, and cell growth inhibition. Even though no liver toxicity was observed in the AffiDC study [14], it is possible that prolonged treatment regimens using higher doses could constitute a problem, and minimization of liver uptake is thus desirable.

In the initial AffiDC study [14], an attempt to decrease liver uptake was performed by pretreating mice with a several-fold excess of the non-MC-DM1-conjugated, HER2-targeting affibody molecule, $Z_{HER2:342}$, to block available HER2 receptors. However, the hepatic uptake of AffiDC was not reduced by this pretreatment strategy. As mentioned above, the uptake of the AffiDC in liver was significantly higher compared to previously reported HER2-targeting affibody constructs lacking MC-DM1 [16,17]. A possible explanation is that the elevated hepatic uptake is mediated, at least in part, by the presence of the relatively lipophilic MC-DM1. It is known that hydrophobic compounds may facilitate greater reticuloendothelial system clearance and, therefore, increased uptake by the liver. Such effect of drug hydrophobicity on tissue distribution was observed earlier for ADCs, especially at high DARs [22].

In this study, we hypothesized that incorporation of a hydrophilic glutamate-based spacer adjacent to MC-DM1 would reduce hepatic uptake by counteracting the hydrophobic nature of the drug. To test this hypothesis, we designed AffiDCs containing either a triglutamate spacer–(($Z_{HER2:2891}$)$_2$–ABD–E_3–MC-DM1) or a hexaglutamate–spacer–(($Z_{HER2:2891}$)$_2$–ABD–E_6–MC-DM1) (Figure 1A).

These two drug conjugates were compared, in vitro, with the previously evaluated AffiDC, ($Z_{HER2:2891}$)$_2$–ABD–MC-DM1, containing no spacer. The conjugates were also radiolabeled with ^{99m}Tc ($T_{1/2}$ = 6 h, $E\gamma$ = 140 keV), through the N-terminally localized HEHEHE-tag (Scheme 1 in Supplementary Figure S1), and the influence of the glutamate spacer on hepatic uptake and overall biodistribution in a HER2-overexpressing preclinical murine tumor model was investigated.

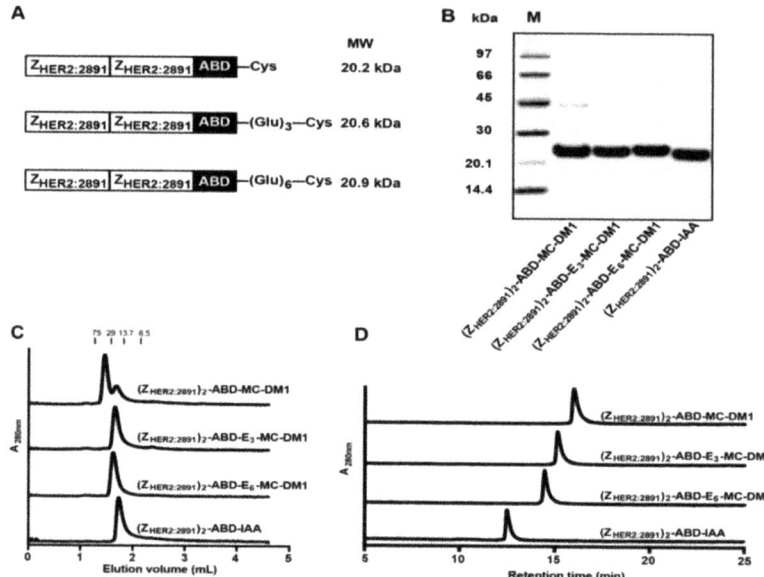

Figure 1. Production and initial biochemical characterization of the conjugates. (**A**) Schematic representation of the proteins. (**B**) Conjugates after final RP-HPLC purification were analyzed on a 4%–12% SDS-PAGE gel under reducing conditions. The numbers to the left are the molecular weight (kDa) of the marker proteins in lane M. (**C**) Analytical size-exclusion chromatography profiles of the conjugates. The numbers above the chromatograms are the molecular weight (kDa) of protein standards. (**D**) RP-HPLC analysis of the conjugates during a 20 min linear gradient from 30% to 60% acetonitrile in water with 0.1% TFA.

2. Results

2.1. Production and Biochemical Characterization of the Affibody–MC-DM1 Conjugates

The affibody constructs, schematically represented in Figure 1A, were recombinantly expressed and purified, and MC-DM1 was conjugated to a C-terminal cysteine. A construct lacking MC-DM1 was used ((Z$_{HER2:2891}$)$_2$–ABD–IAA) as a control, where the C-terminal cysteine was instead alkylated by 2-iodoacetamide (IAA). The purified conjugates were analyzed by SDS-PAGE under reducing conditions, and the gel showed pure proteins with essentially the expected molecular weights (Figure 1B). A weak contaminating band in the lane of (Z$_{HER2:2891}$)$_2$–ABD–MC-DM1 was visible with a molecular weight of approximately 45 kDa, and could thus constitute a dimer. The conjugates were further analyzed by size-exclusion chromatography under native conditions. The chromatogram from (Z$_{HER2:2891}$)$_2$–ABD–MC-DM1 showed that the protein was eluted as a double-peak, where the major peak had a retention time corresponding to a dimer and the minor peak had a retention time corresponding to a monomer. The other three conjugates were eluted as a single symmetrical peak with a retention time corresponding to a monomer (Figure 1C). The molecular weights were measured by ESI-TOF (Table 1) and the results showed conjugates matching exactly the molecular weight of monomeric proteins with a drug-to-affibody ratio of 1. The conjugates were further analyzed by passage through a C18 column using a linear gradient of acetonitrile in water in an RP-HPLC setup (Figure 1D). The recorded chromatograms showed that (Z$_{HER2:2891}$)$_2$–ABD–E$_6$–MC-DM1 was eluted first, followed by (Z$_{HER2:2891}$)$_2$–ABD–E$_3$–MC-DM1 and (Z$_{HER2:2891}$)$_2$–ABD–MC-DM1, suggesting that incorporation of glutamate residues reduced the hydrophobicity of the conjugates by shielding the MC-DM1 part from interaction with the C18 column. The control (Z$_{HER2:2891}$)$_2$–ABD–IAA, lacking

MC-DM1, was eluted even earlier than the other three, further suggesting a profound increase in hydrophobicity of the conjugates by addition of MC-DM1.

Table 1. Biochemical characterization of the conjugates.

Conjugates	Purity (%) [a]	Calc. Mw (Da)	Found Mw (Da) [b]
$(Z_{HER2:2891})_2$–ABD–MC-DM1	>95	21,006.3	21,005.8
$(Z_{HER2:2891})_2$–ABD–E_3–MC-DM1	>95	21,393.6	21,393.0
$(Z_{HER2:2891})_2$–ABD–E_6–MC-DM1	>95	21,781.0	21,780.1
$(Z_{HER2:2891})_2$–ABD–IAA	>95	20,219.9	20,219.5

[a] Determined by analytical RP-HPLC; [b] Mass spectrometry was used to determine the molecular weight (Mw) of the conjugates. Deconvolution was performed to determine the monoisotopic molecular weight of the proteins.

2.2. Binding Specificity and Affinity Determination of Affibody–MC-DM1 Conjugates

To investigate if MC-DM1 conjugation and glutamic acid insertion would affect the affinity of $Z_{HER2:2891}$ to HER2, a dilution series of the conjugates were injected into a biosensor over three different surfaces with different levels of immobilized extracellular domain of HER2 (Figure 2). Since each construct contains two affibody molecules, a potential avidity effect could occur if the HER2 receptor molecules are too closely spaced and allow simultaneous interaction with both. The interaction was analyzed assuming a 1:1 interaction, and consistent on- and off-rates were determined from the recorded sensorgrams for the three surfaces, indicating a lack of avidity effect and that a 1:1 interaction occurred. The equilibrium dissociation constant (K_D) for the interactions were determined from the on- and off-rates and are displayed in Table 2. The K_D values were found to be similar for the three MC-DM1 conjugates and the control, and ranged from 17 to 28 nM. The ability of the conjugates to interact with human serum albumin (HSA) and mouse serum albumin (MSA) was investigated by injection of a dilution series over a chip with immobilized HSA or MSA (Figure 3). The kinetic constants were derived from the sensorgrams (Table 3). The affinities (K_D) for HSA ranged from 0.57 to 1.2 nM. The affinities for MSA were slightly weaker and ranged from 2.5 to 8.0 nM.

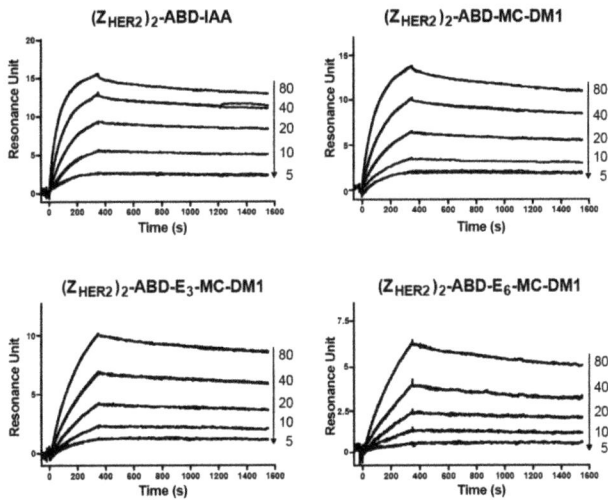

Figure 2. Biosensor analysis of the interactions between the conjugates and HER2. Dilution series of the conjugates were sequentially injected over flow cells with immobilized extracellular domain of HER2. All experiments were repeated once and each panel is an overlay of all concentrations, in duplicates, for each conjugate. The numbers to the right of each panel indicate the concentrations of the injected conjugates (nM) corresponding to each sensorgram.

Table 2. Affinity constants for conjugates interacting with HER2.

Measurement	$(Z_{HER2:2891})_2$–ABD–IAA	$(Z_{HER2:2891})_2$–ABD–MC-DM1	$(Z_{HER2:2891})_2$–ABD–E_3–MC-DM1	$(Z_{HER2:2891})_2$–ABD–E_6–MC-DM1
k_a (1/M·s)	3.0×10^5	7.9×10^4	5.6×10^4	5.5×10^4
k_d (1/s)	9.6×10^{-5}	1.4×10^{-4}	1.3×10^{-4}	1.5×10^{-4}
K_D (M)	3.2×10^{-10}	1.7×10^{-9}	2.4×10^{-9}	2.8×10^{-9}

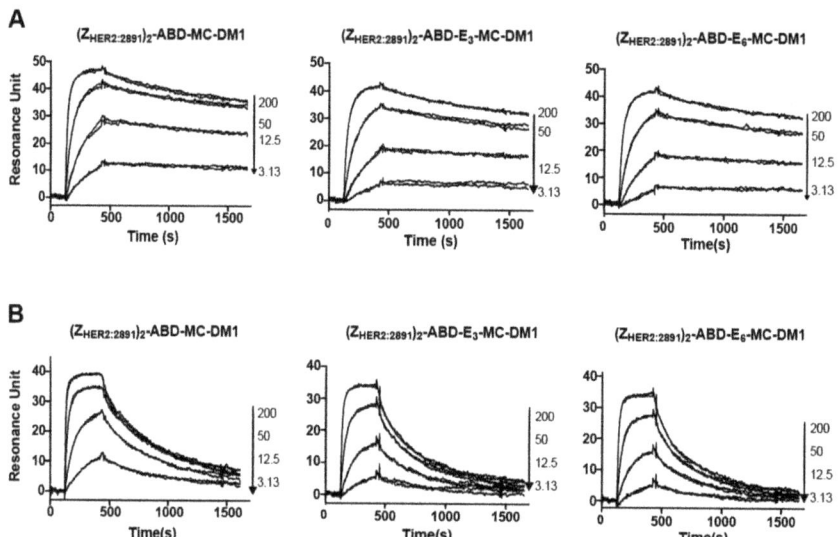

Figure 3. Biosensor analysis of the interactions between the conjugates and serum albumin. Serial dilutions of the conjugates were injected over a flow cell with immobilized HSA (**A**) or mouse serum albumin (MSA) (**B**). All experiments were repeated once, and each panel is an overlay of all concentrations in duplicates for each conjugate. The numbers to the right of each panel indicate the concentrations of the injected conjugates (nM) corresponding to each sensorgram.

Table 3. Affinity constants for conjugates interacting with serum albumin.

Measurement	$(Z_{HER2:2891})_2$–ABD–MC-DM1		$(Z_{HER2:2891})_2$–ABD–E_3–MC-DM1		$(Z_{HER2:2891})_2$–ABD–E_6–MC-DM1	
	HSA	MSA	HSA	MSA	HSA	MSA
k_a (1/M·s)	3.3×10^5	6.0×10^5	1.7×10^5	2.8×10^5	1.6×10^5	3.0×10^5
k_d (1/s)	1.9×10^{-4}	1.5×10^{-3}	2.0×10^{-4}	2.0×10^{-3}	1.9×10^{-4}	2.4×10^{-3}
K_D (M)	5.7×10^{-10}	2.5×10^{-9}	1.2×10^{-9}	7.2×10^{-9}	1.2×10^{-9}	8.0×10^{-9}

2.3. In Vitro Cytotoxicity Analysis

The cytotoxicity of the affibody–MC-DM1 conjugates was measured by treating AU565 (high HER2 expression), SKBR3 (high HER2 expression), SKOV3 (high HER2 expression), A549 (moderate HER2 expression), and MCF7 (low HER2 expression) cells, with serial dilutions of the conjugates followed by measurement of cell viability (Figure 4, Table 4). Two controls were also included, the nontoxic control $(Z_{HER2:2891})_2$–ABD–IAA lacking MC-DM1, and the nontarget control $(Z_{Taq})_2$–ABD–MC-DM1. The nontarget control was a size matched control where $Z_{HER2:2891}$ had been replaced with Z_{Taq}, an affibody molecule that specifically binds to DNA polymerase from *Thermus aquaticus*, and was thus not expected to bind to any protein of human origin [14]. $(Z_{Taq})_2$–ABD–MC-DM1 was previously characterized and was found to be a homogenous protein of the expected molecular weight with a purity >95% [14]. It was found not to interact with the HER2 receptor and did not induce cell death in cells overexpressing the HER2 receptor [14]. The targeting drug conjugates demonstrated subnanomolar IC_{50} values on AU565 and SKBR-3 cell lines. For AU565 cells, the IC_{50} values ranged from 0.22 to 0.48 nM, and for SKBR3 cells from 0.14 to 0.38 nM. For SKOV3, the IC_{50} values ranged from 47 to 116 nM. The nontoxic control $(Z_{HER2:2891})_2$–ABD–IAA showed a slight inhibition of cell growth on the AU565 and SKBR3 cell lines at higher concentrations (>10^{-9} M). For SKOV3 cells, a slight growth-promoting effect was observed at the highest concentration. All conjugates demonstrated a substantially weaker cytotoxic effect on A549 and MCF7 cells. The IC_{50} could not be measured at the concentrations used, but from Figure 4, it is evident that they were weaker than 10^{-6} M in all cases. For all five cell lines, the nontarget control $(Z_{Taq})_2$–ABD–MC-DM1 required high concentrations to affect cell viability. The IC_{50} values could not be determined from the concentration range used, except for SKOV3 cells (IC_{50} 350 nM). From Figure 4, it is evident that the IC_{50} value is 2 to 3 orders of magnitude weaker for the high expressing cell lines. The nontarget control $(Z_{Taq})_2$-ABD-MC-DM1 had a cytotoxic potential similar to the $Z_{HER2:2891}$-containing conjugates on A549 and MCF7 cells.

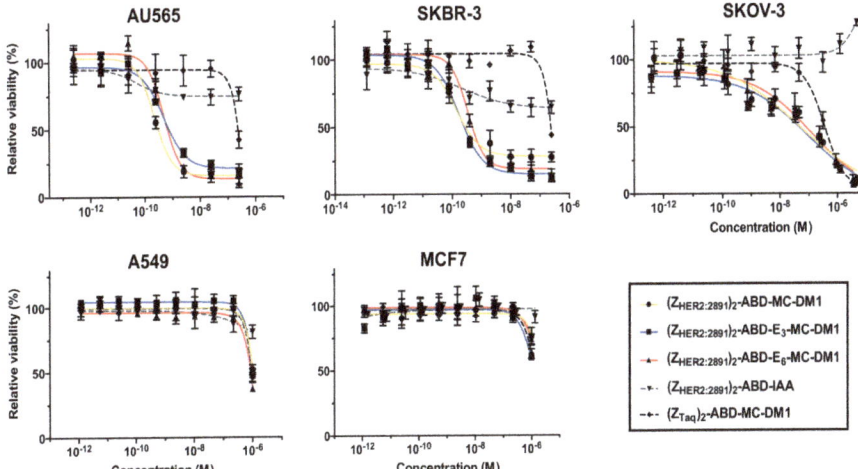

Figure 4. In vitro cytotoxicity of the conjugates. The cytotoxicity was determined by incubating serial dilutions of the conjugates with the cell lines indicated above the panels. The concentration ranges were 0.25–250 nM (AU565), 0.13–250 nM (SKBR3), 0.4 nM–5 µM (SKOV3), 1.2 nM–1 µM (A549), and 1.2 nM–1.35 µM (MCF7). The relative viability of the cells is plotted on the Y-axis as a function of the compound concentration on the X-axis. The relative viability of cells cultivated in medium was used as reference (100%). Each datapoint corresponds to the average of four independent experiments and the error bars correspond to 1 SD.

Table 4. In vitro cytotoxicity of the conjugates.

	IC_{50} (nM)				
Cell Line	$(Z_{HER2:2891})_2$–ABD–MC-DM1	$(Z_{HER2:2891})_2$–ABD–E_3–MC-DM1	$(Z_{HER2:2891})_2$–ABD–E_6–MC-DM1	$(Z_{HER2:2891})_2$–ABD–IAA	$(Z_{Taq})_2$–ABD–MC-DM1
AU565	0.22 (0.16–0.26) [a]	0.48 (0.38–0.70)	0.48 (0.33–0.69)	NM [b]	NM
SKBR-3	0.14 (0.10–0.19)	0.17 (0.13–0.23)	0.38 (0.27–0.43)	NM	NM
SKOV-3	47.0	82.8	116	NM	350

[a] Ranges in parenthesis correspond to 95% confidence interval; [b] Not measured.

2.4. Radiolabeling and Stability Test of Radiolabeled Constructs

For further in vitro characterization and to facilitate in vivo comparison, the conjugates were site-specifically radiolabeled with ^{99m}Tc through the N-terminally localized HEHEHE-tag. Data concerning the labeling yield, radiochemical purity, and stability of the conjugates are presented in Table 5. All three AffiDCs were efficiently labeled with ^{99m}Tc (radiochemical yield = 58%–61%). The radiochemical purity after purification by size-exclusion chromatography was >99%. Incubation with a 5000-fold molar excess of histidine showed that most of the activity (>97%) was still bound to the AffiDCs even after 24 h (Table 5).

Table 5. Labeling yield and radiochemical purity of ^{99m}Tc-labeled AffiDCs.

Conjugate	Yield [a] (%)	Radiochemical Purity (%) [b]	Stability Under Histidine Challenge (%)			
			Histidine 5000×		Control	
			4 h	24 h	4 h	24 h
^{99m}Tc-($Z_{HER2:2891}$)$_2$–ABD–MC-DM1	63 ± 15	99.5 ± 0.6	98.6 ± 0.2	98.4 ± 1.1	100 ± 0.2	98.8 ± 0.8
^{99m}Tc-($Z_{HER2:2891}$)$_2$–ABD–E$_3$–MC-DM1	61 ± 14	99.7 ± 0.3	99.2 ± 0.4	98 ± 1	99.9 ± 0.1	99.5 ± 0.1
^{99m}Tc-($Z_{HER2:2891}$)$_2$–ABD–E$_6$–MC-DM1	58 ± 16	99.8 ± 0.3	98.9 ± 0.1	97.3 ± 1.1	99.3 ± 0.3	99.1 ± 0.1

[a] Yield is calculated as % of conjugate-bound radioactivity from total added radioactivity determined by iTLC;
[b] Radiochemical purity is calculated as proportion of conjugate-bound radioactivity from total radioactivity after purification.

2.5. In Vitro Specificity and Internalization

To evaluate the integrity and cell interaction capability of the radiolabeled constructs, a specificity test was conducted. SKOV3 cells were incubated with the conjugates, with or without preincubation with a 500-fold molar excess of nonradiolabeled anti-HER2 affibody molecule $Z_{HER2:342}$ to block available HER2 receptors. $Z_{HER2:342}$ binds to the same epitope as $Z_{HER2:2891}$ [23]. The three constructs could bind to SKOV3 cells in a HER2-dependent manner, since the cell-associated radioactivity was reduced significantly when HER2-receptors were presaturated with $Z_{HER2:342}$ (Figure 5).

The internalization of the three AffiDCs by SKOV3 cells (high HER2 expression) was performed using a continuous incubation assay (Figure 6). The cell-associated radioactivity showed a continuous growth for the three AffiDCs up to 6 h of incubation, but at slightly different rates. The internalization of the three AffiDCs also increased over time but, again, at different rates. The construct with no glutamate spacer ($Z_{HER2:2891}$)$_2$–ABD–MC-DM1 demonstrated the highest rate of internalization compared to the glutamate spacer-containing variants ($Z_{HER2:2891}$)$_2$–ABD–E$_3$–MC-DM1 and ($Z_{HER2:2891}$)$_2$–ABD–E$_6$–MC-DM1 at all studied timepoints. The internalized fraction after 6 h incubation accounted for 36.5% ± 1.2%, 26.4% ± 1.3%, and 22.3% ± 2.3% of the total cell-associated radioactivity for ($Z_{HER2:2891}$)$_2$–ABD–MC-DM1, ($Z_{HER2:2891}$)$_2$–ABD–E$_3$–MC-DM1, and ($Z_{HER2:2891}$)$_2$–ABD–E$_6$–MC-DM1, respectively (Figure 6).

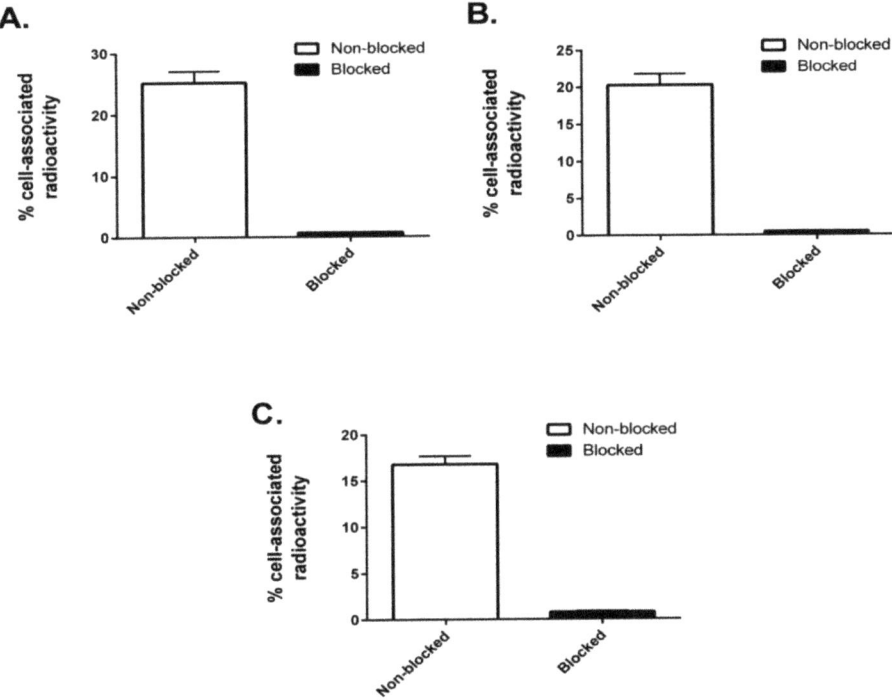

Figure 5. In vitro specificity. Specificity of binding of ^{99m}Tc-labeled $(Z_{HER2:2891})_2$–ABD–MC-DM1 (**A**), $(Z_{HER2:2891})_2$–ABD–E$_3$–MC-DM1 (**B**), and $(Z_{HER2:2891})_2$–ABD–E$_6$–MC-DM1 (**C**) to HER2-expressing SKOV-3 cells in vitro. Each bar shows the mean of the values measured in 3 dishes and the error bars correspond to SD.

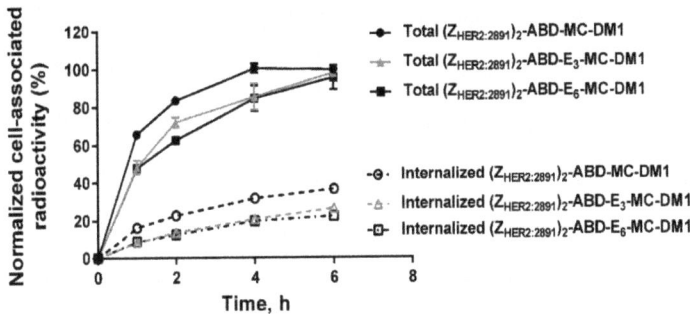

Figure 6. In vitro internalization. Internalization of ^{99m}Tc-labeled $(Z_{HER2:2891})_2$–ABD–MC-DM1 (circle), $(Z_{HER2:2891})_2$–ABD–E$_3$–MC-DM1 (triangle), and $(Z_{HER2:2891})_2$–ABD–E$_6$–MC-DM1 (square) by HER2-expressing SKOV-3 cells at 37 °C. Each datapoint is the average of three individual experiments ± 1 SD.

2.6. Biodistribution and In Vivo Tumor Targeting

Data concerning in vivo biodistribution and tumor targeting of ^{99m}Tc-labeled $(Z_{HER2:2891})_2$–ABD–MC–DM1, $(Z_{HER2:2891})_2$–ABD–E$_3$–MC–DM1, and $(Z_{HER2:2891})_2$–ABD–E$_6$–MC–DM1 at 4, 24, and 46 h post injection (p.i.) in BALB/c-nu/nu mice bearing HER2-expressing SKOV-3 xenografts are displayed in Figure 7. There was no significant difference in the residence in circulation between the AffiDCs at all studied timepoints. The tumor uptake of the three AffiDCs was comparable at all studied timepoints and showed better retention with time compared to uptake in other organs. By 46 h p.i., the tumor uptake of all three AffiDCs (5.2%–6.5% ID/g) was higher than the uptake in any other organ except the kidneys. The tumor uptake at 46 h p.i. in mice bearing RAMOS lymphoma xenografts (HER2 negative) was 6–10-fold lower compared to that in SKOV-3 xenografts: 0.9% ± 0.1%, 0.6% ± 0.1%, and 0.6% ± 0.2% ID/g for $(Z_{HER2:2891})_2$–ABD–MC–DM1, $(Z_{HER2:2891})_2$–ABD–E$_3$–MC–DM1, and $(Z_{HER2:2891})_2$–ABD–E$_6$–MC–DM1, respectively (Figure S2).

There was no significant difference in activity concentration in most organs, and it generally followed the kinetics in the blood. However, a striking difference in the uptake in the liver was observed. The activity uptake of $(Z_{HER2:2891})_2$–ABD–E$_3$–MC–DM1 and $(Z_{HER2:2891})_2$–ABD–E$_6$–MC–DM1 was significantly lower compared to $(Z_{HER2:2891})_2$–ABD–MC–DM1 at 4 h p.i. (8.7% ± 0.2% and 8.6% ± 0.9% vs. 13.4% ± 0.9 % ID/g) and at 24 h p.i. (6.3% ± 1.8% and 5.7% ± 0.3% vs. 9.3% ± 0.7% ID/g). This difference in hepatic uptake disappeared by 46 h p.i. (6.5% ± 1.8% and 5.4% ± 1.3% vs. 5.2% ± 0.9% ID/g). Interestingly, there was no significant difference in radioactivity uptake in the gastrointestinal tract and kidneys, in connection with the reduction in hepatic uptake.

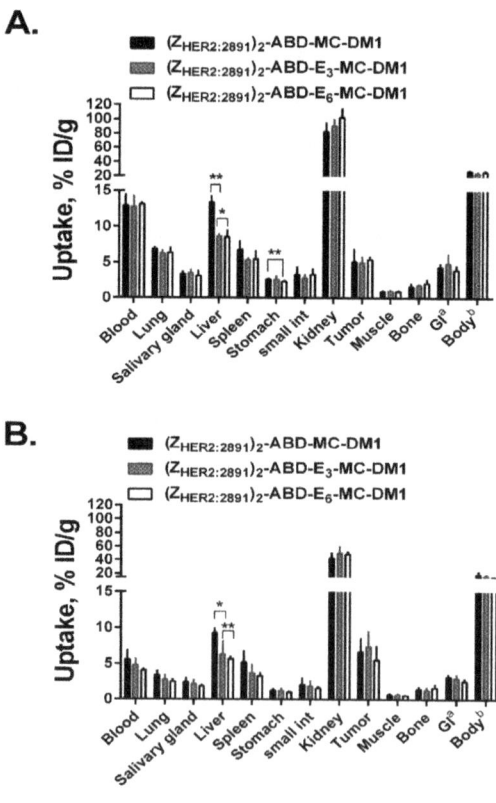

Figure 7. *Cont.*

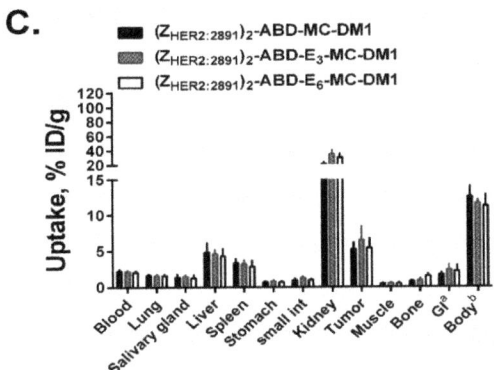

Figure 7. In vivo biodistribution. Comparative biodistribution of ^{99m}Tc-labeled DM1 conjugates expressed as % ID/g and presented as an average value from 4 animals ± 1 SD at 4 (**A**), 24 (**B**), and 46 (**C**) h post i.v. injection in female BALB/c nude mice bearing SKOV-3 xenografts. a,b Data are presented as % ID per whole sample. Data were assessed by one-way ANOVA with Bonferroni's post hoc multiple comparisons test in order to determine significant differences between groups ($p < 0.05$) at the same timepoint.

3. Discussion

In this study, the aim has been to investigate if hepatic uptake of AffiDCs could be reduced by incorporation of a hydrophilic glutamate-based spacer adjacent to site of MC-DM1 attachment. Hepatotoxicity is one of the most common reasons for drug development failures and withdrawal of drugs from the market [24,25]. In the field of ADCs, several reports have found a link between treatment and drug-induced liver injuries. For example, it was observed that T-DM1 therapy was associated with serious grade 3 or greater adverse events in some patients, including hepatotoxicity [18–20]. Similarly, several patients treated with the prostate-specific membrane antigen-directed ADC, MLN2704, have experienced elevated dose-dependent levels of hepatic transaminases [26]. Many drug development programs therefore include development of methods aiming to identify potential liver toxicities and their mechanisms [20,21,24,25]. Despite those efforts, hepatotoxicity still remains to be one of the most complex and poorly understood areas of human toxicity. For example, Yan and coworkers tried to understand the molecular basis for hepatotoxicity induced by T-DM1 [21]. This group concluded that HER2-mediated uptake of T-DM1 by hepatocytes is directly linked to DM1-associated liver toxicity.

We have earlier reported on the development of an AffiDC, $(Z_{HER2:2891})_2$–ABD–MC-DM1, targeting HER2. The AffiDC demonstrated relatively high hepatic uptake in mice post i.v. injection. The accumulation in liver of AffiDC was several-fold higher compared to other ABD-fused affibody molecules [16,17]. As mentioned above, Yan et al. reported earlier that T-DM1 induced liver toxicity through a HER2-mediated uptake of the ADC by hepatocytes. We tested this assumption by preinjecting mice with >100-fold molar excess of parental HER2-targeting affibody molecule to potentially block available HER2 receptors [14]. We found that there was no reduction in hepatic uptake of AffiDC after HER2-blocking, suggesting an unspecific liver uptake of AffiDC [14]. The main difference between AffiDC and other reported ABD-fused affibody molecules [16,17] is the presence of the drug DM1. Such drug-induced hepatic uptake has also been observed for MAbs after addition of the drug molecules [27,28]. Several groups have hypothesized that the increased hepatic uptake of ADCs may result from an increase in overall hydrophobicity of the conjugate after addition of lipophilic linkers or drug molecules [22,27,28]. Based on this, it would therefore be reasonable to suspect that the relatively high hepatic uptake of AffiDC is mainly a drug-mediated effect. We hypothesized that the incorporation of a hydrophilic spacer consisting of glutamic acid residues next to the cysteine used for MC-DM1 conjugation would lead to a decrease in hepatic uptake.

Comparison of $(Z_{HER2:2891})_2$–ABD–MC-DM1 and the nondrug-conjugated $(Z_{HER2:2891})_2$–ABD–IAA showed that addition of MC-DM1 increased the retention time during passage through a RP-HPLC column (Figure 1C). This represents evidence of the increased hydrophobicity conferred by MC-DM1. Further comparison of $(Z_{HER2:2891})_2$–ABD–MC-DM1 with the newly designed polyglutamate spacer-containing variants, $(Z_{HER2:2891})_2$–ABD–E_3–MC-DM1 and $(Z_{HER2:2891})_2$–ABD–E_6–MC-DM1, showed that addition of glutamic acid residues decreased the retention time, suggesting a shielding effect on the interaction with the C18 ligand in the column.

The newly designed AffiDCs demonstrated high binding affinity as well as specificity to HER2 receptors (Figure 2). Retaining the capacity to bind HER2 with high affinity is essential for efficient targeting. The setup in the biosensor with immobilized receptor only allows for determination of an apparent affinity since the affinity of the two affibody domains in the AffiDC for HER2 could be different, and we would thus record a mixture of the signal obtained from affibody one and affibody two interacting with HER2. However, since the kinetic constants were similar for the AffiDC/HER2 interaction on three surfaces with different HER2 density, only one of them are engaged with HER2 at any given time, and an avidity in the interaction is between the analyte and the surface is negligible. The setup with immobilized HER2 rather than immobilized AffiDC was chosen since it better mimics the cell experiments where HER2 is part of the plasma membrane and the AffiDC is free in solution. The albumin-binding function was also retained as demonstrated by the biosensor analysis of the interactions between the conjugates and serum albumin (Figure 3). All tested conjugates demonstrated a sub- to single-digit nanomolar affinity (K_D value) for both HSA and MSA. These K_D values are similar to results obtained previously for several affibody-based ABD-fused targeting agents [14,16,17,29,30]. The biodistribution experiments confirmed the capacity of ABD to extend AffiDC circulation time. The three AffiDCs demonstrated comparable retention in the blood at all studied timepoints. The blood associated radioactivity was 13% ± 1%, 5% ± 1%, and 2% ± 0.2% ID/g at 4, 24, and 46 h p.i. of the ^{99m}Tc-labeled AffiDCs. Affibody molecules, by themselves or as head-to-tail dimers, are generally cleared almost completely from blood within 1 h [31]. For example, in a similarly conducted biodistribution experiment, the blood activity 4 h p.i. of an anti-HER2 monomeric Z and dimeric ZZ affibody molecules (lacking an ABD) was only 1.5% ± 0.2% and 2.5% ± 0.2 % ID/g, respectively.

Being a natural amino acid, inserted glutamates were not expected to affect the degradation of affibody–MC-DM1 conjugates in the lysosomes during the process of cell intoxication. The results from the in vitro toxicity study demonstrated clearly the cytotoxicity potential of the newly designed AffiDCs with IC_{50} values similar to the parental $(Z_{HER2:2891})_2$–ABD–MC-DM1 (Figure 4 and Table 4). This cell killing potential is also comparable to that of the clinically approved trastuzumab emtansine, as was demonstrated earlier [14]. It is evident that HER2 specificity is important for efficient cytotoxic activity of the AffiDCs. The sensitivity of the low-HER2-expressing MCF-7 cells and the moderate-HER2-expressing A549 cells for AffiDCs was almost 3 orders of magnitude lower than the sensitivity of the high-HER2-expressing SKOV3, SKBR3, and AU565 cell lines. Surprisingly, there was a big discrepancy between the sensitivity of the high-HER2-expressing cell lines to our AffiDCs. The measured IC_{50} values were in the range of 47 to 116 nM in SKOV-3 cells while it was ca. 300-fold lower in SKBR3 and AU565 (Table 4). As the level of HER2 in the three cell lines is comparable, the difference may be attributed to other factors known to decrease sensitivity to drug conjugates. These may include, among others, differences in the expression level of multidrug resistance transporters, impairment of receptor internalization, and dysfunction of lysosomal degradation mechanisms [32–34].

An unexpected finding of this study was the growth-promoting effect for SKOV-3 cells observed after incubation with the non-DM1-containing $(Z_{HER2:2891})_2$–ABD–IAA affibody. We may speculate that it might be caused by HER2 dimerization, mediated by the two affibody domains in the construct, followed by an increase in intracellular signaling by the receptor. It is possible that the increased proliferation observed during incubation with a high concentration of $(Z_{HER2:2891})_2$–ABD–IAA could enhance the cytotoxic activity of DM1, since the drug is strongly acting/selective towards rapidly dividing cells through prevention of microtubule formation.

The three AffiDCs were site-specifically labeled with ^{99m}Tc through the N-terminally localized HEHEHE-tag (Table 5). After histidine challenge for 24 h, most (>97%) of the radioactivity was still associated with the conjugates. Stable labeling of the conjugates is a perquisite for accurate in vivo evaluation. It is important to mention that the spacer in $(Z_{HER2:2891})_2$–ABD–E_3–MC–DM1 and $(Z_{HER2:2891})_2$–ABD–E_6–MC–DM1 could potentially offer an alternative weak-chelating pocket for ^{99m}Tc, due to the electron-donating properties of glutamate sidechains [35]. However, the minimal activity release in the presence of competing histidines revealed that this is not the case for these conjugates.

The three radiolabeled AffiDCs demonstrated HER2-mediated binding to SKOV-3 cells in vitro (Figure 5). This clearly showed that site-specific radiolabeling had no negative influence on the HER2-binding properties. There was an apparent influence of the spacer on the internalization rate of the conjugates where both conjugates containing a polyglutamate spacer demonstrated a slower internalization rate compared to $(Z_{HER2:2891})_2$–ABD–MC–DM1 at all studied timepoints (Figure 6). Nonetheless, the internalization experiment clearly showed that both $(Z_{HER2:2891})_2$–ABD–E_3–MC–DM1 and $(Z_{HER2:2891})_2$–ABD–E_6–MC–DM1 are still efficiently internalized and should thus be capable of targeted delivery of the drug DM1 to kill tumor cells similar to the previously evaluated $(Z_{HER2:2891})_2$–ABD–MC–DM1.

The biodistribution data of the three AffiDCs in BALB/c nu/nu mice were in a good agreement with the data reported earlier for $(Z_{HER2:2891})_2$–ABD–MC–DM1 [14]. The AffiDCs clearly demonstrated the capacity to bind to tumor xenografts in vivo in a HER2-dependent manner (Figure 7 and Figure S2). The results of the biodistribution experiment confirmed the relation between the hydrophobicity of the DM1-containing AffiDC and liver accumulation. Incorporation of the hydrophilic polyglutamate spacer enabled modulation of liver accumulation. The hydrophilized $(Z_{HER2:2891})_2$–ABD–E_3–MC–DM1 and $(Z_{HER2:2891})_2$–ABD–E_6–MC–DM1 AffiDCs had nearly 1.5-fold ($p < 0.05$) lower liver accumulation than that of the parental $(Z_{HER2:2891})_2$–ABD–MC–DM1 (Figure 7). Several overlapping factors may be associated with the selective accumulation of drug conjugates in the liver [36]. These factors include affinity between the construct and the hepatocellular transport proteins residing outside of the cells, the potential to trigger endocytosis, the release from the endosomes or lysosomes inside the hepatic cells, and the rate at which the linker between the targeting agent and the drug is cleaved. Moreover, the affinity between the construct and its catabolites to the hepatocellular efflux transporters might also play a role in hepatic accumulation. It is important to mention that the radiolabel and the drug DM1 are located at different ends of the AffiDCs. This makes it difficult to link any observed differences in hepatic accumulation to the nature of DM1–catabolites formed after lysosomal degradation. The most plausible explanation for the observed difference in hepatic accumulation of radioactivity, stems from the difference in uptake of the three AffiDCs—having different degree of hydrophilicity—by hepatocytes. This is based on earlier findings, where reduction of overall hydrophobicity of targeting agents was found to suppress hepatic uptake [29,37–39]. Decreasing overall hydrophobicity by incorporation of hydrophilic groups or linkers has also resulted in better in vivo targeting properties for bulky ADCs, particularly reduction of hepatic accumulation [22,28]. Since the AffiDCs are approximately 10 times smaller than ADCs, it is expected that the influence of hydrophilization on liver uptake should be more profound for AffiDCs. Surprisingly, the effect on hepatic accumulation was not directly proportional to the number of incorporated glutamate residues and no significant difference in liver accumulation between $(Z_{HER2:2891})_2$–ABD–E_3–MC–DM1 and $(Z_{HER2:2891})_2$–ABD–E_6–MC–DM1 was found at any of the timepoints (Figure 7). Regardless of the underlying reason, a reduction in hepatic uptake could have a positive impact on the maximum tolerated dose of AffiDC.

4. Materials and Methods

All chemicals were purchased from Sigma-Aldrich (St. Louis, MO, USA) or Merck (Darmstadt, Germany) unless otherwise stated. Restriction enzymes were from New England Biolabs (Ipswitch, MA, USA).

4.1. Construction of Genes Encoding Affibody Constructs

Genes encoding $(Z_{HER2:2891})_2$–ABD–Cys and $(Z_{Taq})_2$–ABD–Cys were constructed previously [14]. Genes encoding $(Z_{HER2:2891})_2$–ABD–E_3–Cys, $(Z_{HER2:2891})_2$–ABD–E_6–Cys flanked by NdeI and BamHI restriction sites were synthesized by Thermo Fisher Scientific (Waltham, MA, USA). They were subcloned into the pET-21a(+) plasmid vector (Novagen, Madison, WI, USA) using NdeI and BamHI restriction enzymes.

4.2. Expression and Purification of Affibody Constructs

The affibody constructs were expressed at 37 °C in shake flask cultures of Escherichia coli BL21 Star (DE3) (New England Biolabs). When OD_{600} was between 0.6 and 1, protein expression was induced by addition of 1 mM isopropyl β-D-1-thiogalactopyranoside (Appolo Scientific, Stockport, UK). Protein production was carried out for 3 h, after which the cells were harvested by centrifugation and lysed by sonication. The supernatants were clarified by centrifugation and filtration through a 0.45 μm Acrodisc syringe filter (Pall, Port Washington, NY, USA). The recombinantly expressed affibody constructs were purified by affinity chromatography on a HiTrap NHS sepharose column (GE Healthcare, Uppsala, Sweden) with immobilized human serum albumin (HSA) using an ÄKTA system (GE Healthcare), essentially as previously described [14] including elution with 50 mM acetic acid. The fractions containing affibody constructs were pooled and lyophilized.

4.3. Conjugation with MC-DM1

The lyophilized proteins were dissolved in PBS at pH 6.5 to a final concentration of 0.1 mM and incubated with 5 mM tris(2-carboxyethyl) phosphine (TCEP) for 30 min at room temperature., to reduce the sulfur on the C-terminal cysteine of the constructs, which could potentially have been oxidized during protein production and purification. Freshly prepared MC-DM1 (Levena Biopharma, San Diego, CA, USA), dissolved in DMSO (20 mM), was mixed with the affibody constructs at a molar ratio of 2:1, and the conjugation mixture was incubated overnight at r.t. The conjugation reaction mixture was diluted with HPLC buffer A (0.1% trifluoroacetic acid in H_2O) and then loaded on a Zorbax C18 SB column (Agilent, Santa Clara, CA, USA). Bound material was eluted by a 25 min gradient from 20% or 30% to 60% or 80% buffer B (0.1% trifluoroacetic acid in acetonitrile). The fractions containing affibody–MC-DM1 conjugates were pooled followed by lyophilization.

Capping of the C-terminal cysteine to create the nontoxic control $(Z_{HER2:2891})_2$–ABD–IAA was carried out with 2-iodoacetamide. Lyophilized $(Z_{HER2:2891})_2$–ABD–Cys was dissolved in alkylation buffer (6M urea, 0.1 M NH_4HCO_3) after which dithiothreitol was added to a final concentration of 4 mM, followed by incubation for 30 min at 37 °C to reduce any potentially oxidized cysteine residues. 2-Iodoacetamide was added to a final concentration of 10 mM followed by incubation for 30 min at r.t. to alkylate the cysteines. The capped proteins were purified by RP-HPLC as described above for the affibody–MC-DM1 conjugates, followed by lyophilization.

The lyophilized proteins were dissolved in sterile PBS buffer and stored at −20 °C until use. Purified proteins (5 μg in each sample) were analyzed by SDS-PAGE (Biorad, Hercules, CA, USA) under reducing conditions. The molecular weight of purified affibody–MC-DM1 conjugates was measured by ESI-TOF mass spectrometry (Agilent).

4.4. Binding Specificity and Affinity Determination

A Biacore T200 and a Biacore 3000 instrument (GE Healthcare) were used for biosensor analysis. The extracellular domain of HER2 (HER2$_{ECD}$) (Sino Biological, Beijing, China) was immobilized to 210, 310, and 456 RUs on three different flow cells on a CM5 chip by amine coupling in sodium acetate buffer, pH 4.5. A reference flow cell was created by activation and deactivation. On a second CM-5 chip, HSA (Novozymes, Bagsvaerd, Denmark), MSA (Sigma-Aldrich, St. Louis, MO, USA), and BSA (Merck Millipore) were immobilized in the same way. The final immobilization levels were 869, 584, and 779 RUs, respectively. HBS-EP (10 mM HEPES, 150 mM NaCl, 3 mM EDTA, 0.05% Tween 20, pH 7.4) was used as running buffer and for dilution of the analytes. All experiments were performed at 25 °C with a flow rate of 50 µL/min. The chips were regenerated by injection of 15 mM HCl for 30 s. The binding kinetics was analyzed by the Biacore evaluation software using the one-to-one kinetics model.

4.5. In Vitro Cytotoxicity Analysis

AU565, SKBR-3, SKOV-3, A549, and MCF7 cell lines were obtained from American Type Culture Collection (American Type Culture Collection, ATCC via LGC Promochem, Borås, Sweden) and were grown in McCoy's 5A (SKOV-3, SKBR-3), RPMI-1640 (AU565), or Dulbecco's modified Eagle medium (A549 and MCF7) (Flow, Irvine, UK) supplemented with 10% FBS (Sigma-Aldrich, St. Louis, MO, USA) in a humidified incubator at 37 °C in 5% CO_2 atmosphere. Approximately 5000 cells/well (2000 cells/well for SKOV-3) were seeded in a 96-well plate and allowed to attach for 24 h. Subsequently, the medium was replaced with fresh medium containing serial dilutions of affibody–MC-DM1 conjugates or 2-iodoacetamide-capped nontoxic control followed by incubation for 72 h. Cell viability was determined using Cell Counting Kit-8 (CCK-8; Sigma-Aldrich) according to the manufacturer's protocol with measurement of A_{450} in each well. The obtained absorbance values were analyzed by GraphPad Prism using a log(inhibitor) vs. response-variable slope (four parameters) model (GraphPad Software, Inc., La Jolla, CA, USA).

4.6. Radiolabeling and Stability Test of Radiolabeled Constructs

Site-specific radiolabeling of AffiDCs (($Z_{HER2:2891}$)$_2$–ABD–MC-DM1, ($Z_{HER2:2891}$)$_2$–ABD–E$_3$–MC-DM1, and ($Z_{HER2:2891}$)$_2$–ABD–E$_6$–MC-DM1) with ^{99m}Tc using (^{99m}Tc(CO)$_3$(H$_2$O)$_3$) + precursor was performed as previously described [14]. In brief, eluted pertechnetate, ^{99m}TcO$_4^-$, (400–500 µL) from ^{99}Mo/^{99m}Tc generator was added to a CRS kit (PSI, Villigen, Switzerland) to generate the (^{99m}Tc(CO)$_3$(H$_2$O)$_3$) + (tricarbonyl technetium) precursor. The mixture was vortexed carefully and incubated at 100 °C for 20 min. After incubation, 20 µL of the tricarbonyl technetium solution was added to a tube containing 55 µg of the respective AffiDC in 100 µL of PBS and incubated for 60 min at 60 °C. To isolate the radiolabeled AffiDCs, the mixture was passed through a NAP-5 size-exclusion column (GE Healthcare) pre-equilibrated and eluted with 2% BSA in PBS. Radiochemical yield and purity of the conjugates were determined using silica-impregnated ITLC strips (150–771 DARK GREEN Tec-Control Chromatography strips (Biodex Medical Systems, Shirley, NY, USA) eluted with PBS and measured using the Cyclone Storage Phosphor System (PerkinElmer, Waltham, MA, USA). To evaluate the stability of the radiolabeled AffiDCs, they were incubated with a 5000-fold molar excess of histidine at 37 °C for up to 4 and 24 h, respectively. The percentage of protein-bound radioactivity after histidine challenge was determined using radio-ITLC as mentioned above.

4.7. In vitro Specificity and Internalization

To confirm the specificity of binding of ^{99m}Tc-radiolabeled AffiDCs to HER2-expressing cells in vitro, SKOV-3 cells (5–7.5 × 10^5) were incubated with 2 nM of each conjugate at 37 °C for 60 min (n = 3). For blocking, another set of dishes containing SKOV-3 cells were preincubated with 500-fold molar excess of nonlabeled anti-HER2 affibody molecule $Z_{HER2:342}$ prior to the addition of radiolabeled AffiDCs. Thereafter, both medium and cells were collected from each dish and measured for radioactivity using an automated γ-spectrometer (1480 Wizard; Wallac Oy, Turku, Finland). Data are presented as mean values from three cell dishes with standard deviation.

The internalization of ^{99m}Tc-radiolabeled AffiDCs by HER2-expressing cells was studied using a method described earlier by Altai et al. [14]. For this, four groups of dishes (n = 3) containing SKOV-3 cells (5–7.5 × 10^5 cells/dish) were incubated with 2 nM (per dish) of the respective conjugate at 37 °C. At determined timepoints (1, 2, 4, and 6 h) after incubation, a group of dishes (n = 3) was removed from the incubator. Media was then discarded, and cells were washed with 1 mL of serum-free media. Thereafter, cells were incubated with 0.5 mL urea–glycine buffer pH 2.5 (acid wash) for 5 min on ice. This acid wash was then collected. An additional 0.5 mL of the acid wash was also used to wash the cells, and this fraction was collected immediately. Cells were then incubated with 0.5 mL 1 M NaOH solution for at least 30 min at 37 °C to lysate the cells (base wash). Cells were additionally washed with 0.5 mL base wash. Both acid and base washes were measured for radioactivity using automated γ-spectrometer.

4.8. Biodistribution and In Vivo Targeting

The animal experiments were planned and performed in accordance with national legislation on laboratory animal protection. The animal studies were approved by the local ethics committee for animal research in Uppsala, Sweden (C85/15).

Comparative biodistribution studies of ^{99m}Tc-labeled $(Z_{HER2:2891})_2$–ABD–MC-DM1, $(Z_{HER2:2891})_2$–ABD–E_3–MC-DM1, and $(Z_{HER2:2891})_2$–ABD–E_6–MC-DM1 were performed in female BALB/c nude mice (Scanbur A/S, Karlslunde, Denmark). Two weeks before the start of the experiment, 36 mice (6–8 weeks old) were injected with 10 × 10^6 SKOV-3 cells/per mouse (HER2+) in the right hind leg. The mice (18.4 ± 1.4 g) were randomized to nine groups, with four mice in each group. Animals were injected intravenously with 6 µg (of each conjugate) per animal in 100 µL PBS containing 2% BSA. The injected radioactivity was calculated to give 30 kBq per mouse by the time of dissection. At predetermined timepoints (4, 24, and 46 h p.i.) mice were euthanized by overdosing of anesthesia (Ketalar (ketamine): 10 mg/mL, Pfizer AB, Sweden; Rompun (xylazine): 1 mg/mL, Bayer AG, Leverkusen, Germany) followed by heart puncture and exsanguination. Organs and tissue samples were collected and weighed, and the radioactivity was measured using an automated γ-spectrometer.

To demonstrate the specific delivery of ^{99m}Tc-labeled $(Z_{HER2:2891})_2$–ABD–MC-DM1, $(Z_{HER2:2891})_2$–ABD–E_3–MC-DM1, and $(Z_{HER2:2891})_2$–ABD–E_6–MC-DM1 to HER2-expressing tumors, an in vivo specificity study was performed. For this, an additional 12 BALB/c nude mice were xenografted with 5 × 10^6 RAMOS (HER2) lymphoma cells in the right hind leg. Each group of four mice (n = 4) were i.v. injected with 6 µg (30 kBq) of the respective conjugate in 100 µL PBS containing 2% BSA. Mice were euthanized at 46 h p.i. and treated as mentioned above.

5. Conclusions

In conclusion, this study demonstrated that insertion of a polyglutamate spacer is an effective strategy to decrease hepatic uptake of affinity protein drug conjugates. The use of the hydrophilic and negatively charged glutamate spacer provided, by far, the lowest level of hepatic uptake for AffiDCs. Accumulation in other organs and tissues was also low, and no influence on the HER2-mediated tumor uptake was observed. We believe that the approach described here represents a means for the development of other targeting affinity protein drug conjugates for treatment of disseminated cancers and to facilitate their clinical translatability.

Supplementary Materials: The following are available online at http://www.mdpi.com/2072-6694/11/8/1168/s1, Figure S1: Scheme 1: Structures of the ^{99m}Tc(CO)$_3$ chelated by HEHEHE tag, Figure S2: In vivo specificity.

Author Contributions: H.D. and M.A. contributed equally to this study. H.D., M.A., V.T., A.O. and T.G. conceived and designed the experiments. H.D., M.A., S.R., A.V., V.T., A.O. and T.G. performed the experiments and analyzed the data. H.D., M.A. and T.G. wrote the paper. All authors agreed with the accuracy and integrity of all parts of the work.

Funding: This research was funded by the Swedish Cancer Society (grants CAN 2018/824 (T.G.), CAN 2017/425 (A.O.) and CAN2015/350 (V.T.)), the Swedish Research Council (2015-02509 (A.O.) and 2015-02353 (V.T.)), an ESCAPE Cancer grant from the Swedish Agency for Innovation VINNOVA (2016-04060 and 2019-00104 A.O.), and the Swedish Society for Medical Research (M.A.).

Conflicts of Interest: V.T. and A.O. own shares in Affibody AB. M.A., H.D., A.V., S.R. and T.G. declare no conflict of interest.

References

1. Zhuang, C.; Guan, X.; Ma, H.; Cong, H.; Zhang, W.; Miao, Z. Small molecule-drug conjugates: A novel strategy for cancer-targeted treatment. *Eur. J. Med. Chem.* **2019**, *163*, 883–895. [CrossRef] [PubMed]
2. Richards, D.A. Exploring alternative antibody scaffolds: Antibody fragments and antibody mimics for targeted drug delivery. *Drug Discov. Today Technol.* **2018**, *30*, 35–46. [CrossRef] [PubMed]
3. Abdollahpour-Alitappeh, M.; Lotfinia, M.; Gharibi, T.; Mardaneh, J.; Farhadihosseinabadi, B.; Larki, P.; Faghfourian, B.; Sepehr, K.S.; Abbaszadeh-Goudarzi, K.; Abbaszadeh-Goudarzi, G.; et al. Antibody-drug conjugates (ADCs) for cancer therapy: Strategies, challenges, and successes. *J. Cell. Physiol.* **2019**, *234*, 5628–5642. [CrossRef] [PubMed]
4. Leal, A.D.; Krishnamurthy, A.; Head, L.; Messersmith, W.A. Antibody drug conjugates under investigation in phase I and phase II clinical trials for gastrointestinal cancer. *Expert Opin. Investig. Drugs* **2018**, *27*, 901–916. [CrossRef]
5. Hedrich, W.D.; Fandy, T.E.; Ashour, H.M.; Wang, H.; Hassan, H.E. Antibody–Drug Conjugates: Pharmacokinetic/Pharmacodynamic Modeling, Preclinical Characterization, Clinical Studies, and Lessons Learned. *Clin. Pharmacokinet.* **2018**, *57*, 687–703. [CrossRef] [PubMed]
6. Beck, A.; Goetsch, L.; Dumontet, C.; Corvaïa, N. Strategies and challenges for the next generation of antibody–drug conjugates. *Nat. Rev. Drug Discov.* **2017**, *16*, 315–337. [CrossRef]
7. Yamada, K.; Ito, Y. Recent Chemical Approaches for Site-specific Conjugation of Native Antibodies: Technologies toward Next Generation Antibody-Drug Conjugates. *Chembiochem* **2019**. [CrossRef] [PubMed]
8. Axup, J.Y.; Bajjuri, K.M.; Ritland, M.; Hutchins, B.M.; Kim, C.H.; Kazane, S.A.; Halder, R.; Forsyth, J.S.; Santidrian, A.F.; Stafin, K.; et al. Synthesis of site-specific antibody-drug conjugates using unnatural amino acids. *Proc. Natl. Acad. Sci. USA* **2012**, *109*, 16101–16106. [CrossRef] [PubMed]
9. Adem, Y.T.; Schwarz, K.A.; Duenas, E.; Patapoff, T.W.; Galush, W.J.; Esue, O. Auristatin Antibody Drug Conjugate Physical Instability and the Role of Drug Payload. *Bioconjug. Chem.* **2014**, *25*, 656–664. [CrossRef] [PubMed]
10. Simeon, R.; Chen, Z. In vitro-engineered non-antibody protein therapeutics. *Protein Cell* **2018**, *9*, 3–14. [CrossRef] [PubMed]
11. Ståhl, S.; Gräslund, T.; Eriksson Karlström, A.; Frejd, F.Y.; Nygren, P.-Å.; Löfblom, J. Affibody Molecules in Biotechnological and Medical Applications. *Trends Biotechnol.* **2017**, *35*, 691–712. [CrossRef] [PubMed]
12. Löfblom, J.; Feldwisch, J.; Tolmachev, V.; Carlsson, J.; Ståhl, S.; Frejd, F.Y. Affibody molecules: Engineered proteins for therapeutic, diagnostic and biotechnological applications. *FEBS Lett.* **2010**, *584*, 2670–2680. [CrossRef] [PubMed]
13. Fleetwood, F.; Andersson, K.G.; Ståhl, S.; Löfblom, J. An engineered autotransporter-based surface expression vector enables efficient display of Affibody molecules on OmpT-negative E. coli as well as protease-mediated secretion in OmpT-positive strains. *Microb. Cell Fact.* **2014**, *13*, 179. [CrossRef]
14. Altai, M.; Liu, H.; Ding, H.; Mitran, B.; Edqvist, P.-H.; Tolmachev, V.; Orlova, A.; Gräslund, T. Affibody-derived drug conjugates: Potent cytotoxic molecules for treatment of HER2 over-expressing tumors. *J. Control. Release* **2018**, *288*, 84–95. [CrossRef] [PubMed]
15. Thurber, G.M.; Schmidt, M.M.; Wittrup, K.D. Factors determining antibody distribution in tumors. *Trends Pharmacol. Sci.* **2008**, *29*, 57–61. [CrossRef]

16. Tolmachev, V.; Orlova, A.; Pehrson, R.; Galli, J.; Baastrup, B.; Andersson, K.; Sandstrom, M.; Rosik, D.; Carlsson, J.; Lundqvist, H.; et al. Radionuclide Therapy of HER2-Positive Microxenografts Using a 177Lu-Labeled HER2-Specific Affibody Molecule. *Cancer Res.* **2007**, *67*, 2773–2782. [CrossRef] [PubMed]
17. Orlova, A.; Jonsson, A.; Rosik, D.; Lundqvist, H.; Lindborg, M.; Abrahmsen, L.; Ekblad, C.; Frejd, F.Y.; Tolmachev, V. Site-specific radiometal labeling and improved biodistribution using ABY-027, a novel HER2-targeting affibody molecule-albumin-binding domain fusion protein. *J. Nucl. Med.* **2013**, *54*, 961–968. [CrossRef] [PubMed]
18. Krop, I.E.; LoRusso, P.; Miller, K.D.; Modi, S.; Yardley, D.; Rodriguez, G.; Guardino, E.; Lu, M.; Zheng, M.; Girish, S.; et al. A phase II study of trastuzumab emtansine in patients with human epidermal growth factor receptor 2-positive metastatic breast cancer who were previously treated with trastuzumab, lapatinib, an anthracycline, a taxane, and capecitabine. *J. Clin. Oncol.* **2012**, *30*, 3234–3241. [CrossRef] [PubMed]
19. Verma, S.; Miles, D.; Gianni, L.; Krop, I.E.; Welslau, M.; Baselga, J.; Pegram, M.; Oh, D.-Y.; Diéras, V.; Guardino, E.; et al. Trastuzumab Emtansine for HER2-Positive Advanced Breast Cancer. *N. Engl. J. Med.* **2012**, *367*, 1783–1791. [CrossRef]
20. Diéras, V.; Harbeck, N.; Budd, G.T.; Greenson, J.K.; Guardino, A.E.; Samant, M.; Chernyukhin, N.; Smitt, M.C.; Krop, I.E. Trastuzumab emtansine in human epidermal growth factor receptor 2-positive metastatic breast cancer: An integrated safety analysis. *J. Clin. Oncol.* **2014**, *32*, 2750–2757. [CrossRef]
21. Yan, H.; Endo, Y.; Shen, Y.; Rotstein, D.; Dokmanovic, M.; Mohan, N.; Mukhopadhyay, P.; Gao, B.; Pacher, P.; Wu, W.J. Ado-Trastuzumab Emtansine Targets Hepatocytes Via Human Epidermal Growth Factor Receptor 2 to Induce *Hepatotoxicity*. *Mol. Cancer Ther.* **2016**, *15*, 480–490. [CrossRef]
22. Boswell, C.A.; Mundo, E.E.; Zhang, C.; Bumbaca, D.; Valle, N.R.; Kozak, K.R.; Fourie, A.; Chuh, J.; Koppada, N.; Saad, O.; et al. Impact of Drug Conjugation on Pharmacokinetics and Tissue Distribution of Anti-STEAP1 Antibody–Drug Conjugates in Rats. *Bioconjug. Chem.* **2011**, *22*, 1994–2004. [CrossRef]
23. Feldwisch, J.; Tolmachev, V.; Lendel, C.; Herne, N.; Sjöberg, A.; Larsson, B.; Rosik, D.; Lindqvist, E.; Fant, G.; Höidén-Guthenberg, I.; et al. Design of an Optimized Scaffold for Affibody *Molecules*. *J. Mol. Biol.* **2010**, *398*, 232–247. [CrossRef] [PubMed]
24. Hewitt, M.; Enoch, S.J.; Madden, J.C.; Przybylak, K.R.; Cronin, M.T.D. Hepatotoxicity: A scheme for generating chemical categories for read-across, structural alerts and insights into mechanism(s) of action. *Crit. Rev. Toxicol.* **2013**, *43*, 537–558. [CrossRef] [PubMed]
25. Schuster, D.; Laggner, C.; Langer, T. Why Drugs Fail—A Study on Side Effects in New Chemical Entities. *Curr. Pharm. Des.* **2005**, *11*, 3545–3559. [CrossRef] [PubMed]
26. Galsky, M.D.; Eisenberger, M.; Moore-Cooper, S.; Kelly, W.K.; Slovin, S.F.; DeLaCruz, A.; Lee, Y.; Webb, I.J.; Scher, H.I. Phase I trial of the prostate-specific membrane antigen-directed immunoconjugate MLN2704 in patients with progressive metastatic castration-resistant prostate cancer. *J. Clin. Oncol.* **2008**, *26*, 2147–2154. [CrossRef] [PubMed]
27. Herbertson, R.A.; Tebbutt, N.C.; Lee, F.-T.; Macfarlane, D.J.; Chappell, B.; Micallef, N.; Lee, S.-T.; Saunder, T.; Hopkins, W.; Smyth, F.E.; et al. Cancer Therapy: Clinical Phase I Biodistribution and Pharmacokinetic Study of Lewis Y-Targeting Immunoconjugate CMD-193 in Patients with Advanced Epithelial Cancers. *Clin. Cancer Res.* **2009**, *15*, 6709–6715. [CrossRef]
28. Lyon, R.P.; Bovee, T.D.; Doronina, S.O.; Burke, P.J.; Hunter, J.H.; Neff-LaFord, H.D.; Jonas, M.; Anderson, M.E.; Setter, J.R.; Senter, P.D. Reducing hydrophobicity of homogeneous antibody-drug conjugates improves pharmacokinetics and therapeutic index. *Nat. Biotechnol.* **2015**, *33*, 733–735. [CrossRef]
29. Altai, M.; Liu, H.; Orlova, A.; Tolmachev, V.; Gräslund, T. Influence of molecular design on biodistribution and targeting properties of an Affibody-fused HER2-recognising anticancer toxin. *Int. J. Oncol.* **2016**, *49*, 1185–1194. [CrossRef]
30. Altai, M.; Leitao, C.; Rinne, S.; Vorobyeva, A.; Atterby, C.; Ståhl, S.; Tolmachev, V.; Löfblom, J.; Orlova, A.; Altai, M.; et al. Influence of Molecular Design on the Targeting Properties of ABD-Fused Mono- and Bi-Valent Anti-HER3 Affibody Therapeutic Constructs. *Cells* **2018**, *7*, 164. [CrossRef]
31. Cheng, Z.; De Jesus, O.P.; Kramer, D.J.; De, A.; Webster, J.M.; Gheysens, O.; Levi, J.; Namavari, M.; Wang, S.; Park, J.M.; et al. 64Cu-Labeled Affibody Molecules for Imaging of HER2 Expressing Tumors. *Mol. Imaging Biol.* **2010**, *12*, 316–324. [CrossRef]

32. Kovtun, Y.V.; Audette, C.A.; Mayo, M.F.; Jones, G.E.; Doherty, H.; Maloney, E.K.; Erickson, H.K.; Sun, X.; Wilhelm, S.; Ab, O.; et al. Antibody-Maytansinoid Conjugates Designed to Bypass Multidrug Resistance. *Cancer Res.* **2010**, *70*, 2528–2537. [CrossRef]
33. von Schwarzenberg, K.; Lajtos, T.; Simon, L.; Müller, R.; Vereb, G.; Vollmar, A.M. V-ATPase inhibition overcomes trastuzumab resistance in breast cancer. *Mol. Oncol.* **2014**, *8*, 9–19. [CrossRef]
34. Barok, M.; Joensuu, H.; Isola, J. Trastuzumab emtansine: Mechanisms of action and drug resistance. *Breast Cancer Res.* **2014**, *16*, 3378. [CrossRef]
35. Oroujeni, M.; Andersson, K.G.; Steinhardt, X.; Altai, M.; Orlova, A.; Mitran, B.; Vorobyeva, A.; Garousi, J.; Tolmachev, V.; Löfblom, J. Influence of composition of cysteine-containing peptide-based chelators on biodistribution of 99mTc-labeled anti-EGFR affibody molecules. *Amino Acids* **2018**, *50*, 981–994. [CrossRef]
36. Hosseinimehr, S.J.; Tolmachev, V.; Orlova, A. Liver uptake of radiolabeled targeting proteins and peptides: Considerations for targeting peptide conjugate design. *Drug Discov. Today* **2012**, *17*, 1224–1232. [CrossRef]
37. Decristoforo, C.; Mather, S.J. 99m-Technetium-labelled peptide-HYNIC conjugates: Effects of lipophilicity and stability on biodistribution. *Nucl. Med. Biol.* **1999**, *26*, 389–396. [CrossRef]
38. Lin, K.S.; Luu, A.; Baidoo, K.E.; Hashemzadeh-Gargari, H.; Chen, M.K.; Brenneman, K.; Pili, R.; Pomper, M.; Carducci, M.A.; Wagner, H.N., Jr. A New High Affinity Technetium-99m-Bombesin Analogue with Low Abdominal Accumulation. *Bioconjug. Chem.* **2005**, *16*, 43–50. [CrossRef]
39. Hofström, C.; Orlova, A.; Altai, M.; Wangsell, F.; Gräslund, T.; Tolmachev, V. Use of a HEHEHE purification tag instead of a hexahistidine tag improves biodistribution of affibody molecules site-specifically labeled with 99mTc, 111In, and 125I. *J. Med. Chem.* **2011**, *54*, 3817–3826. [CrossRef]

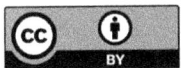

© 2019 by the authors. Licensee MDPI, Basel, Switzerland. This article is an open access article distributed under the terms and conditions of the Creative Commons Attribution (CC BY) license (http://creativecommons.org/licenses/by/4.0/).

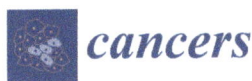

Article

IL3RA-Targeting Antibody–Drug Conjugate BAY-943 with a Kinesin Spindle Protein Inhibitor Payload Shows Efficacy in Preclinical Models of Hematologic Malignancies

Dennis Kirchhoff [1,*], Beatrix Stelte-Ludwig [2], Hans-Georg Lerchen [2], Antje Margret Wengner [1], Oliver von Ahsen [1], Pascale Buchmann [2], Stephan Märsch [2], Christoph Mahlert [2], Simone Greven [2], Lisa Dietz [2], Michael Erkelenz [1], Ruprecht Zierz [1], Sandra Johanssen [1], Dominik Mumberg [1] and Anette Sommer [1]

[1] Bayer AG, Pharmaceuticals, Research & Development, 13342 Berlin, Germany; antje.wengner@bayer.com (A.M.W.); oliver.vonahsen@bayer.com (O.v.A.); michael.erkelenz@bayer.com (M.E.); ruprecht.zierz@bayer.com (R.Z.); sandra.johanssen@bayer.com (S.J.); dominik.mumberg@bayer.com (D.M.)

[2] Bayer AG, Pharmaceuticals, Research & Development, 42096 Wuppertal, Germany; beatrix.stelte-ludwig@bayer.com (B.S.-L.); hans-georg.lerchen@bayer.com (H.-G.L.); pascale.buchmann@bayer.com (P.B.); stephanmaersch@hotmail.com (S.M.); christoph.mahlert@bayer.com (C.M.); simone.greven@bayer.com (S.G.); lisa.dietz@bayer.com (L.D.)

* Correspondence: dennis.kirchhoff@bayer.com; Tel.: +49-30-468193479

Received: 26 October 2020; Accepted: 17 November 2020; Published: 20 November 2020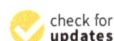

Simple Summary: IL3RA (alpha subunit of the interleukin 3 receptor) is a cell membrane protein frequently expressed in acute myeloid leukemia (AML) and Hodgkin lymphoma; therefore, it is a promising therapeutic target for cancer treatment. Here, we introduce BAY-943, a novel IL3RA-targeting antibody–drug conjugate that shows potent and selective efficacy in IL3RA-positive AML and Hodgkin lymphoma cell lines. In IL3RA-positive AML mouse models, BAY-943 improved survival and reduced tumor burden. Impressively, treatment with BAY-943 induced complete tumor remission in 12 out of 13 mice in an IL3RA-positive HL model. BAY-943 showed a favorable safety profile without any signs of toxicity in rats and monkeys. Overall, these preclinical results support the further development of BAY-943 for the treatment of IL3RA-positive hematologic malignancies.

Abstract: IL3RA (CD123) is the alpha subunit of the interleukin 3 (IL-3) receptor, which regulates the proliferation, survival, and differentiation of hematopoietic cells. IL3RA is frequently expressed in acute myeloid leukemia (AML) and classical Hodgkin lymphoma (HL), presenting an opportunity to treat AML and HL with an IL3RA-directed antibody–drug conjugate (ADC). Here, we describe BAY-943 (IL3RA-ADC), a novel IL3RA-targeting ADC consisting of a humanized anti-IL3RA antibody conjugated to a potent proprietary kinesin spindle protein inhibitor (KSPi). In vitro, IL3RA-ADC showed potent and selective antiproliferative efficacy in a panel of IL3RA-expressing AML and HL cell lines. In vivo, IL3RA-ADC improved survival and reduced tumor burden in IL3RA-positive human AML cell line-derived (MOLM-13 and MV-4-11) as well as in patient-derived xenograft (PDX) models (AM7577 and AML11655) in mice. Furthermore, IL3RA-ADC induced complete tumor remission in 12 out of 13 mice in an IL3RA-positive HL cell line-derived xenograft model (HDLM-2). IL3RA-ADC was well-tolerated and showed no signs of thrombocytopenia, neutropenia, or liver toxicity in rats, or in cynomolgus monkeys when dosed up to 20 mg/kg. Overall, the preclinical results support the further development of BAY-943 as an innovative approach for the treatment of IL3RA-positive hematologic malignancies.

Keywords: acute myeloid leukemia; antibody-drug conjugate; CD123; IL3RA; kinesin spindle protein inhibitor

1. Introduction

Interleukin 3 receptor subunit alpha (IL3RA; also known as CD123) is the α subunit of the heterodimeric IL-3 receptor. Together with the β subunit, it forms a functional high-affinity receptor for IL-3 [1–3]. IL-3 is a pleiotropic cytokine that is mainly produced by activated T lymphocytes, and it regulates the function and production of hematopoietic and immune cells [4]. IL3RA is expressed at high levels in ≈80% of acute myeloid leukemias (AML) [1,2,5], 59–100% of classical Hodgkin lymphomas (cHL), and the majority of blastic plasmacytoid dendritic cell neoplasms (BPDCN) [6–10]. It is also expressed by close to 100% of myelodysplastic syndrome (MDS) patients, but the expression intensity may vary [11–14]. Importantly, IL3RA overexpression on AML blasts has been associated with an increased number of leukemic blast cells at diagnosis and with a negative prognosis [15]. IL3RA is also expressed in basophils and plasmacytoid dendritic cells [5,16].

Several studies have indicated that IL-3 and its receptor play important roles in the progression of AML [3,17], and indeed, experiments with a monoclonal antibody that blocks the binding of IL-3 to IL3RA have shown increased survival in AML mouse models [18]. Characterization of hematologic malignancies has demonstrated increased IL3RA expression in $CD34^+CD38^-$ AML blasts as compared to expression in normal cells. Furthermore, these IL3RA-overexpressing cells have been shown to be able to initiate and maintain the leukemic process in immuno-deficient mice and thus act as leukemic stem cells [3,19]. Consequently, IL3RA has been shown to be a very useful biomarker for the detection of minimal residual disease, thereby predicting relapse in AML patients [20,21]. Taken together, these results suggest that IL3RA is a very attractive target for an antibody–drug conjugate (ADC) approach for the treatment of AML and other IL3RA-positive hematologic malignancies [10].

Here, we exploited a novel pyrrole subclass payload that potently inhibits the kinesin spindle protein (KSP/KIF11/Eg5) in biochemical and cellular assays to develop an ADC to target IL3RA on cancer cells [22–25]. KSP is a motor protein responsible for an essential event in mitosis, the segregation of duplicated centrosomes during spindle formation in the G2/M phase of the cell cycle, and therefore, it is required for productive cell divisions [26]. High expression of KSP in hematologic indications such as AML blasts and diffuse large B-cell lymphoma (DLBCL) [27] and in solid cancers such as breast, bladder, and pancreatic cancer has been linked to poorer prognosis [28], and thus, KSP presents an attractive target for cancer treatment.

KSP is active in all proliferating cells and therefore, KSP inhibitors (KSPi) representing various structural classes have resulted in neutropenia, mucositis, and stomatitis in clinical trials [28–32]. However, ADCs that combine a cancer cell-targeting antibody and a cytotoxic payload via a linker can deliver a cytotoxic payload specifically to target-expressing cancer cells. This approach could protect healthy tissue from exposure to the cytotoxic compound, thus decreasing overall side effects especially on highly proliferative tissues, thereby expanding the therapeutic window.

To generate the IL3RA-ADC BAY-943, a non-cell-permeable KSPi was conjugated randomly to the lysine residues of a humanized derivative of the anti-IL3RA antibody 7G3 [33], TPP-9476, via a novel protease-cleavable peptide linker [24]. IL3RA-ADC was efficacious in IL3RA-positive AML and HL cell lines in vitro, as well as in IL3RA-expressing AML and HL cell line and patient-derived xenograft (PDX) models in vivo. IL3RA-ADC was well-tolerated in the mouse, rat, and cynomolgus monkey. No signs of neutropenia, mucositis, or stomatitis, the typical side effects of small molecule KSPis, were observed in safety studies performed in rat and cynomolgus monkey. Taken together, these data support the further development of the compound as a novel therapy option for patients with AML or other hematologic malignancies expressing IL3RA.

2. Results

2.1. Characterization of the IL3RA-Targeting Antibody TPP-9476 and IL3RA-ADC BAY-943

The binding affinity of the IL3RA-targeting antibody TPP-9476 (IL3RA-Ab) to human and cynomolgus monkey IL3RA was assessed by surface plasmon resonance (SPR) and flow cytometry. IL3RA-Ab showed high affinity to both the human and the cynomolgus monkey IL3RA protein with dissociation constants (KD) of 11 nmol/L and 16 nmol/L, respectively, as determined by SPR. No binding to murine IL3RA was observed. Furthermore, IL3RA-Ab bound specifically to the IL3RA-expressing human hematologic cancer cell lines MOLM-13, MV-4-11, and KG-1 as determined by flow cytometry (Figure 1A).

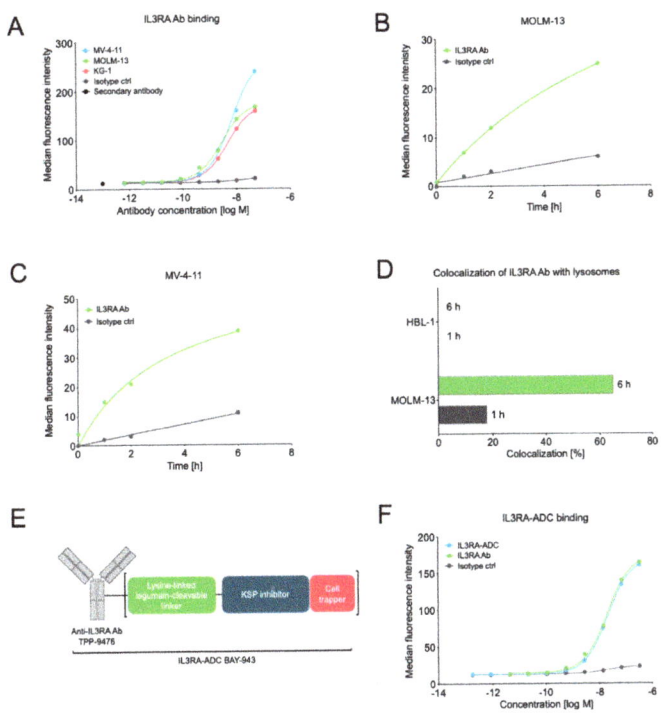

Figure 1. Characterization of the interleukin 3 receptor subunit alpha (IL3RA) antibody TPP-9476 and schematic representation of the IL3RA antibody–drug conjugate (ADC) BAY-943. (**A**) The binding of the IL3RA-targeting antibody (IL3RA Ab) TPP-9476 to IL3RA-positive hematologic cell lines as determined by flow cytometry. The obtained EC$_{50}$ values were 2.73×10^{-9} M for MOLM-13, 6.53×10^{-9} M for MV-4-11, and 4.54×10^{-9} M for KG-1 cells. (**B,C**) The internalization of the IL3RA Ab TPP-9476 and an isotype control antibody into IL3RA-positive MOLM-13 (**B**) and MV-4-11 (**C**) cells as determined by flow cytometry-based imaging. (**D**) The colocalization of the IL3RA Ab TPP-9476 in lysosomes in the IL3RA-positive MOLM-13 and IL3RA-negative HBL-1 cells. (**E**) Schematic representation of the IL3RA-ADC BAY-943. TPP-9476 represents the IL3RA-Ab. The "cell trapper" functionality indicates a non-cell-permeable payload metabolite that enables maximal retention in target cells after cleavage. (**F**) The binding of the IL3RA-ADC BAY-943 to IL3RA-positive MOLM-13 cells as determined by flow cytometry. The obtained EC$_{50}$ values were 20.4×10^{-9} M for ILRA3A-ADC and 18.7×10^{-9} M for ILRA3A Ab, respectively.

As the prerequisite for ADC activity is to effectively deliver the cytotoxic payload into the cells, we next studied the ability of IL3RA-Ab to internalize upon target binding. The fluorescently labeled IL3RA-Ab showed highly specific, target-dependent internalization in the IL3RA-positive MOLM-13 and MV-4-11 cell lines with >3.5-fold enhancement as compared with the non-specific internalization of the isotype control antibody (Figure 1B,C). In flow cytometry-based imaging, IL3RA-Ab showed lysosomal colocalization in the IL3RA-positive MOLM-13 but not in the IL3RA-negative HBL-1 cell line (Figure 1D). The lysosomal colocalization of IL3RA-Ab indicates that when incorporated into an ADC, it allows the release of the payload metabolite. This can occur via the cleavage of the linker by a lysosomal protease that is active at acidic pH (such as legumain) and/or by proteolytic degradation of the antibody.

Since IL3RA-Ab demonstrated the essential properties of an effective ADC antibody, we conjugated a non-cell permeable KSPi to the lysine residues of the IL3RA-Ab TPP-9476 via a novel legumain-cleavable peptide linker [24] to produce the IL3RA-targeting ADC BAY-943 (IL3RA-ADC; Figure 1E). IL3RA-ADC showed high stability in human plasma (Supplementary Figure S1C) and a comparable binding affinity to the IL3RA-Ab (half-maximal effective concentration, EC_{50} 18–21 nmol/L in MOLM-13 cells; Figure 1F), indicating that the attachment of the KSPi payload linker does not impact the binding affinity of the ADC antibody moiety. Furthermore, the active payload metabolite of IL3RA-ADC, BAY-716, showed poor permeability across Caco-2 cells (apparent permeability, Papp A-B = 1.8 nm/s, Papp B-A = 2.7 nm/s) with an efflux ratio (Papp B-A/Papp A-B) of 1.6, indicating that no active efflux takes place in Caco-2 cells. The poor permeability from B-A in Caco-2 cells indicates a long residence time after intracellular release of the active KSPi metabolite BAY-716 in tumor cells. As Caco-2 cells express the efflux transporter P-gP (P-glycoprotein), it also suggests that BAY-716 is a poor substrate for the efflux transporter P-gP.

2.2. IL3RA-ADC Shows Potent and Selective Efficacy In Vitro

The in vitro cytotoxicity of the IL3RA-ADC BAY-943 was assessed in a panel of human tumor cell lines with different IL3RA expression levels (Table 1). IL3RA-ADC demonstrated potent antiproliferative activity with half-maximal inhibitory concentration (IC_{50}) values at the subnanomolar to nanomolar range in the IL3RA-positive AML (MV-4-11, MOLM-13) and HL (HDLM-2, L-428) derived cell lines, whereas little activity was observed in the tumor cell lines with low levels of or negative for IL3RA membrane expression (NCI-H292, HT). Moreover, in IL3RA-positive AML and HL cell lines, a 10 to 100-fold higher sensitivity to IL3RA-ADC compared to the non-targeted isotype control ADC was observed (Table 2), demonstrating that the activity of IL3RA-ADC is target-dependent. Furthermore, IL3RA-ADC was found to induce apoptosis specifically in IL3RA-positive cells, as demonstrated by caspase 3/7 activation in MV-4-11 with an EC_{50} of 4.33 nmol/L, but not in the IL3RA-negative MDA-MB-231 cells (EC_{50} > 300 nmol/L; Supplementary Figure S2), further supporting the selectivity of IL3RA-ADC.

2.3. IL3RA-ADC Improves Survival in the MOLM-13 and MV-4-11 Xenograft Models

The antitumor efficacy of the IL3RA-ADC BAY-943 was tested in two IL3RA-positive, systemic (intravenous transplantation) cell line-derived xenografts: MOLM-13 human AML and MV-4-11 human biphenotypic leukemia models in mice. Both the MOLM-13 and MV-4-11 cell lines harbor *FLT3-ITD* mutations shown to be associated with an unfavorable prognosis in AML [34]. The median survival time (MST) for the vehicle and isotype control ADC was 22.5 and 46, respectively (Figure 2). By contrast, in the MOLM-13 model, 80–100% of the mice treated with 10 mg/kg IL3RA-ADC survived without signs of leukemia until day 123, when the study was terminated (Figure 2B), while all mice treated with the isotype control ADC were sacrificed due to signs of disease by day 67 after tumor cell inoculation. In the MV-4-11 model, the administration of IL3RA-ADC once weekly (Q7D), every two weeks (Q14D), or every three weeks (Q21D) resulted in a potent and sustained antitumor effect with MSTs of 120.5, 145.5, and 105 at the IL3RA-ADC dose of 2.5 mg/kg (Figure 2C) and 162, 153, and 140 days at the IL3RA-ADC dose of 10 mg/kg, respectively (Figure 2D). The MST for the vehicle and the isotype control ADC was 48 and 148, respectively. No significant differences in efficacy between the tested treatment schedules were observed in either of the models.

Table 1. The antiproliferative activity of IL3RA-ADC in a panel of tumor cells.

Cell Line	Provider (Catalog No.)	Date Obtained	Date Authenticated	Origin	Anti-IL3RA ABC	IL3RA-ADC IC$_{50}$ (M)
MV-4-11	ATCC (CRL 9591)	5/5/2008	02/05/2019	Biphenotypic B myelomonocytic leukemia	≈26,700	1.58×10^{-10}
MOLM-13	DSMZ (ACC 554)	5/2/2008	02/05/2019	Acute myeloid leukemia	≈15,100 [a]	6.37×10^{-10}
HDLM-2	DSMZ (ACC 17)	19/02/2015	06/05/2015	Pleural effusion of Hodgkin lymphoma	≈74,300	1.97×10^{-9}
L-428	origin unknown	1996	17/04/2013	Pleural effusion of Hodgkin lymphoma	≈111,300	3.97×10^{-10}
THP-1	ATCC (TIB 202)	15/02/2006	19/03/2014	Acute monocytic leukemia	≈21,100	2.92×10^{-9}
KG-1	ATCC (CCL 246)	28/10/2010	24/03/2011	Acute myelogenous leukemia	≈7200	8.34×10^{-9}
HT	DSMZ (ACC567)	12/09/2013	19/03/2014	Diffuse mixed lymphoma	≈350	$>3.00 \times 10^{-7}$
NCI-H292	ATCC (CRL 1848)	13/08/2009	07/02/2012	Non-small cell lung cancer	≈500	$>3.00 \times 10^{-7}$
HBL-1	Charité (Prof. Lenz)	15/04/2011	03/11/2017	Diffuse B cell lymphoma	n.d.	n.d.
Kasumi-3	DSMZ (ACC 714)	20/04/2017	05/09/2017	Acute myeloid leukemia	23,500	6.89×10^{-9} [b]
Rec-1	ATCC (CRL-3004)	24/02/2014	23/08/2018	Mantle cell lymphoma	n.d.	1.03×10^{-7}
OVCAR-8	NCI (NCI-60 panel)	20/10/2008	02/05/2019	Ovarian cancer	n.d.	1.47×10^{-7}
MDA-MB-231	ATCC HTB-26	05/04/2006	15/10/2019	Breast cancer	≈890	$>3.00 \times 10^{-7}$
Ramos	ATCC CRL 1596	08/03/2011	06/0572015	Burkitt's lymphoma	n.d. [a]	n.d.

In vitro cytotoxicity (CellTiter-Glo®, Promega) of the IL3RA-ADC BAY-943 in cancer cell lines with different levels of anti-IL3RA antibody bound per cell (ABC) as determined by quantitative flow cytometry. The mean IC$_{50}$ values from up to six individual assays are shown. n.d., not determined. [a] IL3RA expression analyzed by IHC on paraffin-embedded cell pellets; [b] IC$_{50}$ determined at 144 h (at 72 h for the other cell lines).

Table 2. The selectivity of IL3RA-ADC compared to the isotype control ADC.

		Cytotoxicity, IC$_{50}$ (M)				
Compound	DAR	MV-4-11 (IL3RA ≈26,700)	MOLM-13 (IL3RA ≈15,100)	HDLM-2 (IL3RA ≈74,300)	THP-1 (IL3RA ≈21,100)	NCI-H292 (IL3RA ≈500)
IL3RA-ADC	6.3	1.58×10^{-10}	6.37×10^{-10}	1.29×10^{-9}	2.92×10^{-9}	$>3.00 \times 10^{-7}$
Control ADC	7	$>3.00 \times 10^{-7}$	2.18×10^{-9}	1.52×10^{-7}	1.48×10^{-8}	2.12×10^{-7}
IL3RA-Ab	n.a.	$>3.00 \times 10^{-7}$	$>3.00 \times 10^{-7}$	$>3.00 \times 10^{-7}$	$>3.00 \times 10^{-7}$	$>3.00 \times 10^{-7}$
KSPi SMOL	n.a.	9.05×10^{-11}	8.95×10^{-11}	1.00×10^{-10}	3.07×10^{-10}	2.16×10^{-10}

In vitro cytotoxicity (CellTiter-Glo®, Promega) of the IL3RA-ADC BAY-943, isotype control ADC BAY-229, IL3RA antibody TPP-9476, and small molecule KSP inhibitor BAY-331 in the IL3RA-positive AML cell lines MV-4-11, MOLM-13, HDLM-2, THP-1 and in the IL3RA-low expressing NSCLC cell line NCI-H292 after 72 h incubation time. Anti-IL3RA ABC levels as determined by quantitative flow cytometry are indicated in the parentheses after each cell line. Ab, antibody; ADC, antibody–drug conjugate; DAR, drug-to-antibody ratio; n.a., not applicable; NSCLC, non-small-cell lung carcinoma; SMOL, small molecule.

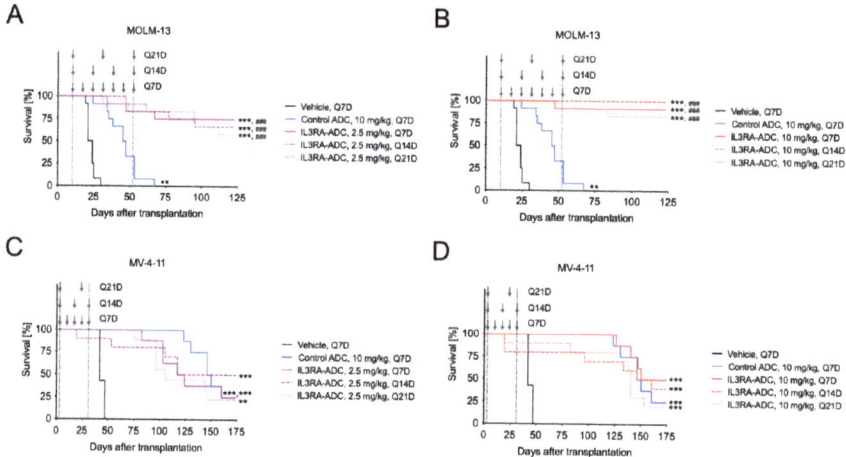

Figure 2. Antitumor efficacy of the IL3RA-ADC BAY-943 in the systemic MOLM-13 and MV-4-11 leukemia xenograft models. A-B. Kaplan–Meier survival plots of mice transplanted with the MOLM-13 human acute myeloid leukemia (AML) cells and treated intravenously (i.v.) with the isotype control ADC (10 mg/kg, Q7D) or IL3RA-ADC at 2.5 mg/kg (**A**) or 10 mg/kg (**B**); Q7D, Q14D, or Q21D. C-D. Kaplan–Meier survival plots of mice transplanted with the MV-4-11 human biphenotypic leukemia cells and treated i.v. with the isotype control ADC (10 mg/kg, Q7D) or IL3RA-ADC at 2.5 mg/kg (**C**) or 10 mg/kg (**D**); Q7D, Q14D or Q21D. The vertical dashed gray lines delineate the treatment period, and the arrows indicate time of treatment. Data were analyzed using the Cox proportional hazards model and corrected for family-wise error rate using Sidak's method. Asterisks and hashtags indicate statistical significance in comparison to the vehicle (** $p < 0.01$, *** $p < 0.001$) or isotype control ADC (### $p < 0.001$).

In the vehicle and the isotype control ADC groups, nearly all mice had symptoms of leukemia, i.e., splenomegaly and paralysis of hind limbs. In addition, the mean body weights decreased in these treatment groups, indicating that the mice suffered from leukemia (Supplementary Figure S3). However, no treatment-related side effects or abnormalities were observed during the study or at gross necropsy in the IL3RA-ADC-treated groups.

The antitumor efficacy of IL3RA-ADC was also tested in the subcutaneous MOLM-13 and MV-4-11 xenograft models in mice. Repetitive dosing with IL3RA-ADC resulted in a significant suppression of tumor growth in both models compared to the isotype control ADC, while the standard-of-care cytarabine showed no activity in these models (Supplementary Figure S4). Furthermore, in the MV-4-11 model, treatment with the unconjugated IL3RA-Ab TPP-9476 at 5 mg/kg, Q7D×2 showed no tumor growth inhibition (Supplementary Figure S4C,D), indicating that the antitumor activity of IL3RA-ADC is conveyed by the targeted delivery of the KSPi payload and not the IL3RA-Ab.

2.4. IL3RA-ADC Suppresses Tumor Burden and Improves Survival in Systemic AM7577 and AML11655 PDX Models

The efficacy of IL3RA-ADC was further evaluated in the systemic AM7577 and AML11655 patient-derived AML xenograft models in mice. These PDX models showed high IL3RA protein expression (Supplementary Figure S5) and harbor a typical AML genotype with mutations in genes including *NMP1*, *FLT3-ITD*, *IDH1*, *IDH2*, and *DNMT3A* (Supplementary Table S1).

In the AM7577 PDX model, IL3RA-ADC administered at 10 mg/kg intraperitoneally (i.p.) reduced tumor burden compared to the vehicle or isotype control ADC, as indicated by a decreased number of human CD45 (hCD45)/human IL3RA (hIL3RA)-positive cells in blood on day 56 (both $p < 0.001$;

Figure 3A). Furthermore, treatment with IL3RA-ADC resulted in improved survival with the MST of 69 days at the dose of 2.5 + 10 mg/kg and 82 days at the dose of 10 mg/kg. The MST for the vehicle and the isotype control ADC was 62 and 64 days, respectively (Figure 3B).

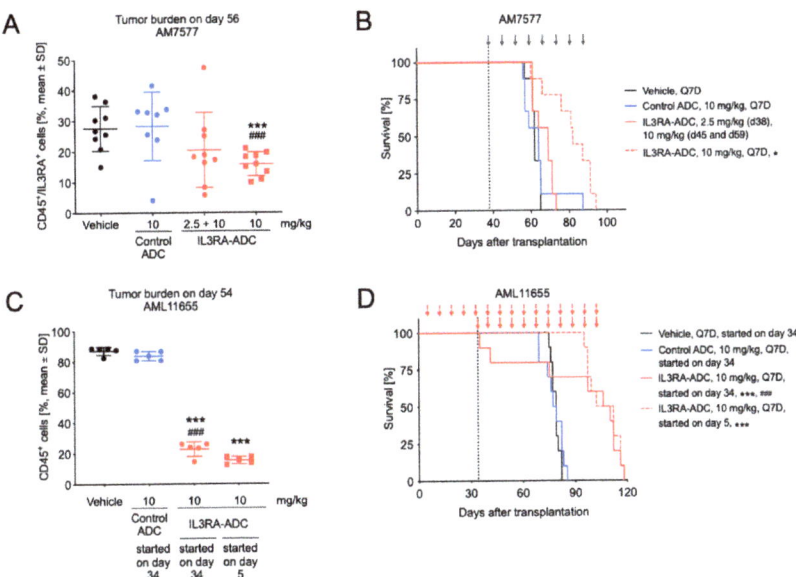

Figure 3. Antitumor efficacy of the IL3RA-ADC BAY-943 in the patient-derived AM7577 and AML11655 AML xenograft models. (**A**) Tumor burden on day 56 in mice transplanted with AM7577 cells and treated i.p. with the isotype control ADC (10 mg/kg, Q7D) and IL3RA-ADC (2.5 + 10 mg/kg or 10 mg/kg, Q7D). In the 2.5 + 10 mg/kg IL3RA-ADC treatment group, the first dose was 2.5 mg/kg (day 38) and the two subsequent doses (on days 45 and 59) 10 mg/kg. (**B**) Kaplan–Meier survival plots of mice described in panel A. Treatment days in all groups except for the 2.5 + 10 mg/kg IL3RA-ADC treatment group are indicated with gray arrows. (**C**) Tumor burden on day 54 in mice transplanted with AML11655 cells. Intraperitoneal treatments with the isotype control ADC (10 mg/kg, Q7D) were initiated on day 34 and with IL3RA-ADC (10 mg/kg, Q7D) on day 5 (preventive setting) or 34 (therapeutic setting). (**D**) Kaplan–Meier survival plots of mice described in panel C. Treatment days are indicated with red arrows. The data were analyzed using the Cox proportional-hazards model and corrected for family-wise error rate using Sidak's method. Asterisks and hashtags indicate statistical significance in comparison to vehicle (* $p < 0.05$, *** $p < 0.001$) and the isotype control ADC (### $p < 0.001$).

In the AML11655 mouse xenograft model, IL3RA-ADC was administered i.p. using either a preventive (treatment started on day 5) or a therapeutic (treatment started on day 34) setting. IL3RA-ADC administered at 10 mg/kg inhibited the growth of IL3RA-positive AML cells, as indicated by temporarily reduced numbers of hCD45-positive cells in blood compared to vehicle or isotype control ADC in both settings (Figure 3C,D; all $p < 0.001$). In addition, treatment with IL3RA-ADC using either the preventive or therapeutic setting resulted in prolonged MSTs of 107 or 108 days, respectively (Figure 3D). The MST for the vehicle and the isotype control ADC was 79 and 78 days, respectively.

2.5. IL3RA-ADC Demonstrates Antitumor Efficacy in Subcutaneous HDLM-2 Hodgkin Lymphoma Xenograft Model

Finally, the antitumor efficacy of the IL3RA-ADC BAY-943 was tested in a subcutaneous HDLM-2 Hodgkin lymphoma xenograft model in mice. This model showed a high IL3RA antigen density with ≈74,300 anti-IL3RA antibodies bound per cell (Table S1), which is in line with the literature [8]. In the

HDLM-2 model, the i.p. injection of IL3RA-ADC at 5 or 10 mg/kg resulted in a strong reduction of tumor growth compared to the vehicle (both $p < 0.001$; Figure 4). This effect was comparable with the clinically studied KSPi ispinesib administered at 10 mg/kg in the same model. In the two IL3RA-ADC treatment groups, total tumor eradication was observed in twelve mice out of thirteen (92%) at the end of the study.

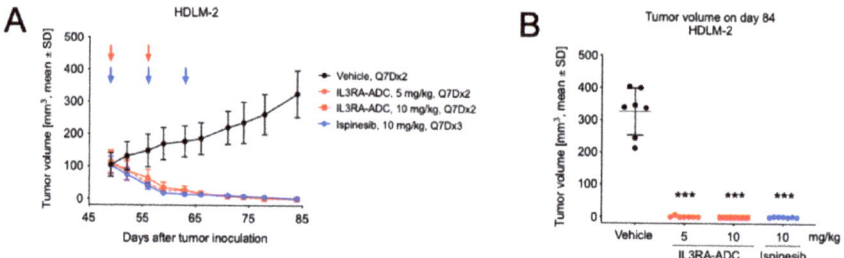

Figure 4. Antitumor efficacy of the IL3RA-ADC BAY-943 in the subcutaneous HDLM-2 Hodgkin lymphoma xenograft model. Mice were transplanted with HDLM-2 cells and treatments with IL3RA-ADC (5 or 10 mg/kg, Q7D×2, i.p.) or ispinesib (10 mg/kg, Q7D×3, i.v.) were initiated on day 49. (**A**) Tumor growth curves. ADC treatment days are indicated with red arrows and ispinesib administration is indicated with blue arrows. (**B**) Tumor volume on day 84. Statistical analyses were performed using a linear mixed-effects model with random intercepts and slopes for each subject (n = 6–7). Mean comparisons between the treatment and control groups were performed using the estimated linear mixed-effects model and corrected for family-wise error rate using Sidak's method. Asterisks indicate statistical significance in comparison to vehicle (*** $p < 0.001$).

2.6. IL3RA-ADC Is Well-Tolerated

The safety, including possible changes in the hematologic cell populations, of IL3RA-ADC was evaluated in the cynomolgus monkey in two range-finding studies with single or repeated dosing. IL3RA-ADC was well-tolerated without adverse events typically observed with ADCs containing other payload classes, such as thrombocytopenia, neutropenia, or signs of liver toxicity. In addition, mucositis, a dose-limiting toxicity for small molecule KSP inhibitors in clinical studies [35], was not observed. A single dose of IL3RA-ADC up to 20 mg/kg or three repeated doses of IL3RA-ADC up to 10 mg/kg given every three weeks resulted in a transient reduction of IL3RA-positive basophils and plasmacytoid dendritic cells (pDCs), indicating targeting of the IL3RA-ADC to antigen-positive cells (data not shown). Furthermore, the administration of IL3RA-ADC showed no obvious changes in the percentage of the CD34$^+$Lin$^-$ bone marrow cell population containing the hematopoietic stem cells, as analyzed by flow cytometry (data not shown).

The effect of the toxophore metabolite BAY-716 was also analyzed after a single dose of 0.25 mg/kg in rats (data not shown). No laboratory or histopathology findings were observed, indicating that this non-cell-permeable toxophore metabolite does not induce toxic effects thereby underlining the good safety profile of IL3RA-ADC.

3. Discussion

Despite the recent progress in the treatment of AML, clinical outcomes have improved only minimally over the past three decades. Therefore, novel therapeutic agents with a larger therapeutic window and a favorable tolerability profile are urgently needed to improve the therapeutic outcome for AML patients. Increasing evidence indicates that IL3RA is highly expressed in leukemic stem cells but not in normal hematopoietic stem cells, and it associates in AML with treatment response, minimal residual disease detection, and prognosis [3,15,17]. Consequently, several IL3RA-targeting approaches, such as an anti-IL3RA antibody enhanced for antibody-dependent cell-mediated cytotoxicity, anti-IL3RA-ADCs with highly potent payloads of the pyrrolobenzodiazepine (PBD) or indolinobenzodiazepine pseudodimer (IGN) class, various bispecific T cell recruiting antibodies, or chimeric antigen receptor T cell (CAR-T) therapies are currently under preclinical or clinical development [10,28,36–39].

Here, we explored a novel concept to improve the therapeutic window and safety of KSP inhibition by targeting a non-cell-permeable KSP inhibitor as ADC to AML cells, and thereby, sparing fast-dividing healthy cells from KSP inhibition. This provides a payload with a novel mode of action and would be a new therapeutic option for the treatment of IL3RA-positive malignancies. The investigated IL3RA-targeting ADC (BAY-943, IL3RA-ADC) consists of a humanized anti-IL3RA antibody conjugated with a stable lysine linkage to a potent proprietary KSPi via a protease-cleavable linker, producing a non-cell-permeable payload metabolite.

KSP is an ATP-dependent plus-end directed motor protein, which generates force and moves along microtubules, and it is involved in the separation of the centrosomes, the generation of the bipolar spindle, and thereby plays an important role in mitosis [26]. The inhibition of KSP with small molecules such as monastrol or small interfering RNA (siRNA)-mediated knockdown results in the formation of monopolar spindles (termed a "monoaster"), which lead to aberrant mitotic arrest and apoptosis [30,40]. Thus, KSP presents a convincing target for the development of an anti-mitotic approach for cancer treatment. Accordingly, several allosteric KSP inhibitors such as ispinesib, litronesib, and filanesib (ARRY-520) have been or are in clinical trials [35,41–44]. Filanesib has also been explored in a Phase I clinical trial in AML [43], and clinical studies are ongoing in relapsed refractory multiple myeloma (rrMM). The antitumor activity of filanesib has previously been shown in AML cells in vitro and in xenograft mouse models [27]. The most common side effects of KSP inhibitors with different chemical scaffolds are neutropenia, mucositis, and stomatitis [35]. This has been explained by the inhibition of KSP in highly proliferative cells such as neutrophils and cells lining the mucosa and the stoma, respectively, thus limiting their therapeutic efficacy due to a small therapeutic window.

Antibody–drug conjugates (ADCs) are one solution that has been proposed to mitigate the toxic side effects of anti-mitotic therapies and to broaden their therapeutic window. In fact, currently more than 60 ADCs against multiple targets in solid and hematologic tumors are in clinical trials [45,46], and eight ADCs have meanwhile been approved [47]. The payload classes currently used are confined to microtubule destabilizers (e.g., auristatin, dolastatin, maytansinoid, tubulysine), DNA interacting agents (e.g., calicheamicin, duocarmycin, PBD, IGN), and topoisomerase inhibitors (e.g., camptothecin derivative SN-38, exatecan). Many of these permeable payloads and/or highly potent DNA-interacting payloads have safety issues and therefore result in an insufficient therapeutic window. For example, the clinical trials for the CD33-targeting SGN-CD33A and the IL3RA-targeting SGN-CD123A [38,39] both with a PBD payload were terminated in 2017 and 2018, respectively. Recently, the first IL3RA-targeting therapy was approved for BPDCN [9]. However, the fusion protein tagraxofusp-erzs (formerly called SL-401), which consists of the ligand IL3 fused to a truncated diphtheria toxin, has been reported to cause capillary leak syndrome as a common side effect in more than 55% of patients [10]. This further underlines that efficacious therapies with acceptable safety profiles are still urgently required for targeting IL3RA-positive malignancies.

The IL3RA-ADC BAY-943 demonstrated the capability of delivering a novel cytotoxic payload to IL3RA-positive cells. The IL3RA antibody TPP-9476 to which the KSP inhibitor payload is linked via a legumain-cleavable peptide linker showed high binding affinity and specificity to IL3RA and bound specifically to IL3RA-expressing human AML and HL cell lines. The IL3RA antibody internalized into the lysosomes of IL3RA-positive MOLM-13 and MV-4-11 AML cell lines, and IL3RA-ADC demonstrated high cytotoxic potency in IL3RA-positive MV-4-11 and MOLM-13 AML and HDLM-2 and L-428 HL derived cell lines. Furthermore, in the IL3RA-positive cell lines tested, IL3RA-ADC showed 10 to 1000-fold cytotoxicity compared with the isotype control ADC, indicating high target selectivity. The less prominent selectivity observed in MOLM-13 and THP-1 cells may be explained by a non-specific uptake of the isotype control ADC to AML cells differentiated along the macrophage lineage.

In an in vivo setting, IL3RA-ADC administered at 10 mg/kg increased survival in both the IL3RA-positive MOLM-13 and MV-4-11 cell line-derived and IL3RA-positive AM7577 and AML11655 patient-derived AML xenograft models harboring molecular alterations associated with poor prognosis in AML. The increased survival was accompanied by a reduction in the growth of IL3RA-positive AML cells and tumor size in the systemic and subcutaneous models, respectively. In the IL3RA-positive HDLM-2 subcutaneous Hodgkin lymphoma model, IL3RA-ADC treatment also resulted in significant antitumor efficacy with most animals being tumor-free at the end of the study.

The body weights of the animals decreased over the course of the study, indicating that they suffered from leukemia. However, no IL3RA-ADC treatment-related body weight losses were observed, suggesting good tolerability (Supplementary Figures S3 and S6), particularly in comparison to the small molecule KSPi ispinesib, which induced a transient body weight loss in mice after the second treatment (Supplementary Figure S6C). The treatments with IL3RA-ADC in the HDLM-2 subcutaneous Hodgkin lymphoma model were also well-tolerated.

The good tolerability of the IL3RA-ADC was confirmed by repeated dose safety and immunotoxicity assessments in the cynomolgus monkey with no changes in the portion of the $CD34^+Lin^-$ cell population, and transient decreases in basophils and IL3RA-positive basophils. Importantly, liver toxicity, thrombocytopenia, and neutropenia, which are frequently observed with ADCs in the clinic and in cynomolgus monkey preclinical studies [48,49], were not apparent, which was most likely due to the fact that the IL3RA-ADC toxophore metabolite is non-cell permeable. In addition, neutropenia and mucositis, which were the dose-limiting toxicities for small molecule KSP inhibitors in the clinic, were not observed. Furthermore, the IL3RA-ADC metabolite BAY-716 showed poor permeability across Caco-2 cells, indicating that the metabolite is trapped in tumor cells after its intracellular release. This "cell trapper" functionality enables a long-lasting exposure and at the same time potentially reduces off-target toxicities through the low permeability of KSPi into normal cells.

4. Materials and Methods

4.1. Cell Lines

Cell lines were acquired from DSMZ (German Collection of Microorganisms and Cell Cultures GmbH; Braunschweig, Germany) unless otherwise noted and cultured according to the provider's instructions. Human MDA-MB-231 breast cancer, NCI-H292 non-small cell lung cancer, MV-4-11 and THP-1 acute monocytic leukemia, KG-1 acute myelogenous leukemia, Rec-1 mantle cell lymphoma, and Ramos Burkitt's lymphoma cells were obtained from ATCC (American Type Culture Collection; Manassas, VA, USA). Human OVCAR-8 ovarian cancer cells were acquired from the NCI-60 Human Tumor Cell Line Panel (National Cancer Institute, Rockville, MD, USA). The human diffuse B cell lymphoma cell line HBL-1 was obtained from Dr. Georg Lenz (Charité Universitätsklinikum, Berlin, Germany) and cultivated in RPMI 1640 supplemented with 10% fetal calf serum (FCS). The human Hodgkin lymphoma cell line L-428 (source not known) was cultivated in RPMI 1640 supplemented with 10% FCS. Cancer cell lines were obtained between 2002 and 2012, authenticated using short tandem repeat DNA fingerprinting at DSMZ (Table 1), and subjected frequently to mycoplasma testing.

4.2. Compounds

The anti-IL3RA antibodies TPP-9476 and TPP-8988 (recognizes a different epitope in the extracellular domain of IL3RA than TPP-9476) and the isotype control antibody TPP-754, the IL3RA-ADC BAY-943, the isotype control ADC BAY-229 (with TPP-754), the non-cell-permeable toxophore metabolite BAY-716 (active toxophore metabolite of IL3RA-ADC), and the cell-permeable small molecule KSPi BAY-331 were manufactured at Bayer AG. Ispinesib (SYNT1009) was purchased from Syncom (a contract research organization in organic chemistry, www.syncom.eu; Groningen, the Netherlands), cytarabine (HT0476) from Accord Healthcare GmbH (Neutraubling, Germany), and staurosporine (#S4400) from Sigma-Aldrich (Saint Louis, MO, USA).

The IL3RA-specific hIgG1 antibody (IL3RA-Ab, TPP-9476) was generated by humanization of the murine anti-IL3RA antibody 7G3 [33] as described in Lerchen et al. [22]. During a protein engineering process, which is meant to bring the amino acid sequence as close as possible to the next human germline [50], multiple variants were tested. The final version, TPP-9476, comprises several amino acid exchanges in the light and heavy chain that resulted in enhanced internalization.

The generation and characterization of the IL3RA-Ab is described in the Supplementary Methods. The IL3RA-targeting ADC BAY-943 (IL3RA-ADC) was generated by conjugating the KSPi to the lysine residues of IL3RA-Ab via a protease-cleavable linker [24]. The characterization of IL3RA-ADC is described in the Supplementary Methods. In the in vivo efficacy studies, IL3RA-ADC BAY-943 with a drug-to-antibody ratio (DAR) of 6.3 as determined by mass spectrometry was used. At a DAR of 6.3, no aggregation of the IL3RA-ADC was observed (Supplementary Figure S1)

4.3. Internalization and Lysosomal Colocalization of IL3RA-Ab

Internalization and colocalization experiments were performed in MOLM-13 and MV-4-11 AML cell lines using flow cytometry-based imaging. The IL3RA-specific antibody TPP-9476, IL3RA-ADC BAY-943, corresponding isotype control antibody TPP-754, and isotype control ADC BAY-229 were lysine-conjugated with a ten-fold molar excess of CypHer 5E mono NHS ester (GE Healthcare, Chicago, IL, USA) at pH 8.3. The reaction mixture was purified by chromatography (PD10 desalting column, GE Healthcare, Chicago, IL, USA), followed by centrifugation (Vivaspin 500, Sartorius Stedim Biotech, Aubagne, France). Alexa 488 (Jackson ImmunoResearch, West Grove, PA, USA) was utilized as a constitutive dye. The fluorescence was measured using the Amnis® FlowSight® or the Guava easyCyte™ flow cytometers (Luminex Corporation, Austin, TX, USA) and analyzed using the IDEAS® software or the guavaSoft 2.6 software (Luminex Corporation, Austin, TX, USA).

For the internalization assay, the tumor cells (5×10^4/well) were incubated with the labeled antibodies (10 µg/mL) at 37 °C, 5% CO_2 for 0, 1, 2, and 6 h. The fluorescence was measured using the Amnis® FlowSight® or the Guava easyCyte™ flow cytometers and analyzed using the IDEAS® or the guavaSoft 2.6 software. The kinetics of the internalization were determined based on the analysis of the median fluorescence intensity (MFI) over time.

For the colocalization studies, MOLM-13 and MV-4-11 tumor cells (5×10^4/well) were incubated with the labeled antibodies (20 µg/mL) at 37 °C, 5% CO_2 for 0 h, 0.5 h, 2 h, and 6 h. The lysosomal compartment marker CytoPainter LysoGreen (1:2000; Abcam, Cambridge, UK) was added 30 min before the end of the incubation period. After incubation, the cells were washed and resuspended in ice-cold FACS (fluorescence-activated cell sorting) buffer consisting of phosphate-buffered saline (PBS) and 3% FCS. The lysosomal colocalization was analyzed with FACS image analysis using the IDEAS® software.

The assessment of the stability of the IL3RA-ADC BAY-943 in human plasma and the permeability of the KSPi toxophore metabolite BAY-716 in Caco-2 cells are described in the Supplementary Methods.

4.4. In Vitro Cytotoxicity of IL3RA-ADC

The antiproliferative activity of IL3RA-ADC was determined in a panel of human tumor cell lines using the CellTiter-Glo® assay (Promega Madison, WI, USA). Cells (2000–5000 cells/well) were incubated at 37 °C, 5% CO_2 for 24 h and the compounds were added at concentrations of 3×10^{-11}–3×10^{-7} M (or 3×10^{-12}–3×10^{-8} M, depending on the cell line tested) in triplicates. Cell viability was determined at the beginning (day 0) and after 72 h incubation in the presence or absence of ADCs. The IC_{50} of the growth inhibition was calculated in comparison to day 0. The IL3RA antigen density was determined with the QIFI (Dako, Glostrup, Denmark) quantitative flow cytometry assay using the murine anti-IL3RA antibody clone 7G3 (Becton Dickinson, Franklin Lakes, NJ, USA).

4.5. In Vivo Studies

All animal experiments were conducted in accordance with the German Animal Welfare Law and approved by Berlin authorities (Landesamt für Arbeitsschutz, Gesundheitsschutz und technische Sicherheit Berlin, LAGetSi; code number A0378/12). When a body weight loss of >10% was observed, treatment was ceased until recovery. In the systemic models, mice were sacrificed individually when signs of leukemia were observed (>20–30% body weight loss, hind leg paralysis, or general deterioration of health status). The molecular alterations of the tested in vivo models are described in Supplementary Table S1.

For the systemic MOLM-13 and MV-4-11 models, female CB17-SCID (Janvier Labs, Le Genest-Saint-Isle, France) or NOD SCID (Taconic, Køge, Denmark) mice were injected intravenously (i.v.) with 200 µL of 7.5×10^6 or 5×10^6 cancer cells in 0.9% NaCl, respectively. The mice were treated with i.p. injection of IL3RA-ADC at 2.5 or 10 mg/kg once weekly (Q7D), every two weeks (Q14D), or every three weeks (Q21D). In the MOLM-13 model, treatments were started on day 10, and the study was terminated on day 124. In the MV-4-11 model, treatments were started on day 3, and the study was terminated on day 174 after tumor cell injection.

For the systemic AM7577 PDX model, female NOD/SCID mice (Shanghai Lingchang Bio-Technology Co. Ltd., LC, Shanghai, China) were injected i.v. with 100 µL of 1.4×10^6 cancer cells in PBS at CrownBio (Beijing, China). The development of AML was monitored by flow cytometric analysis of the percentage of hCD45 cells in blood. On day 38 after tumor cell injection, when approximately 4% of hCD45-positive cells were present, the mice were randomized, and treatments were started. The mice were treated with i.v. injections of IL3RA-ADC at 2.5 or 10 mg/kg, Q7D or the isotype control ADC at 10 mg/kg, Q7D. In the first IL3RA-ADC treatment group, the initial dose of 2.5 mg/kg, Q7D was increased to 10 mg/kg, Q14D from the second administration onwards (indicated as 2.5 + 10 mg/kg). The study was terminated on day 104 after tumor cell injection.

For the systemic AML11655 PDX model, female CIEA NOG mice® (NOD.Cg-$Prkdc^{scid}$ $Il2rg^{tm1Sug}$/JicTac, Taconic, Køge, Denmark) were injected i.v. with 400 µL of 1×10^7 cancer cells in PBS at EPO Berlin-Buch GmbH (Berlin, Germany). The development of AML was monitored by the percentage of hCD45-positive cells in blood as determined by flow cytometry. Treatments were initiated on day 5 after tumor cell injection (preventive setting) or day 34 after tumor cell injection (therapeutic setting) when approximately 46% of hCD45-positive cells were detected in blood. The mice were treated with i.v. injections of IL3RA-ADC at 10 mg/kg, Q7D or the isotype control ADC at 10 mg/kg, Q7D. The study was terminated on day 118 after tumor cell injection.

For the HDLM-2 Hodgkin lymphoma model, female CB17-SCID mice (Janvier Labs, Le Genest-Saint-Isle, France) were injected subcutaneously (s.c.) with 100 µL of 1×10^7 cancer cells suspended in 30% Matrigel/70% medium. Tumor volume ($0.5 \times$ length $\times$ width^2) was determined based on twice weekly measurement of tumor area by a caliper (length and width). Treatments with IL3RA-ADC (5 or 10 mg/kg, i.p., Q7D×2) or ispinesib (10 mg/kg, i.v., Q7D×3) were started on day 49 when the tumors had reached a mean size of 100 mm^3. The study was terminated on day 84 after tumor cell injection.

The subcutaneous MOLM-13 and MV-4-11 models as well as safety studies are described in the Supplementary Methods.

4.6. Statsitical Analyses

Statistical analyses were performed using R (version 3.3.2 or newer; R Foundation for Statistical Computing, Vienna, Austria) [51]. Flow cytometry and tumor volume data were analyzed using a linear model estimated with generalized least squares that included separate variance parameters for each study group or linear mixed-effects model with random intercepts and slopes for each subject. Mean comparisons between the treatment and control groups were performed using the estimated linear or linear mixed-effects model and corrected for family-wise error rate using Sidak's method. Survival analyses were performed using the Cox proportional-hazards model and corrected for family-wise error rate using Sidak's method. p values < 0.05 were considered significant.

5. Conclusions

The novel IL3RA-ADC with a differentiated mode-of action demonstrates selective binding and internalization to IL3RA-positive cells, which translates into selective and efficacious antitumor activity in IL3RA-positive AML and Hodgkin lymphoma models. By employing a KSP inhibitor, a stable lysine linkage between the payload and the antibody, and a legumain-cleavable linker resulting in a non-cell-permeable payload metabolite, IL3RA-ADC presents a new alternative for the treatment of IL3RA-positive malignancies. Using the KSPi as a payload in an ADC is expected to result in manageable toxicity and a broader therapeutic window compared to that reported for the systemic application of KSPi in clinical trials. Our data support further development of the IL3RA-ADC BAY-943 as an innovative approach for the treatment of patients with IL3RA-positive AML.

Supplementary Materials: The following are available online at http://www.mdpi.com/2072-6694/12/11/3464/s1, Figure S1: Drug-to-antibody ratio (DAR) of the IL3RA-ADC BAY-943, Figure S2: Apoptotic activity of the IL3RA-ADC BAY-943 in IL3RA-positive cells in vitro, Figure S3: Body weights in the systemic MOLM-13 and MV-4-11 leukemia xenograft models, Figure S4: Antitumor efficacy of the IL3RA-ADC BAY-943 in the subcutaneous MOLM-13 human AML and MV-4-11 human biphenotypic leukemia xenograft models, Figure S5: IL3RA expression in the patient-derived AML11655 and AM7577 AML xenografts models and cell line-derived AML and HL models, Figure S6: Time course of relative body weight changes in mouse models, Table S1: Characteristics of the in vivo mouse xenograft models.

Author Contributions: Conceptualization, A.S., D.K., H.-G.L. and B.S.-L.; methodology, D.K., A.M.W., B.S.-L. and H.-G.L.; software, M.E., C.M. and S.G.; validation, H.-G.L., R.Z., S.J. and P.B.; investigation, D.K., B.S.-L., H.-G.L., A.M.W., O.v.A., P.B., S.M., L.D., M.E., R.Z., S.J., S.G., C.M. and A.S.; resources, S.M. and H.-G.L.; data curation, A.S. and L.D.; writing—original draft preparation, A.S. and D.K.; writing—review and editing, A.S. and D.K.; visualization, B.S.-L., A.M.W., D.K., O.v.A. and A.S.; supervision, D.K. and D.M.; project administration, A.S.; funding acquisition, D.M. All authors have read and agreed to the published version of the manuscript.

Funding: This research received no external funding.

Acknowledgments: Birgit Albrecht, Susanne Bendix, Henryk Bubik, Anna DiBetta, Charlene Döring, Lisa Ehresmann, Claudia Gerressen, Nils Guthof, Beate König, Michael Krzemien, Katja Kauffeldt, Petra Leidenfrost, Stefanie Mai, Bettina Muchow, Christine Nieland, Volker Pickard, Maria Ritter, Holger Spiecker, Rukiye Tamm, Frank Tesche, Ulrike Uhlig, Sebastian Wertz, and Dirk Wolter are acknowledged for excellent technical support. We thank Bertolt Kreft and Lars Linden for fruitful discussions. We thank Xin Tang, Lily Tong, Yuandong Wang, and Kira Böhmer at CrownBio and Antje Siegert, Michael Becker, and Jens Hoffmann at EPO Berlin-Buch GmbH for performing the in vivo studies in AML PDX models. Aurexel Life Sciences Ltd. (www.aurexel.com) is acknowledged for medical writing and editorial support funded by Bayer AG.

Conflicts of Interest: All authors are current or former employees of Bayer AG and inventors on Bayer AG patent applications. Anette Sommer, Hans-Georg Lerchen, Stephan Märsch, Michael Erkelenz, and Dominik Mumberg have ownership interest as shares in Bayer AG.

Abbreviations

Ab	antibody
ABC	antibodies bound per cell
ADC	antibody–drug conjugate
AML	acute myeloid leukemia
BPDCN	blastic plasmacytoid dendritic cell neoplasm
CAR-T	chimeric antigen receptor T cell
cHL	classical Hodgkin lymphoma
DAR	drug-to-antibody ratio
DLBCL	diffuse large B-cell lymphoma
EC_{50}	half-maximal effective concentration
FACS	fluorescence-activated cell sorting
FCS	fetal calf serum
hCD45	human CD45

hIL3RA	human IL3RA
HL	Hodgkin lymphoma
IC$_{50}$	half-maximal inhibitory concentration
IGN	indolinobenzodiazepine pseudodimer
IL-3	interleukin 3
IL3RA	interleukin 3 receptor subunit alpha
IL3RA-Ab	IL3RA-targeting antibody
i.p.	intraperitoneal(ly)
i.v.	intravenous(ly)
KD	dissociation constant
KSP	kinesin spindle protein
KSPi	kinesin spindle protein inhibitor
MDS	myelodysplastic syndrome
MFI	median fluorescence intensity
MST	median survival time
Papp	apparent permeability
PBD	pyrrolobenzodiazepine
PBS	phosphate-buffered saline
pDCs	plasmacytoid dendritic cells
PDX	patient-derived xenograft
P-gP	P-glycoprotein
Q7D	once weekly
Q14D	every two weeks
Q21D	every three weeks
rrMM	relapsed refractory multiple myeloma
s.c.	subcutaneous(ly)
siRNA	small interfering RNA
SPR	surface plasmon resonance

References

1. Ehninger, A.; Kramer, M.; Röllig, C.; Thiede, C.; Bornhäuser, M.; von Bonin, M.; Wermke, M.; Feldmann, A.; Bachmann, M.; Ehninger, G.; et al. Distribution and levels of cell surface expression of CD33 and CD123 in acute myeloid leukemia. *Blood Cancer J.* **2014**, *4*, e218. [CrossRef]
2. Muñoz, L.; Nomdedéu, J.F.; Lopez, O.; Carnicer, M.J.; Bellido, M.; Aventín, A.; Brunet, S.; Sierra, J. Interleukin-3 receptor alpha chain (CD123) is widely expressed in hematologic malignancies. *Haematologica* **2001**, *86*, 1261–1269.
3. Testa, U.; Pelosi, E.; Frankel, A. CD 123 is a membrane biomarker and a therapeutic target in hematologic malignancies. *Biomark. Res.* **2014**, *2*, 4. [CrossRef]
4. Lopez, A.F.; Hercus, T.R.; Ekert, P.; Littler, D.R.; Guthridge, M.; Thomas, D.; Ramshaw, H.S.; Stomski, F.; Perugini, M.; D'Andrea, R.; et al. Molecular basis of cytokine receptor activation. *Int. Union Biochem. Mol. Biol. Life* **2010**, *62*, 509–518. [CrossRef] [PubMed]
5. Bras, A.E.; de Haas, V.; van Stigt, A.; Jongen-Lavrencic, M.; Beverloo, H.B.; Te Marvelde, J.G.; Zwaan, C.M.; van Dongen, J.J.M.; Leusen, J.H.W.; van der Velden, V.H.J. CD123 expression levels in 846 acute leukemia patients based on standardized immunophenotyping. *Cytom. Part B Clin. Cytom.* **2019**, *96*, 134–142. [CrossRef] [PubMed]
6. Aldinucci, D.; Poletto, D.; Gloghini, A.; Nanni, P.; Degan, M.; Perin, T.; Ceolin, P.; Rossi, F.M.; Gattei, V.; Carbone, A.; et al. Expression of functional interleukin-3 receptors on Hodgkin and Reed-Sternberg cells. *Am. J. Pathol.* **2002**, *160*, 585–596. [CrossRef]
7. Fromm, J.R. Flow cytometric analysis of CD123 is useful for immunophenotyping classical Hodgkin lymphoma. *Cytom. Part B Clin. Cytom.* **2011**, *80*, 91–99. [CrossRef] [PubMed]
8. Ruella, M.; Klichinsky, M.; Kenderian, S.S.; Shestova, O.; Ziober, A.; Kraft, D.O.; Feldman, M.; Wasik, M.A.; June, C.H.; Gill, S. Overcoming the immunosuppressive tumor microenvironment of Hodgkin lymphoma using chimeric antigen receptor T cells. *Cancer Discov.* **2017**, *7*, 1154–1167. [CrossRef] [PubMed]

9. Kerr, D., II; Zhang, L.; Sokol, L. Blastic plasmacytoid dendritic cell neoplasm. *Curr. Treat. Options Oncol.* **2019**, *20*, 9. [CrossRef]
10. Testa, U.; Pelosi, E.; Castelli, G. CD123 as a therapeutic target in the treatment of hematological malignancies. *Cancers* **2019**, *11*, 1358. [CrossRef]
11. De Smet, D.; Trullemans, F.; Jochmans, K.; Renmans, W.; Smet, L.; Heylen, O.; Bael, A.M.; Schots, R.; Leus, B.; De Waele, M. Diagnostic potential of $CD34^+$ cell antigen expression in myelodysplastic syndromes. *Am. J. Clin. Pathol.* **2012**, *138*, 732–743. [CrossRef] [PubMed]
12. Li, L.J.; Tao, J.L.; Fu, R.; Wang, H.Q.; Jiang, H.J.; Yue, L.Z.; Zhang, W.; Liu, H.; Shao, Z.H. Increased $CD34^+CD38^-CD123^+$ cells in myelodysplastic syndrome displaying malignant features similar to those in AML. *Int. J. Hematol.* **2014**, *100*, 60–69. [CrossRef] [PubMed]
13. Shastri, A.; Will, B.; Steidl, U.; Verma, A. Stem and progenitor cell alterations in myelodysplastic syndromes. *Blood* **2017**, *129*, 1586–1594. [CrossRef] [PubMed]
14. Yue, L.Z.; Fu, R.; Wang, H.Q.; Li, L.J.; Hu, H.R.; Fu, L.; Shao, Z.H. Expression of CD123 and CD114 on the bone marrow cells of patients with myelodysplastic syndrome. *Chin. Med. J. (UK)* **2010**, *123*, 2034–2037.
15. Testa, U.; Riccioni, R.; Militi, S.; Coccia, E.; Stellacci, E.; Samoggia, P.; Latagliata, R.; Mariani, G.; Rossini, A.; Battistini, A.; et al. Elevated expression of IL-3Ralpha in acute myelogenous leukemia is associated with enhanced blast proliferation, increased cellularity, and poor prognosis. *Blood* **2002**, *100*, 2980–2988. [CrossRef]
16. Lantz, C.S.; Boesiger, J.; Song, C.H.; Mach, N.; Kobayashi, T.; Mulligan, R.C.; Nawa, Y.; Dranoff, G.; Galli, S.J. Role for interleukin-3 in mast-cell and basophil development and in immunity to parasites. *Nature* **1998**, *392*, 90–93. [CrossRef]
17. Broughton, S.E.; Dhagat, U.; Hercus, T.R.; Nero, T.L.; Grimbaldeston, M.A.; Bonder, C.S.; Lopez, A.F.; Parker, M.W. The GM-CSF/IL-3/IL-5 cytokine receptor family: From ligand recognition to initiation of signaling. *Immunol. Rev.* **2012**, *250*, 277–302. [CrossRef]
18. Jin, L.; Lee, E.M.; Ramshaw, H.S.; Busfield, S.J.; Peoppl, A.G.; Wilkinson, L.; Guthridge, M.A.; Thomas, D.; Barry, E.F.; Boyd, A.; et al. Monoclonal antibody-mediated targeting of CD123, IL-3 receptor alpha chain, eliminates human acute myeloid leukemic stem cells. *Cell Stem Cell* **2009**, *5*, 31–42. [CrossRef]
19. Jordan, C.T.; Upchurch, D.; Szilvassy, S.J.; Guzman, M.L.; Howard, D.S.; Pettigrew, A.L.; Meyerrose, T.; Rossi, R.; Grimes, B.; Rizzieri, D.A.; et al. The interleukin-3 receptor alpha chain is a unique marker for human acute myelogenous leukemia stem cells. *Leukemia* **2000**, *14*, 1777–1784. [CrossRef]
20. Coustan-Smith, E.; Song, G.; Clark, C.; Key, L.; Liu, P.; Mehrpooya, M.; Stow, P.; Su, X.; Shurtleff, S.; Pui, C.H.; et al. New markers for minimal residual disease detection in acute lymphoblastic leukemia. *Blood* **2011**, *117*, 6267–6276. [CrossRef]
21. Han, L.; Jorgensen, J.L.; Wang, S.A.; Huang, X.; Nogueras González, G.M.; Brooks, C.; Rowinsky, E.; Levis, M.; Zhou, J.; Ciurea, S.O.; et al. Leukemia stem cell marker CD123 (IL-3R alpha) predicts minimal residual disease and relapse, providing a valid target for SL-101 in acute myeloid leukemia with FLT3-ITD mutations. *Blood* **2013**, *122*, 359. [CrossRef]
22. Lerchen, H.G.; Rebstock, A.S.; Cancho-Grande, Y.; Wittrock, S.; Stelte-Ludwig, B.; Kirchhoff, D.; Mahlert, C.; Greven, S.; Märsch, S. Specific Antibody-Drug-Conjugates (ADCs) with KSP Inhibitors and Anti-CD123-Antibodies. Patent WO 2017/216028, 21 December 2017.
23. Lerchen, H.G.; Stelte-Ludwig, B.; Berndt, S.; Sommer, A.; Dietz, L.; Rebstock, A.S.; Johannes, S.; Marx, L.; Jorissen, H.; Mahlert, C.; et al. Antibody-prodrug conjugates with KSP inhibitors and legumain-mediated metabolite formation. *Chemistry* **2019**, *25*, 8208–8213. [CrossRef] [PubMed]
24. Lerchen, H.G.; Stelte-Ludwig, B.; Sommer, A.; Berndt, M.C.; Rebstock, A.-S.; Johannes, S.; Mahlert, C.; Greven, S.; Dietz, L.; Jörissen, H. Tailored linker chemistries for the efficient and selective activation of ADCs with KSPi payloads. *Bioconjugate Chem.* **2020**, *31*, 1893–1898. [CrossRef] [PubMed]
25. Lerchen, H.G.; Wittrock, S.; Stelte-Ludwig, B.; Sommer, A.; Berndt, S.; Griebenow, N.; Rebstock, A.S.; Johannes, S.; Cancho-Grande, Y.; Mahlert, C.; et al. Antibody-drug conjugates with pyrrole-based KSP inhibitors as the payload class. *Angew. Chem. Int. Ed.* **2018**, *57*, 15243–15247. [CrossRef] [PubMed]
26. Myers, S.M.; Collins, I. Recent findings and future directions for interpolar mitotic kinesin inhibitors in cancer therapy. *Future Med. Chem.* **2016**, *8*, 463–489. [CrossRef] [PubMed]
27. Carter, B.Z.; Mak, D.H.; Woessner, R.; Gross, S.; Schober, W.D.; Estrov, Z.; Kantarjian, H.; Andreeff, M. Inhibition of KSP by ARRY-520 induces cell cycle block and cell death via the mitochondrial pathway in AML cells. *Leukemia* **2009**, *23*, 1755–1762. [CrossRef] [PubMed]

28. El-Nassan, H.B. Advances in the discovery of kinesin spindle protein (Eg5) inhibitors as antitumor agents. *Eur. J. Med. Chem.* **2013**, *62*, 614–631. [CrossRef] [PubMed]
29. Ding, S.; Xing, N.; Lu, J.; Zhang, H.; Nishizawa, K.; Liu, S.; Yuan, X.; Qin, Y.; Liu, Y.; Ogawa, O.; et al. Overexpression of Eg5 predicts unfavorable prognosis in non-muscle invasive bladder urothelial carcinoma. *Int. J. Urol.* **2011**, *18*, 432–438. [CrossRef] [PubMed]
30. Mayer, T.U.; Kapoor, T.M.; Haggarty, S.J.; King, R.W.; Schreiber, S.L.; Mitchison, T.J. Small molecule inhibitor of mitotic spindle bipolarity identified in a phenotype-based screen. *Science* **1999**, *286*, 971–974. [CrossRef] [PubMed]
31. Pelosi, E.; Castelli, G.; Testa, U. Targeting LSCs through membrane antigens selectively or preferentially expressed on these cells. *Blood Cells Mol. Dis.* **2015**, *55*, 336–346. [CrossRef] [PubMed]
32. Rath, O.; Kozielski, F. Kinesins and cancer. *Nat. Rev. Cancer* **2012**, *12*, 527–539. [CrossRef] [PubMed]
33. Sun, Q.; Woodcock, J.M.; Rapoport, A.; Stomski, F.C.; Korpelainen, E.I.; Bagley, C.J.; Goodall, G.J.; Smith, W.B.; Gamble, J.R.; Vadas, M.A.; et al. Monoclonal antibody 7G3 recognizes the N-terminal domain of the human interleukin-3 (IL-3) receptor alpha-chain and functions as a specific IL-3 receptor antagonist. *Blood* **1996**, *87*, 83–92. [CrossRef] [PubMed]
34. Quentmeier, H.; Reinhardt, J.; Zaborski, M.; Drexler, H.G. FLT3 mutations in acute myeloid leukemia cell lines. *Leukemia* **2003**, *17*, 120–124. [CrossRef] [PubMed]
35. Wakui, H.; Yamamoto, N.; Kitazono, S.; Mizugaki, H.; Nakamichi, S.; Fujiwara, Y.; Nokihara, H.; Yamada, Y.; Suzuki, K.; Kanda, H.; et al. A phase 1 and dose-finding study of LY2523355 (litronesib), an Eg5 inhibitor, in Japanese patients with advanced solid tumors. *Cancer Chemother. Pharmacol.* **2014**, *74*, 15–23. [CrossRef]
36. Angelova, E.; Audette, C.; Kovtun, Y.; Daver, N.; Wang, S.A.; Pierce, S.; Konoplev, S.N.; Khogeer, H.; Jorgensen, J.L.; Konopleva, M.; et al. CD123 expression patterns and selective targeting with a CD123-targeted antibody-drug conjugate (IMGN632) in acute lymphoblastic leukemia. *Haematologica* **2019**, *104*, 749–755. [CrossRef]
37. Kovtun, Y.; Jones, G.E.; Adams, S.; Harvey, L.; Audette, C.A.; Wilhelm, A.; Bai, C.; Rui, L.; Laleau, R.; Liu, F.; et al. A CD123-targeting antibody-drug conjugate, IMGN632, designed to eradicate AML while sparing normal bone marrow cells. *Blood Adv.* **2018**, *2*, 848–858. [CrossRef]
38. Li, F.; Sutherland, M.K.; Yu, C.; Walter, R.B.; Westendorf, L.; Valliere-Douglass, J.; Pan, L.; Cronkite, A.; Sussman, D.; Klussman, K.; et al. Characterization of SGN-CD123A, a potent CD123-directed antibody-drug conjugate for acute myeloid leukemia. *Mol. Cancer Ther.* **2018**, *17*, 554–564. [CrossRef]
39. Sutherland, M.S.K.; Yu, C.; Walter, R.B.; Westendorf, L.; Valliere-Douglass, J.; Pan, L.; Sussman, D.; Anderson, M.; Zeng, W.; Stone, I.; et al. SGN-CD123A, a pyrrolobenzodiazepine dimer linked anti-CD123 antibody drug conjugate, demonstrates effective anti-leukemic activity in multiple preclinical models of AML. *Blood* **2015**, *126*, 330. [CrossRef]
40. Zhu, C.; Zhao, J.; Bibikova, M.; Leverson, J.D.; Bossy-Wetzel, E.; Fan, J.B.; Abraham, R.T.; Jiang, W. Functional analysis of human microtubule-based motor proteins, the kinesins and dyneins, in mitosis/cytokinesis using RNA interference. *Mol. Biol. Cell* **2005**, *16*, 3187–3199. [CrossRef]
41. Burris, H.A., III; Jones, S.F.; Williams, D.D.; Kathman, S.J.; Hodge, J.P.; Pandite, L.; Ho, P.T.; Boerner, S.A.; Lorusso, P. A phase I study of ispinesib, a kinesin spindle protein inhibitor, administered weekly for three consecutive weeks of a 28-day cycle in patients with solid tumors. *Investig. New Drugs* **2011**, *29*, 467–472. [CrossRef]
42. Gomez, H.L.; Philco, M.; Pimentel, P.; Kiyan, M.; Monsalvo, M.L.; Conlan, M.G.; Saikali, K.G.; Chen, M.M.; Seroogy, J.J.; Wolff, A.A.; et al. Phase I dose-escalation and pharmacokinetic study of ispinesib, a kinesin spindle protein inhibitor, administered on days 1 and 15 of a 28-day schedule in patients with no prior treatment for advanced breast cancer. *Anticancer Drugs* **2012**, *23*, 335–341. [CrossRef] [PubMed]
43. Khoury, H.J.; Garcia-Manero, G.; Borthakur, G.; Kadia, T.; Foudray, M.C.; Arellano, M.; Langston, A.; Bethelmie-Bryan, B.; Rush, S.; Litwiler, K.; et al. A phase 1 dose-escalation study of ARRY-520, a kinesin spindle protein inhibitor, in patients with advanced myeloid leukemias. *Cancer* **2012**, *118*, 3556–3564. [CrossRef] [PubMed]
44. Shah, J.J.; Kaufman, J.L.; Zonder, J.A.; Cohen, A.D.; Bensinger, W.I.; Hilder, B.W.; Rush, S.A.; Walker, D.H.; Tunquist, B.J.; Litwiler, K.S.; et al. A phase 1 and 2 study of filanesib alone and in combination with low-dose dexamethasone in relapsed/refractory multiple myeloma. *Cancer* **2017**, *123*, 4617–4630. [CrossRef] [PubMed]

45. Beck, A.; Goetsch, L.; Dumontet, C.; Corvaia, N. Strategies and challenges for the next generation of antibody-drug conjugates. *Nat. Rev. Drug Discov.* **2017**, *16*, 315–337. [CrossRef]
46. Birrer, M.J.; Moore, K.N.; Betella, I.; Bates, R.C. Antibody-drug conjugate-based therapeutics: State of the science. *J. Natl. Cancer Inst.* **2019**, *111*, 538–549. [CrossRef]
47. Tolcher, A.W. The evolution of antibody-drug conjugates: A positive inflexion point. *Am. Soc. Clin. Oncol. Educ. Book* **2020**, *40*, 1–8. [CrossRef]
48. Donaghy, H. Effects of antibody, drug and linker on the preclinical and clinical toxicities of antibody-drug conjugates. *MAbs* **2016**, *8*, 659–671. [CrossRef]
49. Masters, J.C.; Nickens, D.J.; Xuan, D.; Shazer, R.L.; Amantea, M. Clinical toxicity of antibody drug conjugates: A meta-analysis of payloads. *Investig. New Drugs* **2018**, *36*, 121–135. [CrossRef]
50. Lo, K.M.; Leger, O.; Hock, B. Antibody engineering. *Microbiol. Spectr.* **2014**, *2*, AID-0007-2012. [CrossRef]
51. R Core Team. R: A Language and Environment for Statistical Computing. Available online: https://www.R-project.org/ (accessed on 18 November 2020).

Publisher's Note: MDPI stays neutral with regard to jurisdictional claims in published maps and institutional affiliations.

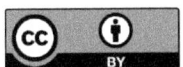

© 2020 by the authors. Licensee MDPI, Basel, Switzerland. This article is an open access article distributed under the terms and conditions of the Creative Commons Attribution (CC BY) license (http://creativecommons.org/licenses/by/4.0/).

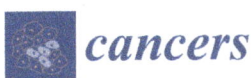

Article

An Antibody Specific for the Dog Leukocyte Antigen DR (DLA-DR) and Its Novel Methotrexate Conjugate Inhibit the Growth of Canine B Cell Lymphoma

Marta Lisowska [1], Magdalena Milczarek [2], Jarosław Ciekot [2], Justyna Kutkowska [2], Wojciech Hildebrand [3], Andrzej Rapak [2,*] and Arkadiusz Miazek [4,5,*]

1. Department of Tumor Immunology, Hirszfeld Institute of Immunology and Experimental Therapy, Polish Academy of Sciences, 53-114 Wroclaw, Poland; marta.lisowska@hirszfeld.pl
2. Department of Experimental Oncology, Hirszfeld Institute of Immunology and Experimental Therapy, Polish Academy of Sciences, 53-114 Wroclaw, Poland; magdalena.milczarek@hirszfeld.pl (M.M.); jaroslaw.ciekot@hirszfeld.pl (J.C.); justyna.kutkowska@hirszfeld.pl (J.K.)
3. Veterinary Clinic NeoVet, 52-225 Wroclaw, Poland; hildek@interia.eu
4. Department of Biochemistry and Molecular Biology, Wroclaw University of Environmental and Life Sciences, 50-375 Wroclaw, Poland
5. Centre of Genetic Engineering, Wroclaw University of Environmental and Life Sciences, 50-366 Wroclaw, Poland
* Correspondence: andrzej.rapak@hirszfeld.pl (A.R.); arkadiusz.miazek@upwr.edu.pl (A.M.); Tel.: +48-71-370-90-00 (ext. 178) (A.R.); +48-71-320-54-36 (A.M.)

Received: 31 July 2019; Accepted: 24 September 2019; Published: 26 September 2019

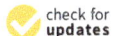

Abstract: Canine B-cell lymphoma (CBL) is an incurable, spontaneous lymphoid malignancy constituting an accurate animal model for testing novel therapeutic strategies in human medicine. Resources of available species-specific therapeutic monoclonal antibodies (mAbs) targeting CBL are scarce. The aim of the present study was to evaluate the therapeutic potential of mAb B5, specific for the dog leukocyte antigen DR (DLA-DR) and its antibody-drug conjugate with methotrexate (B5-MTX). B5 induced caspase-dependent apoptosis of DLA-DR-expressing canine B cell lymphoma/CLBL1 and CLB70 leukemia lines, but not the GL-1 line not expressing DLA-DR. The cytotoxicity of B5-MTX to sensitive cells was further potentiated by a payload of MTX, but without any substantial off-target effects. The infusion of B5 and B5-MTX in a murine model of disseminated, advanced canine lymphoma, mediated >80% and >90% improvement in survival, respectively, and was well tolerated by the animals. Interestingly, the concentrations of soluble DLA-DR (sDLA-DR) antigens present in the blood serum of tumor-bearing mice were found proportional to the tumor burden. On this basis, sDLA-DR levels were evaluated as a potential biomarker using samples from canine lymphoma patients. In summary, the action of B5 and B5-MTX holds promise for further development as an alternative/complementary option for the diagnosis and treatment of canine lymphoma.

Keywords: passive immunotherapy; canine B-cell lymphoma; DLA-DR; HLA-DR; antibody-drug conjugate; ADC; methotrexate

1. Introduction

Canine B cell lymphoma (CBL) is a spontaneous malignancy bearing numerous molecular, histopathological and clinical similarities to human non-Hodgkin lymphoma (NHL) [1]. For this reason, dogs are considered an important animal model for pre-clinical testing of new therapies for human lymphoma [2,3]. CBL is the most frequent hematological malignancy with various histopathological presentations and accounts for over 60% of all diagnosed lymphoma cases in dogs [4]. Around

16,000 to 80,000 dogs owned in the United States alone suffer from hematological malignancies annually [5,6]. Current clinical management of CBL involves combination chemotherapy, but in contrast to human regimens, it employs lower doses of cytostatics and lacks biologicals. Relapses of the disease are usually observed within 10–14 months post-treatment, with less than 25% of dogs surviving two years [2].

The use of a therapeutic anti-CD20 monoclonal antibody (rituximab) has greatly ameliorated NHL treatment, but direct application of rituximab for CBL treatment is impossible due to the lack of amino acid sequence conservation between human and canine CD20 [7]. Efforts to raise therapeutic monoclonal antibodies to canine CD20 have resulted in the development of several candidate reagents [8–10]. Of those, 1E4 and its caninized derivatives showed a therapeutic effect against the CLBL1 canine lymphoma cell line in vitro and in vivo [11].

Major histocompatibility antigen class II antigen DR (MHC II DR) is an attractive and alternative target to CD20 for passive immunotherapy of NHL and CBL [12]. MHC II DR is highly expressed by B cell neoplasms in humans and dogs with mean cell surface levels exceeding those of CD20 [13,14]. Research on mAbs targeting MHC II DR dates back to 1987, when eradication of murine lymphoma in a syngeneic model stimulated the development of similar human strategies [15]. However, a record of limited success in clinical trials and safety concerns related to immune toxicity raised some doubts about further exploration of these therapeutic mAbs [16]. The renaissance of interest in therapeutic HLA-DR targeting came with the characterization of the humanized murine L243 antibody, named IMMU-114, which is specific for a monomorphic determinant on the HLA-DR alpha chain [12]. In preclinical trials, it demonstrated a better efficacy in killing various hematological malignancies than CD20. Moreover, it displayed a promising efficacy in phase I clinical trial in relapsed or refractory NHL and in chronic lymphocytic leukemia (CLL) [17]. With the advent of antibody-drug conjugate (ADC) technology, IMMU-114 has recently been modified to carry a payload of an active irinotecan metabolite. With this payload, therapeutic effects were observed in preclinical models of IMMU-114-resistant tumors such as acute myeloblastic leukemia and malignant melanoma [18]. A good safety profile of IMMU-114 has been reported both in human and canine patients [14]. However, due to the limited cross-reactivity of IMMU-114 with canine DLA-DR [19], a thorough assessment of the full therapeutic potential of this target in dogs is difficult.

In the search for species-specific mAbs for therapeutic targeting of DLA-DR, we have developed a murine mAb, B5. This antibody binds strongly to a conformational epitope of canine DR alpha chain (DLA-DRα), but shows only minimal cross-reactivity with HLA-DRα. We have previously shown that B5 exerts immune-dependent and direct cytotoxic effects in vitro [19].

Here, we extend these studies and report on the generation and pre-clinical testing of the novel B5 ADC with methotrexate (B5-MTX). Methotrexate (MTX) is an inexpensive and pharmacologically well-characterized antimetabolite drug [20]. Canine lymphoma cell lines were found to be 10 times more sensitive to MTX (IC50 values of 2–3 nM) than the human Raji B cell lymphoma and Jurkat T-ALL cell lines [21]. At high doses, MTX is still used in combination with rituximab to treat Burkitt's lymphoma and primary mediastinal B-cell lymphoma [22]. Conjugation of mAbs with MTX changes their mode of entry to target cells [23]. It has been shown in several studies that the MTX payload increases the rate of tumor cell inhibition due to rapid conjugate uptake and an increase in sensitivity to direct cytotoxic effects of therapeutic mAbs [23]. We hypothesized that conjugating mAb B5 with MTX can exert an additive effect of both components and contribute to a better cytotoxicity profile of this ADC against CBL.

We report as well on a novel enzyme-linked immunosorbent assay (ELISA) for the detection of circulating soluble DLA-DR (sDLA-DR) complexes in the blood serum of dogs. Physiologically, soluble circulating MHC II molecules (sMHC II) loaded with self-peptides contribute to the maintenance of self-tolerance [24]. They can be released from antigen-presenting cells or tumor B cells as well and suppress T cell immune-surveillance by directly competing with membrane-bound MHC II ligands [24]. In this report, we aimed at testing the hypothesis that blood serum levels of sDLA-DR could be indicative of tumor burden. We present observations supporting sDLA-DR as a potentially useful biomarker for monitoring the outcome of CBL chemotherapy. Overall, our data indicate the potential therapeutic and diagnostic value of anti-DLA-DR-specific antibodies in CBL.

2. Results

2.1. Characterization of the B5-MTX Conjugate

Crosslinking of MTX anhydride with mAb B5 resulted in >94% homogenous preparation of the B5-MTX antibody-drug conjugate (Figure 1A). Size-exclusion HPLC analysis of unmodified mAb B5 versus B5-MTX revealed a delay in retention times (tr = 25.05 versus tr = 26.3), which was due to the high average drug to antibody substitution ratio (DAR), estimated at 42.6 (Figure 1A). The visible second peak at retention time tr = 46.317 min corresponded to free MTX dissociated from the conjugate. The resulting B5-MTX conjugate demonstrated approximately 49% loss of target binding activity in comparison to unconjugated B5 and had negligible nonspecific binding activity (Figure 1B).

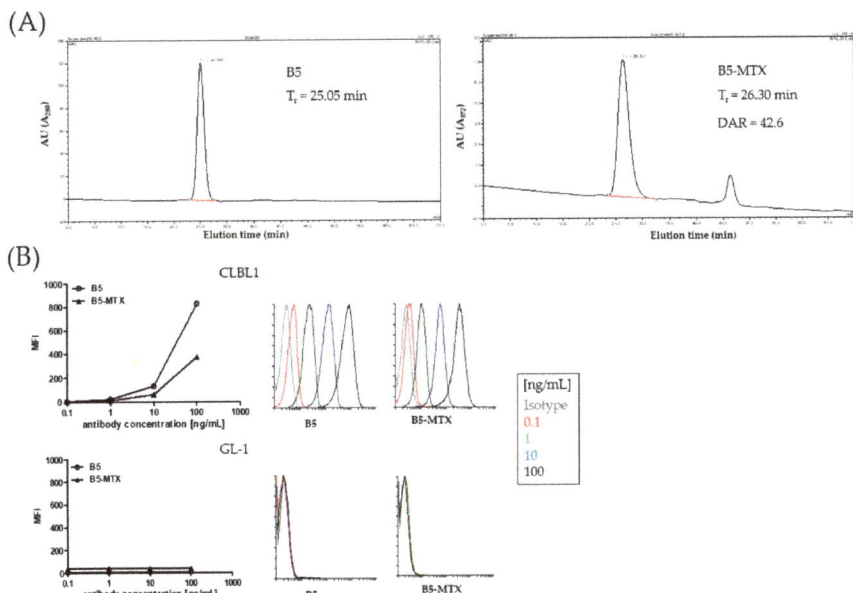

Figure 1. Synthesis of B5-MTX ADC. (**A**) Size-exclusion HPLC of unmodified mAb B5 (top), detected at A280 nm and B5-MTX conjugate (bottom) detected at A372 nm (peak elution absorbance is given in absorbance units—AU) with a molar ratio of MTX to mAb (DAR) of 42.6. The conjugate was >94% pure and monomeric. Retention time (tr) difference of free mAb and B5-MTX resulted from the high substitution rate. (**B**) Flow cytometry assessment of B5 and B5-MTX staining intensity (MFI-mean fluorescence intensity) in DLA-DR expressing CLBL1 and non-expressing GL-1 cell lines. Isotype control mouse IgG2a antibody was used at the concentration of 100ng/mL (grey histogram). Color histograms correspond to signal intensities obtained with the indicated concentrations of antibody or conjugate in [ng/mL].

2.2. Cytotoxicity of B5 and B5-MTX Against Canine Lymphoma/Leukemia Lines In Vitro

To evaluate the cytotoxicity of B5 and B5-MTX, canine B cell lymphoma/leukemia cell lines expressing DLA-DR (CLBL1 and CLB70) and not expressing DLA-DR (GL-1) were exposed to 2 μg/mL of both preparations for 48 h. As previously reported [19], several hallmarks of direct apoptotic cell death, including caspase 3/7 activation, annexin V binding, DNA fragmentation (subG1 DNA content), were observed upon B5 treatment of DLA-DR expressing cell lines (Supplementary Figure S1). In comparison with B5, the B5-MTX conjugate exerted more potency, but also cell-specific cytotoxic effects at the same time, as no significant increase in toxicity against the DLA-DR non-expressing GL-1 cell line was detected. The average percentages of cell death induced by several tested concentrations (0.1–10 µg/mL) of B5 and B5-MTX were used to calculate IC50 and maximum inhibition values of both preparations. B5-MTX showed a higher maximum cytotoxicity (85% to 88% versus 65% to 69%) and lower IC50 values (5–6.25 nM versus 9.53–11.5 nM) against the CLBL1 and CLB70 cell lines than B5 (Table 1).

Table 1. In vitro cytotoxicity of mAb B5 and B5-MTX in canine lymphoma/leukemia cell lines.

Cell Line	B5		[1] B5-MTX	
	IC_{50} nM	Maximum Inhibition (%)	IC_{50} nM	Maximum Inhibition (%)
CLBL1	9.53	69	5	85
CLB70	11.5	65	6.25	88
GL-1	n.d.	<2	n.d.	<1

[1] ADC concentration is given as antibody concentration; n.d.—not determined.

Reportedly, MHC II cross-linking can trigger either caspase-dependent or caspase-independent cell death mechanisms [12]. In order to determine whether B5- and B5-MTX-induced apoptosis was caspase-dependent, cell lines indicated in Figure 2 were pre-incubated with a pan-caspase inhibitor, ZVAD, prior to treatment with individual antibody preparations. On average, a 50% decrease in caspase 3/7 activating cells was detected after ZVAD pretreatment of CLBL1 and CLB70 cells, but without unspecific effects on the GL-1 cell line. Inhibition of apoptosis by ZVAD was minimally lower for the CLB70 cell line treated with B5-MTX than for the similarly treated CLBL1 cell line.

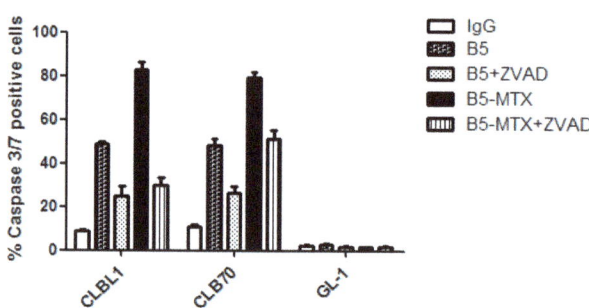

Figure 2. Assessment of caspase 3/7 activation after treatment of individual canine cell lines with B5 and B5-MTX in the presence or absence of a pan-caspase inhibitor (ZVAD). The average percentages of caspase 3/7-activating cells with ±SD were calculated from at least two independent experiments. Every sample was assessed in triplicate.

Together, these data indicated that both B5 and B5-MTX displayed a potent caspase-dependent anti-tumor activity against the CLBL1 and CLB70 cell lines, but not against the GL-1 line in vitro. The MTX payload carried by the B5-MTX conjugate enhanced the specific cytotoxicity compared to B5 alone. The ability of a pan-caspase inhibitor, ZVAD, to strongly interfere with B5- and B5-MTX-induced cell killing supported the caspase-dependent mechanism.

2.3. Therapeutic Efficacy of B5 and B5-MTX in NOD-SCID Mice Xenotransplanted with the CLBL1-Luc Cell Line

To evaluate the efficacy of B5 and B5-MTX treatment in vivo, we established a disseminated disease model in which 1×10^7 cells of the luciferase-expressing CLBL1-derived cell line (CLBL1-Luc) were injected intravenously into immune-deficient NOD-SCID mice. A total of 42 animals were randomly assigned to five groups treated as follows: PBS ($n = 8$), IgG ($n = 8$), MTX ($n = 8$), B5 ($n = 10$), B5-MTX ($n = 8$). Four days after the CLBL1-Luc injection, mice were treated three times a week. On day 15, all mice in PBS, IgG and MTX treatments were sacrificed because of weight loss and signs of morbidity. Five randomly selected mice from the B5 group and five mice from the B5-MTX group, showing no visible symptoms of health deterioration, were sacrificed along with control mice. Blood and organs from sacrificed mice were further analyzed as described below. The remaining animals were treated with B5 and B5-MTX until day 20 and sacrificed once their weight loss exceeded 15% or when they became moribund. On day 15 post-CLBL1-Luc injection, bioluminescence imaging was performed to assess tumor burden. Foci of intense tumor growth in the groups of control mice were located mostly in hind limb bones and in some distant organs. In B5 and B5-MTX treated mice, tumor growth was only localized in the hind limbs of certain mice, whereas other mice had virtually no signs of localized tumor growth (Figure 3A). The intensities of individual bioluminescence measurements for each mouse are plotted in Figure 3B. Groups treated with B5 and B5-MTX presented at least 20 times lower signal intensities than controls.

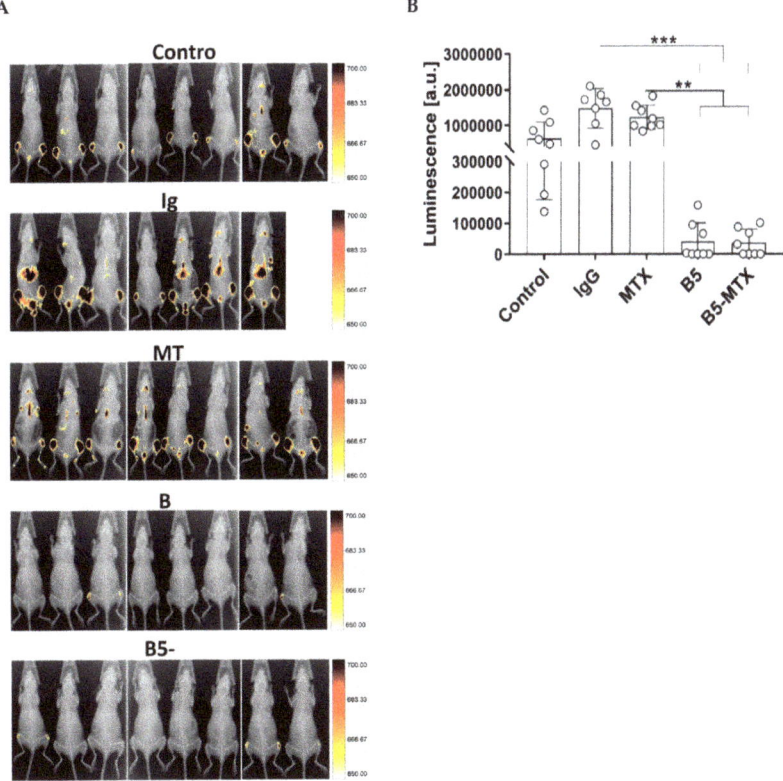

Figure 3. In vivo imaging and quantification of bioluminescence in CLBL1-Luc tumor-bearing mice on day 15 after tumor cell transplantation. (**A**) Control mice were infused with phosphate-buffered saline (Control), isotype-matched mouse IgG immunoglobulin (IgG), free methotrexate (MTX) or were treated with mAb B5 and B5-MTX. Bioluminescence intensity is presented on pseudo-color scales. (†) The IgG group contained seven mice because one mouse was found dead on the day preceding bioluminescence imaging (B) Individual bioluminescence intensities of each mouse were plotted. Statistically significant differences between the groups were marked with an asterisk (*** $p < 0.001$, ** $p < 0.01$).

We sought for more sensitive methods than bioluminescence to quantify tumor cell burden in bone marrows and other tissues of CLBL1-Luc-infused mice. For this purpose, Western blotting and flow cytometry with an anti-pan-DLA-DR antibody, E11 [19], was used. This antibody was chosen because it recognized a different epitope of DLA-DR than B5 and therefore did not interfere with mAbs infused for therapeutic treatment. Tumor burden in tested organs of control, but not B5- and B5-MTX-treated mice, was demonstrated by Western blotting. Specific bands corresponding to DLA-DR were present in all tested tissues except for peripheral blood mononuclear cells, and much weaker bands were found in brains (Figure 4A and Supplementary Figure S2). In bone marrows of control mice (PBS, IgG, MTX) sacrificed on day 15, CLBL1-Luc cell content exceeded 40%, but was less than 10% in the B5- and B5-MTX-treated groups (Figure 4B).

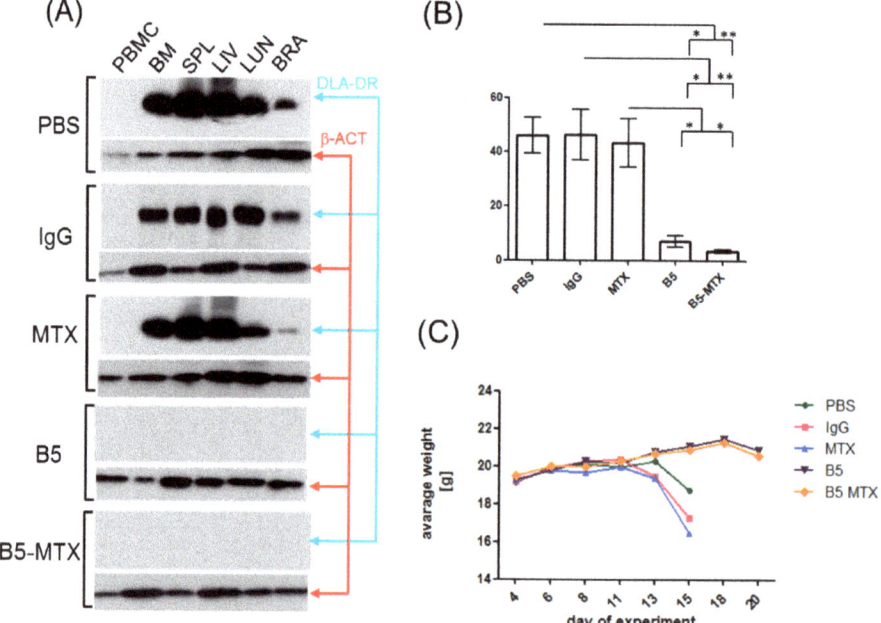

Figure 4. Analysis of tumor cell spread and body weight loss in CLBL-Luc tumor-bearing mice. (**A**) Protein lysates were obtained from the following organs/tissues of tumor-bearing mice: peripheral blood mononuclear cells (PBMC), bone marrow (BM), spleen (SPL), liver (LIV), lung (LUN), brain (BRA). Admixture of CLBL1-Luc cells in the above organs/tissues, reflecting tumor burden, was evaluated by Western blotting with anti-DLA-DR antibody. Protein loading was controlled with an anti-beta actin antibody (β-ACT) (**B**) Cell suspensions of bone marrows were prepared from mice treated with PBS ($n = 8$), IgG ($n = 7$), MTX ($n = 8$), B5 ($n = 5$) and B5-MTX ($n = 5$) and assessed for CLBL1-Luc cell content by flow cytometry with an anti-DLA-DR antibody, E11. (**C**) The average body weights of mice from the indicated experimental groups ($n = 8$ mice per group except for B5, $n = 10$ mice per group) were plotted. Statistically significant differences between the groups were marked with an asterisk (*** $p < 0.001$, ** $p < 0.01$).

All control mice succumbed to the tumor by day 15 post CLBL1-Luc cell injection, whereas mice treated with B5 and B5-MTX experienced an >80% (22.0 ± 2.45 days versus 13.5 ± 0.86 days, $p < 0.001$) and >90% (28.0 ± 8.49 days versus 13.5 ± 0.86 days, $p < 0.05$) delay in time to tumor progression, respectively (Table 2) (TTP parameter is defined in the Materials and Methods section). B5 and B5-MTX treatment was well tolerated by the animals because neither evidence of significant weight loss resulting from off-target toxicity (Figure 4C) nor blood parameter changes (Supplementary Table S1) were noted.

Table 2. Time to tumor progression (TTP) for CLBL1-Luc bearing mice treated with B5 and B5-MTX.

Treatment	N	TTP (Days) ± S.D.	%PR (TF)	(p) B5 versus Others	(p) B5-MTX versus Others
B5-MTX	3	28.0 ± 8.49	100 (1)	n.s.	N.A.
B5	5	22.0 ± 2.45	100 (0)	N.A.	n.s.
MTX	8	14.0 ± 1.00	0	<0.01	n.s.
IgG	8	13.5 ± 0.86	0	<0.001	<0.05
PBS	8	14.7 ± 0.69	0	n.s.	n.s.

%PR—percentage of response to treatment, TF—number of tumor-free animals after day 40, p—probability, N.A.—not applicable, n.s.—not significant.

2.4. Detection of Soluble, Circulating DLA-DR Complexes with A B5-Based Immunoassay

Based on a published report [25], we have hypothesized that canine B cell neoplasms can release soluble DLA-DR molecules in quantities proportional to the tumor burden. Monitoring of soluble DLA-DR levels in the blood serum of CLBL1-Luc bearing mice revealed that B5- and B5-MTX-treated groups had statistically significantly lower values than the control groups (except for the difference between the PBS and B5 groups) (Figure 5A). Therefore, we asked if differences in soluble DLA-DR levels would apply to dogs diagnosed with CBL and subjected to chemotherapy as well. To this end, the blood serum of 18 healthy control dogs, 13 dogs diagnosed with B cell lymphoma (CBL group) and 10 dogs subjected to chemotherapy during remission (CBL + CHOP) was assessed for serum sDLA-DR levels. Detailed clinical data of canine patients whose blood was used in the present study is given in Supplementary Table S2. Analysis of variance showed significant differences between the control group and the CBL group ($p < 0.05$) and between the CBL group and the CBL + CHOP group ($p < 0.01$) (Figure 5B). To further determine immunoassay performance, we analyzed sensitivity, specificity, positive predictive value (PPV) and negative predictive value (NPV) using receiver operating characteristic (ROC) analysis; two separate sets of data were analyzed. First, we sought to determine whether elevated serum sDLA-DR levels could be predictive of CBL. The results shown in Figure 6A suggest that this parameter had a strong positive predictive value of 92%, but at the same time it had a relatively low negative predictive value of 56%, and the area under the curve was 0.835. The set of data in Figure 6B was evaluated to see whether the decrease in sDLA-DR level could be used as a biomarker for successful response to chemotherapy. As shown, 100% of PPV and NPV parameters and the AUC value equal to 1 indicated that this test could reliably predict the response to chemotherapy. However, since the sample size was not pre-defined and no paired blood samples from canine patients before and after chemotherapy were available for this analysis, the above results have to be treated with caution and as preliminary.

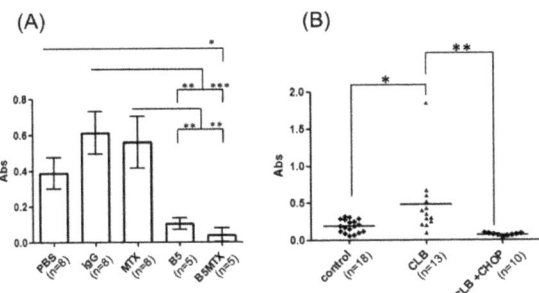

Figure 5. Assessment of soluble DLA-DR levels in blood sera of tumor-bearing NOD-SCID mice (**A**) and healthy dogs or canine lymphoma patients (**B**). Average serum levels (Abs) of DLA-DR in mice in the indicated experimental groups and healthy (control) or diseased dogs upon admission to the veterinary clinic (CBL) or after chemotherapy (CLB + CHOP) were plotted. Statistically significant differences between the groups were marked with asterisk * $p < 0.05$, ** $p < 0.01$, *** $p < 0.001$.

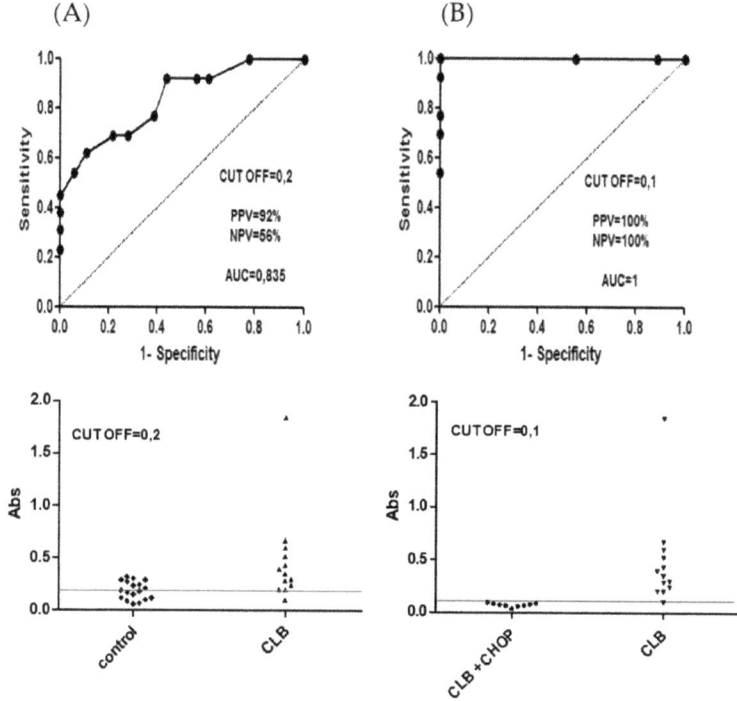

Figure 6. Evaluation of the diagnostic potential of soluble DLA-DR levels in canine CBL patients versus healthy control dogs (**A**), and in CBL patients versus post-chemotherapy patients (**B**). Receiver operating characteristics analysis was used to determine sensitivity, specificity, positive predictive value (PPV), negative predictive value (NPV), area under the curve (AUC) value and cut off (CUT OFF) value for the soluble DLA-DR immunoassay.

3. Discussion

Targeted delivery of cytotoxic drugs using ADC technology improves their therapeutic window and minimizes chemo-associated side effects [26–28]. Methotrexate (MTX), a first-generation anti-folate chemotherapeutic with a narrow therapeutic window, is clinically approved for the treatment of multiple neoplasms [20,29]. It is also one of the very few chemotherapeutics with a fully known clinical profile in human and canine patients [30,31]. Relatively low potency of MTX as a payload can be ameliorated by increasing the drug to antibody ratio (DAR), while maintaining acceptable biological activity of the mAb. Reported DAR values for MTX-based ADCs depend on available lysyl and arginyl side chains in antibody molecules and range from 10 to 14.6 [23,32]. In the present work, an even higher DAR value was obtained by MTX anhydride crosslinking reaction. Despite the considerable loss of binding activity of the B5-MTX conjugate to DLA-DR, in vitro and in vivo data confirmed an increase in specific cytotoxicity against lymphoma cells expressing the target antigen. This was achieved without any substantial unspecific cytotoxicity towards the DLA-DR negative GL-1 cell line. In vivo data indicated that the B5-MTX conjugate not only showed promising anti-tumor activity in a model of advanced, disseminated lymphoma at a relatively low dose (2.5 mg/kg body weight), but had a good safety profile as well.

Signaling through anti-HLA-DR mAbs in tumor B cells activates multiple, pro-survival and pro-apoptotic pathways, but ultimately leads to cell death [12,33,34]. In the current work, we determined that apoptosis induced by B5 and B5-MTX in canine lymphoma/leukemia cell lines followed the intrinsic, caspase-dependent pathway that could partly be inhibited by ZVAD. Despite decades of clinical use, the precise mechanism of MTX cytotoxicity remains largely unknown. Available data on biological effects of MTX released from ADCs indicate a mechanism of cell sensitization [23]. Our data further support these observations, because many hallmarks of apoptotic cell death typical of B5 treatment (e.g., annexin-V binding levels and sub-G1 DNA levels shown in Supplementary Figure S1) were amplified in the case of B5-MTX.

In our hands, the CLBL1 cell line—a canine model of diffuse large B cell lymphoma (DLBCL)—was equally sensitive to the cytotoxic action of B5 and B5-MTX as the CLB70 cell line, with characteristics of chronic lymphocytic leukemia (CLL). This is in line with the observations reported by Stein et al. in models of human DLBLC and CLL cell lines treated with a humanized anti-HLA-DR antibody, IMMU-114 [12]. In this context, evolutionary conservation of death signaling pathways between human and canine hematological malignances opens interesting possibilities for comparative studies.

Both negative and positive associations of soluble HLA-DR levels in the blood serum were reported for patients with malignant melanoma and non-Hodgkin lymphoma, respectively [25,35]. Various strategies of tumor survival could account for the observed variations in sHLA-DR. We speculate that, on the one hand, melanoma cells could down-modulate HLA-DR expression in order to counteract recognition by tumor-specific effector T cells. On the other hand, a massive release of sHLA-DR by B cell neoplasms might induce tolerogenic T cell responses, which could weaken tumor immune-surveillance [24,36]. In order to assess the levels of soluble, circulating DLA-DR molecules (sDLA-DR) in the blood of tumor-bearing NOD-SCID mice undergoing experimental therapy with B5 and B5-MTX, we devised an immune-enzymatic assay based on the use of two species-specific mAbs recognizing different and non-overlapping epitopes of DLA-DR (B5 and E11) [19]. Our results strongly suggested that there was a direct correlation between tumor burden and the serum sDLA-DR levels. We could extend these observations to groups of unrelated canine patients suffering from CBL at the time of diagnosis and during remission. Although these observations offered a possibility of creating tools to help monitor the course of CBL chemotherapy in dogs, more samples, preferentially paired, from patients undergoing chemotherapy are required to fully validate this immunoassay.

4. Materials and Methods

4.1. B5-MTX Conjugate Synthesis

The B5-MTX conjugate was prepared using the method described by Goszczynski et al. [37] Briefly, 1 mg of mAb B5 in bicarbonate buffer pH 8.3 was mixed with MTX anhydride (50-molar excess). The reaction was allowed to proceed for 5 min. Next, the conjugate was separated on a Dionex Ultimate 3000 apparatus equipped (ThermoScientific, Waltham, MA, USA) with a four-component pump, autosampler with a fraction collection and a diode detector using the Superdex 200 10/300 GL resin ((GE Healthcare, Uppsala, Sweden). Isocratic elution was used with 0.1 M sodium bicarbonate at a flow rate of 0.5 mL/min. MTX concentration in conjugate was determined spectrophotometrically using detection at 280 and 372 nm as described by Ciekot, J. et al. [38].

4.2. Cell Lines

The CLBL1 cell line [39] was kindly provided by Dr. Barbara Rutgen (Veterinary University of Vienna, Vienna, Austria). CLB70 [40] was established by us. GL-1 [41] was kindly provided by Drs Y. Fujino and H.Tsujimoto (University of Tokyo, Tokyo, Japan). All cell lines were cultured in RPMI with 15% FBS. The stable luciferase-expressing CLBL1 cell line was generated using premade lentiviral particles (Amsbio LVP434, Abingdon, UK). Lentivirus particles were admixed with cells (1×10^6/mL) at a ratio of 50 µL virus per 0.5 mL of cells. 24 h after transduction, cell culture medium was supplemented with puromycin sulfate (1.5 µg/mL). After one week of antibiotic selection, cell luminescence was validated after D-luciferin addition using a benchtop luminometer (Turner designs, TD-20/20, San Jose, CA, USA).

4.3. In Vitro Cytotoxicity Assays

For in vitro cytotoxicity assays, 1.25×10^5 cells were seeded on a 24-well plate. The cells were preincubated for 2 h with 20 µM ZVAD. Then, 2 µg/mL of B5 or B5-MTX were added to the cells. Cytotoxicity analysis was performed after 48 h of incubation with a CellEvent™ Caspase-3/7 Green Flow Cytometry Assay Kit (Thermo Fischer Scientific, Waltham, MA, USA), according to manufacturer's instructions. Samples were analyzed with a FACSCalibur flow cytometer (Beckton Dickinson, Franklin Lakes, NJ, USA).

To calculate IC50 values, cell lines were exposed to several concentrations of B5 and B5-MTX ranging from 0.1 to 10 µg/mL. Cell viability was determined after 48 h with propidium iodide using flow cytometry. IC50 calculation was performed with an internet tool: MLA—"Quest Graph™ IC50 Calculator." AAT Bioquest, Inc, 25 July, 2019, https://www.aatbio.com/tools/ic50-calculator. Maximal inhibition was determined by propidium iodide staining after 24-h incubation with 10 µg/mL of B5 or B5-MTX.

4.4. In Vivo Monitoring of Anti-Tumor Effects of B5 and B5-MTX

NOD/SCID (NOD.CB17-Prkdcscid/NCrCrl) mice were purchased from Charles River. Mice were housed in IVC cages with a standard sterilized rodent diet and water ad libitum. All experiments using living animals were performed under permission number 117/2017 and 012/2019 from the Local Ethics Committee in Wroclaw (Poland). The anti-tumor activity of the mAb B5 and B5-MTX conjugate was assessed in vivo based on their effect on the growth of CLBL1-Luc cells transplanted intravenously into NOD/SCID mice. Forty-two mice bearing CLBL-1-Luc cells (1×10^7 cells/mouse) were randomly divided into five groups (10 mice in the B5 group and eight animals in other groups). The B5-MTX conjugate, mAb B5, control, isotype matched IgG, MTX alone (0.25 mg/kg body weight) and phosphate-buffered saline (PBS) were administered intra-peritoneally on day 4 post CLBL1-Luc transplantation and repeated every two days. On day 15, all mice from the PBS, IgG and MTX groups were sacrificed because of signs of morbidity along with randomly selected five mice from the B5 group and five mice from the B5-MTX group that did not present any visible signs of disease (no weight loss nor behavioral changes). The remaining five mice from the B5 group and three mice from the B5-MTX group were treated until day 20. B5-MTX and mAb B5 were injected intraperitoneally at a dose of 2.5 mg per kg of body weight. The location of CLBL-1-Luc cells was visualized on day 14 after transplantation using an In-Vivo MS FX PRO system (Bruker INC., Billerica, MA, USA). Twenty minutes before imaging, D-luciferin potassium salt (Synchem, Felsberg, Germany) was administered to each mouse intraperitoneally at a dose of 150 mg/kg. Subsequently, animals were anesthetized with a 3% to 5% (v/v) mixture of isoflurane (Forane, Abbott Laboratories, Lake Bluff, IL, USA) in synthetic air (200 mL/min). Anesthesia was maintained by means of individual masks providing a 1.5% to 2% (v/v) mixture of isoflurane and synthetic air. Visualization was carried out using the following settings: for X-Ray t = 60 s., f-stop = 2.50, FOV = 200.0; for luminescence capture t = 4 min, binning 2×2, f-stop = 2.50, FOV = 200.0. Images were analyzed using Bruker MI software (Bruker INC., USA). The intensity of the luminescent signal is presented as the net intensity of the region of interest and expressed in arbitrary units [a.u.]. Time to progression (TTP) was defined as a day when either body weight loss exceeding 15% or morbidity or limb paralysis were noticed by the operator in any individual mouse.

For Western blotting analysis, mouse organs (brain, liver, lungs, bone marrow, PBMC, spleen) were suspended in a lysis buffer (20 mM Tris-HCl pH 7.5, 50 mM NaCl, 0.5% NP-40 and protease inhibitor set), and sonicated for 10 s on ice. The suspensions were centrifuged at 10,000 rpm at 4 °C for 10 min. Then, non-reducing SDS sample buffer was added to the supernatants and the samples were subjected to a 12% SDS-PAGE gel. The separated proteins were transferred onto a PVDF membrane (Millipore, Burlington, MA, USA) using semi-dry transfer. After transfer, the membrane was blocked with 1% casein in TBS at 4 °C, overnight, and subsequently incubated with 1 µg/mL primary antibody: mab E11 and anti-actin (C-4) (Santa Cruz Biotechnology, Santa Cruz, CAUSA) at room temperature for

1 h, followed by secondary horseradish peroxidase-labeled antibody (DAKO, Agilent, Santa Clara, CA, USA). Bound antibodies were visualized using the ECL blotting detection system (Thermo Fischer Scientific, USA).

4.5. Detection of Soluble DLA-DR Levels in the Blood Serum of Mice and Dogs

Remaining blood serum samples from 41 dogs (18 controls, 13 lymphomas and 10 during CHOP therapy), referred to the "NeoVet" veterinary clinic for periodic blood checks, and blood sera of NOD-SCID mice bearing CLBL1-Luc tumors were used for the detection of soluble DLA-DR levels. In accordance with the provisions of the Act of January 15, 2015, item 266 on the protection of animals used for scientific and educational purposes, the use of blood samples of dogs for clinical veterinary research does not require the consent of local ethics committees.

96 well plates (Nunc) were coated with B5 mAb in PBS (1 µg/mL) overnight at 4 °C. On the next day, the plates were blocked with 5% non-fat milk for 1 h at room temperature (RT), then 20 times diluted blood sera of canine tumor-bearing mice or canine patients were incubated in a 0.5% milk solution at RT for 1 h. Next, biotinylated mAb E11 (1 µg/mL) was added to the solution and incubated for 1 h at RT, followed by the incubation with the Streptavidin-HRP conjugate (1:20,000); after final washes, the 3.3′5.5′-tetramethylbenzidine substrate (Sigma, St. Louis, MO, USA) was added for a 15 to 20-min incubation. The reaction was stopped with 1 N H_2SO_4. The absorbance was measured at 450 nm on a Wallac Victor plate reader (Perkin Elmer, Waltham, MA, USA). Each sample was prepared in triplicate.

4.6. Statistical Analysis

Statistical analysis of in vivo bioluminescence imaging was performed using the non-parametric Kruskal-Wallis test, followed by Dunn's multiple comparison tests (** $p < 0.01$, *** $p < 0.001$). Statistical analysis of all other in vitro assays was performed using one-way ANOVA with Tukey's Multiple Comparison Test. Significance was set at * $p < 0.05$, ** $p < 0.01$, *** $p < 0.001$. Receiver operating characteristic analysis was performed by calculating the shape of the ROC curve. This was done by plotting the values of the sensitivity assay on the y-axis, and the values of false-positive rates (1-specificity) on the x-axis. The area under the curve (AUC) was subsequently calculated.

5. Conclusions

In this report, we tested a novel MTX-based ADC directed against canine lymphoma/leukemia cells. To our knowledge, this is the first pre-clinical study of an ADC designed for veterinary use. The results indicate a significant increase in the specific cytotoxicity of B5-MTX ADC against canine lymphoma/leukemia cell lines in comparison with unmodified mAb in vitro and in vivo. Unlike in humans, DLA-DR antigen, a target of B5 and B5-MTX, is expressed in dogs by both normal B and T cells and by mixed B/T neoplastic cells. Therefore, the use of anti-DLA-DR antibodies in diagnosis or therapy can cover up to 90% of all hematological malignancies in this species. Elevated sensitivity of canine lymphoma/leukemia cell lines to MTX opens up new opportunities for using this antimetabolite as a payload for therapeutic ADCs targeting DLA-DR. Despite the clearly lower potency of MTX in comparison to the second generation cytotoxic payload, such as auristatin, low price, simple conjugation chemistry and lack of intellectual property rights attached to this antimetabolite makes it an interesting option for veterinary use.

In this study, we have shown as well that the observed correlation of soluble DLA-DR levels in the blood serum of canine lymphoma-bearing immune-deficient mice can be further studied in the context of translation into a diagnostic test for monitoring the efficiency of chemotherapy in canine lymphoma.

Supplementary Materials: The following are available online at http://www.mdpi.com/2072-6694/11/10/1438/s1, Figure S1: Analysis of B5 and B5-MTX induced apoptosis in canine cell lines, Figure S2: Cytotoxicity plots used for calculating IC50 and maximum inhibition values of B5 and B5-MTX, Figure S3: Distribution of individual weight measurement of mice used for in vivo studies, Figure S4: Original scans of Western blots with densitometry analysis, Table S1: Haematological analysis of the whole blood of tumor-bearing NOD-SCID mice, Table S2: Clinical description of oncologic canine patients, Table S3: raw absorbance data of anti-sDLA-DR ELISA used for the ROC analysis.

Author Contributions: Conceptualization: A.M. and A.R.; methodology: M.L., J.C., M.M.; software: M.L., M.M., J.C.; validation: M.M., M.L. and J.K.; formal analysis: M.L., M.M., J.C., J.K., W.H.; investigation: M.L., M.M., A.R.; resources: M.L., A.R.; data curation: M.L., M.M., W.H.; writing—original draft preparation: A.M.; writing—review and editing: A.M., A.R., M.M., M.L.; visualization: A.M., M.L.; supervision: A.M.; project administration: A.R., M.L., A.M.; funding acquisition: A.R., M.L., A.M.

Funding: This research was funded by the National Science Center, Poland, under grant number Preludium/2016/21/N/NZ5/01942 (to M.L.); the National Centre for Research and Development, Poland, under grant number TANGO2/340428/NCBR/2017 (to A.R.); and the Wroclaw Centre of Biotechnology, The Leading National Research Centre (KNOW) program for years 2014 to 2018 (to A.M.).

Conflicts of Interest: The authors declare no conflict of interest.

References

1. Richards, K.L.; Suter, S.E. Man's best friend: What can pet dogs teach us about non-Hodgkin's lymphoma? *Immunol. Rev.* **2015**, *263*, 173–191. [CrossRef] [PubMed]
2. Zandvliet, M. Canine lymphoma: A review. *Vet. Q.* **2016**, *36*, 76–104. [CrossRef] [PubMed]
3. Ito, D.; Frantz, A.M.; Modiano, J.F. Canine lymphoma as a comparative model for human non-Hodgkin lymphoma: Recent progress and applications. *Vet. Immunol. Immunopathol.* **2014**, *159*, 192–201. [CrossRef] [PubMed]
4. Dobson, J.M.; Samuel, S.; Milstein, H.; Rogers, K.; Wood, J.L.N. Canine neoplasia in the UK: Estimates of incidence rates from a population of insured dogs. *J. Small Anim. Pract.* **2002**, *43*, 240–246. [CrossRef] [PubMed]
5. Dorn, C.R.; Taylor, D.O.N.; Frye, F.L.; Hibbard, H.H. Survey of animal neoplasms in alameda and contra costa counties, california. i. methodology and description of cases. *J. Natl. Cancer Inst.* **1968**, *40*, 295–305. [PubMed]
6. Yau, P.P.Y.; Dhand, N.K.; Thomson, P.C.; Taylor, R.M. Retrospective study on the occurrence of canine lymphoma and associated breed risks in a population of dogs in NSW (2001–2009). *Aust. Vet. J.* **2017**, *95*, 149–155. [CrossRef] [PubMed]
7. Jubala, C.M.; Wojcieszyn, J.W.; Valli, V.E.; Getzy, D.M.; Fosmire, S.P.; Coffey, D.; Bellgrau, D.; Modiano, J.F. CD20 expression in normal canine B cells and in canine non-Hodgkin lymphoma. *Vet. Pathol.* **2005**, *42*, 468–476. [CrossRef] [PubMed]
8. Ito, D.; Brewer, S.; Modiano, J.F.; Beall, M.J. Development of a novel anti-canine CD20 monoclonal antibody with diagnostic and therapeutic potential. *Leuk. Lymphoma* **2015**, *56*, 219–225. [CrossRef] [PubMed]
9. Jain, S.; Aresu, L.; Comazzi, S.; Shi, J.; Worrall, E.; Clayton, J.; Humphries, W.; Hemmington, S.; Davis, P.; Murray, E.; et al. The Development of a Recombinant scFv Monoclonal Antibody Targeting Canine CD20 for Use in Comparative Medicine. *PLoS ONE* **2016**, *11*, e0148366. [CrossRef]
10. Rue, S.M.; Eckelman, B.P.; Efe, J.A.; Bloink, K.; Deveraux, Q.L.; Lowery, D.; Nasoff, M. Identification of a candidate therapeutic antibody for treatment of canine B-cell lymphoma. *Vet. Immunol. Immunopathol.* **2015**, *164*, 148–159. [CrossRef]
11. Weiskopf, K.; Anderson, K.L.; Ito, D.; Schnorr, P.J.; Tomiyasu, H.; Ring, A.M.; Bloink, K.; Efe, J.; Rue, S.; Lowery, D.; et al. Eradication of Canine Diffuse Large B-Cell Lymphoma in a Murine Xenograft Model with CD47 Blockade and Anti-CD20. *Cancer Immunol. Res.* **2016**, *4*, 1072–1087. [CrossRef] [PubMed]
12. Stein, R.; Gupta, P.; Chen, X.; Cardillo, T.M.; Furman, R.R.; Chen, S.; Chang, C.H.; Goldenberg, D.M. Therapy of B-cell malignancies by anti-HLA-DR humanized monoclonal antibody, IMMU-114, is mediated through hyperactivation of ERK and JNK MAP kinase signaling pathways. *Blood* **2010**, *115*, 5180–5190. [CrossRef] [PubMed]
13. Appelbaum, F.R.; Sale, G.E.; Storb, R.; Charrier, K.; Deeg, H.J.; Graham, T.; Wulff, J.C. Phenotyping of canine lymphoma with monoclonal antibodies directed at cell surface antigens: Classification, morphology, clinical presentation and response to chemotherapy. *Hematol. Oncol.* **1984**, *2*, 151–168. [CrossRef] [PubMed]

14. Stein, R.; Balkman, C.; Chen, S.; Rassnick, K.; McEntee, M.; Page, R.; Goldenberg, D.M. Evaluation of anti-human leukocyte antigen-DR monoclonal antibody therapy in spontaneous canine lymphoma. *Leuk. Lymphoma* **2011**, *52*, 273–284. [CrossRef] [PubMed]
15. Bridges, S.H.; Kruisbeek, A.M.; Longo, D. Selective in vivo antitumor effects of monoclonal anti-I-A antibody on B cell lymphoma. *J. Immunol.* **1987**, *139*, 4242–4249. [PubMed]
16. Lin, T.S.; Stock, W.; Xu, H.; Phelps, M.A.; Lucas, M.S.; Guster, S.K.; Briggs, B.R.; Cheney, C.; Porcu, P.; Flinn, I.W.; et al. A phase I/II dose escalation study of apolizumab (Hu1D10) using a stepped-up dosing schedule in patients with chronic lymphocytic leukemia and acute leukemia. *Leuk. Lymphoma* **2009**, *50*, 1958–1963. [CrossRef]
17. Subcutaneous Injections of IMMU-114 (Anti-HLA-DR IgG4 Monoclonal Antibody): Initial Results of a Phase I First-in-Man Study in Hematologic Malignancies. *Blood* **2015**, *126*, 2740.
18. Cardillo, T.M.; Govindan, S.V.; Zalath, M.B.; Rossi, D.L.; Wang, Y.; Chang, C.-H.; Goldenberg, D.M. IMMU-140, a Novel SN-38 Antibody-Drug Conjugate Targeting HLA-DR, Mediates Dual Cytotoxic Effects in Hematologic Cancers and Malignant Melanoma. *Mol. Cancer Ther.* **2018**, *17*, 150–160. [CrossRef]
19. Lisowska, M.; Pawlak, A.; Kutkowska, J.; Hildebrand, W.; Ugorski, M.; Rapak, A.; Miazek, A. Development of novel monoclonal antibodies to dog leukocyte antigen DR displaying direct and immune-mediated cytotoxicity toward canine lymphoma cell lines. *Hematol. Oncol.* **2018**, *36*, 554–560. [CrossRef]
20. Jolivet, J.; Cowan, K.H.; Curt, G.A.; Clendeninn, N.J.; Chabner, B.A. The Pharmacology and Clinical Use of Methotrexate. *N. Engl. J. Med.* **1983**, *309*, 1094–1104. [CrossRef]
21. Pawlak, A.; Kutkowska, J.; Obmińska-Mrukowicz, B.; Rapak, A. Methotrexate induces high level of apoptosis in canine lymphoma/leukemia cell lines. *Res. Vet. Sci.* **2017**, *114*, 518–523. [CrossRef] [PubMed]
22. Pohlen, M.; Gerth, H.; Liersch, R.; Koschmieder, S.; Mesters, R.M.; Kessler, T.; Appelmann, I.; Müller-Tidow, C.; Berdel, W.E. Primary mediastinal large B-cell and Burkitt's/Burkitt-like lymphoma: Efficacy and toxicity of a rituximab and methotrexate based regimen (GMALL B-ALL/NHL 2002 protocol). *Onkologie* **2011**, *34*, 69–70.
23. Smyth, M.J.; Pietersz, G.A.; McKenzie, I.F.C. The mode of action of Methotrexate-monoclonal antibody conjugates. *Immunol. Cell Biol.* **1987**, *65*, 189–200. [CrossRef]
24. Bakela, K.; Kountourakis, N.; Aivaliotis, M.; Athanassakis, I. Soluble MHC-II proteins promote suppressive activity in CD4+ T cells. *Immunology* **2015**, *144*, 158–169. [CrossRef] [PubMed]
25. Hassan, N.; Idris, S.-Z.; Lee, L.J.; Dhaliwal, J.S.; Mohd Ibrahim, H.; Osman, R.; Abdullah, M. Increased soluble HLA-DRB1 in B-cell acute lymphoblastic leukaemia. *Malays. J. Pathol.* **2015**, *37*, 83–90. [PubMed]
26. Dan, N.; Setua, S.; Kashyap, V.K.; Khan, S.; Jaggi, M.; Yallapu, M.M.; Chauhan, S.C. Antibody-drug conjugates for cancer therapy: Chemistry to clinical implications. *Pharmaceuticals* **2018**, *11*, 32.
27. Stein, R.; Mattes, M.J.; Cardillo, T.M.; Hansen, H.J.; Chang, C.H.; Burton, J.; Govindan, S.; Goldenberg, D.M. CD74: A new candidate target for the immunotherapy of B-cell neoplasms. *Clin. Cancer Res.* **2007**, *13*, 5556s–5563s. [CrossRef]
28. Fuenmayor, J.; Montaño, R.F. Novel antibody-based proteins for cancer immunotherapy. *Cancers* **2011**, *3*, 3370–3393. [CrossRef] [PubMed]
29. Walling, J. From methotrexate to pemetrexed and beyond. A review of the pharmacodynamic and clinical properties of antifolates. *Investig. New Drugs* **2006**, *24*, 37–77. [CrossRef]
30. Morrison, W.B. Cancer Chemotherapy: An Annotated History. *J. Vet. Intern. Med.* **2010**, *24*, 1249–1262. [CrossRef]
31. Longo-Sorbello, G.S.A.; Bertino, J.R. Current understanding of methotrexate pharmacology and efficacy in acute leukemias. Use of newer antifolates in clinical trials. *Haematologica* **2001**, *86*, 121–127. [PubMed]
32. Rowland, A.J.; Harper, M.E.; Wilson, D.W.; Griffiths, K. The effect of an anti-membrane antibody-methotrexate conjugate on the human prostatic tumour line pc3. *Br. J. Cancer* **1990**, *61*, 702–708. [CrossRef] [PubMed]
33. Mone, A.P.; Huang, P.; Pelicano, H.; Cheney, C.M.; Green, J.M.; Tso, J.Y.; Johnson, A.J.; Jefferson, S.; Lin, T.S.; Byrd, J.C. Hu1D10 induces apoptosis concurrent with activation of the AKT survival pathway in human chronic lymphocytic leukemia cells. *Blood* **2004**, *103*, 1846–1854. [CrossRef] [PubMed]
34. Drénou, B.; Blancheteau, V.; Burgess, D.H.; Fauchet, R.; Charron, D.J.; Mooney, N.A. A caspase-independent pathway of MHC class II antigen-mediated apoptosis of human B lymphocytes. *J. Immunol.* **1999**, *163*, 4115–4124.

35. Rebmann, V.; Ugurel, S.; Tilgen, W.; Reinhold, U.; Grosse-Wilde, H. Soluble HLA-DR is a potent predictive indicator of disease progression in serum from early-stage melanoma patients. *Int. J. Cancer* **2002**, *100*, 580–585. [CrossRef] [PubMed]
36. Bakela, K.; Athanassakis, I. Soluble major histocompatibility complex molecules in immune regulation: Highlighting class II antigens. *Immunology* **2018**, *153*, 315–324. [CrossRef]
37. Goszczyński, T.M.; Filip-Psurska, B.; Kempińska, K.; Wietrzyk, J.; Boratyński, J. Hydroxyethyl starch as an effective methotrexate carrier in anticancer therapy. *Pharmacol. Res. Perspect.* **2014**, *2*, e00047. [CrossRef]
38. Ciekot, J.; Goszczyński, T.; Boratyński, J. Methods for methotrexate determination in macromolecular conjugates drug carrier. *Acta Pol. Pharm. Drug Res.* **2012**, *69*, 1342–1346.
39. Rutgen, B.C.; Hammer, S.E.; Gerner, W.; Christian, M.; de Arespacochaga, A.G.; Willmann, M.; Kleiter, M.; Schwendenwein, I.; Saalmuller, A. Establishment and characterization of a novel canine B-cell line derived from a spontaneously occurring diffuse large cell lymphoma. *Leuk. Res.* **2010**, *34*, 932–938. [CrossRef]
40. Pawlak, A.; Rapak, A.; Drynda, A.; Poradowski, D.; Zbyryt, I.; Dzimira, S.; Suchanski, J.; Obminska-Mrukowicz, B. Immunophenotypic characterization of canine malignant lymphoma: A retrospective study of cases diagnosed in Poland Lower Silesia, over the period 2011–2013. *Vet. Comp. Oncol.* **2016**, *14* (Suppl. 1), 52–60. [CrossRef]
41. Nakaichi, M.; Taura, Y.; Kanki, M.; Mamba, K.; Momoi, Y.; Tsujimoto, H.; Nakama, S. Establishment and characterization of a new canine B-cell leukemia cell line. *J. Vet. Med. Sci.* **1996**, *58*, 469–471. [CrossRef] [PubMed]

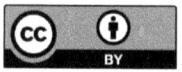

© 2019 by the authors. Licensee MDPI, Basel, Switzerland. This article is an open access article distributed under the terms and conditions of the Creative Commons Attribution (CC BY) license (http://creativecommons.org/licenses/by/4.0/).

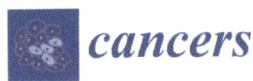

Communication

The Risks and Benefits of Immune Checkpoint Blockade in Anti-AChR Antibody-Seropositive Non-Small Cell Lung Cancer Patients

Koichi Saruwatari [1,†], Ryo Sato [1,†], Shunya Nakane [2,3], Shinya Sakata [1], Koutaro Takamatsu [2], Takayuki Jodai [1], Remi Mito [1], Yuko Horio [1], Sho Saeki [1], Yusuke Tomita [1,*] and Takuro Sakagami [1]

[1] Department of Respiratory Medicine, Graduate School of Medical Sciences, Kumamoto University, Honjo 1-1-1, Chuo-ku, Kumamoto-shi, Kumamoto 860–8556, Japan; rmkqq751@ybb.ne.jp (K.S.); ryosato.1981@gmail.com (R.S.); sakata-1027@hotmail.co.jp (S.Sak.); jojojojody@gmail.com (T.J.); candypinkcolor@yahoo.co.jp (R.M.); yu1980327@yahoo.co.jp (Y.H.); saeshow@wg7.so-net.ne.jp (S.Sae.); stakuro@kumamoto-u.ac.jp (T.S.)

[2] Department of Neurology, Graduate School of Medical Sciences, Kumamoto University, Honjo 1-1-1, Chuo-ku, Kumamoto-shi, Kumamoto 860–8556, Japan; nakaneshunya@gmail.com (S.N.); takamakt@gmail.com (K.T.)

[3] Department of Molecular Neurology and Therapeutics, Kumamoto University Hospital, Honjo 1-1-1, Chuo-ku, Kumamoto-shi, Kumamoto 860–8556, Japan

* Correspondence: y-tomita@kumadai.jp; Tel.: +81-96-373-5012; Fax: +81-96-373-5328
† The authors contributed equally to this work.

Received: 30 December 2018; Accepted: 21 January 2019; Published: 24 January 2019

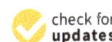

Abstract: Background: Anti-programmed cell death 1 (PD-1) monoclonal antibodies (Abs) unleash an immune response to cancer. However, a disruption of the immune checkpoint function by blocking PD-1/PD-ligand 1(PD-L1) signaling may trigger myasthenia gravis (MG) as a life-threatening immune-related adverse event. MG is a neuromuscular disease and is closely associated with being positive for anti-acetylcholine receptor (anti-AChR) Abs, which are high specific and diagnostic Abs for MG. Methods: A 72-year-old man was diagnosed with chemotherapy-refractory lung squamous cell carcinoma and nivolumab was selected as the third-line regimen. We describe the first report of an anti-AChR Ab-seropositive lung cancer patient achieving a durable complete response (CR) to an anti-PD-1 antibody therapy. To further explore this case, we performed multiplex immunofluorescence analysis on a pretreatment tumor. Results: The patient achieved a durable CR without developing MG. However, the levels of anti-AChR Abs were elevated during two years of anti-PD-1 antibody therapy. The tumor of the subclinical MG patient had high PD-L1 expression and an infiltrated–inflamed tumor immune microenvironment. Conclusions: This study suggests that immune checkpoint inhibitors can be safely used and provide the benefits for advanced cancer patients with immunologically 'hot' tumor even if anti-AChR Abs are positive. Although careful monitoring clinical manifestation in consultation with neurologist is needed, immune checkpoint inhibitors should be considered as a treatment option for asymptomatic anti-AChR Ab-seropositive cancer patients.

Keywords: anti-PD-1 monoclonal antibodies; anti-acetylcholine receptor (AChR) antibody; B cell; immune checkpoint blockade; immune-related adverse events (irAEs); myasthenia gravis (MG); non-small-cell lung cancer (NSCLC); nivolumab; programmed cell death ligand 1 (PD-L1); T cell

1. Introduction

Monoclonal antibodies (Abs) acting against programmed cell death 1 (PD-1) such as nivolumab and pembrolizumab are a class of drugs called immune checkpoint inhibitors that inhibit the interaction between PD-1 and programmed cell death ligand 1 (PD-L1) and unleash an immune response to cancer in contrast with chemotherapies that exert direct cytotoxic effects on tumor cells. The development of immune checkpoint blockade therapy has recently led to a paradigm shift in non-small-cell lung cancer (NSCLC) treatment and dramatically changed the treatment landscape of NSCLC patients [1–3].

For patients with advanced NSCLC, the immune checkpoint inhibitors have shown significant and long-lasting clinical responses in addition to a more favorable toxicity profile and improved tolerability than chemotherapy, and is currently a standard of care [2–7]. However, a disruption of the immune checkpoint function caused by blocking PD-1/PD-L1 signaling can lead to imbalances in immune homeostasis and self-tolerance, which results in an unfavorable immune response to normal tissues, which are termed immune-related adverse events (irAEs) [8,9]. The irAEs that emerge with immune checkpoint blockade therapy share clinical features with autoimmune diseases. The irAEs are usually reversible. However, in rare cases, they can be severe and life-threatening [8,10,11]. In addition, as clinical experience with immune checkpoint inhibitors increases, unexpected severe irAEs have emerged in the real-world clinical practice [10–13]. Thus, elucidating mechanisms of irAEs is urgently needed to improve their early diagnosis and develop more precise treatments for irAEs [8,9].

Myasthenia gravis (MG) is an autoimmune neuromuscular disease that is characterized by muscle weakness and fatigue, and is closely associated with a positive result for the anti-acetylcholine receptor (AChR) antibody directed against the AChR at the neuromuscular junction [14]. Anti-PD-1/PD-L1 monoclonal Abs have been known to trigger the onset of MG as one of the life-threatening irAEs [8,9,15]. Anti-AChR Abs is high specific and diagnostic antibody for MG, and the positivity of anti-AChR Abs has been reported to align with the onset of MG as an irAE in cancer patients, which discourages clinicians from using immune checkpoint inhibitors for cancer patients with pre-existing anti-AChR Abs [8,15,16]. Although several studies highlight the severity of MG as an irAE and the risks of the use of immune checkpoint inhibitors for the cancer patients with pre-existing MG or subclinical MG (asymptomatic anti-AChR Ab-seropositive cancer patients), the benefits and safety of immune checkpoint inhibitors in asymptomatic patients with pre-existing anti-AChR Abs, have not been studied [9,14–17].

In this case, we show a case of anti-AChR Ab-seropositive NSCLC patients achieving a durable complete response (CR) to an anti-PD-1 monoclonal antibody therapy (nivolumab) without developing MG. To further explore this case, we performed multiplex immunofluorescence analysis on a pretreatment tumor sample. This study provides new insights into the use of immune checkpoint monoclonal Abs for cancer patients with pre-existing anti-AChR Abs.

2. Results

2.1. An Anti-AChR Antibody-Seropositive NSCLC Patient Achieving a Durable Complete Response to an Anti-PD-1 Monoclonal Antibody without Developing MG

A 72-year-old man was diagnosed with lung squamous cell carcinoma and had left upper lobectomy and lymph node resection (pathological T2aN2M0 stage IB, PD-L1 tumor proportion score $\geq$ 50%). He had a 90 pack-year history of cigarette smoking. He received S-1 monotherapy as postoperative adjuvant chemotherapy for two years. However, he was diagnosed with recurrence of lung squamous carcinoma with right cervical and mediastinal lymph node metastases. He had pulmonary metastases and enlargement of the lymph node metastases after receiving four cycles of carboplatin plus nab-paclitaxel as the first-line chemotherapy regimen and one cycle of docetaxel as the second-line chemotherapy regimen. Thus, an anti-PD-1 monoclonal antibody, nivolumab, was selected as the third-line regimen.

Screening tests for autoimmune diseases including disease-specific autoantibodies were done before administration of nivolumab. He had no history of thymic epithelial tumor and autoimmune disease. He had no symptom associated with autoimmune or neuromuscular diseases. His performance status was 0. Creatine kinase was not elevated. However, he was positive for serum anti-AChR Abs (0.8 nM, normal upper limit, 0.2 nM). The potential risks and benefits of an anti-PD-1 antibody therapy for the anti-AChR Ab-seropositive advanced NSCLC patient were carefully evaluated in consultation with neurologists. Then, after obtaining informed consent, nivolumab was administered 3 mg/kg every two weeks with careful monitoring of clinical symptoms and levels of anti-AChR Abs by neurologists. Following four cycles of nivolumab, he had hypothyroidism as an irAE and hormone replacement therapy was initiated. The common irAEs such as pyrexia, rash, interstitial pneumonia, hepatitis, and colitis were not observed. After 17 cycles of nivolumab, a fluorodeoxyglucose (FDG)-positron emission tomography-computed tomography (PET/CT) scan revealed a remarkable shrinkage of metastatic lesions of lung and lymph nodes and he achieved a CR (see Figure 1A,B). Importantly, the patient achieved a durable CR without developing MG even though the levels of anti-AChR Abs were elevated (0.8–1.80 nM) during two years of anti-PD-1 antibody therapy (Figure 1C).

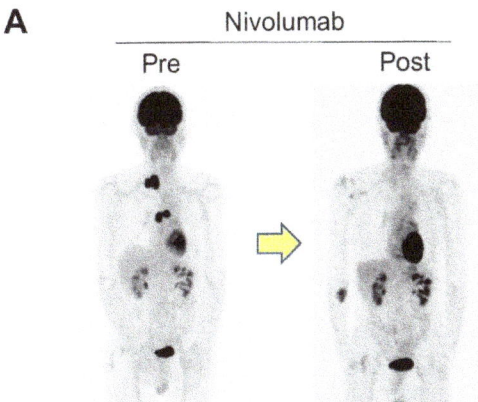

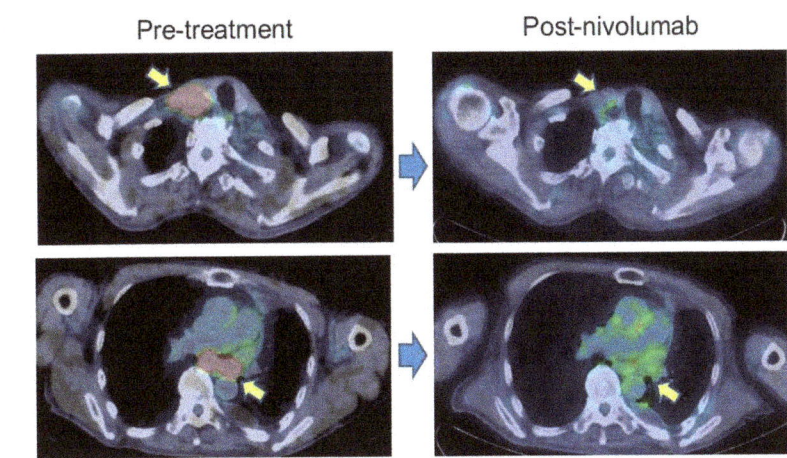

Figure 1. *Cont.*

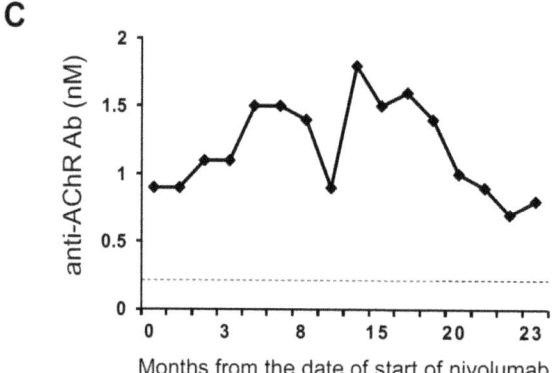

Figure 1. Key imaging and longitudinal analysis of the levels of anti-AChR Abs in asymptomatic anti-AChR Ab-seropositive patient who had a complete response to an anti-PD-1 antibody therapy. Panel (**A**) and (**B**) show FDG-PET/CT imaging pre-nivolumab and post-nivolumab. Arrows in panel (**B**) indicate supraclavicular lymph node (upper panels) and mediastinal lymph node (lower panels) metastases. Panel (**C**) shows the longitudinal analysis of serum concentrations of anti-AChR Ab (nM) before and after nivolumab. The dashed line indicates a normal upper limit of the concentrations of anti-AChR Abs.

2.2. The Tumor of Subclinical MG Patient with a Durable Complete Response to an Anti-PD-1 Antibody Therapy had an Immunologically 'Hot' Tumor Microenvironment

To further explore this case, we investigated the immune contexture of pretreatment lung tumor of the anti-AChR Ab-seropositive NSCLC patient who achieved a CR to nivolumab by fluorescent multiplex immunohistochemistry (mIHC). The mIHC analysis has been shown to capture multidimensional data related to tissue architecture, spatial distribution of multiple cell phenotypes, and co-expression of signaling [18,19]. A high density of tumor-infiltrating CD8+ T cells and CD20+ B cells has been shown to correlate with prolonged survival in patients with a wide variety of human cancers including lung cancer [20–22]. Regulatory T cells (Tregs) have immunosuppressive activity and play a critical role in maintaining immune homeostasis and negatively regulating anti-tumor immune responses [23–25]. Thus, a pretreatment tumor sample from the patient was analyzed for tumor-infiltrating CD8+ T cells, CD20+ B cells, and Tregs (FOXP3+ CD3+ T cells) by fluorescent mIHC. Pan-cytokeratin of tumor cells and PD-L1 were simultaneously stained to evaluate the complex relationship among tissue architecture, spatial distribution of immune cells, and expression of PD-L1.

PD-L1 immunohistochemistry using PD-L1 22C3 pharmDx revealed the tumor PD-L1 tumor proportion score $\geq$ 50% (Figure 2A,B). CD8+ T cells were infiltrated into both tumor stroma and tumor cell nests (Figure 2). CD20+ B cells were mainly localized to the tumor stroma rather than tumor cell nests and infiltrated at the invasive tumor margin (Figure 3). Tregs were infiltrated into both tumor stroma and tumor cell nests (Figure 4), but the number of tumor-infiltrating Tregs was fewer than conventional T cells (FOXP3-negative CD3+ T cells) or CD8+ T cells (Figures 2 and 4). Altogether, these results demonstrate that an anti-AChR Ab-seropositive NSCLC patient who achieved a CR to nivolumab had an infiltrated–inflamed tumor immune micro-environment and immunologically 'hot' tumor [26,27]. The immunologically 'hot' tumor micro-environment might associate with the benefits of immune checkpoint blockade therapy without developing MG.

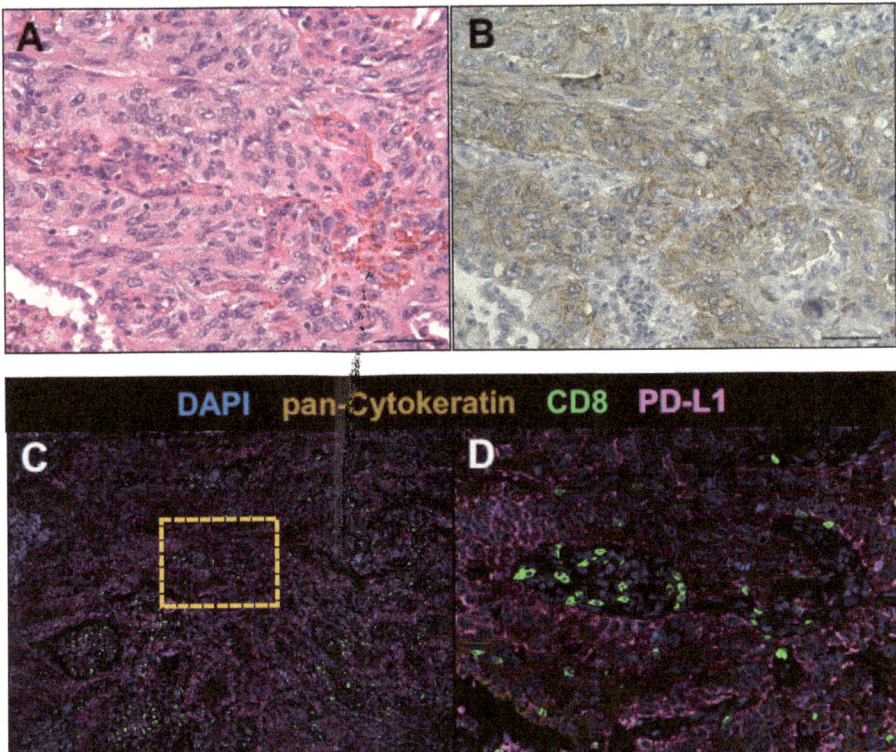

Figure 2. CD8+ T cells infiltrate pretreatment lung tumor of the anti-AChR Ab-seropositive NSCLC patient who achieved a CR to nivolumab. The surgically resected tumor was analyzed by fluorescent multiplex immuno-histochemistry. Serial formalin-fixed paraffin-embedded (FFPE) sections of the tumor sample were stained with Haematoxylin and Eosin (**A**), PD-L1 IHC 22C3 pharmDx (**B**) and analyzed by fluorescent multiplex immunohistochemistry (**C,D**). The panel (**D**) shows the boxed region in the panel (**C**) at high magnification. CD8+ T cells (green) were infiltrated into both tumor stroma and pan-Cytokeratin positive tumor cell nests (dark yellow). The tumor expressed PD-L1 (magenta). Nuclei were stained with DAPI (blue). Scale bars, 50 μm (**A**, **B**, and **D**) and 200 μm (**C**), are shown in each panel.

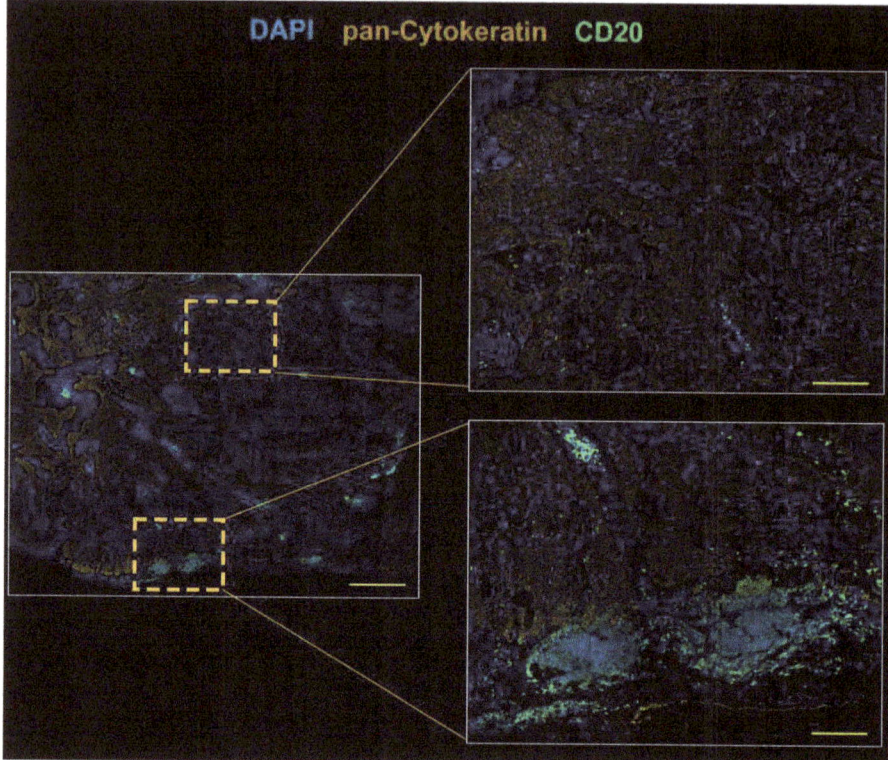

Figure 3. CD20+ B cells infiltrate pretreatment lung tumor at the invasive tumor margin. Serial FFPE sections were stained with antibodies against CD20 (green) and pan-Cytokeratin, and analyzed by fluorescent multiplex immunohistochemistry. The right panels show the boxed regions in the left panel at high magnification. CD20+ B cells (green) were infiltrated at the invasive tumor margin rather than tumor cell nests. Scale bars, 1000 µm (left panel), or 200 µm (right panels) are shown in each panel.

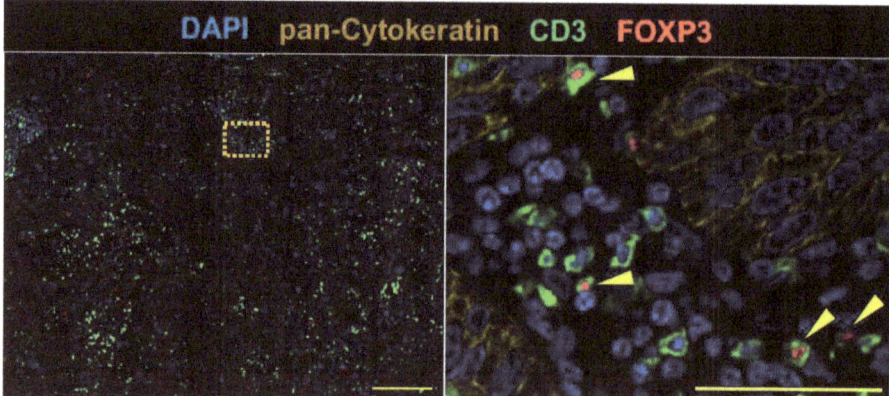

Figure 4. FOXP3+ CD3+ T cells (Tregs) sparsely infiltrate pretreatment lung tumor. Serial FFPE sections were stained with antibodies against CD3 (green), FOXP3 (red), and pan-Cytokeratin. The right panel show the boxed region in the left panel at high magnification. Tregs were sparsely infiltrated in this tumor tissue. Scale bars, 200 µm (left panel), and 50 µm (right panel) are shown in each panel.

3. Discussion

Anti-PD-1 monoclonal Abs block the interaction between PD-1 and its ligand, PD-L1, which unleashes the anti-tumor immune response [1,5,26]. However, the disruption of immune checkpoint signaling can lead to imbalances in immunologic tolerance and result in an unfavorable immune response, which clinically manifest as irAEs [9,11,12,28]. A unique set of inflammatory and autoimmune side effects known as irAEs was quickly recognized in clinical trials in association with the nature of immune checkpoint inhibitors impacting systemic immunity of cancer patients [9,29]. Although the common irAEs are rash, endocrinopathies, interstitial pneumonia, hepatitis, and colitis, rare but serious irAEs have been identified during post-marketing surveillance [8–11,13]. The pathophysiology underlying these irAEs has not been fully understood, which elucidates mechanisms of irAEs. This is urgently needed to improve their early diagnosis and develop more precise treatments for irAEs [8].

As the use of anti-PD-1/PD-L1 monoclonal Abs is extending to various malignancies with unprecedented speed, there is also an unmet need to identify risks and benefits of immune checkpoint blockade therapy in cancer patients with a history of autoimmune disease [8,29]. Most of the evidence regarding irAEs comes from prospective clinical trials, but cancer patients with concurrent autoimmune disease have been excluded from most of the clinical trials because of concerns that these individuals potentially have an elevated risk for developing serious irAEs. Therefore, the safety of anti-PD-1/PD-L1 monoclonal Abs in cancer patients with a history of autoimmune disease is less clear [8,29]. Recent retrospective studies of immune checkpoint blockade in patients with NSCLC and pre-existing autoimmune disease have shown that adverse events were generally manageable and infrequently led to the discontinuation of immunotherapy. The retrospective studies have also shown that anti-PD-1/PD-L1 monoclonal Abs can achieve clinical benefit in those patients. However, the risks and benefits of immune checkpoint inhibitors in asymptomatic patients with pre-existing disease-specific autoantibodies remain unclear [8,15–17,29].

In the current study, we have shown that an anti-AChR Ab-seropositive NSCLC patient achieved a durable CR to an anti-PD-1 monoclonal antibody therapy without developing MG (Figure 1). Makarious et al. showed that the specific MG-related mortality is high (30.4%) in immune checkpoint antibody therapies even though immune checkpoint inhibitor-associated MG is rare [16]. Among the 23 reported cases of irAEs manifesting as MG, 72.7% were de novo, 18.2% were pre-existing MG exacerbations, and only 9.1% ($n = 2$) were exacerbations of subclinical MG (asymptomatic anti-AChR Ab-seropositive cancer patients before administration of immune checkpoint blockade) [16]. One out of the two exacerbations of subclinical MG patients died (the mortality of exacerbations of subclinical MG, 50%). In a study of two-year safety databases based on post-marketing surveys, Suzuki et al. reported that 12 among 9869 cancer patients treated with nivolumab developed MG (0.12%). The nivolumab-induced MG was severe and two MG patients died (MG-related mortality, 17%) [15]. In this study, two cases of exacerbations of subclinical MG have been reported. These studies highlight the importance of recognizing MG as a life-threatening irAE. However, little is known about the potential benefits and the safety of immune checkpoint blockade for subclinical MG [14–16].

Understanding the complex tumor microenvironment offers the opportunity to make better prognostic evaluations and select optimum treatments [26,27,30]. Accumulating evidence suggests that a high density of tumor-infiltrating CD8+ T cells and CD20+ B cells strongly associates with positive clinical outcomes in various cancer types [20–22,31]. However, the immune contexture of anti-AChR Ab-seropositive tumor response to immune checkpoint inhibitors without developing MG remains unknown. Thus, we analyzed pretreatment tissue of the patient. Infiltrated–inflamed tumor immune micro-environments are considered to be immunologically 'hot' tumors and are characterized by high immune infiltrations including CD8+ T cells, B cells, and tumor cells expressing PD-L1 [26,27]. In the current study, the tumor of the subclinical MG patient had high PD-L1 expression and an infiltrated–inflamed tumor immune microenvironment, which suggests similar cases may respond to immune checkpoint blockade therapy without developing MG.

Although anti-PD-1/PD-L1 monoclonal Abs are selectively targeting the PD-1/PD-L1 pathway, the antibodies do not selectively target the PD-1/PD-L1 signaling between tumor antigen-specific T cells and tumor cells. Furthermore, both PD-1 and PD-L1 are expressed not only on effector CD8+ T cells called "killer T cells", but also on a variety of immune subsets including other T cell subsets and B cells [11,13,32–34]. Thus, administered anti-PD-1/PD-L1 monoclonal Abs may bind to the various non-tumor-specific immune subsets and induce the unwanted activation of the immune system, which may disturb the balance established between tolerance and autoimmunity and lead to irAEs such as MG (Figure 5).

A concept of "immune normalization" for the class of drugs called immune checkpoint inhibitors has recently been proposed [1,5]. However, immune checkpoint inhibitors do not always change the immune balance toward a favorable direction for anti-tumor immunity. MG is a B cell–mediated autoimmune disease in which the target auto-antigen is AChR at the neuromuscular junction and also has been known as one of the life-threatening irAEs associated with immune checkpoint blockade for malignancies [14–16,35]. PD-1 expresses on activated B cells as well as activated T cells [33,36,37], which indicates that there is a potential risk of triggering B cell–mediated autoimmune disease such as MG by the blockade of the interaction between PD-1 and PD-L1. The evidence suggests that blocking PD-1/PD-L1 signaling may shift the systemic immune balance from the T cell-mediated immune response (cellular immune response) to the B-cell mediated immune response (humoral immune response) [33,36,37] which enhances pre-existing anti-AChR antibody, and may lead to the onset of MG as an irAE (Figure 5A).

CD4+ T cells include T helper type 1 (Th1), which drives the cellular immune responses, and CD4+ T helper 2 (Th2), which promotes humoral immune responses. Th2 cells enhance B-cell mediated immunity and promote antibody production [38,39]. PD-1 expresses on Th2 cells as well as Th1 cells and CD8+ T cells. Therefore, the blockade of PD-1/PD-L1 signaling has been shown to promote Th2 cell responses and Th2-type inflammations [13,40], which suggests that immune checkpoint blockade has the potential to modulate the balance between cellular immune response and humoral immune response and may lead to the onset of MG (Figure 5B).

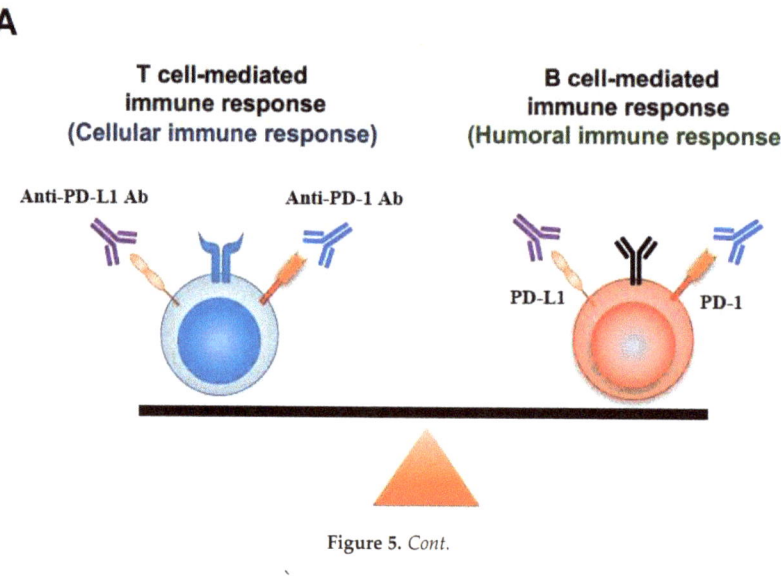

Figure 5. Cont.

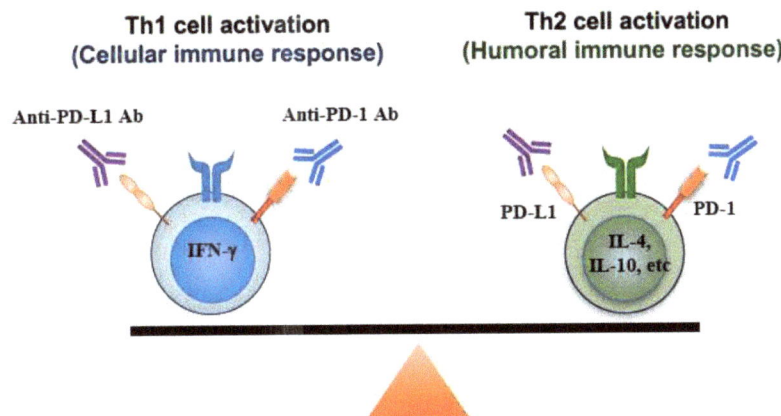

Figure 5. Underlying mechanisms of humoral immune response-associated irAEs. Panel (**A**) shows a model demonstrating the immune balance between a T cell-mediated immune response and a B cell-mediated immune response. Immune checkpoint inhibitors can activate both T cells (cellular immune response) and B cells (humoral immune response), and have the potential to modulate the balance between cellular immune response and humoral immune response, since PD-1/PD-L1 express on both T cells and B cells. Panel (**B**) shows a model demonstrating immune balance between the Th1 cell and the Th2 cell. Immune checkpoint inhibitors can activate both Th1 cells (cellular immune response) and Th2 cells (humoral immune response), and have the potential to modulate the balance between cellular immune response and humoral immune response, since PD-1/PD-L1 express on both Th1 cells and Th2 cells.

There is no evidence of the safety of anti-PD-1 Ab therapy for cancer patients who are positive for anti-AChR Abs. [15,16]. Although we demonstrated that an anti-AChR-seropositive lung cancer patient had immunologically 'hot' tumor and achieved a durable CR to an anti-PD-1 monoclonal antibody therapy without developing MG, our study could not uncover enough evidence to explain the reason why the present case did not develop MG. It is conceivable that the patient might have not been susceptible to an increased anti-AChR antibodies by chance. Thus, clinicians should be cautious to use immune checkpoint blockade for cancer patients with subclinical MG.

Because MG as irAE is life-threatening and closely associated with positive for anti-AChR Ab, the pre-existing serum anti-AChR Ab in cancer patients discourages clinicians from using immune checkpoint inhibitors [14–16]. However, the present study indicates that avoiding use of immune checkpoint inhibitors for cancer patients with subclinical MG potentially lead to losing the chance to cure advanced cancers.

4. Materials and Methods

4.1. Patinet

The Kumamoto University Institutional Review Board approved the study (IRB number, 2287, Approval Date, 23 January 2018).

4.2. PD-L1 Staining

PD-L1 expression in the lung cancer specimen was analyzed by immunohistochemical staining using the PD-L1 IHC 22C3 pharmDx antibody (clone 22C3 (Dako North America, Inc., Carpinteria,

CA, USA)). The antibody was applied according to DAKO-recommended detection methods. PD-L1 expression in tumor cells was scored as the percentage of stained cells.

4.3. Fluorescent Multiplex Immunohistochemistry

Fluorescent multiplex immunohistochemistry was performed with OPAL Multiplex Fluorescent Immunohistochemistry Reagents (PerkinElmer, Waltham, MA, USA) following the manufacturer's protocol. As outlined in the Table 1, formalin-fixed paraffin-embedded (FFPE) sections were stained by one of the three sequences of primary antibodies, PD-L1, pan-Cytokeratin and CD8, pan-Cytokeratin and CD20, or pan-Cytokeratin, FOXP3, and CD3, respectively, using the tyramide signal amplification (TSA) system with Opal dye reagents. Each labeling step consisted of the following at room temperature. Sections of formalin-fixed, paraffin-embedded tissue were depleted of paraffin and were then hydrated and processed for antigen retrieval by treatment with 10 mM citrate antigen buffers (pH 6.0) via microwave radiation (except for PD-L1 which was processed by pH 9.0 citrate buffer via autoclave). The sections were incubated with 3% H_2O_2 for 5 min to inhibit endogenous peroxidase activity, washed with 0.05% Tween in TBS (TBST), exposed to blocking buffer (5% goat serum, 0.5% bovine serum albumin in PBS) for 20 min at room temperature, and incubated for 60 min at room temperature with primary antibodies. They were then washed with TBST, incubated with anti-mouse or anti-rabbit HRP polymer conjugated secondary antibodies (Nichirei, Tokyo, Japan) for 10 min at room temperature except for PD-L1 (incubated for 30 min at room temperature), and washed again, after which immune complexes were detected with Opal reagents. Nuclei were counterstained with 4',6-diamidino-2-phenylindole dihydrochloride (DAPI) (DOJINDO, Kumamoto, Japan) in water, and whole sections were mounted in ProLong Diamond (Thermo Fisher Scientific, Waltham, MA, USA). Multiplexed slides were observed with a fluorescence microscope (BZ-X700, Keyence, Osaka, Japan). The antibodies used for fluorescent multiplex immunohistochemistry analysis are listed below.

Table 1. The list of antibodies used for fluorescent multiplex immunohistochemistry analysis.

Figure	Antibody	Clone (Host)/Company	Dilution	Incubation	TSA Dyes
	CD8	C8/144B (mouse)/Nichirei	undiluted	60 min	520
2	pan-Cytokeratin	AE1/AE3 + 5D3 (mouse)/abcam	1:200	60 min	570
	PD-L1	E1L3N (rabbit)/Cell Signaling	1:100	60 min	650
3	CD20	L26 (mouse)/abcam	1:50	60 min	520
	pan-Cytokeratin	AE1/AE3 + 5D3 (mouse)/abcam	1:200	60 min	570
	CD3	SP7 (rabbit)/abcam	1:100	60 min	520
4	FOXP3	236A/E7 (mouse)/abcam	1:100	60 min	570
	pan-Cytokeratin	AE1/AE3 + 5D3 (mouse)/abcam	1:200	60 min	650

5. Conclusions

In conclusion, to the best of our knowledge, this is the first report of an anti-AChR antibody-seropositive cancer patient achieving a durable CR to immune checkpoint blockade therapy without developing MG. This study suggests that immune checkpoint inhibitors can be safely used and provide benefits for advanced cancer patients with an immunologically 'hot' tumor even if the anti-AChR antibody are positive. Although careful monitoring clinical manifestation in consultation with a neurologist is needed, immune checkpoint blockade therapy should be considered as a treatment option for asymptomatic anti-AChR Ab-seropositive cancer patients. This study not only provides new insights into the use of immune checkpoint monoclonal Abs for cancer patients with pre-existing disease-specific auto-antibodies, but also may improve our understanding of the pathophysiology underlying irAEs and MG.

Author Contributions: Conception and design: K.S., R.S., S.N., S.S. (Shinya Sakata), S.S. (Sho Saeki), and Y.T. Acquisition of clinical data and patient care: K.S., R.S., S.N., S.S. (Shinya Sakata), K.T., T.J., R.M., Y.H., S.S.

(Sho Saeki), T.S., and Y.T. Acquisition, analysis, and interpretation of biological data: K.S., R.S., S.N., S.S. (Shinya Sakata), K.T., and Y.T. Writing, review, and/or revision of the manuscript: K.S., R.S., S.N., Y.H., T.S., and Y.T. Study supervision: K.S., R.S., S.N., T.S., and Y.T.

Funding: This work was supported by the Takeda Science Foundation and JSPS KAKENHI Grant Number JP18K15928.

Acknowledgments: We thank the Departments of Thoracic Surgery and Department of Respiratory Medicine, National Hospital Organization Kumamoto Minami Hospital, for their assistance in obtaining the tissue from the patient and thank Misako Takahashi (Department of Respiratory Medicine, Kumamoto University) for technical assistance in fluorescent multiplex immunohistochemistry analysis. We are very grateful to our patient for his participation in this study.

Conflicts of Interest: The authors declare no conflict of interest.

References

1. Wei, S.C.; Duffy, C.R.; Allison, J.P. Fundamental Mechanisms of Immune Checkpoint Blockade Therapy. *Cancer Discov.* **2018**, *8*, 1069–1086. [CrossRef] [PubMed]
2. Ribas, A.; Wolchok, J.D. Cancer immunotherapy using checkpoint blockade. *Science* **2018**, *359*, 1350–1355. [CrossRef] [PubMed]
3. Abdin, S.M.; Zaher, D.M.; Arafa, E.A.; Omar, H.A. Tackling Cancer Resistance by Immunotherapy: Updated Clinical Impact and Safety of PD-1/PD-L1 Inhibitors. *Cancers* **2018**, *10*, 32. [CrossRef] [PubMed]
4. Dugger, S.A.; Platt, A.; Goldstein, D.B. Drug development in the era of precision medicine. *Nat. Rev. Drug Discov.* **2018**, *17*, 183–196. [CrossRef] [PubMed]
5. Sanmamed, M.F.; Chen, L. A Paradigm Shift in Cancer Immunotherapy: From Enhancement to Normalization. *Cell* **2018**, *175*, 313–326. [CrossRef] [PubMed]
6. Borghaei, H.; Paz-Ares, L.; Horn, L.; Spigel, D.R.; Steins, M.; Ready, N.E.; Chow, L.Q.; Vokes, E.E.; Felip, E.; Holgado, E.; et al. Nivolumab versus Docetaxel in Advanced Nonsquamous Non-Small-Cell Lung Cancer. *N. Engl. J. Med.* **2015**, *373*, 1627–1639. [CrossRef] [PubMed]
7. Brahmer, J.; Reckamp, K.L.; Baas, P.; Crino, L.; Eberhardt, W.E.; Poddubskaya, E.; Antonia, S.; Pluzanski, A.; Vokes, E.E.; Holgado, E.; et al. Nivolumab versus Docetaxel in Advanced Squamous-Cell Non-Small-Cell Lung Cancer. *N. Engl. J. Med.* **2015**, *373*, 123–135. [CrossRef] [PubMed]
8. Postow, M.A.; Sidlow, R.; Hellmann, M.D. Immune-Related Adverse Events Associated with Immune Checkpoint Blockade. *N. Engl. J. Med.* **2018**, *378*, 158–168. [CrossRef] [PubMed]
9. Brahmer, J.R.; Lacchetti, C.; Schneider, B.J.; Atkins, M.B.; Brassil, K.J.; Caterino, J.M.; Chau, I.; Ernstoff, M.S.; Gardner, J.M.; Ginex, P.; et al. Management of Immune-Related Adverse Events in Patients Treated With Immune Checkpoint Inhibitor Therapy: American Society of Clinical Oncology Clinical Practice Guideline. *J. Clin. Oncol.* **2018**, *36*, 1714–1768. [CrossRef] [PubMed]
10. Horio, Y.; Takamatsu, K.; Tamanoi, D.; Sato, R.; Saruwatari, K.; Ikeda, T.; Nakane, S.; Nakajima, M.; Saeki, S.; Ichiyasu, H.; et al. Trousseau's syndrome triggered by an immune checkpoint blockade in a non-small cell lung cancer patient. *Eur. J. Immunol.* **2018**, *48*, 1764–1767. [CrossRef] [PubMed]
11. Tomita, Y.; Sueta, D.; Kakiuchi, Y.; Saeki, S.; Saruwatari, K.; Sakata, S.; Jodai, T.; Migiyama, Y.; Akaike, K.; Hirosako, S.; et al. Acute coronary syndrome as a possible immune-related adverse event in a lung cancer patient achieving a complete response to anti-PD-1 immune checkpoint antibody. *Ann. Oncol.* **2017**, *28*, 2893–2895. [CrossRef] [PubMed]
12. Suresh, K.; Naidoo, J.; Lin, C.T.; Danoff, S. Immune Checkpoint Immunotherapy for Non-Small Cell Lung Cancer: Benefits and Pulmonary Toxicities. *Chest* **2018**, *154*, 1416–1423. [CrossRef] [PubMed]
13. Jodai, T.; Yoshida, C.; Sato, R.; Kakiuchi, Y.; Sato, N.; Iyama, S.; Kimura, T.; Saruwatari, K.; Saeki, S.; Ichiyasu, H.; et al. A potential mechanism of the onset of acute eosinophilic pneumonia triggered by an anti-PD-1 immune checkpoint antibody in a lung cancer patient. *Immun. Inflamm. Dis.* **2018**. [CrossRef] [PubMed]
14. Gilhus, N.E.; Verschuuren, J.J. Myasthenia gravis: Subgroup classification and therapeutic strategies. *Lancet Neurol.* **2015**, *14*, 1023–1036. [CrossRef]
15. Suzuki, S.; Ishikawa, N.; Konoeda, F.; Seki, N.; Fukushima, S.; Takahashi, K.; Uhara, H.; Hasegawa, Y.; Inomata, S.; Otani, Y.; et al. Nivolumab-related myasthenia gravis with myositis and myocarditis in Japan. *Neurology* **2017**, *89*, 1127–1134. [CrossRef] [PubMed]

16. Makarious, D.; Horwood, K.; Coward, J.I.G. Myasthenia gravis: An emerging toxicity of immune checkpoint inhibitors. *Eur. J. Cancer* **2017**, *82*, 128–136. [CrossRef] [PubMed]
17. Toi, Y.; Sugawara, S.; Sugisaka, J.; Ono, H.; Kawashima, Y.; Aiba, T.; Kawana, S.; Saito, R.; Aso, M.; Tsurumi, K.; et al. Profiling Preexisting Antibodies in Patients Treated With Anti-PD-1 Therapy for Advanced Non-Small Cell Lung Cancer. *JAMA Oncol.* **2018**. [CrossRef] [PubMed]
18. Remark, R.; Merghoub, T.; Grabe, N.; Litjens, G.; Damotte, D.; Wolchok, J.D.; Merad, M.; Gnjatic, S. In-depth tissue profiling using multiplexed immunohistochemical consecutive staining on single slide. *Sci. Immunol.* **2016**, *1*, aaf6925. [CrossRef] [PubMed]
19. Forde, P.M.; Chaft, J.E.; Smith, K.N.; Anagnostou, V.; Cottrell, T.R.; Hellmann, M.D.; Zahurak, M.; Yang, S.C.; Jones, D.R.; Broderick, S.; et al. Neoadjuvant PD-1 Blockade in Resectable Lung Cancer. *N. Engl. J. Med.* **2018**, *378*, 1976–1986. [CrossRef] [PubMed]
20. Ho, K.H.; Chang, C.J.; Huang, T.W.; Shih, C.M.; Liu, A.J.; Chen, P.H.; Cheng, K.T.; Chen, K.C. Gene landscape and correlation between B-cell infiltration and programmed death ligand 1 expression in lung adenocarcinoma patients from The Cancer Genome Atlas data set. *PLoS ONE* **2018**, *13*, e0208459. [CrossRef] [PubMed]
21. Tsou, P.; Katayama, H.; Ostrin, E.J.; Hanash, S.M. The Emerging Role of B Cells in Tumor Immunity. *Cancer Res.* **2016**, *76*, 5597–5601. [CrossRef] [PubMed]
22. Linnebacher, M.; Maletzki, C. Tumor-infiltrating B cells: The ignored players in tumor immunology. *Oncoimmunology* **2012**, *1*, 1186–1188. [CrossRef] [PubMed]
23. Spolski, R.; Li, P.; Leonard, W.J. Biology and regulation of IL-2: From molecular mechanisms to human therapy. *Nat. Rev. Immunol.* **2018**, *18*, 648–659. [CrossRef] [PubMed]
24. Magnuson, A.M.; Kiner, E.; Ergun, A.; Park, J.S.; Asinovski, N.; Ortiz-Lopez, A.; Kilcoyne, A.; Paoluzzi-Tomada, E.; Weissleder, R.; Mathis, D.; et al. Identification and validation of a tumor-infiltrating Treg transcriptional signature conserved across species and tumor types. *Proc. Natl. Acad. Sci. USA* **2018**, *115*, E10672–E10681. [CrossRef] [PubMed]
25. Shang, B.; Liu, Y.; Jiang, S.J.; Liu, Y. Prognostic value of tumor-infiltrating FoxP3+ regulatory T cells in cancers: A systematic review and meta-analysis. *Sci. Rep.* **2015**, *5*, 15179. [CrossRef] [PubMed]
26. Binnewies, M.; Roberts, E.W.; Kersten, K.; Chan, V.; Fearon, D.F.; Merad, M.; Coussens, L.M.; Gabrilovich, D.I.; Ostrand-Rosenberg, S.; Hedrick, C.C.; et al. Understanding the tumor immune microenvironment (TIME) for effective therapy. *Nat. Med.* **2018**, *24*, 541–550. [CrossRef]
27. Joyce, J.A.; Fearon, D.T. T cell exclusion, immune privilege, and the tumor microenvironment. *Science* **2015**, *348*, 74–80. [CrossRef] [PubMed]
28. Naidoo, J.; Page, D.B.; Li, B.T.; Connell, L.C.; Schindler, K.; Lacouture, M.E.; Postow, M.A.; Wolchok, J.D. Toxicities of the anti-PD-1 and anti-PD-L1 immune checkpoint antibodies. *Ann. Oncol.* **2015**, *26*, 2375–2391. [CrossRef]
29. Leonardi, G.C.; Gainor, J.F.; Altan, M.; Kravets, S.; Dahlberg, S.E.; Gedmintas, L.; Azimi, R.; Rizvi, H.; Riess, J.W.; Hellmann, M.D.; et al. Safety of Programmed Death-1 Pathway Inhibitors Among Patients With Non-Small-Cell Lung Cancer and Preexisting Autoimmune Disorders. *J. Clin. Oncol.* **2018**, *36*, 1905–1912. [CrossRef]
30. Hegde, P.S.; Karanikas, V.; Evers, S. The Where, the When, and the How of Immune Monitoring for Cancer Immunotherapies in the Era of Checkpoint Inhibition. *Clin. Cancer Res.* **2016**, *22*, 1865–1874. [CrossRef]
31. Varn, F.S.; Wang, Y.; Cheng, C. A B cell-derived gene expression signature associates with an immunologically active tumor microenvironment and response to immune checkpoint blockade therapy. *Oncoimmunology* **2019**, *8*, e1513440. [CrossRef]
32. Mahoney, K.M.; Rennert, P.D.; Freeman, G.J. Combination cancer immunotherapy and new immunomodulatory targets. *Nat. Rev. Drug Discov.* **2015**, *14*, 561–584. [CrossRef]
33. Thibult, M.L.; Mamessier, E.; Gertner-Dardenne, J.; Pastor, S.; Just-Landi, S.; Xerri, L.; Chetaille, B.; Olive, D. PD-1 is a novel regulator of human B-cell activation. *Int. Immunol.* **2013**, *25*, 129–137. [CrossRef] [PubMed]
34. Elsner, R.A.; Hastey, C.J.; Baumgarth, N. CD4+ T cells promote antibody production but not sustained affinity maturation during Borrelia burgdorferi infection. *Infect. Immun.* **2015**, *83*, 48–56. [CrossRef] [PubMed]
35. Ragheb, S.; Lisak, R.; Lewis, R.; Van Stavern, G.; Gonzales, F.; Simon, K. A potential role for B-cell activating factor in the pathogenesis of autoimmune myasthenia gravis. *Arch. Neurol.* **2008**, *65*, 1358–1362. [CrossRef] [PubMed]

36. Page, D.B.; Postow, M.A.; Callahan, M.K.; Allison, J.P.; Wolchok, J.D. Immune modulation in cancer with antibodies. *Annu. Rev. Med.* **2014**, *65*, 185–202. [CrossRef] [PubMed]
37. Okazaki, T.; Maeda, A.; Nishimura, H.; Kurosaki, T.; Honjo, T. PD-1 immunoreceptor inhibits B cell receptor-mediated signaling by recruiting src homology 2-domain-containing tyrosine phosphatase 2 to phosphotyrosine. *Proc. Natl. Acad. Sci. USA* **2001**, *98*, 13866–13871. [CrossRef]
38. Knosp, C.A.; Johnston, J.A. Regulation of CD4+ T-cell polarization by suppressor of cytokine signalling proteins. *Immunology* **2012**, *135*, 101–111. [CrossRef]
39. Lambrecht, B.N.; Hammad, H. The immunology of asthma. *Nat. Immunol.* **2015**, *16*, 45–56. [CrossRef] [PubMed]
40. Zhou, S.; Jin, X.; Li, Y.; Li, W.; Chen, X.; Xu, L.; Zhu, J.; Xu, Z.; Zhang, Y.; Liu, F.; et al. Blockade of PD-1 Signaling Enhances Th2 Cell Responses and Aggravates Liver Immunopathology in Mice with Schistosomiasis japonica. *PLoS Negl. Trop. Dis.* **2016**, *10*, e0005094. [CrossRef]

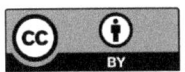

© 2019 by the authors. Licensee MDPI, Basel, Switzerland. This article is an open access article distributed under the terms and conditions of the Creative Commons Attribution (CC BY) license (http://creativecommons.org/licenses/by/4.0/).

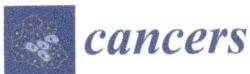

Review

Structure and Optimization of Checkpoint Inhibitors

Sarah L. Picardo [1,*], Jeffrey Doi [2] and Aaron R. Hansen [1]

1 Department of Medical Oncology, Princess Margaret Cancer Centre, 700 University Avenue, Toronto, ON M5G 1X6, Canada; aaron.hansen@uhn.ca
2 Department of Pharmacy, Princess Margaret Cancer Centre, 610 University Avenue, Toronto, ON M5G 2M9, Canada; jeffrey.doi@uhn.ca
* Correspondence: sarah.picardo@uhn.ca

Received: 20 November 2019; Accepted: 16 December 2019; Published: 21 December 2019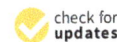

Abstract: With the advent of checkpoint inhibitor treatment for various cancer types, the optimization of drug selection, pharmacokinetics and biomarker assays is an urgent and as yet unresolved dilemma for clinicians, pharmaceutical companies and researchers. Drugs which inhibit cytotoxic T-lymphocyte associated protein-4 (CTLA-4), such as ipilimumab and tremelimumab, programmed cell death protein-1 (PD-1), such as nivolumab and pembrolizumab, and programmed cell death ligand-1 (PD-L1), such as atezolizumab, durvalumab and avelumab, each appear to have varying pharmacokinetics and clinical activity in different cancer types. Each drug differs in terms of dosing, which becomes an issue when drug comparisons are attempted. Here, we examine the various checkpoint inhibitors currently used and in development. We discuss the antibodies and their protein targets, their pharmacokinetics as measured in various tumor types, and their binding affinities to their respective antigens. We also examine the various dosing regimens for these drugs and how they differ. Finally, we examine new developments and methods to optimize delivery and efficacy in the field of checkpoint inhibitors, including non-fucosylation, prodrug formations, bispecific antibodies, and newer small molecule and peptide checkpoint inhibitors.

Keywords: checkpoint inhibitors 1; protein structure 2; pharmacokinetics 3; drug optimization 4

---

1. Introduction

Checkpoint inhibitors (CPIs) induce an anti-tumor immune response by antagonizing suppressive immune checkpoint regulatory pathways. The recognized function of these immune checkpoints is to modulate or prevent autoimmune responses and or auto-inflammation. The advent of antibodies targeting programmed cell death protein-1 (PD-1), programmed cell death protein ligand-1 (PD-L1) and cytotoxic T-lymphocyte associated protein-4 (CTLA-4) has led to the development of drugs targeting these pathways in the last 10 years. However, their variable pharmacokinetics and response rates has led to efforts to optimize these drugs, as well as to develop new drugs targeting other checkpoint pathways. Here we examine the structure and mechanism of action of these drugs and human pharmacokinetics in terms of their binding affinities, clearance, and the significance of dosing regimens. In addition, we describe efforts to enhance the delivery and formulation of CPIs, while attempting to minimize the immune-related adverse events (irAEs) associated with these treatments.

2. CTLA-4, PD-1 and PD-L1 Proteins and Antibodies

2.1. Proteins

2.1.1. CTLA-4

CTLA-4 was first described in 1987 as "a new member of the immunoglobulin superfamily" [1]. It is a 223 amino acid protein which is expressed on activated T cells co-expressing CD28 [2] and has extracellular, transmembrane and intracellular components. Its ligands are CD80 (B7-1) and CD86 (B7-2), found on antigen presenting cells and T-regulatory (T-reg) cells, with binding causing downregulation of activated T cell activity and upregulation of suppressive T-reg function. The importance of CTLA-4 is demonstrated in CTLA-4-knockout mice, who develop early and catastrophic immune hyperactivation causing myocarditis and pancreatitis, and die by 3–4 weeks of age [3].

2.1.2. PD-1 and PD-L1

The PD-1 protein is a 288 amino acid protein which is primarily expressed on T cells, but also on other immune cells, such as B cells, natural killer T cells, and monocytes. It was first identified at a gene level in murine cell lines and was initially thought to be involved in apoptosis, as its expression was induced when thymocyte cell death was induced [4]. Subsequently, it was found to suppress immune responses, and, in particular, it is hypothesized that PD-1 suppresses anti-self-responses [5,6]. This theory is supported by the fact that PD-1 induction is suppressed in the presence of "foreign" antigens such as lipopolysaccharide (LPS) and a stimulatory CpG-containing oligodeoxynucleotide CpG1826 [7]. The protein itself has an intracellular domain, a hydrophobic transmembrane domain and an extracellular immunoglobulin domain which is folded into a β-strand "sandwich" connected by a disulphide bridge. The intracellular domain, or cytoplasmic tail, contains an N-terminal sequence which forms an immunoreceptor tyrosine-based inhibition motif, as well as a C-terminal sequence which forms an immunoreceptor tyrosine-based switch motif. The murine and human forms of PD-1 share a 62% identical sequence, but there are significant differences in the ligand-binding sites, including alterations in size, polarity and charge [8].

The PD-1 protein has two major ligands—PD-L1 and PD-L2. Both ligands contain an N-terminal domain, which binds to PD-1, and a C-terminal domain, the function of which is as yet unknown. Both domains have an immunoglobulin-like fold forming a β-strand sandwich similar to that of PD-1 and are joined by a short linker. Nuclear magnetic resonance characterization suggests that PD-L1 proteins form homodimers, exposing the hydrophobic PD-1 binding sites, although whether this occurs in vivo remains unclear [8–10]. The PD-L2 molecule has a similar structure, with two immunoglobulin domains and a linker region, with most of the residues in the binding interfaces of both ligands conserved [11].

The binding of human PD-1 and PD-L1 proteins forms a 1:1 complex and induces a conformational change in PD-1, with the closure of the CC' loop around PD-L1 and formation of hydrogen bonds, which are hypothesized to stabilize the complex and cause re-arrangements of the PD-1 protein [10,12]. The binding regions contain both hydrophobic and polar sites, with the majority of the interaction occurring in the front strands of both proteins using the large hydrophobic surfaces of the immunoglobulin-V-type domains; the complex between PD-1 and PD-L2 is thought to be similar, although much of this work is only in murine proteins [11].

2.1.3. Significance in Cancer Immunity

CTLA-4 was the first checkpoint molecule targeted in cancer treatment, initially in melanoma with dramatic results, and subsequently in other cancer types. Its significance in anti-tumor immunity was described over 20 years ago in murine models where blockade of CTLA-4 caused tumor rejection both in established tumors and with secondary exposure to tumor cells [13]. PD-1 is mainly expressed on immune cells, in particular T lymphocytes, as well as B lymphocytes, NK cells, dendritic cells and monocytes, and its expression can be induced by many factors, including interleukins, infectious agents and LPS [14–16]. As described above, its main function is in immune suppression; therefore, in tumors, it can have the detrimental effect of decreasing anti-tumor immunity, particularly because many cancers develop the capability to express the PD-L1 ligand. On presentation of an antigen to a T lymphocyte, a typical T-cell response involves binding the antigen to the specific T-cell receptor, expansion of this T cell clone and, finally, an effector phase of the response. The co-receptors CD28 and CD3 are involved in the induction of this response. Specifically, in the tumor microenvironment, neoantigens from cancer cells are released, captured and processed by antigen-presenting cells. Antigen presentation to T cells must be accompanied by a secondary signal mechanism in order for T cells to be primed and activated. This secondary signal can be via cytokines, such as IL-12 and type 1 interferon, factors released by dying cancer cells or via the gut microbiota [17,18]. Both CTLA-4 and PD-1 suppress CD28-mediated pathways; PD-1 does this by the activation of phosphatidylinositol-3-kinase which in turn inhibits Akt phosphorylation, thereby suppressing T-cell activation, and also inhibits glycolytic pathways, thereby decreasing cellular metabolism [19]. CTLA-4 binds to its B7 ligands with a much higher affinity than CD28, preventing T-cell stimulation.

Tumor cells in many cancer types express PD-L1 and therefore can activate this pathway to escape immune surveillance. The expression of PD-L1 by tumor cells may be an adaptive response to anti-tumor immune response, with PD-L1 expression co-localized with tumor-infiltrating lymphocytes and IFN-δ, an inflammatory cytokine [20]. However, the clinical significance of PD-L1 expression is tumor histology-specific, with some cancers demonstrating improved outcomes with high PD-L1 expression, while, in other tumors, PD-L1 expression does not correlate with better survival [21–26]. The expression of PD-1 and PD-L1 in tumors may also be heterogeneous both intra-tumorally and between primary and metastatic tumor sites [27–30].

2.2. Monoclonal Antibodies

2.2.1. Anti-CTLA-4

Ipilimumab, which binds to CTLA-4, was the first CPI to be licensed in 2011, and was initially used for the treatment of metastatic melanoma but is now indicated in multiple tumor types. It has a high surface area at its binding site and has a dissociation constant of 5.25 nM, with a large surface area buried at its binding surface with CTLA-4 [31] (Table 1). Tremelimumab is another monoclonal antibody targeting CTLA-4 but has not yet been licensed for any indication, although it has orphan drug status for treatment of mesothelioma. Tremelimumab is an IgG2 antibody; this subtype is thought to have less complement activation and antibody-dependent cell-mediated cytotoxicity [32]. It is currently in ongoing clinical trials, in particular in combination with durvalumab [33].

Table 1. Checkpoint inhibitors, their pharmacokinetic and dosing profiles and indications.

Agent	Type	Antigen	Clearance	Dissociation Constant/ Binding Affinity	Half-Life	Indications	Companion/Complementary Diagnostic Assay	Dosing	Year First Licensed	Pharmaceutical Company
Ipilimumab	IgG1 human antibody	CTLA-4	Stable clearance over doses 0.3–10 mg/kg	Dissociation constant 5.25 nM	15.4 days	Melanoma, renal cell carcinoma, MSI-high colorectal carcinoma	None	Weight-based dosing (1–10 mg/kg)	2011	Bristol Myers Squibb
Tremelimumab	IgG2 human antibody	CTLA-4	Stable clearance over doses 10–15 mg/kg	Binding affinity 0.28 nM	22 days	None as yet	None	Weight-based dosing (3–15 mg/kg) or fixed dosing (75 mg)	Not yet licensed	AstraZeneca
Nivolumab	IgG4 human antibody	PD-1	Linear clearance over doses of 0.1–20 mg/kg	Dissociation constant 1.45 nM	25 days	Melanoma, non-small cell lung cancer, renal cell carcinoma, small cell lung cancer, head and neck cancer, hepatocellular carcinoma, Hodgkin lymphoma, urothelial cancer, MSI-high or mismatch repair-deficient colorectal cancer	Dako 28-8 Pharm Dx assay (complementary)	Weight-based dosing (1–3 mg/kg) or flat dosing (240 mg)	2014	Bristol Myers Squibb
Pembrolizumab	IgG4 human antibody	PD-1	Linear clearance over doses 1–10 mg/kg	Dissociation constant 29 pM	22 days	Melanoma, non-small cell lung cancer, renal cell carcinoma, small cell lung cancer, Hodgkin lymphoma, primary mediastinal large B-cell lymphoma, Merkel cell carcinoma, hepatocellular carcinoma, gastric cancer, renal cell carcinoma, endometrial carcinoma, cervical cancer, head and neck cancers, urothelial carcinoma, gastric/GEJ/esophageal cancers, mismatch repair deficient tumors	Dako 22C3 Pharm Dx (companion for non-small cell lung cancer, gastric or gastroesophageal junction adenocarcinoma, cervical cancer, urothelial carcinoma, head and neck squamous cell carcinoma, and esophageal squamous cell carcinoma)	Fixed dosing (200 mg)	2014	Merck
Atezolizumab	IgG1 human antibody	PD-L1	Linear clearance over doses 1–20 mg/kg	Binding affinity 971 Å2	27 days	Urothelial carcinoma, non-small cell lung cancer, triple-negative breast cancer, small cell lung cancer	Ventana SP142 (companion for urothelial carcinoma and triple-negative breast carcinoma)	Fixed dosing (840 mg, 1200 mg, 1680 mg)	2016	Genentech
Avelumab	IgG1 human antibody	PD-L1	Linear clearance over doses 1–20 mg/kg	Binding affinity 875.4 Å2	6 days	Merkel cell carcinoma, urothelial carcinoma, renal cell carcinoma	None	Fixed dosing (800 mg) or weight-based dosing (10 mg/kg) (not Food and Drug Administration (FDA) approved)	2017	EMD Serono/Pfizer
Durvalumab	IgG1 human antibody	PD-L1	Linear clearance at doses higher than 3 mg/kg	Dissociation constant 667 pM	18 days	Urothelial carcinoma, non-small cell lung cancer	Ventana SP263 (complementary)	Weight-based dosing (10 mg/kg) or fixed dosing (1500 mg) (not FDA-approved)	2017	AstraZeneca

2.2.2. Anti-PD-1/PD-L1

The first two anti-PD-1 CPIs licensed were nivolumab and pembrolizumab, based on their anti-tumor activity in phase I studies [34–36]. Pembrolizumab is an IgG4 human antibody; these antibodies have a low affinity for C1q and Fc receptors compared to other IgG molecules, making them a good antibody choice for immunotherapy, with the lowest chance of host immunity stimulation [37]. Most IgG4 antibodies are capable of a process called Fab arm exchange, in which half-molecules (a heavy chain and attached light chain) can be exchanged between IgG4 molecules [38]; pembrolizumab has a hinge region containing a S288P mutation, which prevents Fab arm exchange due to a conformational change [39,40]. The structure of nivolumab is very similar; it is an IgG4 antibody which differs from pembrolizumab only in the variable region of epitope binding-pembrolizumab binds to the C′D loop and nivolumab binds to the N-terminal loop on the PD-1 molecule [41].

Atezolizumab was the first anti-PD-L1 antibody licensed in the US. Atezolizumab and the other licensed anti-PD-L1 antibodies avelumab and durvalumab are IgG1 antibodies, which bind to the front beta-sheet of PD-L1. The heavy chain and light chain regions of these antibodies are involved in binding, with varying buried surface areas on each molecule which may affect their binding affinities [42,43]. These three antibodies have been noted to use all three complementarity determining regions from their heavy chains and two from the light chains [43,44].

After ipilimumab was licensed for the treatment of metastatic melanoma in 2011, the anti-PD-1 and anti-PD-L1 CPIs were subsequently approved for the treatment of many other cancer types, in the metastatic, adjuvant and neo-adjuvant settings. Initial approvals were for refractory/advanced melanoma and non-small cell lung cancer (NSCLC) for the anti-PD-1 CPIs, with subsequent licensing for their use in head and neck cancers, renal cell carcinoma, Hodgkin lymphoma and urothelial carcinomas [45]. Interestingly, the anti-PD-1 antibody pembrolizumab was the first oncologic therapy to be approved for use on the basis of a genetic alteration, with FDA approval granted in 2017 for its use in any tumor demonstrating microsatellite instability (MSI) [46]. The anti-PD-L1 antibodies are used in urothelial, kidney, lung and Merkel cell carcinoma, with many further studies ongoing. The presence of high tumor mutational burden (TMB) (the number of somatic tumor mutations per megabase of sequenced DNA) may identify tumors that are more likely to respond to CPI, such as those tumors that are microsatellite-unstable; however, to date, high TMB is not used to select therapy for patients [47]. Interestingly, responses to CPIs can be durable, with subsets of patients achieving long-lasting complete responses in some disease types, although, for many others, immune escape mechanisms develop, allowing tumors to evade the response primed by CPIs [48]. These treatments generally have a high tolerability, although the main toxicities, which are immune-related inflammatory effects, may be serious in a subset of patients.

2.2.3. Binding Affinities and Pharmacokinetics

Nivolumab has a binding affinity to the PD-1 protein of 3.06 nM, while pembrolizumab has an even higher affinity, with a dissociation constant of 27 pM, possibly due to its extensive binding sites to PD-1, which include hydrogen bonds, specifically water-mediated hydrogen bonds, and salt bridges [41,49,50]. Interestingly, pembrolizumab has a much lower affinity for mouse PD-1, which may be explained by specific amino acid substitutions (Asp^{85} to Gly^{85}) which, when mutated in human PD-1, abolish pembrolizumab binding. Atezolizumab has a high binding affinity of 0.4 nM, utilizing specific hot-spot residues on the protein binding surface [42,51], while avelumab and durvalumab have dissociation constants of 42.1 pM [43] and 667 pM [52], respectively.

Studies have shown moderate inter-individual variability (IIV) in pharmacokinetics of CPIs. Ipilimumab has stable clearance over dose ranges from 0.3 to 10 mg/kg, with a half-life of 14.7 days and IIV largely influenced by body weight and baseline LDH value, while age, gender, renal and hepatic function do not affect clearance [53]. The steady state trough concentration of ipilimumab is a predictor of response, with higher trough concentrations (in patients receiving higher doses) resulting in improved complete response rates and higher overall survival (OS), but also in increased rates of irAEs [54,55]. Both the anti-PD-1 antibodies nivolumab and pembrolizumab have linear clearance over dose ranges of 0.1–20 mg/kg and 1–10 mg/kg respectively, with both demonstrating a time-dependent decline in clearance rates, although the decline did not appear to impact clinical outcomes [56–58]. For the anti-PD-L1 antibodies atezolizumab, avelumab and durvalumab, linear clearance is seen again over wide ranges of doses. For atezolizumab, which is usually used at a fixed dose of 1200 mg, clearance was stable at doses between 1–20 mg/kg and rates were affected by body weight and serum albumin [59]. Avelumab has a similar linear clearance, but interestingly, time-dependent clearance changes differed between tumor types, with Merkel cell carcinoma and head and neck squamous cell carcinoma patients having clearance declines of 24–32%, while all other tumor types had minimal decline in clearance over time [60]. Durvalumab had linear clearance at doses higher than 3 mg/kg, with numerous factors influencing clearance including albumin, body weight, cancer type and gender [61]. Interestingly, a factor that influences clearance in all three anti-PD-L1 antibodies is the development of anti-drug antibodies, which develop in 31.7%, 4.16% and 3.1% respectively for atezolizumab, avelumab and durvalumab, but are unlikely to be clinically relevant as they did not affect clearance to a meaningful degree.

The antitumor effect of pembrolizumab is driven by the reactivation of adaptive immune response by inhibiting PD-1 expressed on T-cells. Once the PD-1 on T-cells are fully saturated by pembrolizumab, the shape of the exposure–response relationship within the dose range of 2–10 mg/kg or 200 mg (exposure at 2 mg/kg every three weeks is similar to exposure at 200 mg every three weeks) is flat, as demonstrated in multiple indications [62]. Available pharmacokinetics (PK) results in participants with various indications (melanoma, NSCLC, HNSCC, and MSI-H) supporting a lack of meaningful difference in PK among tumor types. Therefore, the selection of the 200 mg every three weeks dosing for pembrolizumab was supported as an appropriate dose for multiple tumor types.

Similarly, nivolumab, dosed at a fixed dose of either 240 mg every two weeks or 480 mg every four weeks results in a similar time-averaged steady state exposure and safety as 3 mg/kg every two weeks across multiple tumor types in numerous clinical trials, and is approved at a fixed dosing for most indications [63–65]. Peripheral PD-1 receptor occupancy is saturated at doses ≥ 0.3 mg/kg after eight weeks treatment, again supporting minimizing the doses administered, although the degree of intra-tumoral receptor occupancy is not yet known [66]. Some regulatory authorities have suggested weight-based dosing for patients less than 80 kg and fixed dosing above, to avoid unnecessarily high doses for lower-weight patients [67]. Avelumab is currently approved at a weight-based dosing of 10 mg/kg, but simulations suggested that similar risk/benefit profiles would result from fixed dosing at 800 mg, leading to FDA approval of this fixed dose [68]. Issues with cost and drug wastage are also improved with flat dosing [69]; these results are leading to a move towards fixed dosing in many CPI indications and trials, as evidence from the majority of CPIs demonstrates that exposure, efficacy and safety are similar to weight-based dosing.

2.2.4. Immune-Related Adverse Events

A full discussion of the irAEs associated with CPIs is beyond the scope of this review, but, briefly, these side effects are due to off-target activation or dysregulation of the immune system, which can affect any body organ or system. Common organs affected include the bowel, causing colitis, which can be severe, the lungs, causing pneumonitis, the thyroid gland, which can cause both overproduction or underproduction of the thyroid hormone, the adrenal or pituitary glands, the liver and the skin [70]. There appear to be some patterns to the frequency of irAEs with various CPIs, with colitis and hypophysitis more common with the anti-CTLA-4 antibodies and pneumonitis and hypothyroidism more frequently seen with anti-PD-1 therapies [71]. Deaths from irAEs are rare but do occur, with the most common causes being severe colitis and pneumonitis [71]. Rates of grade 3–4 irAEs increase with combination treatment compared with single agent treatment; for example, treatment of metastatic melanoma with ipilimumab and nivolumab resulted in 59% grade 3–4 AEs, compared with 21% for nivolumab alone and 28% for ipilimumab alone [72]. The management of irAEs includes use of steroids for less severe cases, and immunosuppression for more severe cases, using agents such as infliximab and mycophenolate [73].

3. Optimization of Checkpoint Inhibitors

While CPIs are part of standard of care in multiple tumor types, efforts to optimize these antibodies to improve their efficacy and safety are currently underway.

3.1. Non-Fucosylated Antibodies

Non-fucosylated antibodies have been modified so that the glycans in the Fc binding portion of the antibody are not fucose-bound. This modification enhances the antibody-dependent cell-mediated cytotoxicity (ADCC) via the enrichment of Fc-gamma-receptor-expressing effector cells and depletion of T-regulatory cells [74–77]. A non-fucosylated variant of ipilimumab has been constructed, and, in mice, demonstrated increased anti-tumor activity, peripheral T-cell activation and T-reg depletion compared with standard ipilimumab, and also enhanced T-cell-mediated vaccine responses in macaques [76,78]. A modified molecule, similar to atezolizumab but with reduced core fucosylation, demonstrated increased binding to Fc-gamma-receptor-IIIa and enhanced ADCC against PD-L1-expressing tumor cells in a cell-line model [79]. Knockout of the fucosyltransferase gene FUT8 or the pharmacologic inhibition of this gene, which decreased fucosylation, resulted in decreased PD-1 expression and increased T-cell activation in mice, again supporting this as a potential mechanism to enhance the activity of checkpoint inhibitors [80]. Phase I trials of non-fucosylated ipilimumab are enrolling.

3.2. Pro-Drug Formulations

Prodrug formulations of antibodies utilize a masking peptide that binds to the antigen-binding site of the CPI which reduces systemic activity. When the antibody reaches the tumor site, proteases cleave the masking peptide and the antibody becomes fully functional, allowing tumor-targeted activity and theoretically reducing off-target systemic adverse effects. Prodrug versions of ipilimumab have been developed and demonstrate equivalent anti-tumor and immune activity and reduced lymphohistiocytic inflammation in the gastrointestinal tract and kidneys compared with standard ipilimumab [76,78]. The result is an improved safety profile. Probody^{TM} therapeutics are protease-activated antibodies which have shown pre-clinical efficacy targeting PD-L1 with minimal systemic auto-immunity [81,82]; the Probody drug CX-072 is now in phase I/II clinical trial for solid tumors and lymphoma [NCT03013491].

3.3. Bispecific Antibodies

Another method to optimize CPIs is to fuse them to another antibody which can then simultaneously bind another target molecule. These molecules then have the extracellular domains of two separate antibodies, both of which can bind to their respective ligands and retain their signaling activity. An example of this type of protein is the PD1-Fc-OX40L molecule, which, on testing, retained its high affinity binding for both PD-L1/L2 and OX40, caused T-cell activation and also demonstrated an improved anti-tumor immune response compared with single antibody treatment or the combination of the two separate PD-1 and OX40 antibodies [83]. A bispecific antibody to CTLA-4 and OX40 has also been effective in pre-clinical models, reducing tumor growth and enhancing response to PD-1 targeted therapy, and is now in phase I clinical trials [NCT03782467] [84]. The RANK/RANKL pathway is usually associated with bone homeostasis and is targeted using bone-protective agents, such as denosumab in patients with metastatic bony lesions and with osteoporosis [85]. However, this pathway is also involved in the tumor-associated immune response, with increased RANKL expression seen in tumor-infiltrating T-cells and RANK expression on dendritic cells and immunosuppressive M2 macrophages [86]. While trials are underway combining CPIs with denosumab, bispecific antibodies targeting the PD-1/PD-L1 and RANK/RANKL pathways have been developed, and show significant anti-tumor activity in mouse models, in particular those of colon and lung cancer [87]. This activity was dependent on CD8+ T cells and IFN-γ, and could be increased further by combining the bispecific antibody with an anti-CTLA4 antibody.

Bispecific antibodies have already entered early phase clinical trials. A fusion protein consisting of an anti-PD-L1 antibody fused to the extracellular domain of TGF-β receptor II, M7824, showed excellent pre-clinical activity, suppressing metastases, inducing long-term anti-tumor immunity and improving OS in mouse models of breast and colon cancer, both as a single agent and in combination with a therapeutic cancer vaccine [88,89]. It is currently in phase I/II trials in many cancer types including breast, prostate, lung, biliary tract and colorectal, with an early biliary tract cancer trial showing an overall response rate of 27% [PMC6421177, PMC6421170]. Another bispecific antibody, MGD013, which targets PD-L1 and LAG-3, another CPI, has shown pre-clinical activity and is in phase I trials in solid tumors [NCT03219268] [90,91]. Issues that arise with bispecific antibodies include the potential for increased immunogenicity and therefore more adverse events, as well as difficulties with safety assessments in animal models. There are many other bispecific antibodies in pre-clinical development, combining immune checkpoint blockade with other tumor-specific protein binding.

4. New Agents Targeting Immune Checkpoints

4.1. Small Molecule Checkpoint Inhibitors

While there has been considerable progress in the development of antibodies targeting the PD-1/PD-L1 pathway, interest has been growing in attempts to block this axis using small molecules. The purported benefits of using small molecules rather than antibodies include potentially better oral bioavailability, fewer immune-related adverse events, improved tumor penetration and a lower production cost. The initial molecules shown to inhibit this pathway were sulfamonomethoxine and sulfamethizole, which could rescue PD-1-mediated inhibition of IFN-g production, a process which was dependent on PD-L2 [92]. Substituting particular rings in the structure of the sulfamethizole compound, such as a phenyl ring instead of a pyridyl ring, improved the efficacy of the compound in restoring IFN-γ expression. While, ultimately, research into these compounds was not continued, they provided proof of concept for the small molecule inhibition of the PD-1/PD-L1 pathway.

Several other small molecule compounds that inhibit PD-L1 have been patented [93]. These molecules have been shown to bind directly to each dimer of PD-L1 and can dissociate the PD-1/PD-L1 complex, and certain "hot spots" on the PD-L1 molecule, which are targetable by small molecules, have been identified using in vitro studies of these compounds [94,95]. However, one of the major problems with small molecule inhibitors to date has been their large molecular weight, which impairs adequate absorption and distribution in the human body.

The only small molecule currently in human clinical trials is a molecule called Ca-170, which inhibits both the PD-L1 pathway and the V-domain Ig suppressor of the T-cell activation (VISTA) pathway. Pre-clinical work has demonstrated that in mice, this molecule can inhibit tumor growth, enhance peripheral T cell activation and increase activation of tumor-infiltrating CD8+ T-cells [96,97]. Oral bioavailability in mice was 40%, but in monkeys was <10%, again raising the issue of oral administration of these compounds. Ca-170 is in phase 1 clinical trials in patients with advanced solid tumors and lymphoma, and also in phase II trials, with a clinical benefit rate of 59.5% reported, and higher response rates seen at lower doses [98]. Interestingly, a recent study examining the mechanism of binding of Ca-170 has shown that there is no direct binding between the compound and the PD-L1 molecule, suggesting there may be an alternative mechanism of action [99]. To date, the majority of small molecule inhibitors of PD-L1 do not appear to be ready for widespread clinical usage and further pre-clinical work is needed to optimize their formulation and use.

4.2. Peptide Checkpoint Inhibitors

As described above, the crystal structure of the PD-1 and PD-L1 molecules and the mechanism by which they bind has been clearly defined, and, therefore, interest has grown in designing a peptide inhibitor that could bind to one of these binding sites. With this data, the first peptide antagonist, (D)PPA-1, was described in 2015, and designed using a mirror-image phage display method, binding to PD-L1 and blocking the PD-1/PD-L1 interaction and decreasing tumor growth in vivo [100]. Replacing the L-amino acids with D-amino acids can improve the stability and oral bioavailability of these drugs. Another more recently developed peptide, PL120131, was designed to interact with the PD-1 molecule, based on the interacting residues on PD-L1 from the amino acid glycine at position 120 to asparagine at position 131 [101]. PL120131 was shown to act as a competitive inhibitor of PD-L1 by associating with the binding groove on PD-1, and to reverse the apoptotic signal induced by soluble PD-L1 in Jurkat cells and primary lymphocytes. Another class of peptides are the macrocyclic peptides, which bind to the PD-1-binding site on the PD-L1 molecule, and can restore T-cell function in vitro [102].

To date, none of the peptide inhibitors of the PD-1/PD-L1 pathway have been used in human trials. The peptide molecule TPP-1 has a high affinity for human PD-L1, and, in a mouse model, could decrease tumor growth by 56% compared with control peptide-treated mice, by re-activating T cells through blocking the PD-1/PD-L1 interaction [103]. A compound called UNP-12 demonstrated a 44% reduction in tumor growth in mice [104,105]. More recently, NP-12, which also inhibits the PD-1/PD-L1 interaction and can inhibit tumor growth and metastases in colon and melanoma mouse models, demonstrated improved efficacy when combined with tumor vaccination or cyclophosphamide [106]. The peptide inhibitors are still in early phases of development but may provide an alternative method through which to inhibit immune checkpoints.

5. Conclusions

CPIs have changed the landscape of cancer treatment in recent years, with a small proportion of patients with a variety of tumors experiencing deep and durable responses. Understanding the pharmacokinetics of many CPIs has led to a switch from weight-based to fixed dosing, which is likely to continue as more studies of the efficacy and PK of fixed dosing are completed. IrAEs and heterogeneity in responses has led to efforts to optimize existing CPIs and to develop new methods by which to inhibit checkpoint molecules. Understanding the structure of CPIs and their ligands can help in the further enhancement of these therapeutic agents.

Funding: This research received no external funding.

Conflicts of Interest: The authors declare no conflict of interest

Abbreviations

Abb.	Full Name
Å-2	angstrom-2
ADCC	antibody-dependent cell-mediated cytotoxicity
CPI	checkpoint inhibitors
CTLA-4	cytotoxic T-lymphocyte associated protein-4
IgG	immunoglobulin G
IIV	interindividual variability
IL-12	interleukin-12
irAE	immune-related adverse event
nM	nanomolar
OS	overall survival
PD-1	programmed cell death protein-1
PD-L1	programmed cell death protein ligand-1
PD-L2	programmed cell death protein ligand-2
pM	picomolar
RANK	Receptor activator of nuclear factor kappa-B
RANKL	Receptor activator of nuclear factor kappa-B ligand
T-reg	T-regulatory

References

1. Brunet, J.F.; Denizot, F.; Luciani, M.F.; Roux-Dosseto, M.; Suzan, M.; Mattei, M.-G.; Golstein, P. A new member of the immunoglobulin superfamily—Ctla-4. *Nature* **1987**, *328*, 267–270. [CrossRef] [PubMed]
2. Lindsten, T.; Lee, K.P.; Harris, E.S.; Petryniak, B.; Craighead, N.; Reynolds, P.J.; Lombard, D.B.; Freeman, G.J.; Nadler, L.M.; Gray, G.S.; et al. Characterization of CTLA-4 structure and expression on human T cells. *J. Immunol.* **1993**, *151*, 3489–3499. [PubMed]
3. Tivol, E.A.; Borriello, F.; Schweitzer, A.N.; Lynch, W.P.; Bluestone, J.A.; Sharpe, A.H. Loss of CTLA-4 leads to massive lymphoproliferation and fatal multiorgan tissue destruction, revealing a critical negative regulatory role of CTLA-4. *Immunity* **1995**, *3*, 541–547. [CrossRef]
4. Ishida, Y.; Agata, Y.; Shibahara, K.; Honjo, T. Induced expression of PD-1, a novel member of the immunoglobulin gene superfamily, upon programmed cell death. *EMBO J.* **1992**, *11*, 3887–3895. [CrossRef]
5. Nishimura, H.; Nose, M.; Hiai, H.; Minato, N.; Honjo, T. Development of lupus-like autoimmune diseases by disruption of the PD-1 gene encoding an ITIM motif-carrying immunoreceptor. *Immunity* **1999**, *11*, 141–151. [CrossRef]
6. Nishimura, H.; Okazaki, T.; Tanaka, Y.; Nakatani, K.; Hara, M.; Matsumori, A.; Sasayama, S.; Mizoguchi, A.; Hiai, H.; Minato, N.; et al. Autoimmune dilated cardiomyopathy in PD-1 receptor-deficient mice. *Science* **2001**, *291*, 319–322. [CrossRef]
7. Zhong, X.; Bai, C.; Gao, W.; Strom, T.B.; Rothstein, T.L. Suppression of expression and function of negative immune regulator PD-1 by certain pattern recognition and cytokine receptor signals associated with immune system danger. *Int. Immunol.* **2004**, *16*, 1181–1188. [CrossRef]
8. Zak, K.M.; Grudnik, P.; Magiera, K.; Domling, A.; Dubin, G.; Holak, T.A. Structural Biology of the Immune Checkpoint Receptor PD-1 and Its Ligands PD-L1/PD-L2. *Structure* **2017**, *25*, 1163–1174. [CrossRef]
9. Guzik, K.; Zak, K.M.; Grudnik, P.; Magiera, K.; Musielak, B.; Törner, R.; Skalniak, L.; Dömling, A.; Dubin, G.; Holak, T.A. Small-Molecule Inhibitors of the Programmed Cell Death-1/Programmed Death-Ligand 1 (PD-1/PD-L1) Interaction via Transiently Induced Protein States and Dimerization of PD-L1. *J. Med. Chem.* **2017**, *60*, 5857–5867. [CrossRef]
10. Zak, K.M.; Kitel, R.; Przetocka, S.; Golik, P.; Guzik, K.; Musielak, B.; Dömling, A.; Dubin, G.; Holak, T.A. Structure of the Complex of Human Programmed Death 1, PD-1, and Its Ligand PD-L1. *Structure* **2015**, *23*, 2341–2348. [CrossRef]
11. Lazar-Molnar, E.; Yan, Q.; Cao, E.; Ramagopal, U.; Nathenson, S.G.; Almo, S.C. Crystal structure of the complex between programmed death-1 (PD-1) and its ligand PD-L2. *Proc. Natl. Acad. Sci. USA* **2008**, *105*, 10483–10488. [CrossRef] [PubMed]
12. Lin, D.Y.; Tanaka, Y.; Iwasaki, M.; Gittis, A.G.; Su, H.P.; Mikami, B.; Okazaki, T.; Honjo, T.; Minato, N.; Garboczi, D.N. The PD-1/PD-L1 complex resembles the antigen-binding Fv domains of antibodies and T cell receptors. *Proc. Natl. Acad. Sci. USA* **2008**, *105*, 3011–3016. [CrossRef] [PubMed]
13. Leach, D.R.; Krummel, M.F.; Allison, J.P. Enhancement of antitumor immunity by CTLA-4 blockade. *Science* **1996**, *271*, 1734–1736. [CrossRef] [PubMed]
14. Watanabe, T.; Bertoletti, A.; Tanoto, T.A. PD-1/PD-L1 pathway and T-cell exhaustion in chronic hepatitis virus infection. *J. Viral Hepat.* **2010**, *17*, 453–458. [CrossRef] [PubMed]
15. Kinter, A.L.; Godbout, E.J.; McNally, J.P.; Sereti, I.; Roby, G.A.; O'Shea, M.A.; Fauci, A.S. The common gamma-chain cytokines IL-2, IL-7, IL-15, and IL-21 induce the expression of programmed death-1 and its ligands. *J. Immunol.* **2008**, *181*, 6738–6746. [CrossRef] [PubMed]
16. Nam, S.; Lee, A.; Lim, J.; Lim, J.S. Analysis of the Expression and Regulation of PD-1 Protein on the Surface of Myeloid-Derived Suppressor Cells (MDSCs). *Biomol. Ther.* **2019**, *27*, 63–70. [CrossRef] [PubMed]
17. Guram, K.; Kim, S.S.; Wu, V.; Sanders, P.D.; Patel, S.; Schoenberger, S.P.; Cohen, E.E.W.; Chen, S.Y.; Sharabi, A.B. A Threshold Model for T-Cell Activation in the Era of Checkpoint Blockade Immunotherapy. *Front. Immunol.* **2019**, *10*, 491. [CrossRef]
18. Sanchez-Paulete, A.R.; Teijeira, A.; Cueto, F.J.; Garasa, S.; Pérez-Gracia, J.L.; Sánchez-Arráez, A.; Sancho, D.; Melero, I. Antigen cross-presentation and T-cell cross-priming in cancer immunology and immunotherapy. *Ann. Oncol.* **2017**, *28*, xii44–xii55. [CrossRef]

19. Parry, R.V.; Chemnitz, J.M.; Frauwirth, K.A.; Lanfranco, A.R.; Braunstein, I.; Kobayashi, S.V.; Linsley, P.S.; Thompson, C.B.; Riley, J.L. LCTLA-4 and PD-1 receptors inhibit T-cell activation by distinct mechanisms. *Mol. Cell. Biol.* **2005**, *25*, 9543–9553. [CrossRef]
20. Taube, J.M.; Anders, R.A.; Young, G.D.; Xu, H.; Sharma, R.; McMiller, T.L.; Chen, S.; Klein, A.P.; Pardoll, D.M.; Topalian, S.L.; et al. Colocalization of inflammatory response with B7-h1 expression in human melanocytic lesions supports an adaptive resistance mechanism of immune escape. *Sci. Transl. Med.* **2012**, *4*, 127ra37. [CrossRef]
21. Sabatier, R.; Finetti, P.; Mamessier, E.; Adelaide, J.; Chaffanet, M.; Ali, H.R.; Viens, P.; Caldas, C.; Birnbaum, D.; Bertucci, F. Prognostic and predictive value of PDL1 expression in breast cancer. *Oncotarget* **2015**, *6*, 5449–5464. [CrossRef] [PubMed]
22. Rahn, S.; Kruger, S.; Mennrich, R.; Goebel, L.; Wesch, D.; Oberg, H.H.; Vogel, I.; Ebsen, M.; Röcken, C.; Helm, O.; et al. POLE Score: A comprehensive profiling of programmed death 1 ligand 1 expression in pancreatic ductal adenocarcinoma. *Oncotarget* **2019**, *10*, 1572–1588. [CrossRef] [PubMed]
23. Velcheti, V.; Schalper, K.A.; Carvajal, D.E.; Anagnostou, V.K.; Syrigos, K.N.; Sznol, M.; Herbst, R.S.; Gettinger, S.N.; Chen, L.; Rimm, D.L. Programmed death ligand-1 expression in non-small cell lung cancer. *Lab. Invest.* **2014**, *94*, 107–116. [CrossRef] [PubMed]
24. Muenst, S.; Schaerli, A.R.; Gao, F.; Däster, S.; Trella, E.; Droeser, R.A.; Muraro, M.G.; Zajac, P.; Zanetti, R.; Gillanders, W.E.; et al. Expression of programmed death ligand 1 (PD-L1) is associated with poor prognosis in human breast cancer. *Breast Cancer Res. Treat.* **2014**, *146*, 15–24. [CrossRef]
25. Daud, A.I.; Wolchok, J.D.; Robert, C.; Hwu, W.J.; Weber, J.S.; Ribas, A.; Hodi, F.S.; Joshua, A.M.; Kefford, R.; Hersey, P.; et al. Programmed Death-Ligand 1 Expression and Response to the Anti-Programmed Death 1 Antibody Pembrolizumab in Melanoma. *J. Clin. Oncol.* **2016**, *34*, 4102–4109. [CrossRef]
26. Macek Jilkova, Z.; Aspord, C.; Decaens, T. Predictive Factors for Response to PD-1/PD-L1 Checkpoint Inhibition in the Field of Hepatocellular Carcinoma: Current Status and Challenges. *Cancers* **2019**, *11*, 1554. [CrossRef]
27. Munari, E.; Zamboni, G.; Marconi, M.; Sommaggio, M.; Brunelli, M.; Martignoni, G.; Terzi, A. PD-L1 expression heterogeneity in non-small cell lung cancer: Evaluation of small biopsies reliability. *Oncotarget* **2017**, *8*, 90123–90131. [CrossRef]
28. Munari, E.; Zamboni, G.; Lunardi, G.; Sommaggio, M.; Brunelli, M.; Martignoni, G.; Netto, G.J.; Moretta, F.; Mingari, M.C.; Salgarello, M.; et al. PD-L1 expression comparison between primary and relapsed non-small cell lung carcinoma using whole sections and clone SP263. *Oncotarget* **2018**, *9*, 30465–30471. [CrossRef]
29. Callea, M.; Albiges, L.; Gupta, M.; Cheng, S.C.; Genega, E.M.; Fay, A.P.; Song, J.; Carvo, I.; Bhatt, R.S.; Atkins, M.B.; et al. Differential expression of PD-L1 between primary and metastatic sites in clear-cell renal cell carcinoma. *Cancer Immunol. Res.* **2015**, *3*, 1158–1164. [CrossRef]
30. Madore, J.; Vilain, R.E.; Menzies, A.M.; Kakavand, H.; Wilmott, J.S.; Hyman, J.; Yearley, J.H.; Kefford, R.F.; Thompson, J.F.; Long, G.V.; et al. PD-L1 expression in melanoma shows marked heterogeneity within and between patients: Implications for anti-PD-1/PD-L1 clinical trials. *Pigment Cell Melanoma Res.* **2015**, *28*, 245–253. [CrossRef]
31. Ramagopal, U.A.; Liu, W.; Garrett-Thomson, S.C.; Bonanno, J.B.; Yan, Q.; Srinivasan, M.; Wong, S.C.; Bell, A.; Mankikar, S.; Rangan, V.S.; et al. Structural basis for cancer immunotherapy by the first-in-class checkpoint inhibitor ipilimumab. *Proc. Natl. Acad. Sci. USA* **2017**, *114*, E4223–E4232. [CrossRef] [PubMed]
32. Strome, S.E.; Sausville, E.A.; Mann, D. A mechanistic perspective of monoclonal antibodies in cancer therapy beyond target-related effects. *Oncologist* **2007**, *12*, 1084–1095. [CrossRef] [PubMed]
33. Camacho, L.H.; Antonia, S.; Sosman, J.; Kirkwood, J.M.; Gajewski, T.F.; Redman, B.; Pavlov, D.; Bulanhagui, C.; Bozon, V.A.; Gomez-Navarro, J.; et al. Phase I/II trial of tremelimumab in patients with metastatic melanoma. *J. Clin. Oncol.* **2009**, *27*, 1075–1081. [CrossRef] [PubMed]
34. Brahmer, J.R.; Drake, C.G.; Wollner, I.; Powderly, J.D.; Picus, J.; Sharfman, W.H.; Stankevich, E.; Pons, A.; Salay, T.M.; McMiller, T.L.; et al. Phase I study of single-agent anti-programmed death-1 (MDX-1106) in refractory solid tumors: Safety, clinical activity, pharmacodynamics, and immunologic correlates. *J. Clin. Oncol.* **2010**, *28*, 3167–3175. [CrossRef] [PubMed]
35. Hamid, O.; Robert, C.; Daud, A.; Hodi, F.S.; Hwu, W.J.; Kefford, R.; Wolchok, J.D.; Hersey, P.; Joseph, R.W.; Weber, J.S.; et al. Safety and tumor responses with lambrolizumab (anti-PD-1) in melanoma. *N. Engl. J. Med.* **2013**, *369*, 134–144. [CrossRef]

36. Topalian, S.L.; Hodi, F.S.; Brahmer, J.R.; Gettinger, S.N.; Smith, D.C.; McDermott, D.F.; Powderly, J.D.; Carvajal, R.D.; Sosman, J.A.; Atkins, M.B.; et al. Safety, activity, and immune correlates of anti-PD-1 antibody in cancer. *N. Engl. J. Med.* **2012**, *366*, 2443–2454. [CrossRef]
37. Jefferis, R.; Lund, J. Interaction sites on human IgG-Fc for FcgammaR: Current models. *Immunol. Lett.* **2002**, *82*, 57–65. [CrossRef]
38. Van der Neut Kolfschoten, M.; Schuurman, J.; Losen, M.; Bleeker, W.K.; Martínez-Martínez, P.; Vermeulen, E.; De Baets, M.H. Anti-inflammatory activity of human IgG4 antibodies by dynamic Fab arm exchange. *Science* **2007**, *317*, 1554–1557. [CrossRef]
39. Angal, S.; King, D.J.; Bodmer, M.W.; Turner, A.; Lawson, A.D.; Roberts, G.; Pedley, B.; Adair, J.R. A single amino acid substitution abolishes the heterogeneity of chimeric mouse/human (IgG4) antibody. *Mol. Immunol.* **1993**, *30*, 105–108. [CrossRef]
40. Scapin, G.; Yang, X.; Prosise, W.W.; McCoy, M.; Reichert, P.; Johnston, J.M.; Kashi, R.S.; Strickland, C. Structure of full-length human anti-PD1 therapeutic IgG4 antibody pembrolizumab. *Nat. Struct. Mol. Biol.* **2015**, *22*, 953–958. [CrossRef]
41. Tan, S.; Zhang, H.; Chai, Y.; Song, H.; Tong, Z.; Wang, Q.; Qi, J.; Wong, G.; Zhu, X.; Liu, W.J.; et al. An unexpected N-terminal loop in PD-1 dominates binding by nivolumab. *Nat. Commun.* **2017**, *8*, 14369. [CrossRef] [PubMed]
42. Zhang, F.; Qi, X.; Wang, X.; Wei, D.; Wu, J.; Feng, L.; Cai, H.; Wang, Y.; Zeng, N.; Xu, T.; et al. Structural basis of the therapeutic anti-PD-L1 antibody atezolizumab. *Oncotarget* **2017**, *8*, 90215–90224. [CrossRef] [PubMed]
43. Liu, K.; Tan, S.; Chai, Y.; Chen, D.; Song, H.; Zhang, C.W.; Shi, Y.; Liu, J.; Tan, W.; Lyu, J.; et al. Structural basis of anti-PD-L1 monoclonal antibody avelumab for tumor therapy. *Cell Res.* **2017**, *27*, 151–153. [CrossRef] [PubMed]
44. Lee, H.T.; Lee, J.Y.; Lim, H.; Lee, S.H.; Moon, Y.J.; Pyo, H.J.; Ryu, S.E.; Shin, W.; Heo, Y.S. Molecular mechanism of PD-1/PD-L1 blockade via anti-PD-L1 antibodies atezolizumab and durvalumab. *Sci. Rep.* **2017**, *7*, 5532. [CrossRef]
45. Ribas, A.; Wolchok, J.D. Cancer immunotherapy using checkpoint blockade. *Science* **2018**, *359*, 1350–1355. [CrossRef]
46. Le, D.T.; Durham, J.N.; Smith, K.N.; Wang, H.; Bartlett, B.R.; Aulakh, L.K.; Lu, S.; Kemberling, H.; Wilt, C.; Luber, B.S.; et al. Mismatch repair deficiency predicts response of solid tumors to PD-1 blockade. *Science* **2017**, *357*, 409–413. [CrossRef]
47. Klempner, S.J.; Fabrizio, D.; Bane, S.; Reinhart, M.; Peoples, T.; Ali, S.M.; Sokol, E.S.; Frampton, G.; Schrock, A.B.; Anhorn, R.; et al. Tumor mutational burden as a predictive biomarker for response to immune checkpoint inhibitors: A review of current evidence. *Oncologist* **2019**. [CrossRef]
48. Sharma, P.; Hu-Lieskovan, S.; Wargo, J.A.; Ribas, A. Primary, adaptive, and acquired resistance to cancer immunotherapy. *Cell* **2017**, *168*, 707–723. [CrossRef]
49. Na, Z.; Yeo, S.P.; Bharath, S.R.; Bowler, M.W.; Balıkçı, E.; Wang, C.I.; Song, H. Structural basis for blocking PD-1-mediated immune suppression by therapeutic antibody pembrolizumab. *Cell Res.* **2017**, *27*, 147–150. [CrossRef]
50. Horita, S.; Nomura, Y.; Sato, Y.; Shimamura, T.; Iwata, S.; Nomura, N. High-resolution crystal structure of the therapeutic antibody pembrolizumab bound to the human PD-1. *Sci. Rep.* **2016**, *6*, 35297. [CrossRef]
51. Herbst, R.S.; Soria, J.C.; Kowanetz, M.; Fine, G.D.; Hamid, O.; Gordon, M.S.; Sosman, J.A.; McDermott, D.F.; Powderly, J.D.; Gettinger, S.N.; et al. Predictive correlates of response to the anti-PD-L1 antibody MPDL3280A in cancer patients. *Nature* **2014**, *515*, 563–567. [CrossRef] [PubMed]
52. Tan, S.; Liu, K.; Chai, Y.; Zhang, C.W.; Gao, S.; Gao, G.F.; Qi, J. Distinct PD-L1 binding characteristics of therapeutic monoclonal antibody durvalumab. *Protein Cell* **2018**, *9*, 135–139. [CrossRef] [PubMed]
53. Feng, Y.; Masson, E.; Dai, D.; Parker, S.M.; Berman, D.; Roy, A. Model-based clinical pharmacology profiling of ipilimumab in patients with advanced melanoma. *Br. J. Clin. Pharmacol.* **2014**, *78*, 106–117. [CrossRef] [PubMed]
54. Feng, Y.; Roy, A.; Masson, E.; Chen, T.T.; Humphrey, R.; Weber, J.S. Exposure-response relationships of the efficacy and safety of ipilimumab in patients with advanced melanoma. *Clin. Cancer Res.* **2013**, *19*, 3977–3986. [CrossRef]

55. Bertrand, A.; Kostine, M.; Barnetche, T.; Truchetet, M.E.; Schaeverbeke, T. Immune related adverse events associated with anti-CTLA-4 antibodies: Systematic review and meta-analysis. *BMC Med.* **2015**, *13*, 211. [CrossRef] [PubMed]
56. Elassaiss-Schaap, J.; Rossenu, S.; Lindauer, A.; Kang, S.P.; de Greef, R.; Sachs, J.R.; de Alwis, D.P. Using model-based "learn and confirm" to reveal the pharmacokinetics-pharmacodynamics relationship of pembrolizumab in the KEYNOTE-001 trial. *CPT Pharmacomet. Syst. Pharmacol.* **2017**, *6*, 21–28. [CrossRef]
57. Bajaj, G.; Wang, X.; Agrawal, S.; Gupta, M.; Roy, A.; Feng, Y. Model-Based population pharmacokinetic analysis of nivolumab in patients with solid tumors. *CPT Pharmacomet. Syst. Pharmacol.* **2017**, *6*, 58–66. [CrossRef]
58. Li, H.; Yu, J.; Liu, C.; Liu, J.; Subramaniam, S.; Zhao, H.; Blumenthal, G.M.; Turner, D.C.; Li, C.; Ahamadi, M.; et al. Time dependent pharmacokinetics of pembrolizumab in patients with solid tumor and its correlation with best overall response. *J. Pharmacokinet. Pharmacodyn.* **2017**, *44*, 403–414. [CrossRef]
59. Stroh, M.; Winter, H.; Marchand, M.; Claret, L.; Eppler, S.; Ruppel, J.; Abidoye, O.; Teng, S.L.; Lin, W.T.; Dayog, S.; et al. Clinical pharmacokinetics and pharmacodynamics of atezolizumab in metastatic urothelial carcinoma. *Clin. Pharmacol. Ther.* **2017**, *102*, 305–312. [CrossRef]
60. Wilkins, J.J.; Brockhaus, B.; Dai, H.; Vugmeyster, Y.; White, J.T.; Brar, S.; Bello, C.L.; Neuteboom, B.; Wade, J.R.; Girard, P.; et al. Time-Varying clearance and impact of disease state on the pharmacokinetics of avelumab in merkel cell carcinoma and urothelial carcinoma. *CPT Pharmacomet. Syst. Pharmacol.* **2019**, *8*, 415–427. [CrossRef]
61. Baverel, P.G.; Dubois, V.F.S.; Jin, C.Y.; Zheng, Y.; Song, X.; Jin, X.; Mukhopadhyay, P.; Gupta, A.; Dennis, P.A.; Ben, Y.; et al. Population pharmacokinetics of durvalumab in cancer patients and association with longitudinal biomarkers of disease status. *Clin. Pharmacol. Ther.* **2018**, *103*, 631–642. [CrossRef] [PubMed]
62. Freshwater, T.; Kondic, A.; Ahamadi, M.; Li, C.H.; de Greef, R.; de Alwis, D.; Stone, J.A. Evaluation of dosing strategy for pembrolizumab for oncology indications. *J. Immunother. Cancer* **2017**, *5*, 43. [CrossRef] [PubMed]
63. Long, G.V.; Tykodi, S.S.; Schneider, J.G.; Garbe, C.; Gravis, G.; Rashford, M.; Agrawal, S.; Grigoryeva, E.; Bello, A.; Roy, A.; et al. Assessment of nivolumab exposure and clinical safety of 480 mg every 4 weeks flat-dosing schedule in patients with cancer. *Ann. Oncol.* **2018**, *29*, 2208–2213. [CrossRef] [PubMed]
64. Zhao, X.; Suryawanshi, S.; Hruska, M.; Feng, Y.; Wang, X.; Shen, J.; Vezina, H.E.; McHenry, M.B.; Waxman, I.M.; Achanta, A.; et al. Assessment of nivolumab benefit-risk profile of a 240-mg flat dose relative to a 3-mg/kg dosing regimen in patients with advanced tumors. *Ann. Oncol.* **2017**, *28*, 2002–2008. [CrossRef]
65. Bi, Y.; Liu, J.; Furmanski, B.; Zhao, H.; Yu, J.; Osgood, C.; Ward, A.; Keegan, P.; Booth, B.P.; Rahman, A.; et al. Model-informed drug development approach supporting approval of the 4-week (Q4W) dosing schedule for nivolumab (Opdivo) across multiple indications: A regulatory perspective. *Ann. Oncol.* **2019**, *30*, 644–651. [CrossRef]
66. Agrawal, S.; Feng, Y.; Roy, A.; Kollia, G.; Lestini, B. Nivolumab dose selection: Challenges, opportunities, and lessons learned for cancer immunotherapy. *J. Immunother. Cancer* **2016**, *4*. [CrossRef]
67. De Lemos, M.L.; Kung, C.; Waignein, S. Efficacy of nivolumab four-weekly dosing schedule based on body weight. *J. Oncol. Pharm. Pract.* **2019**, *25*, 961–963. [CrossRef]
68. Novakovic, A.M.; Wilkins, J.J.; Dai, H.; Wade, J.R.; Neuteboom, B.; Brar, S.; Bello, C.L.; Girard, P.; Khandelwal, A. Changing body weight-based dosing to a flat dose for avelumab in metastatic Merkel cell and advanced urothelial carcinoma. *Clin. Pharmacol. Ther.* **2019**. [CrossRef]
69. Ogungbenro, K.; Patel, A.; Duncombe, R.; Nuttall, R.; Clark, J.; Lorigan, P. Dose rationalization of pembrolizumab and nivolumab using pharmacokinetic modeling and simulation and cost analysis. *Clin. Pharmacol. Ther.* **2018**, *103*, 582–590. [CrossRef]
70. Fessas, P.; Possamai, L.A.; Clark, J.; Daniels, E.; Gudd, C.; Mullish, B.H.; Alexander, J.L.; Pinato, D.J. Immunotoxicity from checkpoint inhibitor therapy: Clinical features and underlying mechanisms. *Immunology* **2019**. [CrossRef]
71. Khoja, L.; Day, D.; Wei-Wu Chen, T.; Siu, L.L.; Hansen, A.R. Tumour-and class-specific patterns of immune-related adverse events of immune checkpoint inhibitors: A systematic review. *Ann. Oncol.* **2017**, *28*, 2377–2385. [CrossRef] [PubMed]
72. Wolchok, J.D.; Chiarion-Sileni, V.; Gonzalez, R.; Rutkowski, P.; Grob, J.J.; Cowey, C.L.; Lao, C.D.; Wagstaff, J.; Schadendorf, D.; Ferrucci, P.F.; et al. Overall Survival with Combined Nivolumab and Ipilimumab in Advanced Melanoma. *N. Engl. J. Med.* **2017**, *377*, 1345–1356. [CrossRef] [PubMed]

73. Shivaji, U.N.; Jeffery, L.; Gui, X.; Smith, S.C.L.; Ahmad, O.F.; Akbar, A.; Ghosh, S.; Iacucci, M. Immune checkpoint inhibitor-associated gastrointestinal and hepatic adverse events and their management. *Ther. Adv. Gastroenterol.* **2019**, *12*. [CrossRef] [PubMed]
74. Simpson, T.R.; Li, F.; Montalvo-Ortiz, W.; Sepulveda, M.A.; Bergerhoff, K.; Arce, F.; Roddie, C.; Henry, J.Y.; Yagita, H.; Wolchok, J.D.; et al. Fc-dependent depletion of tumor-infiltrating regulatory T cells co-defines the efficacy of anti-CTLA-4 therapy against melanoma. *J. Exp. Med.* **2013**, *210*, 1695–1710. [CrossRef] [PubMed]
75. Arce-Vargas, F.; Furness, A.J.S.; Litchfield, K.; Joshi, K.; Rosenthal, R.; Ghorani, E.; Solomon, I.; Lesko, M.H.; Ruef, N.; Roddie, C.; et al. Fc Effector Function Contributes to the Activity of Human Anti-CTLA-4 Antibodies. *Cancer Cell* **2018**, *33*, 649–663. [CrossRef] [PubMed]
76. Korman, A.J.; Engelhardt, J.; Loffredo, J.; Valle, J.; Akter, R.; Vuyyuru, R.; Bezman, N.; So, P.; Graziano, R.; Tipton, K.; et al. *Abstract SY09-01: Next-Generation Anti-CTLA-4 Antibodies*; AACR: Philadelphia, PA, USA, 2017; Volume 77.
77. Pereira, N.A.; Chan, K.F.; Lin, P.C.; Song, Z. The "less-is-more" in therapeutic antibodies: Afucosylated anti-cancer antibodies with enhanced antibody-dependent cellular cytotoxicity. *MAbs* **2018**, *10*, 693–711. [CrossRef] [PubMed]
78. Price, K.D.; Simutis, F.; Fletcher, A.; Ramaiah, L.; Srour, R.; Kozlosky, J.; Sathish, J.; Engelhardt, J.; Capozzi, A.; Crona, J.; et al. *Abstract LB-B33: Nonclinical Safety Evaluation of Two Distinct Second Generation Variants of Anti-CTLA4 Monoclonal Antibody, Ipilimumab, in Monkeys*; AACR: Philadelphia, PA, USA, 2018; Volume 17.
79. Goletz, C.; Lischke, T.; Harnack, U.; Schiele, P.; Danielczyk, A.; Rühmann, J.; Goletz, S. Glyco-engineered anti-human programmed death-ligand 1 antibody mediates stronger CD8 T cell activation than its normal glycosylated and non-glycosylated counterparts. *Front. Immunol.* **2018**, *9*, 1614. [CrossRef]
80. Okada, M.; Chikuma, S.; Kondo, T.; Hibino, S.; Machiyama, H.; Yokosuka, T.; Nakano, M.; Yoshimura, A. Blockage of core fucosylation reduces cell-surface expression of PD-1 and promotes anti-tumor immune responses of T cells. *Cell Rep.* **2017**, *20*, 1017–1028. [CrossRef]
81. Wong, C.; Mei, L.; Wong, K.R.; Menendez, E.E.; Vasiljeva, O.; Richardson, J.H.; West, J.W.; Kavanaugh, M.; Irving, B.A. Abstract A081: A PD-L1-targeted Probody provides antitumor efficacy while minimizing induction of systemic autoimmunity. *Cancer Immunol. Res.* **2016**, *4*, A081. [CrossRef]
82. Autio, K.A.; Boni, V.; Humphrey, R.W.; Naing, A. Probody Therapeutics: An Emerging Class of Therapies Designed to Enhance On-target Effects with Reduced Off-tumor Toxicity for Use in Immuno-Oncology. *Clin. Cancer. Res.* **2019**. [CrossRef]
83. Fromm, G.; de Silva, S.; Johannes, K.; Patel, A.; Hornblower, J.C.; Schreiber, T.H. Agonist redirected checkpoint, PD1-Fc-OX40L, for cancer immunotherapy. *J. Immunother. Cancer* **2018**, *6*, 149. [CrossRef] [PubMed]
84. Kvarnhammar, A.M.; Veitonmaki, N.; Hagerbrand, K.; Smith, K.E.; Fritzell, S.; Johansson, M. The CTLA-4 x OX40 bispecific antibody ATOR-1015 induces anti-tumor effects through tumor-directed immune activation. *J. Immunother. Cancer* **2019**, *7*, 103. [CrossRef] [PubMed]
85. Lacey, D.L.; Boyle, W.J.; Simonet, W.S.; Kostenuik, P.J.; Dougall, W.C.; Sullivan, J.K.; San-Martin, J.; Dansey, R. Bench to bedside: Elucidation of the OPG-RANK-RANKL pathway and the development of denosumab. *Nat. Rev. Drug Discov.* **2012**, *11*, 401–419. [CrossRef] [PubMed]
86. Ahern, E.; Smyth, M.J.; Dougall, W.C.; Teng, M.W.L. Roles of the RANKL-RANK axis in antitumour immunity—Implications for therapy. *Nat. Rev. Clin. Oncol.* **2018**, *15*, 676–693. [CrossRef]
87. Dougall, W.C.; Roman Aguilera, A.; Smyth, M.J. Dual targeting of RANKL and PD-1 with a bispecific antibody improves anti-tumor immunity. *Clin. Transl. Immunol.* **2019**, *8*, e01081. [CrossRef]
88. Lan, Y.; Zhang, D.; Xu, C.; Hance, K.W.; Marelli, B.; Qi, J.; Yu, H.; Qin, G.; Sircar, A.; Hernández, V.M.; et al. Enhanced preclinical antitumor activity of M7824, a bifunctional fusion protein simultaneously targeting PD-L1 and TGF-beta. *Sci. Transl. Med.* **2018**, *10*, eaan5488. [CrossRef]
89. Knudson, K.M.; Hicks, K.C.; Luo, X.; Chen, J.Q.; Schlom, J.; Gameiro, S.R. M7824, a novel bifunctional anti-PD-L1/TGFbeta Trap fusion protein, promotes anti-tumor efficacy as monotherapy and in combination with vaccine. *Oncoimmunology* **2018**, *7*, e1426519. [CrossRef]
90. LaMotte-Mohs, R.; Shah, K.; Smith, D.; Gorlatov, S.; Ciccarone, V.; Tamura, J.; Li, H.; Smith, D.; Rillema, J.; Licea, M.; et al. Abstract 3217: MGD013, a bispecific PD-1 x LAG-3 Dual-Affinity Re-Targeting (DART®) protein with T-cell immunomodulatory activity for cancer treatment. *Cancer Res.* **2016**, *76*. [CrossRef]

91. Huang, R.Y.; Eppolito, C.; Lele, S.; Shrikant, P.; Matsuzaki, J.; Odunsi, K. LAG3 and PD1 co-inhibitory molecules collaborate to limit CD8+ T cell signaling and dampen antitumor immunity in a murine ovarian cancer model. *Oncotarget* **2015**, *6*, 27359–27377. [CrossRef]
92. US Patent Application, 2013. 2019. Available online: https://patentimages.storage.googleapis.com/8b/4d/30/d6e970eabaafe5/US20130022629A1.pdf (accessed on 20 November 2019).
93. United States Patent, 2017. 2019. Available online: https://patentimages.storage.googleapis.com/be/e6/87/848fb505a78c89/US9850225.pdf (accessed on 20 November 2019).
94. Zak, K.M.; Grudnik, P.; Guzik, K.; Zieba, B.J.; Musielak, B.; Dömling, A.; Holak, T.A. Structural basis for small molecule targeting of the programmed death ligand 1 (PD-L1). *Oncotarget* **2016**, *7*, 30323–30335. [CrossRef]
95. Incyte Corporation Heterocyclic Compounds as Immunomodulators United States Patent 2017. 2019. Available online: https://patentimages.storage.googleapis.com/71/16/5d/4faf7b71faf81b/WO2017087777A1.pdf (accessed on 20 November 2019).
96. Lazorchak, A.S.; Patterson, T.; Ding, Y.; Sasikumar, P.G.; Sudarshan, N.S.; Gowda, N.M.; Ramachandra, R.K.; Samiulla, D.S.; Giri, S.; Eswarappa, R.; et al. *Abstract A36: CA-170, An Oral Small Molecule PD-L1 and VISTA Immune Checkpoint Antagonist, Promotes T Cell Immune Activation and Inhibits Tumor Growth in Pre-Clinical Models of Cancer*; AACR: Philadelphia, PA, USA, 2017; Volume 5. [CrossRef]
97. Pharmacodynamic effects of CA-170, a First-in-Class Small Molecule Oral Immune Checkpoint Inhibitor (ICI) Dually Targeting V-Domain Ig Suppressor of T-cell Activation (VISTA) and PDL1. 2018. Available online: http://www.curis.com/images/stories/pdfs/posters/SITC2018CA-170RPD961.pdf (accessed on 12 August 2019).
98. Phase 2 trial of CA-170, a Novel Oral Small Molecule Dual Inhibitor of Immune Checkpoints VISTA and PD-1, in Patients with Advanced Solid Tumor and Hodgkin Lymphoma. Available online: http://www.curis.com/images/stories/pdfs/posters/SITC2018CA-170P714ASIAD.pdf (accessed on 12 August 2019).
99. Musielak, B.; Kocik, J.; Skalniak, L.; Magiera-Mularz, K.; Sala, D.; Czub, M.; Plewka, J. CA-170—A Potent Small-Molecule PD-L1 Inhibitor or Not? *Molecules* **2019**, *24*, 2804. [CrossRef] [PubMed]
100. Chang, H.N.; Liu, B.Y.; Qi, Y.K.; Zhou, Y.; Chen, Y.P.; Pan, K.M.; Qi, Y.M. Blocking of the PD-1/PD-L1 Interaction by a D-Peptide Antagonist for Cancer Immunotherapy. *Angew. Chem. Int. Ed.* **2015**, *54*, 11760–11764. [CrossRef] [PubMed]
101. Boohaker, R.J.; Sambandam, V.; Segura, I.; Miller, J.; Suto, M.; Xu, B. Rational design and development of a peptide inhibitor for the PD-1/PD-L1 interaction. *Cancer Lett.* **2018**, *434*, 11–21. [CrossRef] [PubMed]
102. Magiera-Mularz, K.; Skalniak, L.; Zak, K.M.; Musielak, B.; Rudzinska-Szostak, E.; Berlicki, Ł.; Shaabani, S. Bioactive Macrocyclic Inhibitors of the PD-1/PD-L1 Immune Checkpoint. *Angew. Chem. Int. Ed.* **2017**, *56*, 13732–13735. [CrossRef]
103. Li, C.; Zhang, N.; Zhou, J.; Ding, C.; Jin, Y.; Cui, X.; Zhu, Y. Peptide Blocking of PD-1/PD-L1 Interaction for Cancer Immunotherapy. *Cancer Immunol. Res.* **2018**, *6*, 178–188. [CrossRef]
104. AUNP-12—A Novel Peptide Therapeutic Targeting PD-1 Immune Checkpoint Pathway for Cancer Immunotherapy—Structure Activity Relationships & Peptide/Peptidomimetic Analogs. 2014. Available online: http://www.differding.com/page/aunp_12_a_novel_peptide_therapeutic_targeting_pd_1_immune_checkpoint_pathway_for_cancer_immunotherapy/f1.html (accessed on 14 August 2019).
105. Sasikumar, P.; Shrimali, R.; Adurthi, S.; Ramachandra, R.; Satyam, L.; Dhudashiya, A.; Ramachandra, M. A novel peptide therapeutic targeting PD1 immune checkpoint with equipotent antagonism of both ligands and a potential for better management of immune-related adverse events. *J. Immunother. Cancer* **2013**, *1*, 24. [CrossRef]
106. Sasikumar, P.G.; Ramachandra, R.K.; Adurthi, S.; Dhudashiya, A.A.; Vadlamani, S.; Vemula, K.; Vunnum, S.; Satyam, L.K.; Samiulla, D.S.; Subbarao, K.; et al. A Rationally Designed Peptide Antagonist of the PD-1 Signaling Pathway as an Immunomodulatory Agent for Cancer Therapy. *Mol. Cancer Ther.* **2019**, *18*, 1081–1091. [CrossRef]

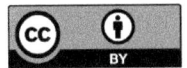

© 2019 by the authors. Licensee MDPI, Basel, Switzerland. This article is an open access article distributed under the terms and conditions of the Creative Commons Attribution (CC BY) license (http://creativecommons.org/licenses/by/4.0/).

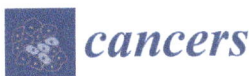

Review

Targeting Negative and Positive Immune Checkpoints with Monoclonal Antibodies in Therapy of Cancer

Katsiaryna Marhelava [1,2], Zofia Pilch [3], Malgorzata Bajor [1], Agnieszka Graczyk-Jarzynka [3] and Radoslaw Zagozdzon [1,4,5,*]

1. Department of Clinical Immunology, Medical University of Warsaw, Nowogrodzka 59 Street, 02-006 Warsaw, Poland; k.marhelava@gmail.com (K.M.); malgorzata.bajor@wum.edu.pl (M.B.)
2. Postgraduate School of Molecular Medicine, Medical University of Warsaw, Trojdena 2a Street, 02-091 Warsaw, Poland
3. Department of Immunology, Medical University of Warsaw, Nielubowicza 5 Street, 02-097 Warsaw, Poland; zofia.pilch@gmail.com (Z.P.); agnieszka.graczyk-jarzynka@wum.edu.pl (A.G.-J.)
4. Department of Immunology, Transplantology and Internal Diseases, Medical University of Warsaw, Nowogrodzka 59 Street, 02-006 Warsaw, Poland
5. Institute of Biochemistry and Biophysics, Polish Academy of Sciences, Pawinskiego 5A Street, 02-106 Warsaw, Poland
* Correspondence: radoslaw.zagozdzon@wum.edu.pl; Tel.: +48-(22)-502-14-72; Fax: +48-(22)-502-21-59

Received: 4 October 2019; Accepted: 6 November 2019; Published: 8 November 2019

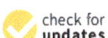

Abstract: The immune checkpoints are regulatory molecules that maintain immune homeostasis in physiological conditions. By sending T cells a series of co-stimulatory or co-inhibitory signals via receptors, immune checkpoints can both protect healthy tissues from adaptive immune response and activate lymphocytes to remove pathogens effectively. However, due to their mode of action, suppressive immune checkpoints may serve as unwanted protection for cancer cells. To restore the functioning of the immune system and make the patient's immune cells able to recognize and destroy tumors, monoclonal antibodies are broadly used in cancer immunotherapy to block the suppressive or to stimulate the positive immune checkpoints. In this review, we aim to present the current state of application of monoclonal antibodies in clinics, used either as single agents or in a combined treatment. We discuss the limitations of these therapies and possible problem-solving with combined treatment approaches involving both non-biological and biological agents. We also highlight the most promising strategies based on the use of monoclonal or bispecific antibodies targeted on immune checkpoints other than currently implemented in clinics.

Keywords: immune checkpoints; monoclonal antibodies; immunotherapy; tumor immunity; combination therapy

1. Introduction

Traditional therapy of disseminated cancer is usually based on systemic treatment with several types of chemotherapy, including molecularly targeted small molecules. However, these kinds of treatment are often not effective enough to defeat cancer due to certain limitations [1]. Even if cancer cells are initially sensitive to standard antitumor modalities, and a rapid diminishment of tumor mass occurs, the eventual recurrence of a refractory cancer is frequent. Importantly, in standard systemic anticancer treatment, the intratumor diversity of cancer cell phenotypes can be a major cause for tumor resistance to the chemotherapeutic agent(s), as some phenotypes can be much more resistant than others to a given therapy. It is exactly the opposite in case of active immunotherapy targeting immune checkpoint molecules with monoclonal antibodies, as the more different the cancer cell is from the host, the stronger immunogenicity it presents. That makes active immunotherapy unique in its concept, as described in detail below. The therapeutic use of the immune checkpoint molecules in cancer treatment has been initiated by targeting the negative checkpoints, but recently growing attention has been paid to the role of positive immune checkpoints as targets for anticancer therapies. This review aims to present the comprehensive look at the current clinical status of both types of therapeutic approaches, and also to describe the most promising recent developments in the field.

2. Immune Checkpoints

Properly functioning human immune system shields our body from pathogens and developing malignancies [2]. However, when overactive and/or malfunctioning, the immune system poses a severe and potentially lethal threat to the human body. Therefore, the activation of the immune system, including its effector cells, such as T lymphocytes and natural killer (NK) cells, is closely monitored. In the case of T lymphocytes, recognition by T cell receptor (TCR) of the specific antigen presented by the major histocompatibility complex (MHC) molecules provides the first signal for activation [3]. This signal stimulates the lymphocytes only briefly and requires co-stimulation, for example from a CD28 molecule recognizing its ligands (CD80 or CD86) on antigen-presenting cell (APC), to introduce T lymphocyte into full activation [4]. This process is additionally regulated by various cytokines acting on the T lymphocyte [5], as well as by the so-called immune checkpoints [6].

Immune checkpoint receptors are membrane molecules, located mainly, but not exclusively, on T lymphocytes and NK cells, which, after recognizing appropriate ligands on the antigen-presenting cells (APC) or the target cells, can play a negative (inhibitory, Figure 1A) or positive (stimulatory, Figure 2A) role in the process of the lymphocyte activation. Immune checkpoints can propagate inhibitory or stimulatory signals via interactions of the checkpoint molecules, i.e., ligands with their cognate receptors located on target and effector cells, respectively (Table 1). Under normal physiological conditions, immune checkpoints are crucial players in maintaining immune homeostasis and preventing autoimmunity [7]. When compared to a motorized vehicle, the TCR-elicited signal would be starting the engine for the T cell, while the negative or positive checkpoints would function as the brake or accelerator, respectively. Setting up the right balance between them is responsible for moving the immune system response into the right direction—tolerance or attack, depending on circumstances.

Table 1. Examples of suppressive (negative) and stimulatory (positive) immune checkpoint ligand–receptor pairs with cellular distribution of these molecules under physiological conditions.

Ligand	Cellular Distribution of the Ligand Expression	Immune Checkpoint Receptor	Cellular Expression of the Receptor Expression
Suppressive (negative) immune checkpoints			
CD80 or CD86	Antigen-presenting cells	CTLA4	Activated T cells, Tregs
PD-L1 (CD274) or PD-L2 (CD273)	DCs, macrophages, peripheral non-lymphoid tissues	PD-1	Activated B and T cells, APCs, NK cells
MHC class II/Lectins	Antigen-presenting cells	LAG3	Activated T cells, Tregs, NK cells, B cells, DCs
CD155/CD112	Normal epithelial, endothelial, neuronal, and fibroblastic cells	TIGIT	Activated T cells, Tregs, NK cells
Galectin 9/ PtdSer /HMGB1	Multiple tissues	TIM3	Activated T cells
VSIG-3	Neurons and glial cells	VISTA	Naïve and activated T cells
CEACAM1	T and NK cells	CEACAM1	Activated T and NK cells

Table 1. Cont.

Ligand	Cellular Distribution of the Ligand Expression	Immune Checkpoint Receptor	Cellular Expression of the Receptor Expression
Stimulatory (positive) immune checkpoints			
B7 molecules: CD80 or CD86	Antigen-presenting cells	CD28	T cells
OX40L	DCs, macrophages, B cells, endothelial cells, smooth muscle cells	OX40	Activated T cells, Tregs, NK cells, neutrophils
CD137L	Antigen-presenting cells	CD137 (4-1BB)	Activated Tcells, NK cells, B cells, DCs, endothelial cells
GITRL	Antigen-presenting cells and endothelium	GITR	T and NK cells, Tregs
ICOSLG	APCs, B cells, DCs and macrophages	ICOS	Naïve and activated T cells
CD70	Activated lymphocytes	CD27	Activated T and NK cells

Checkpoint receptors, such as cytotoxic T-lymphocyte-associated protein 4 (CTLA-4), programmed cell death protein 1 (PD-1), lymphocyte-activation gene 3 protein (LAG-3), T cell immunoglobulin and mucin 3 domain (TIM-3), T cell immunoreceptor with Ig and ITIM domains (TIGIT), and others, are immunosuppressive molecules, as they negatively regulate activation of the immune effector cells [8]. In cancer, these molecules are deemed responsible for immune exhaustion of the effector cells and downregulation of antitumor response [9].

Other checkpoint receptors such as glucocorticoid-induced TNFR-related protein (GITR), CD27, CD40, OX40, and CD137 (4-1BB), which are members of the tumor necrosis factor receptor (TNFR) superfamily, and also checkpoint receptors that belong to the B7-CD28 superfamily, i.e., CD28 itself and inducible T cell co-stimulator (ICOS), are co-stimulating the immune response [10]. Insufficient activity of these molecules in lymphocytes recognizing tumor-related antigens can be one of the causes of the ineffective anticancer immune response. In general, after acquiring the knowledge on the mechanisms of actions of negative and positive immune checkpoints, two main concepts dominate the area of therapies targeting immune checkpoints with monoclonal antibodies. The first is an inhibition (blockade) of negative immune checkpoints with antagonistic antibodies (Figure 1B) and the second is stimulating the positive immune checkpoints with agonistic antibodies (Figure 2B).

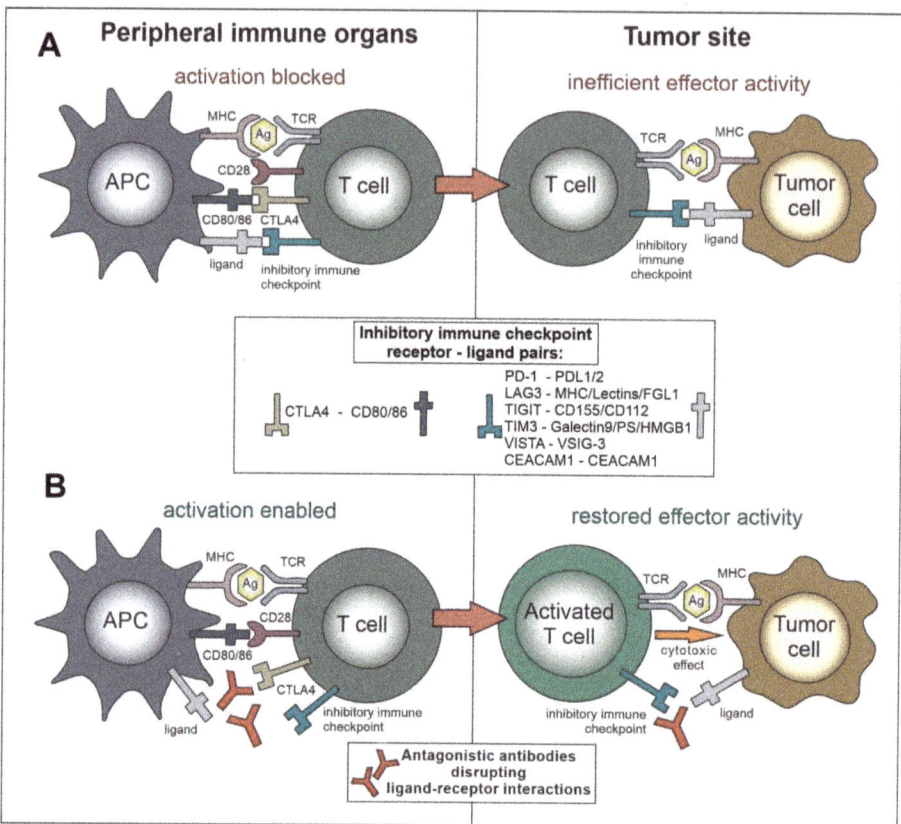

Figure 1. Targeting the negative immune checkpoints with monoclonal antibodies. (**A**) The mechanism of actions of negative immune checkpoints on the example of a T cell. CTLA-4 binds to CD80 and CD86 receptors on the antigen-presenting cells (APCs), outcompeting immuno-stimulatory CD28 binding, and thus dampening the T cell receptor (TCR) signaling. Additionally, some other ligands for inhibitory immune checkpoints on immune cells may be expressed on APCs, and most of them can be overexpressed on tumor cells and/or in tumor microenvironment. Interactions between inhibitory immune checkpoints and their ligands block the activation of immune effector cells and prevent their cytotoxic response towards tumor cells. (**B**) Application of antibodies antagonistic towards the negative immune checkpoint receptors and/or their ligands enables CD80/86 and CD28 immuno-stimulatory signaling and blocks immuno-inhibitory signaling through other negative immune checkpoints. Activated T cells can become capable of overcoming the regulatory mechanisms and elimination of the tumor cells.

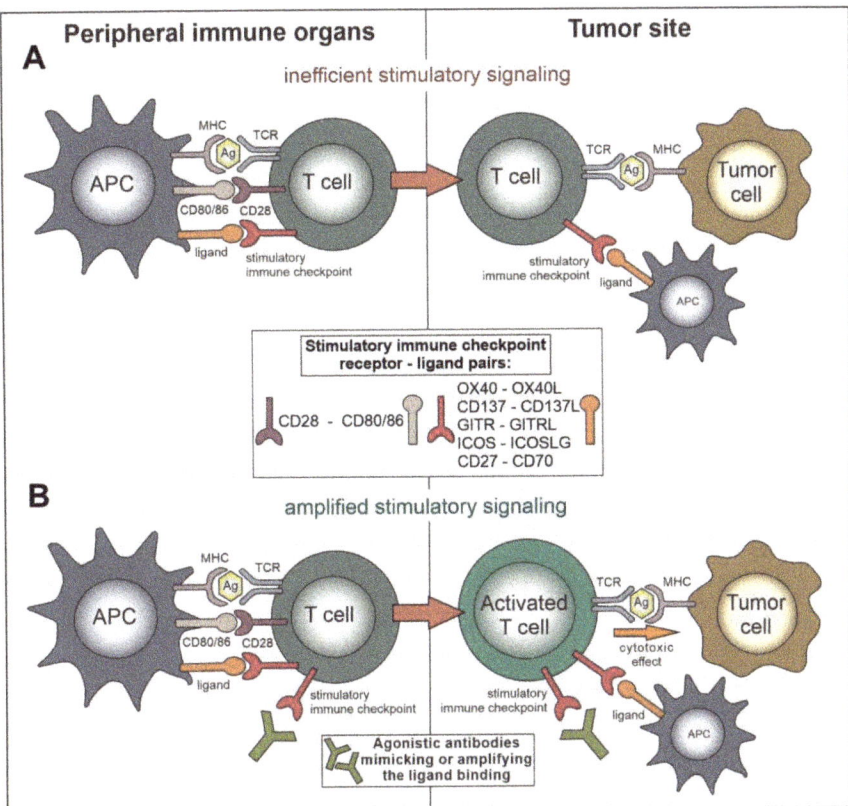

Figure 2. Targeting the positive immune checkpoints with monoclonal antibodies. (**A**) The mechanism of stimulation of a T cell effector function via positive immune checkpoints. The interaction of CD28 with its ligands, CD80 or CD86, follows TCR signaling and co-stimulates immune cell activation. Some of the other stimulatory immune checkpoints may also provide a co-stimulatory signal, but most of them start being expressed on already activated immune cells. In advanced cancer, this positive signaling is, however, often insufficient for eliminating the malignant cells. (**B**) Application of agonistic antibodies mimicking or amplifying binding of the ligands for stimulatory immune checkpoints increases effector activity of T cells towards tumor cells with prospective elimination of cancer cells.

3. Inhibition of Negative Immune Checkpoints in Cancer

3.1. Role of "Classical" Immune Checkpoints—CTLA-4 and PD-L1/PD-1 in Cancer—Early Studies

Discovered in 1987, CTLA-4, is usually referred to as the "classical T cell inhibitory receptor" [11]. The mechanism underlying its immune inhibitory function relies mainly on the competition of CTLA-4 and CD28 in binding to the same ligands—CD80 and CD86 [11]. It is known that high levels of CTLA-4 correlate with reduced activation of T cells primarily in lymph nodes, but also in peripheral tissues and that CTLA-4 expression on T regulatory cells (Tregs) has been shown to be crucial for systemic tolerance [12]. Moreover, it was observed, that *Ctla-4* knockout mice suffer from an expansion of autoreactive and hyperproliferative lymphocytes that eventually take a toll leading to their premature death at the age of 2–3 weeks [13].

Allison et al. have investigated the importance of CTLA-4 signaling in cancer [14]. They revealed that in vivo administration of blocking monoclonal antibodies against CTLA-4 induced tumor rejection and, more importantly, led to the immunity to secondary exposure to tumor cells. This study provided evidence that blockade of CTLA-4 and, therefore, its suppressive activity can enable and potentiate effective immune response against cancer cells in the "brake-off" mechanism [14]. After initial preclinical proof-of-concept studies, in 2000, this strategy was evaluated in patients with advanced cancers. Two fully human CTLA-4–blocking antibodies (ipilimumab and tremelimumab) were used in the first clinical trials [15]. Out of these two antibodies, only ipilimumab received Food and Drug Administration (FDA) approval as the first immune checkpoint inhibitor in cancer treatment in 2011.

Similar to CTLA-4, the role of another "classical" immune checkpoint receptor, i.e., PD-1 in controlling immune tolerance was presented by generating knockout mice [16] by the group of Honjo et al., although the autoimmunity they developed was less severe as compared to CTLA-4 knockout mice. PD-1 expression can be induced on activated B and T cells. Its ligands, programmed death receptor ligand 1 and ligand 2 (PD-L1 and PD-L2), are constitutively expressed at moderate levels in several non-lymphoid tissues, such as heart and lung, with placenta being the most pronounced site for PD-L1 expression [17], but they can also be markedly induced by inflammatory signals in a number of cell types. Thus, the PD-1/PD-L1 axis inhibits T cell activity mostly in the periphery [18].

PD-L1/PD-1 signaling pathway was first linked to tumor immunity in 2002 [19]. Indeed, the overexpression of PD-L1 causes the inhibition of T cell cytolytic activity and thus promoted tumorigenesis, as the effect can be reversed by applying anti-PD-L1 monoclonal antibodies [20]. Several factors can lead to the persistent expression of PD-L1 and/or PD-L2 on tumor cells by, for instance, upregulation by cytokines, chromosomal copy gain [21], disruptions of the PD-L1 3'-untranslated region [22], aberrant activity of pathways mediated by phosphoinositide 3-kinase (PI3K) and protein kinase B (PKB, AKT), epidermal growth factor receptor (EGFR), cyclin-dependent kinase 5 (CDK5), and Janus kinase 2 (JAK2) [21,23], MYC overexpression [24], and viral proteins, e.g., Epstein–Barr virus latent membrane protein 1 (EBV LMP1) [25]. The expression of immunosuppressive PD-L1 molecule can also be induced on other cells presented in the tumor microenvironment (TME), such as endothelial cells, stromal cells, APC, and T cells [26]. Moreover, tumor antigen presentation and TCR triggering are accompanied by interferon-γ (IFN-γ) production, which is a potent stimulator of reactive PD-L1 expression [18]. Therefore, antitumor T cells can be exposed to continuous PD-L1/PD-1 signaling. It causes their exhaustion and inhibits the antitumor cytotoxic T cell response, which can be reversed by anti-PD1/anti-PD-L1 monoclonal antibodies [20].

Currently, the FDA has approved seven monoclonal antibodies targeting classical inhibitory immune checkpoints for the clinical treatment of patients with numerous cancer types: ipilimumab targeting CTLA-4 pathway, and six antibodies targeting PD-L/PD-L1 axis, including atezolizumab, avelumab, durvalumab, nivolumab, cemiplimab, and pembrolizumab. The FDA approval status for each of these antibodies in various cancer types is summarized in Table 2.

Table 2. The list of Food and Drug Administration (FDA)-approved monoclonal antibodies acting as inhibitors of negative checkpoints in human cancer [27].

Checkpoint Inhibitor	Antibody Format	Examples of Types of Cancers with FDA-Approved Use	Year of First Approval
Ipilimumab	Human anti-CTLA4 IgG1	Melanoma, renal cell carcinoma, metastatic colorectal cancer	2011
Pembrolizumab	Humanized anti-PD-1 IgG4	Melanoma, non-small-cell lung cancer, renal cell carcinoma, urothelial bladder cancer, Hodgkin lymphoma, head and neck cancer, Merkel cell carcinoma, microsatellite instability-high cancer, gastric cancer, hepatocellular carcinoma, cervical cancer, primary mediastinal large B-cell lymphoma	2014

Table 2. Cont.

Checkpoint Inhibitor	Antibody Format	Examples of Types of Cancers with FDA-Approved Use	Year of First Approval
Nivolumab	Human anti-PD-1 IgG4	Melanoma, non-small-cell lung cancer, renal cell carcinoma, urothelial bladder cancer, Hodgkin lymphoma, head and neck cancer, colorectal cancer, hepatocellular carcinoma, small cell lung cancer	2014
Atezolizumab	Humanized anti-PD-L1 IgG1	Non-small-cell lung cancer, urothelial bladder cancer, small cell lung cancer, breast cancer	2016
Avelumab	Human anti-PD-L1 IgG1	Merkel cell carcinoma, urothelial bladder cancer	2017
Durvalumab	Human anti-PD-L1 IgG1	Non-small-cell lung cancer, urothelial bladder cancer	2017
Cemiplimab	Human anti-PD-1 IgG4	Cutaneous squamous-cell carcinoma	2018

3.2. Formats of the Anti-Immune Checkpoint Antibodies

The FDA-approved antibodies targeting checkpoints are all the full-size monoclonal antibodies, either human (ipilimubab, nivolumab, avelumab, durvalumab, and cemiplimab) or humanized (pembrolizumab and atezolizumab) of IgG1 or IgG4 subclass (Table 2). All of these antibodies have low or markedly reduced binding to C1q in order to avoid complement-dependent cytotoxicity (CDC) and most of them present reduced binding to Fc receptors in order to diminish the antibody-dependent cellular cytotoxicity (ADCC) (reviewed in [28]). The only exception is avelumab, which is capable of inducing ADCC effect [29]. In experimental settings or early clinical studies, a whole new format of anti-immune checkpoint molecules are the bispecific antibodies (reviewed in [30]), which are described in Section 5 below. Lastly, the antibody-drug conjugate (i.e., anti-PD-L1-doxorubicin) format has also been attempted in preclinical settings [31].

3.3. Clinical Application of Anti-CTLA-4, Anti-PD-1 and Anti-PD-L1 Antibodies

Several biomarkers are used to identify patients more likely to respond to CTLA-4 or PD-1/PD-L1 blockade as well as other immunotherapeutics [32]. PD-L1 expression is evaluated as one of them, though it has some limitations. Across all tumor types, patients with PD-L1-negative tumors respond to anti-PD-1/PD-L1 therapy in 0% to 17%, while those with PD-L1-positive tumors exhibit a response rate from 36% to 100% [33]. However, there is no precise definition of what level of PD-L1 expression is to be considered as positive. Additionally, different detection methods are used and, therefore, standardization is limited. Furthermore, nonmalignant cells within the tumor microenvironment (TME) also can express PD-L1. Thus, several other candidate predictive biomarkers were studied, among them, clinical-pathologic factors, gene and phenotypic alterations, tumor microenvironment, and immune effector cells [34]. The total number of mutations per coding area of a tumor genome, i.e., tumor mutational burden (TMB), turned out to be a promising biomarker for immunotherapies [35]. Higher TMB favors positive response to PD-1/PD-L1 blockade in several types of tumors, e.g., non-small cell lung carcinoma (NSCLC) [36].

It is essential to mention that targeting CTLA-4 and the PD-L1/PD-1 axis simultaneously in cancer patients has produced synergistic effects in numerous cases. Therefore, combinations of ipilimumab with, for instance, nivolumab, have been approved in several types of cancer [37].

3.4. Recent Developments in the Application of Anti-CTLA-4 Antibodies

There is also an ongoing study (NCT03860272) on an improved version of the anti-CTLA-4 monoclonal antibody, AGEN1181, that harbors an engineered Fc domain that increases the stability and half-life of the antibody. This Phase 1 study enrolls patients with refractory, advanced cancer (solid tumors) regardless of diagnosis and prior therapies.

One of the studies has also reported an anti-CTLA-4 antibody that is preferentially released within the tumor microenvironment. Specifically, the CTLA-4 dual variable domain Ig (anti-CTLA-4 DVD) was designed to have the inner CTLA-4-binding domain shielded by an outer tumor-targeting anti-prostate stem cell antigen (PSCA) domain. Once cleaved in the TME, the shield exposes the inner CTLA-4-binding site. The targeted release of anti-CTLA-4 within tumors was found to deplete tumor Tregs, without affecting tissue-resident Tregs, thus not inhibiting their antitumor activities [38].

3.5. Adverse Effects of Immune Checkpoint Inhibition

The grand proportion of patients treated with immune checkpoint inhibitors have experienced drug-induced immune-related adverse events (irAEs). The toxicity of the anti-CTLA-4 antibody was low in most cases, but some patients also experienced severe and life-threatening irAEs [39]. Generally, irAEs are more likely to appear in patients treated with anti-CTLA-4 (60–85%) than anti-PD-1 (16–37%), or anti-PD-L1 (12–24%). However, when the combination of anti-CTLA-4 and anti-PD-1 or anti-PD-L1 was applied, the frequency and severity of irAEs were higher compared to single-agent treatment—up to 60% of patients on combined therapy develop severe side effects that can include autoimmune inflammation in the nervous system [40] and heart [41]. Some studies reported that the frequency may be even higher and appear in even 91% of patients [42]. The most common irAEs include rash, colitis, hepatitis, endocrinopathies, and pneumonitis [43]. Neutrophilic dermatoses are another often an adverse effect of checkpoint inhibitors [44,45]. The management of checkpoint inhibition-induced irAE usually bases on immunosuppression with corticosteroids or other immunosuppressant agents [43].

3.6. Combination Therapies Using Checkpoint Inhibitors

In general, the fundamental problem with the application of immune checkpoint inhibitors is that the presence of T cells in the tumor site is a limiting factor. The lack of effector T cells within the tumor borders makes the elimination of cancer cells via the immune "brake-off" mechanism nearly impossible [46]. Another issue related to the adaptation of cancer cells is checkpoint inhibition by amplification of other negative checkpoint molecules in order to keep the exhausted phenotype of tumor-infiltrating lymphocytes (TILs). The latter phenomenon is being addressed by the application of antibodies inhibiting additional negative checkpoints, as discussed further on.

The problem of initially non-existent tumor infiltrates can be solved by increasing the immunogenicity of the tumor cells, e.g., by induction of the immunogenic cell death by cytotoxic or immuno-stimulatory approaches, or by using the molecularly targeted therapies. Indeed, in order to improve the safety and efficiency of therapies based on immune checkpoint blockade, several combinations are now tested both with non-biological and biological agents. The examples are combined interventions with non-biological approaches are surgery [47], radiation therapy [48], chemotherapy [49], and potentially targeted therapies as well [50]. There is also a substantial number of biological agents for combinatory treatment with immune checkpoint inhibitors either in preclinical or clinical settings, e.g., other therapeutic monoclonal antibodies (NCT02914405), therapeutic vaccines [51], natural or synthetic cytokines [52], anti-cytokine antibodies (NCT03111992), oncolytic virotherapy [53], or immune effector cells used in adoptive therapies [54]. The last one is especially interesting, as the use of lymphocytes guided with natural or synthetic tumor antigen-specific receptors can overcome the problem of non-existent immune cell infiltrates in the tumor. Conversely, as the surrounding microenvironment of solid tumors can use negative checkpoint molecules to hamper the effectiveness of CAR (chimeric antigen receptor)-T-based therapies, the addition of checkpoint blockade can significantly improve the efficacy of adoptive approaches [55,56]. Indeed, several clinical trials of this manner are being currently conducted (e.g., NCT03726515, NCT04003649).

3.7. Antibodies Against Novel Negative Checkpoints

Due to several limitations that appear in therapies based on the use of the anti-CTLA-4, PD-1, or PD-L1 monoclonal antibodies, both as monotherapy or in combination regimens, the additional co-inhibitory pathways are intensively investigated as novel pharmacological targets. Next-generation monoclonal antibodies targeting alternative immune checkpoints in the tumor microenvironment are being explored in clinical trials (reviewed in [57]). The overview of the new target candidates for immune checkpoint inhibition along with the specific antibodies and example clinical trials are presented in Table 3.

Table 3. Inhibitory and stimulatory immune checkpoint molecules with respective anti-receptor antagonistic antibodies and examples of clinical trials.

Receptor	Antagonistic Compounds	Example Clinical Trials (Phase)	Comments
		Inhibitory immune checkpoint molecules	
LAG-3	MGD013 (Anti-PD-1, anti-LAG-3 dual checkpoint inhibitor)	NCT04082364 (Phase 2/3)	HER2-positive gastric cancer or gastroesophageal junction cancer to determine the efficacy of margetuximab combined with anti-HER2 monoclonal antibody and margetuximab combined with anti-HER2 monoclonal antibody or MGD013 and chemotherapy compared to trastuzumab combined with chemotherapy (Cohort B)
	Relatlimab (BMS-986016)	NCT01968109 (Phase 1)	Administered alone and in combination with nivolumab in patients with solid tumors: non-small cell lung cancer, gastric cancer, hepatocellular carcinoma, renal cell carcinoma, bladder cancer, squamous cell carcinoma of the head and neck, and melanoma.
TIGIT	BGB-A1217	NCT04047862 (Phase 2)	Evaluation of anti-tumor effect of BGB-A1217 in combination with tislelizumab in patients with advanced solid tumors.
	BMS-986207	NCT02913313 (Phase 1/2a)	Advanced or spread solid cancers. Administered alone and in combination with nivolumab
TIM-3 (HAVcr2)	Sym023	NCT03489343 (Phase 1)	As a monotherapy in patients with locally advanced/unresectable or metastatic solid tumor malignancies or lymphomas
	TSR-022	NCT02817633 (Phase 1)	As a monotherapy and in combination with an anti-PD-1 antibody and/or an anti-LAG-3 antibody, in patients with advanced solid tumors
	MBG453	NCT03961971 (Phase 1)	MBG453 with stereotactic radiosurgery and spartalizumab in treating patients with recurrent glioblastoma multiforme
		NCT03066648 (Phase 1)	As a monotherapy and in combination with an anti-PD-1 antibody (PDR001) and/or Decitabine in acute myeloid leukemia and high risk myelodysplastic syndromes patients
VISTA	JNJ-61610588	NCT02671955 (Phase 1)	Evaluation the safety and tolerability of JNJ-61610588 in participants with advanced cancer—study terminated.
CEACAM1	CM-24 (MK-6018)	NCT02346955	Advanced or recurrent malignancies, administered as monotherapy or in combination with pembrolizumab—study terminated.

Table 3. Cont.

Receptor	Antagonistic Compounds	Example Clinical Trials (Phase)	Comments
Stimulatory immune checkpoint molecules			
CD28	Theralizumab (TAB08)	NCT03006029 (Phase 1)	Metastatic or unresectable advanced solid malignancies
OX40 (CD134)	BMS 986178	NCT03831295 (Phase 1)	Advanced solid malignancies, combination with TLR9 agonist SD-101
	MEDI6469	NCT02274155 (Phase 1)	Head and neck squamous cell carcinoma
	PF-04518600	NCT03971409 (Phase 2)	Triple negative breast cancer, combination with nivolumab
	GSK3174998	NCT02528357 (Phase 1)	Advanced solid tumors, combination with pembrolizumab
	MOXR0916	NCT02219724 (Phase 1)	Locally advanced or metastatic solid tumors
4-1BB (CD137)	Utomilumab (PF-05082566)	NCT03364348 (Phase 1)	Advanced HER2-positive breast cancer, combination with trastuzumab
		NCT02179918 (Phase 1)	Advanced solid tumors, combination with PD-1 inhibitor MK-3475
	Urelumab (BMS-663513) ES101	NCT02534506 (Phase 1)	Advanced malignancies, alone or in combination with nivolumab
		NCT04009460 (Phase 1)	Advanced solid tumors, anti-PD-L1/4-1BB bispecific antibody
GITRL	BMS-986156	NCT02598960 (Phase 1/2)	Advanced solid tumors, alone or with nivolumab
	TRX-518	NCT01239134 (Phase 1)	Solid malignancies
		NCT02628574 (Phase 1)	Advanced solid tumors, in combination with gemcitabine, pembrolizumab, or nivolumab
	AMG 228	NCT02437916 (Phase 1)	Advanced solid tumors
ICOSLG, (CD275)	JTX-2011	NCT02904226 (Phase 1/2)	Advanced solid malignancies, alone or in combination with nivolumab
	GSK3359609	NCT02723955 (Phase 1)	Advanced solid tumors, alone or in combination with pembrolizumab
	BMS-986226	NCT03251924 (Phase 1/2)	Advanced solid tumors, alone or in combination with nivolumab or ipilimumab
	MEDI-570	NCT02520791 (Phase 1)	T-cell lymphomas, antagonistic antibody
CD27	Varlilumab (CDX-1127)	NCT04081688 (Phase 1) NCT02335918 (Phase 1/2)	Non-small cell lung carcinoma, combination with atezolizumab and radiation therapy Five types of solid tumors, combination with nivolumab

LAG-3 is a negative checkpoint receptor that effectively suppresses T cells activation and cytokines secretion, thereby maintaining immune homeostasis [58]. LAG-3 is expressed primarily on activated effector T cells and Tregs, but also other types of immune cells. The precise molecular mechanisms for inhibitory LAG-3 signaling remain unclear. MHC II is considered to be a canonical ligand for LAG-3, however there is a lack of direct evidence for the protein–protein interaction between these two molecules. Recent studies have reported that fibrinogen-like protein 1 (FGL1) may be a major functional ligand of LAG-3, especially on target cells. The expression levels of both FGL1 mRNA and protein are limited to the liver and pancreas in normal conditions, but has been shown to be upregulated in human solid tumors including lung cancer, prostate cancer, melanoma, and colorectal cancer compared to normal tissues [59]. What is apparent, however, is that LAG-3 shows a strong synergy with PD-1 in multiple settings [60]. Indeed, it was observed that dual LAG-3/PD-1 blockade has a much more significant result on resolving the issue of T cell exhaustion, as compared to only LAG-3 blockade. Moreover, tumor growth was more likely to be reduced in both LAG-3- and PD-1-deficient mice, that when the single knockout of one of these molecules was performed [61]. A similar effect was observed in models of colon adenocarcinoma, fibrosarcoma, ovarian tumors, melanomas, lymphomas, and multiple myelomas, where the mice were treated with one antibody or with combination targeting LAG-3/PD-1 compounds. In all these in vivo studies, increased survival and tumor regression appeared mainly due to the restored $CD8^+$ T cell function and increased cytokine production. Additionally, the blockade of LAG-3 on $CD4^+$ T cells increased their production of interleukin (IL)-2, IL-4, IFN-γ and tumor necrosis factor-alpha (TNF-α) [62]. There are currently several LAG-3-modulating treatments tested in different phases of clinical trials (e.g., NCT03489369, NCT02658981, NCT03311412, NCT03662659). Importantly, the combination of anti-LAG-3 (BMS-986016) and anti-PD-1 (nivolumab) antibodies has been shown to be effective in melanoma patients resistant to anti-PD-1/PD-L1 therapy [63], and is currently being tested in other tumor types (NCT04082364, NCT01968109).

TIGIT is an inhibitory checkpoint receptor that has a role resembling the PD-1/PD-L1-mediated signal in tumor immunity and is upregulated in many types of cancers [64,65]. TIGIT is expressed in both NK cells and T cells (activated, memory, and regulatory) and has a role in their activation and maturation, among others by inducing the generation of mature immuno-regulatory dendritic cells [66]. TIGIT binds as a competitor to the same set of ligands as the CD226 (DNAM-1) receptor: CD155 (poliovirus receptor, PVR) with high affinity and CD112 (Nectin-2 or poliovirus receptor-related 2, PVRL2) with lower affinity [66]. Anti-TIGIT antibodies (e.g., BGB-A1217 and BMS-986207) were shown to act synergistically with inhibition of the anti-PD-1/PD-L1 axis in pre-clinical models [67] and are currently being tested in clinical trials in patients with advanced solid tumors (NCT04047862, NCT02913313).

TIM3 (also known as Hepatitis A Virus Cellular Receptor 2, HAVCR2) also contributes to immune tolerance by providing negative regulation of lymphocyte activation [68]. It is expressed on multiple immune cells, including conventional T cells (activated, memory, and exhausted), Tregs, and innate immune cells [69]. In cancer, chronic stimulation induces TIM3 upregulation in tumor antigen-specific T lymphocytes, especially in $CD8^+$ TILs, and, at the same time, peripheral T cells show minimal TIM3 expression. Similar to the PD-1/PD-L1 axis, TIM3 plays a role in T cell exhaustion during chronic immune stimulation [70], and especially in trimming the Th1-type immune responses [69]. Blocking the TIM3 pathway stimulates tumor antigen-specific T cell proliferation and cytotoxic functions, inhibits the activity of Tregs [71], and decreases the presence of myeloid-derived suppressor cells (MDSCs) in tumors [72]. The inhibition of TIM3 by mAbs is currently evaluated in at least 10 ongoing Phase 1 clinical trials, as a single blockade, with combination strategies (as presented in Table 2), or with bispecific antibodies (e.g., NCT03708328 with RO7121661 compound or NCT03752177 with LY3415244).

What is of importance for generation of anti-TIM3 antibodies for immunomodulatory purposes is the fact that at least several different surface molecules have been presented as ligands for TIM3, including galectin-9, phosphatidylserine (PtdSer), high mobility group protein 1 (HMGB1), and perhaps the carcinoembryonic antigen-related cell adhesion molecule 1 (CEACAM1) [73]. These ligands bind to the extracellular portion of the TIM3 molecule at distinct sites. Thus, the question arises which of the TIM-3 epitopes should be targeted by monoclonal antibodies in order to disrupt specific binding of the ligand(s) responsible for the immunosuppressive actions of this receptor. The study by Sabatos-Peyton et al. suggested that targeting the PtdSer and CEACAM1 binding sites is a shared property of anti-TIM-3 antibodies with demonstrated immunomodulatory functions [73]; however, this topic needs further research. An additional argument for the importance of anti-TIM3 antibodies was given by recent studies on a mouse model of lung adenocarcinoma. It was observed that mice and also some patients, who develop adaptive resistance to anti-PD-1 treatment after an initial response, may show a TIM-3 upregulation. Using anti-TIM3 antibodies in these cases can contribute to improved efficacy of the treatment [74].

Targeting negative checkpoints with monoclonal antibodies does not always lead to noticeable beneficial effects in humans, despite promising results in preclinical models, and examples of such developmental paths are V-domain Ig suppressor of T cell activation (VISTA) and CEACAM1 checkpoint receptors, as described below.

VISTA is a membrane receptor constitutively expressed on the immune cells, primarily in myeloid cells, but also detected in T cells and to some extent in NK cells [75]. VISTA presence is more pronounced on the surface of tumor infiltrating myeloid cells and on Tregs within the tumor mass as compared to those in the peripheral tissues [76]. In mouse models, it has been shown that blocking VISTA with monoclonal antibodies decreases MDSCs infiltration in tumors, and in parallel, it increases the presence of immune effector infiltrates. VISTA can also be expressed by tumor cells and induce regulation of T cell function [77] and anti-VISTA antibody had positive effects on the survival of tumor-bearing mice [77]. Therefore, the anti-VISTA antibody (Onvatilimab, JNJ-61610588) was introduced into the Phase 1 clinical trial in 2016 (NCT02671955), but the study was terminated due to the manufacturer's decision. Despite that, VISTA remains in the focus of cancer studies, as VISTA expressed on intratumor CD68-positive in pancreatic cancer has recently been indicated as an important role player the resistance of these tumors to immune checkpoint inhibitors [78].

CEACAM1 is another recently characterized immune checkpoint. CEACAM1 is expressed at high levels on T cells activated by stimulation with IL-2 or anti-CD3 antibodies or activated NK cells, but also can be expressed on tumor cells and act in homophylic interactions with CEACAM1 on the immune cells [79]. CEACAM1-L, the dominant isoform expressed in most T cells and NK cells, acts as an inhibitory receptor downregulating activation of these cells, e.g., in malignant melanoma [80]. In early preclinical settings, anti-CEACAM1 antibody (CC1) combined with anti-TIM3 intervention generated a robust therapeutic efficacy in mouse intracranial glioma model [81]. Also, CM-24 (MK-6018), a humanized anti-CEACAM1 IgG4 antibody, was demonstrated to increase the cytotoxic activity of lymphocytes against cancer cells in various in vitro and in vivo models [82]. A first clinical trial utilizing CM-24 was initiated in 2015 (NCT02346955) either with CM-24 administered alone or in combination with pembrolizumab, but the study was terminated in 2017, as no efficacy was observed. Subsequently, the anti-mouse CEACAM1 antibody (CC1) has been shown to induce no or minimal antitumor effects in vivo, as a monotherapy or in combination with anti-PD-1 treatment in three mouse models of solid tumors [83]. Interestingly, however, the significant efficacy of another CEACAM1-targeting antibody (MG1124) has recently been reported in combination with pembrolizumab in humanized mice xenografted with human lung cancer cells [84]. The current view is that CEACAM1 plays a multifaceted role as a checkpoint molecule in the human immune system, with either positive or negative effects depending on the circumstances, which might be attributed to the occurrence of various splicing forms of this molecule [85].

4. Application of Agonistic Compounds towards Positive Immune Checkpoints in Cancer

The counterbalance for negative immune checkpoints are the stimulatory (positive) checkpoint molecules, also acting mostly in a ligand-receptor manner. Here, the approach in cancer treatment is to use agonistic antibodies that increase signaling from the stimulatory immune checkpoints and thus positively regulate activation of the immune system against cancer (Figure 2). Although, in theory, this is just an opposite intervention as compared to the negative checkpoint blockade, there is a fundamental difference between these two kinds of approaches. Specifically, while the beneficial effects of inhibiting a negative checkpoint can be seen only if this particular checkpoint is used by the tumor to evade the immune system, the activation of a positive immune checkpoint should be stimulating lymphocytes more broadly, regardless of the particular defenses raised by the tumor. This notion is of importance in the stimulatory approach, as it provides broader universality of treatment, but also a higher risk of adverse effects.

The latter phenomenon has been a reason for a spectacular failure of a treatment attempt with an antibody activating the CD28 molecule, the most powerful of the stimulatory immune checkpoints on T lymphocytes. The interaction of CD28 with its cognate ligands, CD80 or CD86, provides the so-called "the second signal" for activation of the T lymphocyte following the recognition by TCR of specific MHC-antigen complex. The agonistic antibody binding to this receptor, theralizumab (also known as TGN1412, CD28-SuperMAB, or TAB08) was initially designed to treat B cell chronic lymphocytic leukemia (B-CLL) [86]. It was found safe in preclinical studies and, therefore, applied to six trial participants in Phase 1 clinical trial in 2006. Unexpectedly, in all cases, theralizumab induced a severe cytokine release syndrome with a high proportion of multiple organ failure [87]. This incident caused the temporary withdrawal of this anti-CD28 agonistic antibody from further studies in humans and led to a revision of European guidelines for first-in-man phase-1 clinical trials for biologic agents [88]. Despite the initial failure of theralizumab, the Phase 1 trial in patients with advanced neoplasms was initiated in December 2016 (NCT03006029) and is ongoing.

Other positive immune checkpoints are also seen as promising targets in anticancer treatment. The list of the clinical trials with the respective agonistic compound are presented in Table 2. The main difference between CD28 and other stimulatory receptors is that CD28 is present on naïve T cells, while the rest are being expressed mostly following stimulation of the lymphocytes. This increases the safety level of agonistic antibodies against such receptors as OX40, CD137, GITR, ICOS, or CD27.

OX40 (CD134, TNFRSF4) belongs to the superfamily of TNFR and can be detected on the surface of activated $CD4^+$ and $CD8^+$ T cells, and also on Tregs, NK cells, and neutrophils. The expression of its natural ligand, OX40L (CD52), can be induced by proinflammatory cytokines on dendritic cells (DCs), macrophages, B lymphocytes, and also endothelial or smooth muscle cells. OX40 is detected on lymphocytes 24 to 72 h after activation [89]. Stimulation via OX40 has been shown to overcome the negative effects induced by CTLA-4 in T lymphocytes and also to antagonize the suppressive effects of Tregs on the activation of the effector cells [90]. Thus, agonistic antibodies or Fc fusion proteins against OX40, such as BMS986178, GSK3174998, PF-04518600, MEDI6383, MEDI6469, or MOXR0916, have been generated for use against a range of malignancies (reviewed in [90]). Generally, these antibodies are well tolerated in cancer patients and have a mild toxicity profile. Interestingly, the application of anti-OX40 stimulatory compounds (MEDI6383 or MEDI6469) was shown to induce activation and proliferation of T cell populations in cancer patients [91], but also resulted in upregulation of PD-L1 in tumor cells, occurring between 12 and 19 days following the infusion (NCT02274155). This indicates the potential synergism of agonistic anti-OX40 compounds with anti-PD-1/PD-L1 blocking antibodies. Indeed, such combinations, e.g., PF-04518600 with avelumab (NCT03971409) or GSK3174998 with pembrolizumab (NCT02528357), are being tested in clinical trials. In recent preclinical studies, spectacular effects against a range of malignancies have been reported in the combination of anti-OX40 agonist (BMS 986178) with TLR9 agonist SD-101 [92]. This combination is currently tested in Phase 1 clinical trial in advanced cancers (NCT03831295).

CD137 (4-1BB, TNFRSF9) can be primarily detected on activated $CD8^+$ and $CD4^+$ T cells but following induction with proinflammatory stimuli also appears on other cell types, including NK cells, B cells and dendritic cells, or endothelial cells following induction with pro-inflammatory stimuli [93]. CD137 ligand (4-1BBL, CD252) is expressed on various antigen-presenting cells. Ligation of CD137 results in a pro-stimulatory signal, enhancing among others the tumor-selective cytotoxicity of $CD8^+$ T lymphocytes and NK cells and secretion of IFN-γ [94]. The examples of agonistic anti-CD137 antibodies are utomilumab (PF-05082566) and urelumab (BMS-663513). These antibodies are being assessed in numerous clinical trials in cancer patients, mainly in combinations with other immunomodulatory compounds. Notably, urelumab, as an agonist for CD137, appears to act with higher potency than utomilumab [95], which is attributed to different epitopes bound by these antibodies on CD137 molecule [96]. Therefore, a somewhat higher frequency of adverse effects has been reported with urelumab. Similarly to OX-40, anti-CD137 antibodies act in synergy with the inhibitors of PD-1/PD-L1 axis [95], and such combinations are being evaluated in clinical trials. In line with this tendency, a recombinant PD-L1/4-1BB bispecific antibody, ES101, has recently been developed and subjected to Phase 1 clinical trial in advanced solid malignancies (NCT04009460).

GITR (TNFRSF18), also known as activation-inducible tumor necrosis factor receptor (AITR), is another member of the TNFR family, the expression of which is increased upon activation on T and NK cells, and also the $CD4^+CD25^+$ regulatory T cells. GITR ligand (GIRTL) is primarily expressed on antigen-presenting cells and endothelium. Stimulation of GITR has been shown to increase the effector activity of T cells and decrease the immunosuppressive effects elicited by Tregs. Numerous agonistic anti-GITR antibodies have been developed, for instance BMS-986156, TRX-518, AMG 228, INCAGN01876, MEDI1873, MK-4166, and GWN323, all of which are currently being tested in clinical trials in solid or hematological malignancies. Generally, the application of these antibodies is considered safe, with only relatively mild adverse effects [97]. However, most of these antibodies produce quite modest immunostimulatory effects or clinical response rates so far [97]. That indicates that anti-GITR antibodies may be better candidates for combined approaches rather than to be used in monotherapy [98].

ICOS (CD278), unlike most of the costimulatory receptors on T cells, belongs to the superfamily of CD28-type molecules. ICOS is expressed at low levels on naïve T cells, but its expression is significantly increased following activating stimuli and plays a role in T cell activation and governing Th1-, Th2-, and Th17-type responses [99]. The ligand of ICOS (ICOSLG, B7-H2, CD275) appears mostly on APC, including B cells, dendritic cells, and macrophages, and also on non-immune cells following stimulation with lipopolysaccharide [99]. ICOS is also considered a target for agonistic approach in anticancer therapies [100], and therefore several agonistic (such as JTX-2011, GSK3359609, BMS-986226) antibodies were generated, but also an antagonistic (MEDI-570) antibody, as well. Interestingly, the ICOS–ICOSL pathway can sometimes exhibit pro-tumorigenic effects due to the inducing generation and function of Tregs [101], and in particular cases, an inhibitory approach to ICOS signaling might be of preference [100].

CD27 is another member of the TNFR superfamily. Its ligand, CD70, is expressed on highly activated lymphocytes, but also in T- and B-cell lymphomas [102]. Varlilumab (CDX-1127) is an anti-CD27 agonistic antibody that has been and is being evaluated in several clinical trials in solid malignancies (e.g., NCT04081688, NCT02335918). An interesting fact is that CD70 is currently under investigation as a target for the ARGX-110 antibody in the treatment of hematological malignancies (NCT03030612), and the previous study in solid tumors (NCT02759250) has shown promising signs of its biological activity.

5. Perspectives in Immune Checkpoint Targeting—Bispecific Antibodies

The most significant challenge of immunomodulation is balancing between the potency of antitumor effects and the severity of autoimmune and/or inflammatory adverse events. The potential solution for this problem may rely on choosing the appropriate combination of immunomodulatory compounds and potentially other anticancer modalities in order to tip this balance towards the antitumor effectiveness. A derivative of such an approach is using multivalent (e.g., bispecific) antibodies, that combine the beneficial effects of multiple checkpoint targets.

Bispecific antibodies (bsAb) are engineered antibody-derived fusion proteins designed to bind two epitopes (usually on two different antigens) simultaneously. The global development of bsAb is thriving. Currently, there are numerous (>20) technology platforms commercialized for bsAb formation and development, and more than 85 bsAb are in clinical development with two of them already marketed [103]. The most pronounced advantage of bsAb over the combinations of full-size format mAb is that bsAb can bring their targets into close proximity. Also, the amount of balance between both binding arms of bsAb is always 1:1 at the site of destination, while for combinations of full-size mAb, it can be severely shifted in either way depending on circumstances. From the perspective of immune checkpoint targeting, three functional formats of bsAb are applicable [30]:

- Redirectors of cytotoxic effector cells—these bsAb bind to the tumor-associated antigen (a checkpoint molecule in this case) and the molecule responsible for activation of the effector cells (e.g., CD3 on T/NKT cells or CD16 on NK/NKT cells). Such bsAb are also referred to as bi-specific T cell engager (BiTE) or bi-specific killer cell engager (BiKE);
- Dual immunomodulators—the principle of action of these bsAb is to bind two checkpoint molecules simultaneously, usually on the same cell.

- Tumor-associated antigen-targeted immunomodulators—these bsAb bind to the tumor-associated antigen (on cancer cell) and a checkpoint molecule (e.g., a positive immune checkpoint on the effector cell). The difference between these bsAb and redirectors of cytotoxic effector cells is that they would not discriminate between the effector cell type, as long as the positive immune checkpoint molecule is expressed.

The examples of bsAb at various phases of preclinical or early clinical development are presented in Table 4.

Table 4. Examples of bispecific antibodies targeted against immune checkpoint molecules.

Antigens	Name	Cancer Type	Reference or Clinical Trial No.
Redirectors of cytotoxic effector cells			
Anti-PD-L1/CD3		PD-L1-positive human cancers	Preclinical [104]
Dual immunomodulators			
Anti-PD-1/TIM3	LY3415244	Advanced solid tumors	NCT03752177 (Phase 1)
Anti-PD-1/TIM3	RO7121661	Metastatic Melanoma Non-small Cell Lung Cancer (NSCLC) Small Cell Lung Cancer (SCLC)	NCT03708328 (Phase 1)
Anti-PD-1/PD-L1	LY3434172	Advanced solid tumors	NCT03936959 (Phase 1)
Anti-PD-1/CTLA-4	AK104	Gastric Adenocarcinoma Advanced Solid Tumors Gastroesophageal Junction Adenocarcinoma	NCT03852251 (Phase 1/2)
		Advanced Cancer	NCT03261011 (Phase 1)
Anti-CTLA-4/OX40	ATOR-1015	Advanced and/or Refractory Solid Malignancies	NCT03782467 (Phase 1)
Anti-LAG-3/PD-L1	FS118	Advanced Cancer Metastatic Cancer	NCT03440437 (Phase 1)
Tumor-associated antigen-targeted immunomodulators			
Anti-Her2/4-1BB	PRS343	HER2-positive Solid Tumors	NCT03330561 (Phase 1)

6. Summary and Future Directions

Multiple lines of evidence suggest that modulation of the intrinsic antitumor response by using antagonistic compounds towards negative immune checkpoints and agonistic factors stimulating positive immune checkpoints is a highly promising strategy in cancer treatment. The chemical assembly of such immunomodulatory agents is most often based on antibody structure or an antibody derivative. Numerous cancer patients have already achieved long-term remissions from malignancies, that would be lethal prior to the immunotherapy era. Nevertheless, the immunomodulatory approach to cancer treatment is far from perfect. Another solution might be an attempt to mimic as close as possible the natural course of activation of T cells, which should be localized and limited to the site(s) of disease rather than systemic. This effect can be potentially achieved by the intratumoral application of a given immunomodulator with hope for inducing an abscopal effect against the remaining tumors. Also, the identification of new antibody-targetable immune checkpoints can allow for a higher percentage of objective responses in cancer patients resistant to current therapies. An ideal expression profile is high and homogeneous antigen expression on the surface of all tumor cells and absent from normal tissue. However, some types of cancers are made up of multiple cancer subtypes that evolve with time. The recently used approaches to solve this problem are using transcriptome analysis of cancer cells [105,106], also integrated with cell-surface proteomic data [107]. Another novel approach is to identify tumor antigens by analyzing antibodies derived from local lymph nodes [108], which could allow one to also identify tumor antigens expressed by individual cancer patients.

Lastly, elaboration of more precise criteria for evaluation immune-modified responses in solid tumors along with properly chosen companion diagnostics would allow for better identification of patients benefiting from the immunomodulatory therapies. Despite the remaining challenges, the application of antibody-based modulators of immune checkpoints has already opened a new pathway for personalized and precise treatment strategies in cancers and is undoubtedly one of the most significant breakthroughs in current medicine.

Funding: This research received no external funding.

Acknowledgments: The work was supported by the grants from the National Science Centre, Poland (2016/23/B/NZ6/02535, R.Z. and 2015/19/B/NZ6/02862, A.G.-J.) and the Polpharma Scientific Foundation (5FPOL8, A.G.-J.).

Conflicts of Interest: Radoslaw Zagozdzon is a scientific consultant for Pure Biologics S.A. (Wroclaw, Poland). The other authors declare no conflict of interest. The sponsoring institution had no role in the design, execution, interpretation, or writing of the study.

References

1. Pento, J.T. Monoclonal Antibodies for the Treatment of Cancer. *Anticancer Res.* **2017**, *37*, 5935–5939. [CrossRef] [PubMed]
2. Natoli, G.; Ostuni, R. Adaptation and memory in immune responses. *Nat. Immunol.* **2019**, *20*, 783–792. [CrossRef] [PubMed]
3. Zinkernagel, R.M.; Doherty, P.C. The discovery of MHC restriction. *Immunol. Today* **1997**, *18*, 14–17. [CrossRef]
4. Somoza, C.; Lanier, L.L. T-cell costimulation via CD28-CD80/CD86 and CD40-CD40 ligand interactions. *Res. Immunol.* **1995**, *146*, 171–176. [CrossRef]
5. Curtsinger, J.M.; Mescher, M.F. Inflammatory cytokines as a third signal for T cell activation. *Curr. Opin. Immunol.* **2010**, *22*, 333–340. [CrossRef]
6. Chen, L.; Flies, D.B. Molecular mechanisms of T cell co-stimulation and co-inhibition. *Nat. Rev. Immunol.* **2013**, *13*, 227–242. [CrossRef]
7. Ceeraz, S.; Nowak, E.C.; Burns, C.M.; Noelle, R.J. Immune checkpoint receptors in regulating immune reactivity in rheumatic disease. *Arthritis Res. Ther.* **2014**, *16*, 469. [CrossRef]
8. Anderson, A.C.; Joller, N.; Kuchroo, V.K. Lag-3, Tim-3, and TIGIT: Co-inhibitory Receptors with Specialized Functions in Immune Regulation. *Immunity* **2016**, *44*, 989–1004. [CrossRef]
9. Zarour, H.M. Reversing T-cell Dysfunction and Exhaustion in Cancer. *Clin. Cancer Res.* **2016**, *22*, 1856–1864. [CrossRef]
10. Donini, C.; D'Ambrosio, L.; Grignani, G.; Aglietta, M.; Sangiolo, D. Next generation immune-checkpoints for cancer therapy. *J. Thorac. Dis.* **2018**, *10*, S1581–S1601. [CrossRef]
11. Krummel, M.F.; Allison, J.P. CD28 and CTLA-4 have opposing effects on the response of T cells to stimulation. *J. Exp. Med.* **1995**, *182*, 459–465. [CrossRef] [PubMed]
12. Wing, K.; Onishi, Y.; Prieto-Martin, P.; Yamaguchi, T.; Miyara, M.; Fehervari, Z.; Nomura, T.; Sakaguchi, S. CTLA-4 control over Foxp3+ regulatory T cell function. *Science* **2008**, *322*, 271–275. [CrossRef] [PubMed]
13. Khattri, R.; Auger, J.A.; Griffin, M.D.; Sharpe, A.H.; Bluestone, J.A. Lymphoproliferative disorder in CTLA-4 knockout mice is characterized by CD28-regulated activation of Th2 responses. *J. Immunol.* **1999**, *162*, 5784–5791. [PubMed]
14. Leach, D.R.; Krummel, M.F.; Allison, J.P. Enhancement of antitumor immunity by CTLA-4 blockade. *Science* **1996**, *271*, 1734–1736. [CrossRef]

15. Ribas, A. Anti-CTLA4 Antibody Clinical Trials in Melanoma. *Update Cancer Ther.* **2007**, *2*, 133–139. [CrossRef]
16. Nishimura, H.; Honjo, T.; Minato, N. Facilitation of beta selection and modification of positive selection in the thymus of PD-1-deficient mice. *J. Exp. Med.* **2000**, *191*, 891–898. [CrossRef]
17. Guleria, I.; Khosroshahi, A.; Ansari, M.J.; Habicht, A.; Azuma, M.; Yagita, H.; Noelle, R.J.; Coyle, A.; Mellor, A.L.; Khoury, S.J.; et al. A critical role for the programmed death ligand 1 in fetomaternal tolerance. *J. Exp. Med.* **2005**, *202*, 231–237. [CrossRef]
18. Freeman, G.J.; Long, A.J.; Iwai, Y.; Bourque, K.; Chernova, T.; Nishimura, H.; Fitz, L.J.; Malenkovich, N.; Okazaki, T.; Byrne, M.C.; et al. Engagement of the PD-1 immunoinhibitory receptor by a novel B7 family member leads to negative regulation of lymphocyte activation. *J. Exp. Med.* **2000**, *192*, 1027–1034. [CrossRef]
19. Iwai, Y.; Ishida, M.; Tanaka, Y.; Okazaki, T.; Honjo, T.; Minato, N. Involvement of PD-L1 on tumor cells in the escape from host immune system and tumor immunotherapy by PD-L1 blockade. *Proc. Natl. Acad. Sci. USA* **2002**, *99*, 12293–12297. [CrossRef]
20. Dong, H.; Zhu, G.; Tamada, K.; Chen, L. B7-H1, a third member of the B7 family, co-stimulates T-cell proliferation and interleukin-10 secretion. *Nat. Med.* **1999**, *5*, 1365–1369. [CrossRef]
21. Ikeda, S.; Okamoto, T.; Okano, S.; Umemoto, Y.; Tagawa, T.; Morodomi, Y.; Kohno, M.; Shimamatsu, S.; Kitahara, H.; Suzuki, Y.; et al. PD-L1 Is Upregulated by Simultaneous Amplification of the PD-L1 and JAK2 Genes in Non-Small Cell Lung Cancer. *J. Thorac. Oncol.* **2016**, *11*, 62–71. [CrossRef] [PubMed]
22. Kataoka, K.; Shiraishi, Y.; Takeda, Y.; Sakata, S.; Matsumoto, M.; Nagano, S.; Maeda, T.; Nagata, Y.; Kitanaka, A.; Mizuno, S.; et al. Aberrant PD-L1 expression through 3'-UTR disruption in multiple cancers. *Nature* **2016**, *534*, 402–406. [CrossRef] [PubMed]
23. Atefi, M.; Avramis, E.; Lassen, A.; Wong, D.J.; Robert, L.; Foulad, D.; Cerniglia, M.; Titz, B.; Chodon, T.; Graeber, T.G.; et al. Effects of MAPK and PI3K pathways on PD-L1 expression in melanoma. *Clin. Cancer Res.* **2014**, *20*, 3446–3457. [CrossRef] [PubMed]
24. Wang, W.G.; Jiang, X.N.; Sheng, D.; Sun, C.B.; Lee, J.; Zhou, X.Y.; Li, X.Q. PD-L1 over-expression is driven by B-cell receptor signaling in diffuse large B-cell lymphoma. *Lab. Invest.* **2019**, *99*, 1418–1427. [CrossRef] [PubMed]
25. Fang, W.; Zhang, J.; Hong, S.; Zhan, J.; Chen, N.; Qin, T.; Tang, Y.; Zhang, Y.; Kang, S.; Zhou, T.; et al. EBV-driven LMP1 and IFN-gamma up-regulate PD-L1 in nasopharyngeal carcinoma: Implications for oncotargeted therapy. *Oncotarget* **2014**, *5*, 12189–12202. [CrossRef] [PubMed]
26. Mazanet, M.M.; Hughes, C.C. B7-H1 is expressed by human endothelial cells and suppresses T cell cytokine synthesis. *J. Immunol.* **2002**, *169*, 3581–3588. [CrossRef] [PubMed]
27. Timeline of Anti-PD-1/L1 Antibody Approvals by the FDA. Available online: https://public.tableau.com/profile/jia.yu7083#!/vizhome/2018-12-07PD-1approvaltimeline/PD-1approvallandscape (accessed on 30 September 2019).
28. Kellner, C.; Otte, A.; Cappuzzello, E.; Klausz, K.; Peipp, M. Modulating Cytotoxic Effector Functions by Fc Engineering to Improve Cancer Therapy. *Transfus. Med. Hemother.* **2017**, *44*, 327–336. [CrossRef]
29. Julia, E.P.; Amante, A.; Pampena, M.B.; Mordoh, J.; Levy, E.M. Avelumab, an IgG1 anti-PD-L1 Immune Checkpoint Inhibitor, Triggers NK Cell-Mediated Cytotoxicity and Cytokine Production Against Triple Negative Breast Cancer Cells. *Front. Immunol.* **2018**, *9*, 2140. [CrossRef]
30. Dahlen, E.; Veitonmaki, N.; Norlen, P. Bispecific antibodies in cancer immunotherapy. *Ther. Adv. Vaccines Immunother.* **2018**, *6*, 3–17. [CrossRef]
31. Sau, S.; Petrovici, A.; Alsaab, H.O.; Bhise, K.; Iyer, A.K. PDL-1 Antibody Drug Conjugate for Selective Chemo-Guided Immune Modulation of Cancer. *Cancers* **2019**, *11*, 232. [CrossRef]
32. Tunger, A.; Sommer, U.; Wehner, R.; Kubasch, A.S.; Grimm, M.O.; Bachmann, M.P.; Platzbecker, U.; Bornhauser, M.; Baretton, G.; Schmitz, M. The Evolving Landscape of Biomarkers for Anti-PD-1 or Anti-PD-L1 Therapy. *J. Clin. Med.* **2019**, *8*, 1534. [CrossRef] [PubMed]
33. Patel, S.P.; Kurzrock, R. PD-L1 Expression as a Predictive Biomarker in Cancer Immunotherapy. *Mol. Cancer Ther.* **2015**, *14*, 847–856. [CrossRef] [PubMed]
34. Havel, J.J.; Chowell, D.; Chan, T.A. The evolving landscape of biomarkers for checkpoint inhibitor immunotherapy. *Nat. Rev. Cancer* **2019**, *19*, 133–150. [CrossRef] [PubMed]
35. Goodman, A.M.; Kato, S.; Bazhenova, L.; Patel, S.P.; Frampton, G.M.; Miller, V.; Stephens, P.J.; Daniels, G.A.; Kurzrock, R. Tumor Mutational Burden as an Independent Predictor of Response to Immunotherapy in Diverse Cancers. *Mol. Cancer Ther.* **2017**, *16*, 2598–2608. [CrossRef] [PubMed]

36. Chen, Y.; Liu, Q.; Chen, Z.; Wang, Y.; Yang, W.; Hu, Y.; Han, W.; Zeng, H.; Ma, H.; Dai, J.; et al. PD-L1 expression and tumor mutational burden status for prediction of response to chemotherapy and targeted therapy in non-small cell lung cancer. *J. Exp. Clin. Cancer Res.* **2019**, *38*, 193. [CrossRef] [PubMed]
37. Rotte, A. Combination of CTLA-4 and PD-1 blockers for treatment of cancer. *J. Exp. Clin. Cancer Res.* **2019**, *38*, 255. [CrossRef] [PubMed]
38. Pai, C.S.; Simons, D.M.; Lu, X.; Evans, M.; Wei, J.; Wang, Y.H.; Chen, M.; Huang, J.; Park, C.; Chang, A.; et al. Tumor-conditional anti-CTLA4 uncouples antitumor efficacy from immunotherapy-related toxicity. *J. Clin. Investig.* **2019**, *129*, 349–363. [CrossRef]
39. Savoia, P.; Astrua, C.; Fava, P. Ipilimumab (Anti-Ctla-4 Mab) in the treatment of metastatic melanoma: Effectiveness and toxicity management. *Hum. Vaccin. Immunother.* **2016**, *12*, 1092–1101. [CrossRef]
40. Vogrig, A.; Fouret, M.; Joubert, B.; Picard, G.; Rogemond, V.; Pinto, A.L.; Muniz-Castrillo, S.; Roger, M.; Raimbourg, J.; Dayen, C.; et al. Increased frequency of anti-Ma2 encephalitis associated with immune checkpoint inhibitors. *Neurol. Neuroimmunol. Neuroinflamm.* **2019**, *6*. [CrossRef]
41. Champion, S.N.; Stone, J.R. Immune checkpoint inhibitor associated myocarditis occurs in both high-grade and low-grade forms. *Mod. Pathol.* **2019**. [CrossRef]
42. Pauken, K.E.; Dougan, M.; Rose, N.R.; Lichtman, A.H.; Sharpe, A.H. Adverse Events Following Cancer Immunotherapy: Obstacles and Opportunities. *Trends Immunol.* **2019**, *40*, 511–523. [CrossRef] [PubMed]
43. Friedman, C.F.; Proverbs-Singh, T.A.; Postow, M.A. Treatment of the Immune-Related Adverse Effects of Immune Checkpoint Inhibitors: A Review. *JAMA Oncol.* **2016**, *2*, 1346–1353. [CrossRef] [PubMed]
44. Ravi, V.; Maloney, N.J.; Worswick, S. Neutrophilic dermatoses as adverse effects of checkpoint inhibitors: A review. *Derm. Ther.* **2019**, e13074. [CrossRef] [PubMed]
45. Bobrowicz, M.; Zagozdzon, R.; Domagala, J.; Vasconcelos-Berg, R.; Guenova, E.; Winiarska, M. Monoclonal Antibodies in Dermatooncology-State of the Art and Future Perspectives. *Cancers* **2019**, *11*, 1420. [CrossRef]
46. D'Errico, G.; Machado, H.L.; Sainz, B., Jr. A current perspective on cancer immune therapy: Step-by-step approach to constructing the magic bullet. *Clin. Transl. Med.* **2017**, *6*, 3. [CrossRef]
47. Elias, A.W.; Kasi, P.M.; Stauffer, J.A.; Thiel, D.D.; Colibaseanu, D.T.; Mody, K.; Joseph, R.W.; Bagaria, S.P. The Feasibility and Safety of Surgery in Patients Receiving Immune Checkpoint Inhibitors: A Retrospective Study. *Front. Oncol.* **2017**, *7*, 121. [CrossRef]
48. Lamichhane, P.; Amin, N.P.; Agarwal, M.; Lamichhane, N. Checkpoint Inhibition: Will Combination with Radiotherapy and Nanoparticle-Mediated Delivery Improve Efficacy? *Medicines* **2018**, *5*, 114. [CrossRef]
49. Wang, C.; Kulkarni, P.; Salgia, R. Combined Checkpoint Inhibition and Chemotherapy: New Era of 1(st)-Line Treatment for Non-Small-Cell Lung Cancer. *Mol. Ther. Oncolytics* **2019**, *13*, 1–6. [CrossRef]
50. Adderley, H.; Blackhall, F.H.; Lindsay, C.R. KRAS-mutant non-small cell lung cancer: Converging small molecules and immune checkpoint inhibition. *EBioMedicine* **2019**, *41*, 711–716. [CrossRef]
51. Geynisman, D.M.; Chien, C.R.; Smieliauskas, F.; Shen, C.; Shih, Y.C. Economic evaluation of therapeutic cancer vaccines and immunotherapy: A systematic review. *Hum. Vaccin. Immunother.* **2014**, *10*, 3415–3424. [CrossRef]
52. Barroso-Sousa, R.; Ott, P.A. Transformation of Old Concepts for a New Era of Cancer Immunotherapy: Cytokine Therapy and Cancer Vaccines as Combination Partners of PD1/PD-L1 Inhibitors. *Curr. Oncol. Rep.* **2018**, *21*, 1. [CrossRef] [PubMed]
53. Friedman, A.; Lai, X. Combination therapy for cancer with oncolytic virus and checkpoint inhibitor: A mathematical model. *PLoS ONE* **2018**, *13*, e0192449. [CrossRef] [PubMed]
54. Mullinax, J.E.; Hall, M.; Prabhakaran, S.; Weber, J.; Khushalani, N.; Eroglu, Z.; Brohl, A.S.; Markowitz, J.; Royster, E.; Richards, A.; et al. Combination of Ipilimumab and Adoptive Cell Therapy with Tumor-Infiltrating Lymphocytes for Patients with Metastatic Melanoma. *Front. Oncol.* **2018**, *8*, 44. [CrossRef] [PubMed]
55. Zych, A.O.; Bajor, M.; Zagozdzon, R. Application of Genome Editing Techniques in Immunology. *Arch. Immunol. Ther. Exp. (Warsz.)* **2018**, *66*, 289–298. [CrossRef]
56. Serganova, I.; Moroz, E.; Cohen, I.; Moroz, M.; Mane, M.; Zurita, J.; Shenker, L.; Ponomarev, V.; Blasberg, R. Enhancement of PSMA-Directed CAR Adoptive Immunotherapy by PD-1/PD-L1 Blockade. *Mol. Ther. Oncolytics* **2017**, *4*, 41–54. [CrossRef]
57. Tundo, G.R.; Sbardella, D.; Lacal, P.M.; Graziani, G.; Marini, S. On the Horizon: Targeting Next-Generation Immune Checkpoints for Cancer Treatment. *Chemotherapy* **2019**, 1–19. [CrossRef]

58. Long, L.; Zhang, X.; Chen, F.; Pan, Q.; Phiphatwatchara, P.; Zeng, Y.; Chen, H. The promising immune checkpoint LAG-3: From tumor microenvironment to cancer immunotherapy. *Genes Cancer* **2018**, *9*, 176–189. [CrossRef]
59. Wang, J.; Sanmamed, M.F.; Datar, I.; Su, T.T.; Ji, L.; Sun, J.; Chen, L.; Chen, Y.; Zhu, G.; Yin, W.; et al. Fibrinogen-like Protein 1 Is a Major Immune Inhibitory Ligand of LAG-3. *Cell* **2019**, *176*, 334–347.e312. [CrossRef]
60. Zelba, H.; Bedke, J.; Hennenlotter, J.; Mostbock, S.; Zettl, M.; Zichner, T.; Chandran, P.A.; Stenzl, A.; Rammensee, H.G.; Gouttefangeas, C. PD-1 and LAG-3 dominate checkpoint receptor-mediated T cell inhibition in renal cell carcinoma. *Cancer Immunol. Res.* **2019**. [CrossRef]
61. Woo, S.R.; Turnis, M.E.; Goldberg, M.V.; Bankoti, J.; Selby, M.; Nirschl, C.J.; Bettini, M.L.; Gravano, D.M.; Vogel, P.; Liu, C.L.; et al. Immune inhibitory molecules LAG-3 and PD-1 synergistically regulate T-cell function to promote tumoral immune escape. *Cancer Res.* **2012**, *72*, 917–927. [CrossRef]
62. Puhr, H.C.; Ilhan-Mutlu, A. New emerging targets in cancer immunotherapy: The role of LAG3. *ESMO Open* **2019**, *4*, e000482. [CrossRef] [PubMed]
63. Ascierto, P.A.; Melero, I.; Bhatia, S.; Bono, P.; Sanborn, R.E.; Lipson, E.J.; Callahan, M.K.; Gajewski, T.; Gomez-Roca, C.A.; Hodi, F.S.; et al. Initial efficacy of anti-lymphocyte activation gene-3 (anti–LAG-3; BMS-986016) in combination with nivolumab (nivo) in pts with melanoma (MEL) previously treated with anti–PD-1/PD-L1 therapy. *J. Clin. Oncol.* **2017**, *35*, 9520. [CrossRef]
64. Manieri, N.A.; Chiang, E.Y.; Grogan, J.L. TIGIT: A Key Inhibitor of the Cancer Immunity Cycle. *Trends Immunol.* **2017**, *38*, 20–28. [CrossRef] [PubMed]
65. Solomon, B.L.; Garrido-Laguna, I. TIGIT: A novel immunotherapy target moving from bench to bedside. *Cancer Immunol. Immunother.* **2018**, *67*, 1659–1667. [CrossRef] [PubMed]
66. Yu, X.; Harden, K.; Gonzalez, L.C.; Francesco, M.; Chiang, E.; Irving, B.; Tom, I.; Ivelja, S.; Refino, C.J.; Clark, H.; et al. The surface protein TIGIT suppresses T cell activation by promoting the generation of mature immunoregulatory dendritic cells. *Nat. Immunol.* **2009**, *10*, 48–57. [CrossRef]
67. Hung, A.L.; Maxwell, R.; Theodros, D.; Belcaid, Z.; Mathios, D.; Luksik, A.S.; Kim, E.; Wu, A.; Xia, Y.; Garzon-Muvdi, T.; et al. TIGIT and PD-1 dual checkpoint blockade enhances antitumor immunity and survival in GBM. *Oncoimmunology* **2018**, *7*, e1466769. [CrossRef]
68. Friedlaender, A.; Addeo, A.; Banna, G. New emerging targets in cancer immunotherapy: The role of TIM3. *ESMO Open* **2019**, *4*, e000497. [CrossRef]
69. Das, M.; Zhu, C.; Kuchroo, V.K. Tim-3 and its role in regulating anti-tumor immunity. *Immunol. Rev.* **2017**, *276*, 97–111. [CrossRef]
70. Sakuishi, K.; Ngiow, S.F.; Sullivan, J.M.; Teng, M.W.; Kuchroo, V.K.; Smyth, M.J.; Anderson, A.C. TIM3(+)FOXP3(+) regulatory T cells are tissue-specific promoters of T-cell dysfunction in cancer. *Oncoimmunology* **2013**, *2*, e23849. [CrossRef]
71. Zhou, G.; Sprengers, D.; Boor, P.P.C.; Doukas, M.; Schutz, H.; Mancham, S.; Pedroza-Gonzalez, A.; Polak, W.G.; de Jonge, J.; Gaspersz, M.; et al. Antibodies Against Immune Checkpoint Molecules Restore Functions of Tumor-Infiltrating T Cells in Hepatocellular Carcinomas. *Gastroenterology* **2017**, *153*, 1107–1119 e1110. [CrossRef]
72. Liu, J.F.; Ma, S.R.; Mao, L.; Bu, L.L.; Yu, G.T.; Li, Y.C.; Huang, C.F.; Deng, W.W.; Kulkarni, A.B.; Zhang, W.F.; et al. T-cell immunoglobulin mucin 3 blockade drives an antitumor immune response in head and neck cancer. *Mol. Oncol.* **2017**, *11*, 235–247. [CrossRef] [PubMed]
73. Sabatos-Peyton, C.A.; Nevin, J.; Brock, A.; Venable, J.D.; Tan, D.J.; Kassam, N.; Xu, F.; Taraszka, J.; Wesemann, L.; Pertel, T.; et al. Blockade of Tim-3 binding to phosphatidylserine and CEACAM1 is a shared feature of anti-Tim-3 antibodies that have functional efficacy. *Oncoimmunology* **2018**, *7*, e1385690. [CrossRef] [PubMed]
74. Koyama, S.; Akbay, E.A.; Li, Y.Y.; Herter-Sprie, G.S.; Buczkowski, K.A.; Richards, W.G.; Gandhi, L.; Redig, A.J.; Rodig, S.J.; Asahina, H.; et al. Adaptive resistance to therapeutic PD-1 blockade is associated with upregulation of alternative immune checkpoints. *Nat. Commun.* **2016**, *7*, 10501. [CrossRef] [PubMed]
75. Lines, J.L.; Pantazi, E.; Mak, J.; Sempere, L.F.; Wang, L.; O'Connell, S.; Ceeraz, S.; Suriawinata, A.A.; Yan, S.; Ernstoff, M.S.; et al. VISTA is an immune checkpoint molecule for human T cells. *Cancer Res.* **2014**, *74*, 1924–1932. [CrossRef]

76. Nowak, E.C.; Lines, J.L.; Varn, F.S.; Deng, J.; Sarde, A.; Mabaera, R.; Kuta, A.; Le Mercier, I.; Cheng, C.; Noelle, R.J. Immunoregulatory functions of VISTA. *Immunol. Rev.* **2017**, *276*, 66–79. [CrossRef]
77. Mulati, K.; Hamanishi, J.; Matsumura, N.; Chamoto, K.; Mise, N.; Abiko, K.; Baba, T.; Yamaguchi, K.; Horikawa, N.; Murakami, R.; et al. VISTA expressed in tumour cells regulates T cell function. *Br. J. Cancer* **2019**, *120*, 115–127. [CrossRef]
78. Blando, J.; Sharma, A.; Higa, M.G.; Zhao, H.; Vence, L.; Yadav, S.S.; Kim, J.; Sepulveda, A.M.; Sharp, M.; Maitra, A.; et al. Comparison of immune infiltrates in melanoma and pancreatic cancer highlights VISTA as a potential target in pancreatic cancer. *Proc. Natl. Acad. Sci. USA* **2019**, *116*, 1692–1697. [CrossRef]
79. Ortenberg, R.; Sapir, Y.; Raz, L.; Hershkovitz, L.; Ben Arav, A.; Sapoznik, S.; Barshack, I.; Avivi, C.; Berkun, Y.; Besser, M.J.; et al. Novel immunotherapy for malignant melanoma with a monoclonal antibody that blocks CEACAM1 homophilic interactions. *Mol. Cancer Ther.* **2012**, *11*, 1300–1310. [CrossRef]
80. Nichita, L.; Zurac, S.; Bastian, A.; Stinga, P.; Nedelcu, R.; Brinzea, A.; Turcu, G.; Ion, D.; Jilaveanu, L.; Sticlaru, L.; et al. Comparative analysis of CEACAM1 expression in thin melanomas with and without regression. *Oncol. Lett.* **2019**, *17*, 4149–4154. [CrossRef]
81. Li, J.; Liu, X.; Duan, Y.; Liu, Y.; Wang, H.; Lian, S.; Zhuang, G.; Fan, Y. Combined Blockade of T Cell Immunoglobulin and Mucin Domain 3 and Carcinoembryonic Antigen-Related Cell Adhesion Molecule 1 Results in Durable Therapeutic Efficacy in Mice with Intracranial Gliomas. *Med. Sci. Monit.* **2017**, *23*, 3593–3602. [CrossRef]
82. Markel, G.; Sapir, Y.; Mandel, I.; Hakim, M.; Shaked, R.; Meilin, E.; McClanahan, T.; Loboda, A.; Hashmueli, S.; Moshe, T.B. Inhibition of the novel immune checkpoint CEACAM1 to enhance anti-tumor immunological activity. *J. Clin. Oncol.* **2016**, *34*, 3044. [CrossRef]
83. McLeod, R.L.; Angagaw, M.H.; Baral, T.N.; Liu, L.; Moniz, R.J.; Laskey, J.; Hsieh, S.; Lee, M.; Han, J.H.; Issafras, H.; et al. Characterization of murine CEACAM1 in vivo reveals low expression on CD8(+) T cells and no tumor growth modulating activity by anti-CEACAM1 mAb CC1. *Oncotarget* **2018**, *9*, 34459–34470. [CrossRef] [PubMed]
84. Kim, J.-H.; Pyo, K.-H.; Jung, M.-J.; Hur, M.; Won, J.; Cho, B.C. Abstract 2266: Efficacy of CEACAM1-targeting immunoglobulin in combination with pembrolizumab in lung cancer. *Cancer Res.* **2019**, *79*, 2266. [CrossRef]
85. Helfrich, I.; Singer, B.B. Size Matters: The Functional Role of the CEACAM1 Isoform Signature and Its Impact for NK Cell-Mediated Killing in Melanoma. *Cancers* **2019**, *11*, 356. [CrossRef] [PubMed]
86. Brown, K.E. Revisiting CD28 Superagonist TGN1412 as Potential Therapeutic for Pediatric B Cell Leukemia: A Review. *Diseases* **2018**, *6*, 41. [CrossRef]
87. Suntharalingam, G.; Perry, M.R.; Ward, S.; Brett, S.J.; Castello-Cortes, A.; Brunner, M.D.; Panoskaltis, N. Cytokine storm in a phase 1 trial of the anti-CD28 monoclonal antibody TGN1412. *N. Engl. J. Med.* **2006**, *355*, 1018–1028. [CrossRef]
88. Stebbings, R.; Poole, S.; Thorpe, R. Safety of biologics, lessons learnt from TGN1412. *Curr. Opin. Biotechnol.* **2009**, *20*, 673–677. [CrossRef]
89. Redmond, W.L.; Ruby, C.E.; Weinberg, A.D. The role of OX40-mediated co-stimulation in T-cell activation and survival. *Crit. Rev. Immunol.* **2009**, *29*, 187–201. [CrossRef]
90. Aspeslagh, S.; Postel-Vinay, S.; Rusakiewicz, S.; Soria, J.C.; Zitvogel, L.; Marabelle, A. Rationale for anti-OX40 cancer immunotherapy. *Eur. J. Cancer* **2016**, *52*, 50–66. [CrossRef]
91. Curti, B.D.; Kovacsovics-Bankowski, M.; Morris, N.; Walker, E.; Chisholm, L.; Floyd, K.; Walker, J.; Gonzalez, I.; Meeuwsen, T.; Fox, B.A.; et al. OX40 is a potent immune-stimulating target in late-stage cancer patients. *Cancer Res.* **2013**, *73*, 7189–7198. [CrossRef]
92. Sagiv-Barfi, I.; Czerwinski, D.K.; Levy, S.; Alam, I.S.; Mayer, A.T.; Gambhir, S.S.; Levy, R. Eradication of spontaneous malignancy by local immunotherapy. *Sci. Transl. Med.* **2018**, *10*, eaan4488. [CrossRef] [PubMed]
93. Chester, C.; Sanmamed, M.F.; Wang, J.; Melero, I. Immunotherapy targeting 4-1BB: Mechanistic rationale, clinical results, and future strategies. *Blood* **2018**, *131*, 49–57. [CrossRef] [PubMed]
94. Yonezawa, A.; Dutt, S.; Chester, C.; Kim, J.; Kohrt, H.E. Boosting Cancer Immunotherapy with Anti-CD137 Antibody Therapy. *Clin. Cancer Res.* **2015**, *21*, 3113–3120. [CrossRef] [PubMed]
95. Perez-Ruiz, E.; Etxeberria, I.; Rodriguez-Ruiz, M.E.; Melero, I. Anti-CD137 and PD-1/PD-L1 Antibodies En Route toward Clinical Synergy. *Clin. Cancer Res.* **2017**, *23*, 5326–5328. [CrossRef]

96. Chin, S.M.; Kimberlin, C.R.; Roe-Zurz, Z.; Zhang, P.; Xu, A.; Liao-Chan, S.; Sen, D.; Nager, A.R.; Oakdale, N.S.; Brown, C.; et al. Structure of the 4-1BB/4-1BBL complex and distinct binding and functional properties of utomilumab and urelumab. *Nat. Commun.* **2018**, *9*, 4679. [CrossRef]
97. Tran, B.; Carvajal, R.D.; Marabelle, A.; Patel, S.P.; LoRusso, P.M.; Rasmussen, E.; Juan, G.; Upreti, V.V.; Beers, C.; Ngarmchamnanrith, G.; et al. Dose escalation results from a first-in-human, phase 1 study of glucocorticoid-induced TNF receptor-related protein agonist AMG 228 in patients with advanced solid tumors. *J. Immunother. Cancer* **2018**, *6*, 93. [CrossRef]
98. Zappasodi, R.; Sirard, C.; Li, Y.; Budhu, S.; Abu-Akeel, M.; Liu, C.; Yang, X.; Zhong, H.; Newman, W.; Qi, J.; et al. Rational design of anti-GITR-based combination immunotherapy. *Nat. Med.* **2019**, *25*, 759–766. [CrossRef]
99. Dong, C.; Juedes, A.E.; Temann, U.A.; Shresta, S.; Allison, J.P.; Ruddle, N.H.; Flavell, R.A. ICOS co-stimulatory receptor is essential for T-cell activation and function. *Nature* **2001**, *409*, 97–101. [CrossRef]
100. Amatore, F.; Gorvel, L.; Olive, D. Inducible Co-Stimulator (ICOS) as a potential therapeutic target for anti-cancer therapy. *Expert Opin. Ther. Targets* **2018**, *22*, 343–351. [CrossRef]
101. Busse, M.; Krech, M.; Meyer-Bahlburg, A.; Hennig, C.; Hansen, G. ICOS mediates the generation and function of CD4+CD25+Foxp3+ regulatory T cells conveying respiratory tolerance. *J. Immunol.* **2012**, *189*, 1975–1982. [CrossRef]
102. Israel, B.F.; Gulley, M.; Elmore, S.; Ferrini, S.; Feng, W.H.; Kenney, S.C. Anti-CD70 antibodies: A potential treatment for EBV+ CD70-expressing lymphomas. *Mol. Cancer* **2005**, *4*, 2037–2044. [CrossRef] [PubMed]
103. Labrijn, A.F.; Janmaat, M.L.; Reichert, J.M.; Parren, P. Bispecific antibodies: A mechanistic review of the pipeline. *Nat. Rev. Drug Discov.* **2019**, *18*, 585–608. [CrossRef] [PubMed]
104. Horn, L.A.; Ciavattone, N.G.; Atkinson, R.; Woldergerima, N.; Wolf, J.; Clements, V.K.; Sinha, P.; Poudel, M.; Ostrand-Rosenberg, S. CD3xPDL1 bi-specific T cell engager (BiTE) simultaneously activates T cells and NKT cells, kills PDL1(+) tumor cells, and extends the survival of tumor-bearing humanized mice. *Oncotarget* **2017**, *8*, 57964–57980. [CrossRef] [PubMed]
105. Labrecque, M.P.; Coleman, I.M.; Brown, L.G.; True, L.D.; Kollath, L.; Lakely, B.; Nguyen, H.M.; Yang, Y.C.; da Costa, R.M.G.; Kaipainen, A.; et al. Molecular profiling stratifies diverse phenotypes of treatment-refractory metastatic castration-resistant prostate cancer. *J. Clin. Investig.* **2019**, *130*, 4492–4505. [CrossRef]
106. Djureinovic, D.; Hallstrom, B.M.; Horie, M.; Mattsson, J.S.M.; La Fleur, L.; Fagerberg, L.; Brunnstrom, H.; Lindskog, C.; Madjar, K.; Rahnenfuhrer, J.; et al. Profiling cancer testis antigens in non-small-cell lung cancer. *JCI Insight* **2016**, *1*, e86837. [CrossRef]
107. Lee, J.K.; Bangayan, N.J.; Chai, T.; Smith, B.A.; Pariva, T.E.; Yun, S.; Vashisht, A.; Zhang, Q.; Park, J.W.; Corey, E.; et al. Systemic surfaceome profiling identifies target antigens for immune-based therapy in subtypes of advanced prostate cancer. *Proc. Natl. Acad. Sci. USA* **2018**, *115*, E4473–E4482. [CrossRef]
108. Young, A.R.; Duarte, J.D.G.; Coulson, R.; O'Brien, M.; Deb, S.; Lopata, A.; Behren, A.; Mathivanan, S.; Lim, E.; Meeusen, E. Immunoprofiling of Breast Cancer Antigens Using Antibodies Derived from Local Lymph Nodes. *Cancers* **2019**, *11*, 682. [CrossRef]

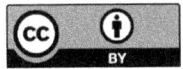

© 2019 by the authors. Licensee MDPI, Basel, Switzerland. This article is an open access article distributed under the terms and conditions of the Creative Commons Attribution (CC BY) license (http://creativecommons.org/licenses/by/4.0/).

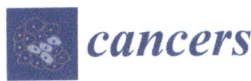

Article

Combination of Baseline LDH, Performance Status and Age as Integrated Algorithm to Identify Solid Tumor Patients with Higher Probability of Response to Anti PD-1 and PD-L1 Monoclonal Antibodies

Maria Silvia Cona [1], Mara Lecchi [2], Sara Cresta [1], Silvia Damian [1], Michele Del Vecchio [1], Andrea Necchi [1], Marta Maria Poggi [1], Daniele Raggi [1], Giovanni Randon [1], Raffaele Ratta [1], Diego Signorelli [1], Claudio Vernieri [1,3], Filippo de Braud [1,4], Paolo Verderio [2] and Massimo Di Nicola [1,*]

[1] Medical Oncology Unit, Fondazione IRCCS, Istituto Nazionale dei Tumori di Milano, Via Giacomo Venezian 1, 20133 Milan, Italy; mariasilvia.cona@istitutotumori.mi.it (M.S.C.); sara.cresta@istitutotumori.mi.it (S.C.); silvia.damian@istitutotumori.mi.it (S.D.); michele.delvecchio@istitutotumori.mi.it (M.D.V.); andrea.necchi@istitutotumori.mi.it (A.N.); martamariapoggi@gmail.com (M.M.P.); daniele.raggi@istitutotumori.mi.it (D.R.); giovanni.randon@istitutotumori.mi.it (G.R.); raffaele.ratta@istitutotumori.mi.it (R.R.); diego.signorelli@istitutotumori.mi.it (D.S.); claudio.vernieri@istitutotumori.mi.it (C.V.); filippo.debraud@istitutotumori.mi.it (F.d.B.)
[2] Bioinformatics and Biostatistics Unit, Fondazione IRCCS, Istituto Nazionale dei Tumori di Milano, Via Giacomo Venezian 1, 20133 Milan, Italy; mara.lecchi@istitutotumori.mi.it (M.L.); paolo.verderio@istitutotumori.mi.it (P.V.)
[3] IFOM (Fondazione Istituto FIRC di Oncologia Molecolare), via Adamello 16, 20139 Milan, Italy
[4] Department of Oncology and Hemato-Oncology, Universita' degli Studi di Milano, 20122 Milan, Italy
* Correspondence: massimo.dinicola@istitutotumori.mi.it

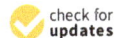

Received: 12 December 2018; Accepted: 12 February 2019; Published: 14 February 2019

Abstract: Predictive biomarkers of response to immune-checkpoint inhibitors (ICIs) are an urgent clinical need. The aim of this study is to identify manageable parameters to use in clinical practice to select patients with higher probability of response to ICIs. Two-hundred-and-seventy-one consecutive metastatic solid tumor patients, treated from 2013 until 2017 with anti- Programmed death-ligand 1 (PD-L1)/programmed cell death protein 1 (PD-1) ICIs, were evaluated for baseline lactate dehydrogenase (LDH) serum level, performance status (PS), age, neutrophil-lymphocyte ratio, type of immunotherapy, number of metastatic sites, histology, and sex. A training and validation set were used to build and test models, respectively. The variables' effects were assessed through odds ratio estimates (OR) and area under the receive operating characteristic curves (AUC), from univariate and multivariate logistic regression models. A final multivariate model with LDH, age and PS showed significant ORs and an AUC of 0.771. Results were statistically validated and used to devise an Excel algorithm to calculate the patient's response probabilities. We implemented an interactive Excel algorithm based on three variables (baseline LDH serum level, age and PS) which is able to provide a higher performance in response prediction to ICIs compared with LDH alone. This tool could be used in a real-life setting to identify ICIs in responding patients.

Keywords: immune-checkpoint inhibitors; LDH; biomarkers

1. Introduction

In the era of immunotherapy, several biological and biochemical factors have been investigated as potential biomarkers of tumor response/resistance to immune-checkpoint inhibitors (ICIs). Select patients is an important clinical need in an attempt to offer them the best therapeutic workup, to avoid unnecessary side effects, and to optimize the use of economic resources. In order to identify a predictive tool of response to ICIs, we evaluated the available and manageable parameters that could ameliorate the selection of patients. In this context, lactate dehydrogenase (LDH) is a potentially interesting, cheap and easy-to-detect biomarker of response [1–4]. Indeed, serum LDH levels are an independent poor prognostic factor in several malignancies, including renal cell [5] and nasopharyngeal carcinoma [6], lymphomas [7], multiple myeloma [8], sarcomas [9] and lung cancer [10,11]. It also seems to be predictive of clinical outcomes in patients treated with anti-PD1 monoclonal antibodies (mAbs) [12]. For instance, it inversely correlates with the probability of achieving a tumor response in metastatic melanoma patients treated with anti- Cytotoxic T-Lymphocyte Antigen 4 (CTLA4) mAbs [13,14]. In previous studies, the link between serum LDH levels and poor patient prognosis has been generally attributed to the fact that high LDH levels reflect a high tumor burden, which is often associated with worse clinical outcomes. However, LDH is an enzyme that catalyses the conversion of pyruvate to lactate in highly glycolytic cancer cells, and its serum levels could be a proxy of tumor metabolic activity and not simply of tumor burden. Of note, recent studies have suggested that enhanced glycolytic activity in human malignancies is associated with an immunosuppressive environment, while glycolysis inhibition reduces tumor infiltration by immunosuppressor myeloid cells (MDSCs), stimulating the infiltration by cytotoxic lymphocytes [15].

Potential biomarkers of response/resistance to immunotherapy other than serum LDH, such as intratumor Programmed death-ligand 1 (PD-L1) expression, tumor microenvironment characteristics, tumor mutational load, mismatch-repair deficiency, and neutrophil-lymphocyte (N/L) ratio in peripheral blood, have been extensively investigated [16]. Unfortunately, no single parameter has been consistently associated with tumor response and clinical outcomes in all types of neoplasms; moreover, many of these biomarkers require specific analyses in tumor specimens, which are not always available. Therefore, cheap and easy-to-measure biochemical and clinical parameters could significantly help in the selection of patients more likely to benefit from ICIs, without increasing costs.

Here, we describe an algorithm based on baseline serum LDH levels, patient Performance Status (PS) and age, which could help clinicians to provide more accurate identification of patient candidates to ICIs.

2. Results

In our study, we enrolled 271 metastatic solid tumor patients treated at Fondazione IRCCS—Istituto Nazionale dei Tumori with anti PD-1 and anti PD-L1 mAbs from April 2013 to August 2017. Patients were evaluated for baseline LDH serum level, PS, age, N/L ratio, type of immunotherapy, number of metastatic sites, histology, and sex. Overall, the population was made up of 43.2% (117) lung cancer, 22.1% (60) melanoma and 34.7% (94) miscellaneous other solid tumors (1 anal, 1 hepatocellular carcinoma (HCC), 1 thyroid, 1 germ cell tumor, 2 gynecologic, 3 gastric, 5 head and neck (H&N), 4 colorectal, 5 sarcoma, 6 biliary tract, 6 mesothelioma, 26 renal, and 33 urothelial). Patient's characteristics of training, validation and overall cohort are reported in Table 1; the number of metastatic sites is defined as the number of involved organs; the PS is evaluated through the Eastern Cooperative Oncology Group (ECOG) criteria [17] and dichotomized as 0 or ≥ 1. All responses were assessed by computed tomography. The categories of response consisted of: complete response (CR), partial response (PR), stable disease (SD), or disease progression (DP) as per RECIST (Response Evaluation Criteria in Solid Tumours) 1.1 criteria [18]. Disease control (DC) was defined as any CR, PR or SD. Overall, 150 (55.35%) patients achieved DC (6 CR, 59 PR, 85 SD) and 121 (44.65%) had DP as their best response.

Table 1. Clinic-pathological characteristics: training, validation and total cohorts.

Characteristics	Training Cohort		Validation Cohort		Total Cohort	
Categorical Variables	Freq	%	Freq	%	Freq	%
Sex						
Female	78	41.71	32	38.1	110	40.59
Male	109	58.29	52	61.9	161	59.41
Tumor Site						
Melanoma	36	19.25	24	28.57	60	22.14
Lung	93	49.73	24	28.57	117	43.17
Others *	58	31.02	36	42.86	94	34.69
Treatment						
PD-1	117	62.57	51	60.71	168	61.99
PD-L1	70	37.43	33	39.29	103	38.01
Line of therapy						
1	8	4.3	37	44.0	45	16.61
2	56	29.9	33	39.3	89	32.84
≥3	123	65.8	14	16.7	137	50.55
Number of Metastatic sites						
1	31	16.6	11	13.1	42	15.5
2	83	44.4	37	44.0	120	44.28
≥3	73	39.0	36	42.9	109	40.22
PS (ECOG)						
0	123	65.78	54	64.29	177	65.31
≥1	64	34.22	30	35.71	94	34.69
Best Response						
DC	104	55.61	46	54.76	150	55.35
DP	83	44.39	38	45.24	121	44.65
Continuos variables	Median	Range	Median	Range	Median	Range
Age, years	61	16; 84	66	34; 83	62	16; 84
N/L ratio	3.44	0.65; 39.50	3.39	0.78; 28.33	3.44	0.65; 39.50
LDH serum level	353.00	152.00; 2048.00	321.50	179.00; 5063.00	343.00	152.00; 5063.00

PS: performance status, DC: disease control, DP: disease progression, N/L ratio: neutrophil to lymphocyte ratio.
* Other solid tumors: 1 anal, 1 HCC, 1 thyroid, 1 germ cell tumor, 2 gynecologic, 3 gastric, 5 H&N, 4 colorectal, 5 sarcoma, 6 biliary tract, 6 mesothelioma, 26 renal, and 33 urothelial.

The evaluation of LDH levels was performed in terms of percentage increase with respect to the upper limit of the specific normality range. This transformed variable was called *LDH normalized*. The median value of *LDH normalized* distribution was −27.7%, the lower quartile −38.48% and the upper −3.96%. A minimum extreme value was observed at −66.96% and a maximum at 954.79%. Figure 1 shows the *LDH normalized* distributions in the training and validation cohorts when considering all patients (Figure 1A) or according to the best response achieved with immunotherapy (Figure 1B).

For all the continuous variables considered in the logistic regression model, we found that a linear relationship between the log odds and their values was satisfied.

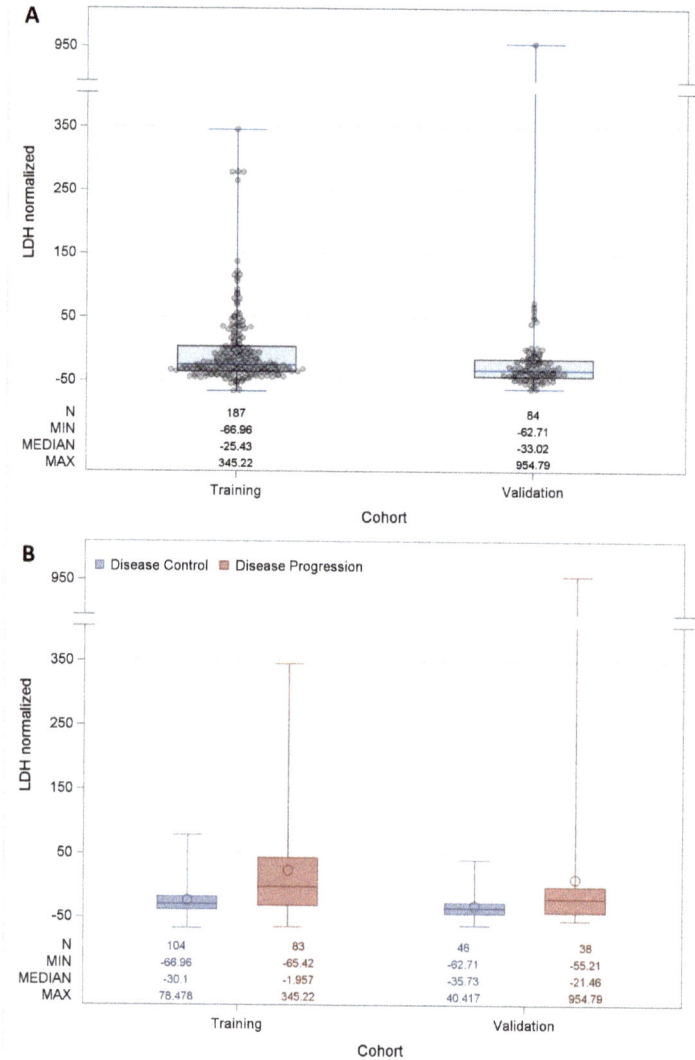

Figure 1. Distribution of lactate dehydrogenase (LDH) *normalized* in the training and validation cohort. (**A**) Boxplots reflecting the distribution of *LDH normalized* for each patient ($n = 271$) distinguished in training and in the validation cohort. Each box indicates the 25th and 75th centiles. The horizontal line inside the box indicates the median, and the whiskers indicate the extreme measured values. Each observation is represented by a grey dot. (**B**) Boxplots reflecting the distribution of *LDH normalized* according to the best response distinguished in training and in the validation cohort. Each box indicates the 25th and 75th centiles. Blue and red colors indicate disease control and disease progression patients, respectively. The horizontal line inside the box indicates the median, and the whiskers indicate the extreme measured values.

Univariate analysis was performed in 104 patients achieving DC and 83 patients undergoing DP (training set); of note, clinical response was significantly associated ($p < 0.0001$) with *LDH normalized*, with an odds ratio estimate (OR) equal to 0.792 for any LDH increment of 10%. We also found a significant positive association between age and tumor response, with an OR of 1.426 for any 10-year increment (p-value: 0.0093), and an inverse association between ECOG PS with an OR equal to 0.530 for 1 vs. 0 score (p-value: 0.0419) or N/L ratio with an OR equal to 0.899 (p-value: 0.014) and tumor response. Then, a logistic multivariate model was built by including these four variables, and a backward selection procedure was performed. Baseline LDH serum levels, age and PS were independently associated with the probability of responding to the treatment, with a statistically significant ($p < 0.05$) or borderline significant (p-value: 0.056 in the case of PS) association; therefore, they were retained in the final model. On the other hand, the N/L ratio was removed because it was not independently associated with the chance of responding (p-value: 0.529). The predictive capability of the final model was evaluated by generating a receive operating characteristic curve (ROC) and using as a pivotal statistic the area under the ROC curve (AUC). A satisfactory predictive capability [19] was observed, showing an AUC of 0.771 (95% Confidence Interval (CI): 0.701;0.842). The contribution of each variable of the final model to the predictive performance is graphically shown in Figure 2, and the differences between AUCs of the *LDH normalized* univariate model and the final one turned out to be significantly different to zero (difference: −0.0585; p-value: 0.0298; 95% CI: −0.111; −0.0057). By applying the training coefficients to the validation set, the model was statistically validated showing a significant AUC of 0.685 (95% CI: 0.569;0.801) (Figure 3). When the validated model was fitted to the totality of 150 patients achieving DC and 121 patients undergoing DP, the impact of these three variables on tumor response remained significant, as shown in Table 2; the overall AUC value, as well as the cross-validated one, were satisfactory (AUC: 0.737 95% CI: 0.675;0.798 and AUC: 0.718 95% CI: 0.654;0.781, respectively). Finally, we implemented an interactive Excel tool like that shown, for feasibility purposes, in the example of Table 3. By inserting for each patient: the upper limit of the normal reference range of the adopted kit for LDH quantification, the baseline LDH serum value, the ECOG PS score (as 0, 1, 2), and the age, it is possible to obtain the corresponding estimated probability of clinical response to ICIs.

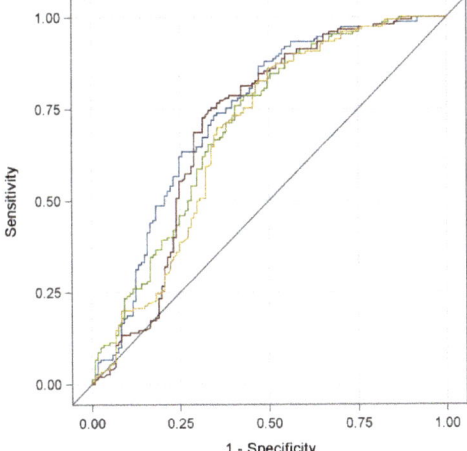

Figure 2. Receive Operating Characteristic (ROC) curves in the training set of the final multivariate model (blue line, Area under the ROC curve (AUC): 0.771), final model without performance status (green line, AUC: 0.749), final model without age (red line, AUC: 0.728), and *LDH normalized* univariate model (yellow line, AUC: 0.713).

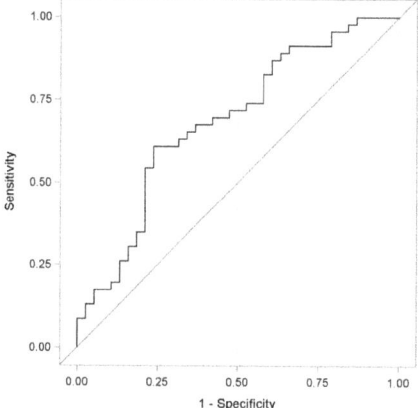

Figure 3. ROC curve of the final multivariate model applied on the validation set with an AUC value of 0.685.

Table 2. Overall Odd Ratio (OR) estimates and 95% Confidence Interval (CI) for each variable of the final model.

Effect	OR	95% CI	
LDH normalized for a 10% increment	0.810	0.744	0.883
Age for a ten-years increment	1.305	1.038	1.641
PS (ECOG) 1 vs. 0 score	0.481	0.274	0.846

OR: Odd Ratio; CI: Confidence Interval; PS: performance status; ECOG: Eastern Cooperative Oncology Group criteria.

Table 3. Example of the excel interactive tool. Grey cells need to be filled; the blue one will show the estimated probability of clinical response.

Variable	Value
Kit Characteristic	
Upper limit of normal reference range	460
Patients Characteristics	
LDH serum value	77
ECOG PS score [17]	1
Age	60
Estimated Probability %	76.39

Finally, we compared the performance (in terms of AUC) of the predictor built starting from the final model, to that derived from the only N/L ratio. As reported in Figure 4, the first classifier, with an AUC equal to 0.737 (95% CI: 0.675; 0.798), showed a higher predictive capability with respect to the N/L ratio classifier characterized by an AUC value of 0.645 (95% CI: 0.579; 0.711). In particular, the AUC values' difference was statistically significant (*p*-value: 0.0220).

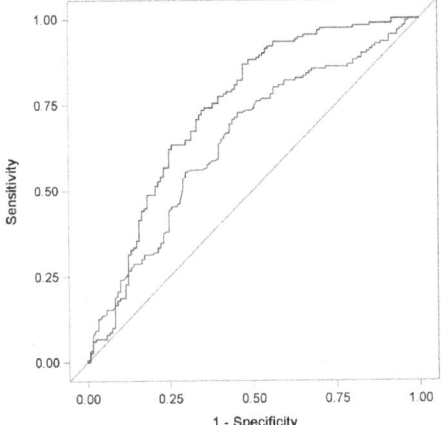

Figure 4. ROC curves of the proposed predictor (red line, AUC: 0.737) and N/L ratio one (blue line, AUC: 0.645).

3. Discussion

The renewed interest for immunotherapy in the last years and the recent introduction of several ICIs in the clinical practice have redefined the therapeutic strategies of different solid tumors. The efficacy of the immunological approach was first proven in advanced melanoma with the anti CTLA-4 mAb Ipilimumab [20]. Thereafter, also anti PD-1/PD-L1 mAbs were tested against tumors that were classically considered to be poorly immunogenic and mostly unresponsive to immunotherapy, such as non-small cell lung cancer (NSCLC); however, these drugs demonstrated impressive and long-lasting anticancer activity in a minority of patients [21–25]. Unfortunately, despite the remarkable clinical efficacy and low toxicity of ICIs, the vast majority of patients with advanced solid cancers fail to achieve durable responses with ICIs. Therefore, predictive biomarkers of clinical benefit from ICIs are urgently needed in order to select patients with a higher probability of response, as well as to optimize the available economic resources. PD-L1 expression, tumor microenvironment (TME) features, mutational load, mismatch-repair deficiency, and N/L ratio in peripheral blood have been extensively investigated [26]. However, a universally recognized biomarker is not available, yet. For example, although high intratumor PD-L1 expression seems to be significantly associated with a better response to PD-1/PD-L1 blockade agents in several tumors [27], the spatial heterogeneity and dynamic changes of expression in the same tumor, together with the lack of reliable detection methods and definite cut-off values, actually limits its widespread use in clinical practice.

In contrast, measuring LDH serum level is a simple and low-cost evaluation that has already been proposed as a biomarker predictive of tumor response/resistance to regorafenib [28], temsirolimus [29], sorafenib [30,31], and anti CTLA-4 mAbs [12] in patients with colorectal, renal, pancreatic cancers, HCC, and melanoma, respectively.

LDH serum levels have been historically considered to reflect the total number of viable and biologically active cancer cells inside a tumor mass; therefore, its inverse association with patient prognosis and/or tumor response to chemotherapy was mainly attributed to the association between serum LDH levels and tumor burden. However, LDH is a metabolic enzyme that takes crucially part to the glycolytic pathway, which is aberrantly activated in several human cancers to fuel tumor bioenergetics and anabolic needs [32,33]. Of note, enhanced glycolysis in cancer masses leads to reduced glucose levels in the TME and, consequently, to glucose starvation in cells of the TME, including cytotoxic lymphocytes that mediate the antitumor immune response. This metabolic competition between cancer cells and immune cells for the use of glucose molecules may be one crucial mechanism through which malignant cells inhibit the activity of cytotoxic lymphocytes.

Therefore, the observed inverse association between serum LDH levels and clinical benefit from ICIs could reflect an impairment of antitumor immunity in highly glycolytic, LDH-overexpressing malignancies. An alternative explanation for the link between tumor glycolytic activity and response to immunotherapy comes from a recently published preclinical study, where the inhibition of glycolysis in different tumor models was associated with reduced secretion of Granulocyte Colony-Stimulating Factor (G-CSF) and Granulocyte-Macrophage Colony-Stimulating Factor (GM-CSF) by cancer cells and lower intratumor infiltration by MDSCs, which restrain the activity of cytotoxic lymphocytes [15]. Therefore, high serum LDH, which reflects tumor glycolytic activity, may also reflect a more immunosuppressive, MDSC-enriched tumor microenvironment.

In order to improve the predictive capability of the LDH serum level, we combined it with other clinical parameters for which a rationale exists to test them as predictive biomarkers. To this aim, we have created an interactive Excel tool based on three variables (baseline LDH, age and PS ECOG score) which is able to provide high accuracy in response prediction to ICIs if compared with LDH alone. Our retrospective analysis confirms that patients with high baseline LDH serum levels have a statistically significant reduced probability of achieving a clinical response during treatment with ICIs, especially in patients who are younger and have poorer performance status.

Since the N/L ratio, which reflects systemic cancer-related inflammatory status, has been proposed as a biomarker of resistance to chemo-immunotherapy, we decided to evaluate its impact on the patient's response to ICIs [34]. We observed that the N/L ratio has a significant predictive role but only in univariate fashion and shows a worse predictive capability than our model. To assess the performance of our algorithm, we tried to test it in three of the four colorectal cancer tissues of whom microsatellite instability (MSI) has been previously evaluated: two out of the three patients scored MSI. It is well known that the MSI subset of colorectal cancer has a greater likelihood of response to ICIs compared to the stable one [35]. It is worth noting that our predictor was able to detect with high accuracy which one between the two MSI patients had a major probability of DC and can really benefit from ICIs (Table 4).

Table 4. Estimated probability of response in colorectal patients according to microsatellite mutational status.

PS (ECOG)	Baseline LDH	Age (years)	Estimated Probability of Response (%)	Best Response	Microsatellite Instability
0	1063	60	8.21	DP	Yes
0	354	67	69.45	SD	Yes
1	925	47	5.29	DP	No

PS: performance status, DP: disease progression, SD: stable disease.

The algorithm that we developed and validated in this study could provide a base to guide physicians in a real-life setting to better plan a therapeutic strategy tailored to patient characteristics and potentially able to identify patients more likely to benefit from ICIs. The clinical relevance of our findings is related to the easy detectability and manageability of the variables tested. Indeed, information about age, baseline LDH serum levels and PS can be collected quickly, already during the medical examination.

The main limits of our study consist in its retrospective nature, the heterogeneity of tumor histologies included, and the relatively small number of patients enrolled. Prospective studies in larger populations and focused on specific tumor types have already started in order to validate our results.

4. Materials and Methods

4.1. Ldh Evaluation

The evaluation of LDH was performed at baseline. All measures were performed in our laboratory, with COBAS® 6000 analyser (Roche Diagnostics, Indianapolis, IN, USA), using a UV-test. The catalytic activity of LDH was determined by the measurement of decreased absorbancy of nicotinamide adenine dinucleotide at 340 nm as a result of catalytic reduction of pyruvate to lactate. From January 2013 to July 2015, the normality reference range was 230–460 Units per liter (U/L); since August 2015, it has changed to 20–480 U/L.

4.2. Statistical Analysis

Discrete variables (line and type of therapy (anti-PD1 vs. anti-PDL1), number of metastatic sites, histology, and sex) were opportunely categorized by taking into consideration their clinical function and according to their distributions. Concerning the continuous variables, age and N/L ratio were used in their original scale, whereas for LDH, an appropriate transformation was applied to the original values in order to normalize levels determined by the UV-test with the two different normal reference ranges. All the analyses were performed in terms of percentage increase with respect to the upper limit of each specific range (*LDH normalized*). In order to investigate the relationship between the clinical response and continuous variables and to detect possible nonlinear effects, we resorted to a logistic regression model based on restricted cubic splines. A training set, consisting of all patients treated before the 1st of January 2016 ($\approx$ 70% of all patients), was used to build models which were tested on a validation set including patients treated since the 1st of January 2016 ($\approx$ 30% of all patients). The relationships between each variable and the clinical response (DC vs. DP) were investigated by resorting to a logistic regression model in both univariate and multivariate fashion. The hypothesis of OR equal to 1 was tested using the Wald Statistic. All the variables resulted statistically significant ($\alpha = 0.05$) in univariate analysis was considered in the initial model of multivariate analysis, and a backward selection procedure was used to obtain the final model. We investigated the predictive capability of the multivariate model by means of the AUC. The nonparametric approach of DeLong and Clarke–Pearson [36] was used to compare the discriminatory performance of different models and evaluate the contribution of each variable of the model. The most satisfactory model was applied on the validation set to statistically validate it and it was fitted overall to obtain the most robust estimates. AUC estimates based on cross-validated predicted probabilities were determined to evaluate the performance of the selected variables in the absence of an independent dataset [37]. All statistical analyses were carried out with SAS software (Version 9.4.; SAS Institute, Inc., Cary, NC, USA) by adopting a significance level of $\alpha = 0.05$. The overall coefficients estimated were used to implement an Excel algorithm that requires the selected clinical variables of the patient and returns the corresponding response probability.

5. Conclusions

Identifying responder patients before starting immunotherapy is an important clinical need in order to define the best therapeutic workup, avoid unnecessary side effects and efficiently use the economic resources. The clinical relevance of our findings is related to the easy detectability and manageability of the variables tested. Indeed, information about age, baseline LDH serum levels and PS can be collected quickly, already during the medical examination.

The main limits of our study consist in its retrospective nature, the heterogeneity of tumor histologies included, and the relatively small number of patients enrolled. Prospective studies in larger populations and focused on specific tumor types have already started in order to validate our results.

Author Contributions: M.S.C.: conceptualization, data curation, methodology, writing–original draft, writing–review and editing. M.L.: formal analysis, data curation, software, methodology, writing–original draft, writing–review and editing. S.C.: data curation, writing–review and editing. S.D.: data curation, writing–review and editing. M.D.V.: data curation, writing–review and editing. A.N.: data curation, writing–review and editing. M.M.P.: data curation. D.R.: data curation, writing–review and editing. G.R.: data curation, writing–review and editing. R.R.: data curation, writing–review and editing. D.S.: data curation, writing–review and editing. C.V.: data curation, writing–review and editing. F.d.B.: conceptualization, methodology, supervision, writing–review and editing. P.V.: formal analysis, data curation, software, methodology, writing–original draft, writing–review and editing. M.D.N.: conceptualization, methodology, supervision, writing–review and editing.

Funding: This research received no external funding.

Conflicts of Interest: The authors declare no conflict of interest.

References

1. Drent, M.; Cobben, N.A.; Henderson, R.F.; Wouters, E.F.; van Dieijen-Visser, M. Usefulness of lactate dehydrogenase and its isoenzymes as indicators of lung damage or inflammation. *Eur. Respir J.* **1996**, *9*, 1736–1742. [CrossRef] [PubMed]
2. Kemp, M.; Donovan, J.; Higham, H.; Hooper, J. Biochemical markers of myocardial injury. *Br. J. Anaesth.* **2004**, *93*, 63–73. [CrossRef] [PubMed]
3. Kato, G.J.; McGowan, V.; Machado, R.F.; Little, J.A.; Taylor, V.I.J.; Morris, C.R.; Nichols, J.S.; Wang, X.; Poljakovic, M.; Morris, S.M.; et al. Lactate dehydrogenase as a biomarker of hemolysis-associated nitric oxide resistance, priapism, leg ulceration, pulmonary hypertension, and death in patients with sickle cell disease. *Blood* **2006**, *107*, 2279–2285. [CrossRef] [PubMed]
4. Vander Heiden, M.G.; Cantley, L.C.; Thompson, C.B. Understanding the Warburg Effect: The Metabolic Requirements of Cell Proliferation. *Science* **2009**, *324*, 1029–1033. [CrossRef] [PubMed]
5. Motzer, R.J.; Escudier, B.; Bukowski, R.; Rini, B.I.; Hutson, T.E.; Barrios, C.H.; Lin, X.; Fly, K.; Matczak, E.; Gore, M.E. Prognostic factors for survival in 1059 patients treated with sunitinib for metastatic renal cell carcinoma. *Br. J. Cancer* **2013**, *108*, 2470–2477. [CrossRef] [PubMed]
6. Wan, X.B.; Wei, L.; Li, H.; Dong, M.; Lin, Q.; Ma, X.K.; Huang, P.Y.; Wen, J.Y.; Li, X.; Chen, J.; et al. High pretreatment serum lactate dehydrogenase level correlates with disease relapse and predicts an inferior outcome in locally advanced nasopharyngeal carcinoma. *Eur. J. Cancer* **2013**, *49*, 2356–2364. [CrossRef]
7. Hagberg, H.; Siegbahn, A. Prognostic level of serum lactic dehydrogenase in non-Hodgkin's lymphoma. *Scand J. Haematol.* **1983**, *31*, 49–56. [CrossRef]
8. Simonsson, B.; Grenning, G.; Källander, C.; Ahre, A. Prognostic level of serum lactic dehydrogenase (S-LDH) in multiple myeloma. *Eur. J. Clin. Investig.* **1987**, *17*, 336–349. [CrossRef]
9. Brereton, H.D.; Simon, R.; Pomeroy, T.C. Pretreatment lactate dehydrogenase predicting metastatic spread in Ewing's sarcoma. *Ann. Intern. Med.* **1975**, *83*, 352–364. [CrossRef]
10. Hermes, A.; Gatzemeier, U.; Waschki, B.; Reck, M. Lactate dehydrogenase as prognostic factor in limited and extensive disease stage small cell lung cancer e A retrospective single institution analysis. *Respir. Med.* **2010**, *104*, 1937–1942. [CrossRef]
11. Giroux Leprieur, E.; Lavole, A.; Ruppert, A.M.; Gounant, V.; Wislez, M.; Cadranel, J.; Milleron, B. Factors associated with long-term survival of patients with advanced non-small cell lung cancer. *Respirology* **2012**, *17*, 134–142. [CrossRef] [PubMed]
12. Diem, S.; Kasenda, B.; Spain, L.; Martin-Liberal, J.; Marconcini, R.; Gore, M.; Larkin, J. Serum lactate dehydrogenase as an early marker for outcome in patients treated with anti-PD-1 therapy in metastatic melanoma. *Br. J. Cancer* **2016**, *114*, 256–261. [CrossRef] [PubMed]
13. Kelderman, S.; Heemskerk, B.; van Tinteren, H.; van den Brom, R.R.; Hospers, G.A.; van den Eertwegh, A.J.; Kapiteijn, E.W.; de Groot, J.W.; Soetekouw, P.; Jansen, R.L.; et al. Lactate dehydrogenase as a selection criterion for ipilimumab treatment in metastatic melanoma. *Cancer Immunol. Immunother.* **2014**, *63*, 449–458. [CrossRef] [PubMed]
14. Manola, J.; Atkins, M.; Ibrahim, J.; Kirkwood, J. Prognostic factors in metastatic melanoma: A pooled analysis of Eastern Cooperative Oncology Group trials. *J. Clin. Oncol.* **2000**, *18*, 3782–3793. [CrossRef] [PubMed]
15. Li, W.; Tanikawa, T.; Kryczek, I.; Xia, H.; Li, G.; Wu, K.; Wei, S.; Zhao, L.; Vatan, L.; Wen, B. Aerobic Glycolysis Controls Myeloid-Derived Suppressor Cells and Tumor Immunity via a Specific CEBPB Isoform in Triple-Negative Breast Cancer. *Cell Metab.* **2018**, *28*, 87–103. [CrossRef] [PubMed]
16. Meng, X.; Huang, Z.; Teng, F.; Xing, L.; Yu, J. Predictive biomarkers in PD-1/PD-L1 checkpoint blockade immunotherapy. *Cancer Treat Rev.* **2015**, *41*, 868–876. [CrossRef] [PubMed]

17. Oken, M.M.; Creech, R.H.; Tormey, D.C.; Horton, J.; Davis, T.E.; McFadden, E.T.; Carbone, P.P. Toxicity and response criteria of the Eastern Cooperative Oncology Group. *Am. J. Clin. Oncol.* **1982**, *5*, 649–655. [CrossRef]
18. Eisenhauer, E.A.; Therasse, P.; Bogaerts, J.; Schwartz, L.H.; Sargent, D.; Ford, R.; Dancey, J.; Arbuck, S.; Gwyther, S.; Mooney, M.; et al. New response evaluation criteria in solid tumours: Revised RECIST guideline (version 1.1). *Eur. J. Cancer* **2009**, *45*, 228–247. [CrossRef]
19. Salvianti, F.; Pinzani, P.; Verderio, P.; Ciniselli, C.M.; Massi, D.; De Giorgi, V.; Grazzini, M.; Pazzagli, M.; Orlando, C. Multiparametric analysis of cell-free DNA in melanoma patients. *PLoS ONE* **2012**, *7*, e49843. [CrossRef]
20. Hodi, F.S.; O'Day, S.J.; McDermott, D.F.; Weber, R.W.; Sosman, J.A.; Haanen, J.B.; Gonzalez, R.; Robert, C.; Schadendorf, D.; Hassel, J.C.; et al. Improved survival with ipilimumab in patients with metastatic melanoma. *N. Engl. J. Med.* **2010**, *363*, 711–723. [CrossRef]
21. Garon, E.B.; Rizvi, N.A.; Hui, R.; Leighl, N.; Balmanoukian, A.S.; Eder, J.P.; Patnaik, A.; Aggarwal, C.; Gubens, M.; Horn, L.; et al. Pembrolizumab for the treatment of non-small-cell lung cancer. *N. Engl. J. Med.* **2015**, *372*, 2018–2028. [CrossRef] [PubMed]
22. Brahmer, J.; Reckamp, K.L.; Baas, P.; Crinò, L.; Eberhardt, W.E.; Poddubskaya, E.; Antonia, S.; Pluzanski, A.; Vokes, E.E.; Holgado, E.; et al. Nivolumab versus docetaxel in advanced squamous-cell non-small-cell lung cancer. *N. Engl. J. Med.* **2015**, *373*, 123–135. [CrossRef] [PubMed]
23. Borghaei, H.; Paz-Ares, L.; Horn, L.; Spigel, D.R.; Steins, M.; Ready, N.E.; Chow, L.Q.; Vokes, E.E.; Felip, E.; Holgado, E.; et al. Nivolumab versus docetaxel in advanced nonsquamous non-small-cell lung cancer. *N. Engl. J. Med.* **2015**, *373*, 1627–1639. [CrossRef]
24. Motzer, R.J.; Escudier, B.; McDermott, D.F.; George, S.; Hammers, H.J.; Srinivas, S.; Tykodi, S.S.; Sosman, J.A.; Procopio, G.; Plimack, E.R.; et al. Nivolumab versus everolimus in advanced renal-cell carcinoma. *N. Engl. J. Med.* **2015**, *373*, 1803–1813. [CrossRef]
25. Balar, A.V.; Galsky, M.D.; Rosenberg, J.E.; Powles, T.; Petrylak, D.P.; Bellmunt, J.; Loriot, Y.; Necchi, A.; Hoffman-Censits, J.; Perez-Gracia, J.L.; et al. Atezolizumab as first-line treatment in cisplatin-ineligible patients with locally advanced and metastatic urothelial carcinoma: A single-arm, multicentre, phase 2 trial. *Lancet* **2017**, *389*, 67–76. [CrossRef]
26. Taube, J.M.; Klein, A.; Brahmer, J.R.; Xu, H.; Pan, X.; Kim, J.H.; Chen, L.; Pardoll, D.M.; Topalian, S.L.; Anders, R.A. Association of PD-1, PD-1 ligands, and other features of the tumor immune microenvironment with response to anti-PD-1 therapy. *Clin. Cancer Res.* **2014**, *20*, 5064–5074. [CrossRef] [PubMed]
27. Daud, A.I.; Wolchok, J.D.; Robert, C.; Hwu, W.J.; Weber, J.S.; Ribas, A.; Hodi, F.S.; Joshua, A.M.; Kefford, R.; Hersey, P.; et al. Programmed Death-Ligand 1 Expression and Response to the Anti-Programmed Death 1 Antibody Pembrolizumab in Melanoma. *J. Clin. Oncol.* **2016**, *34*, 4102–4109. [CrossRef] [PubMed]
28. Del Prete, M.; Giampieri, R.; Loupakis, F.; Prochilo, T.; Salvatore, L.; Faloppi, L.; Bianconi, M.; Bittoni, A.; Aprile, G.; Zaniboni, A.; et al. Prognostic clinical factors in pretreated colorectal cancer patients receiving regorafenib: Implications for clinical management. *Oncotarget* **2015**, *6*, 33982–33992. [CrossRef]
29. Armstrong, A.J.; George, D.J.; Halabi, S. Serum lactate dehydrogenase predicts for overall survival benefit in patients with metastatic renal cell carcinoma treated with inhibition of mammalian target of rapamycin. *J. Clin. Oncol.* **2012**, *30*, 3402–3417. [CrossRef]
30. Faloppi, L.; Bianconi, M.; Giampieri, R.; Sobrero, A.; Labianca, R.; Ferrari, D.; Barni, S.; Aitini, E.; Zaniboni, A.; Boni, C.; et al. The value of lactate dehydrogenase serum levels as a prognostic and predictive factor for advanced pancreatic cancer patients receiving sorafenib. *Oncotarget* **2015**, *6*, 35087–35094. [CrossRef]
31. Faloppi, L.; Scartozzi, M.; Bianconi, M.; Svegliati Baroni, G.; Toniutto, P.; Giampieri, R.; Del Prete, M.; De Minicis, S.; Bitetto, D.; Loretelli, M.; et al. The role of LDH serum levels in predicting global outcome in HCC patients treated with sorafenib: implications for clinical management. *PLoS ONE* **2012**, *7*, e32653. [CrossRef]
32. Martinez-Outschoorn, U.E.; Peiris-Pagés, M.; Pestell, R.G.; Sotgia, F.; Lisanti, M.P. Cancer metabolism: a therapeutic perspective. *Nat. Rev. Clin. Oncol.* **2017**, *14*, 11–31. [CrossRef] [PubMed]
33. Vernieri, C.; Casola, S.; Foiani, M.; Pietrantonio, F.; de Braud, F.; Longo, V. Targeting Cancer Metabolism: Dietary and Pharmacologic Interventions. *Cancer Discov.* **2016**, *6*, 1315–1333. [CrossRef] [PubMed]
34. Mei, Z.; Shi, L.; Wang, B.; Yang, J.; Xiao, Z.; Du, P.; Wang, Q.; Yang, W. Prognostic role of pretreatment blood neutrophil-to-lymphocyte ratio in advanced cancer survivors: A systematic review and meta-analysis of 66 cohort studies. *Cancer Treat. Rev.* **2017**, *58*, 1–13. [CrossRef] [PubMed]

35. Xiao, Y.; Freeman, G.J. The microsatellite instable subset of colorectal cancer is a particularly good candidate for checkpoint blockade immunotherapy. *Cancer Discov.* **2015**, *5*, 16–28. [CrossRef]
36. DeLong, E.R.; DeLong, D.M.; Clarke-Pearson, D.L. Comparing the areas under two or more correlated receiver operating characteristic curves: a nonparametric approach. *Biometrics* **1988**, *44*, 837–845. [CrossRef] [PubMed]
37. Wu, B.; Abbott, T.; Fishman, D.; McMurray, W.; Mor, G.; Stone, K.; Ward, D.; Williams, K.; Zhao, H. Comparison of statistical methods for classification of ovarian cancer using mass spectrometry data. *Bioinformatics* **2003**, *19*, 1636–1643. [CrossRef]

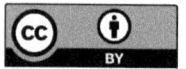

© 2019 by the authors. Licensee MDPI, Basel, Switzerland. This article is an open access article distributed under the terms and conditions of the Creative Commons Attribution (CC BY) license (http://creativecommons.org/licenses/by/4.0/).

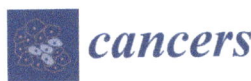

Article

An Fc-Optimized CD133 Antibody for Induction of Natural Killer Cell Reactivity Against Colorectal Cancer

Bastian J. Schmied [1,2,†], Fabian Riegg [1,2,†], Latifa Zekri [1,3], Ludger Grosse-Hovest [3], Hans-Jörg Bühring [4], Gundram Jung [3] and Helmut R. Salih [1,2,*]

1. Clinical Collaboration Unit Translational Immunology, German Cancer Consortium (DKTK) and German Cancer Research Center (DKFZ), Partner site, 72076 Tuebingen, Germany; Bastian.Schmied@med.uni-tuebingen.de (B.J.S.); Fabian.Riegg@med.uni-tuebingen.de (F.R.); l.zekri-metref@dkfz.de (L.Z.)
2. DFG Cluster of Excellence 2180 "Image-guided and Functional Instructed Tumor Therapy (iFIT)", 72076 Tuebingen, Germany
3. Department for Immunology, Eberhard Karls University, 72076 Tuebingen, Germany; grosse-hovest@synimmune.de (L.G.-H.); gundram.jung@uni-tuebingen.de (G.J.)
4. Department of Hematology and Oncology, Eberhard Karls University, 72076 Tuebingen, Germany; hans-joerg.buehring@uni-tuebingen.de
* Correspondence: Helmut.Salih@med.uni-tuebingen.de; Tel.: +49-7071/29-83275
† These authors have contributed equally to this work.

Received: 13 May 2019; Accepted: 5 June 2019; Published: 7 June 2019

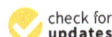

Abstract: The introduction of monoclonal antibodies (mAbs) has largely improved treatment options for cancer patients. The ability of antitumor mAbs to elicit antibody-dependent cellular cytotoxicity (ADCC) contributes to a large extent to their therapeutic efficacy. Many efforts accordingly aim to improve this important function by engineering mAbs with Fc parts that display enhanced affinity to the Fc receptor CD16 expressed, e.g., on natural killer (NK) cells. Here we characterized the CD133 mAb 293C3-SDIE that contains an engineered Fc part modified by the amino acid exchanges S239D/I332E—that reportedly increase the affinity to CD16—with regard to its ability to induce NK reactivity against colorectal cancer (CRC). 293C3-SDIE was found to be a stable protein with favorable binding characteristics achieving saturating binding to CRC cells at concentrations of approximately 1 µg/mL. While not directly affecting CRC cell growth and viability, 293C3-SDIE potently induced NK cell activation, degranulation, secretion of Interferon-γ, as well as ADCC resulting in potent lysis of CRC cell lines. Based on the preclinical characterization presented in this study and the available data indicating that CD133 is broadly expressed in CRC and represents a negative prognostic marker, we conclude that 293C3-SDIE constitutes a promising therapeutic agent for the treatment of CRC and thus warrants clinical evaluation.

Keywords: colorectal cancer; immunotherapy; antibody; NK cells; ADCC; CD133; prominin-1

1. Introduction

The introduction of immunotherapy to induce a specific antitumor immune response constitutes—as monotherapy or combinatorial treatment—A well established option for cancer treatment [1]. Especially monoclonal antibodies (mAbs) have largely improved the treatment options for patients with malignant disease. For example, rituximab and trastuzumab are widely used for therapy of patients with B-cell non-Hodgkin´s lymphoma and human epidermal growth factor receptor 2 (HER2)-positive breast cancer, respectively [2,3]. However, despite their undisputed success, the therapeutic efficacy of these and other antitumor mAbs is still far from satisfactory. While various factors influence the susceptibility of tumor cells to therapeutic mAbs (such as mutant forms of receptors, alternative signaling pathways, genetic variability and receptor shedding; e.g., [4]), one approach to improve efficacy is to enhance the immunostimulatory potency of antitumor mAbs [5]. With regard to mAbs that target tumor cells and mediate their effects (at least in part) via induction of antibody-dependent cellular cytotoxicity (ADCC), one strategy is to modify their Fc part in order to enhance the affinity to the Fc receptor CD16. This improves the recruitment of CD16 expressing immune cells, among which, at least in humans, natural killer (NK) cells are particularly important to induce ADCC [6,7]. The latter constitutes one of the major effector mechanisms by which antitumor mAbs mediate their beneficial effects, at least in hematopoietic malignancies (e.g., [8]). To improve ADCC, Fc parts can be modified either with regard to their glycosylation patterns or by changes in the amino acid sequence. Glyco-optimized mAbs, like obinituzumab, have been approved by the FDA, and others as well as antibodies with Fc parts carrying amino acid substitutions (e.g., S239D/I332E (SDIE) [9]) are currently being evaluated in clinical trials [5].

Recently we reported on the preclinical characterization of Fc-optimized mAbs and antibody-like constructs carrying the SDIE modification for immunotherapy of leukemia [10–14]. Besides an Fc-optimized FLT3 (CD135) mAb that is presently undergoing clinical evaluation (ClinicalTrials.gov ID NCT02789254), this comprised a construct targeting CD133 (prominin-1). The latter is a pentaspan transmembrane glycoprotein and, beyond leukemia, also expressed in various solid tumors [15]. While CD133 has been implicated to play a role, e.g., in chemotherapy resistance and metastasis, its exact biological function remains to be fully elucidated [16]. Particularly in colorectal cancer (CRC), CD133 is frequently expressed and constitutes a negative prognostic marker [17–19]. Since so far immunotherapeutic options for CRC treatment are rather limited, with applications of anti-epidermal growth factor receptor (EGFR) mAbs and checkpoint inhibitors being restricted to the subsets of patients with metastatic disease that display rat sarcoma (RAS) wildtype and microsatellite instability-high/DNA mismatch repair deficiency, respectively, we here set out to evaluate 293C3-SDIE as a potential immunotherapeutic option for CRC.

2. Results

2.1. Binding of Different CD133 mAbs to CRC Cells

Recently we observed pronounced differences in the binding of three different mouse anti-human CD133 mAbs to acute myeloid leukemia (AML) cells. Based on superior binding characteristics, the clone 293C3 was accordingly chosen for construction of our therapeutic construct 293C3-SDIE [14]. To determine whether differential reactivity also occurs in CRC, we first confirmed specific binding using CD133 or control transfected B16F10 cells (Figure 1A). The mouse background of these cells served to exclude that (CD133) cross-reactivity of any of the three anti-human CD133 mAb clones influenced our results. Subsequently, we compared the binding of clone (i) 293C3, (ii) AC133, which is used in other CD133 targeting cancer therapeutics [20], and (iii) W6B3C1 using a panel of five different CRC cell lines that reportedly express CD133 [21–23]. CD133 mRNA expression was observed by quantitative PCR in all CRC cell lines, but with profoundly different levels (Figure 1B). Caco-2 cells, which displayed the highest CD133 mRNA levels, were then employed in dose titration experiments with all three antibodies. Flow cytometric analysis revealed that all three clones achieved saturated binding at approximately 1 µg/mL (Figure 1C). This concentration was then used to comparatively analyze binding in the panel of the five CRC cell lines with different biological characteristics (Table 1; [24,25]). As shown in Figure 1D,E, no marked differences with regard to binding were observed with the different CD133 mAb clones. While this was in contrast to our findings in AML, where clone 293C3 was superior to the other clones [14], and the reason for this discrepancy so far remain elusive, these results warranted the use of our therapeutic construct 293C3-SDIE in further analyses.

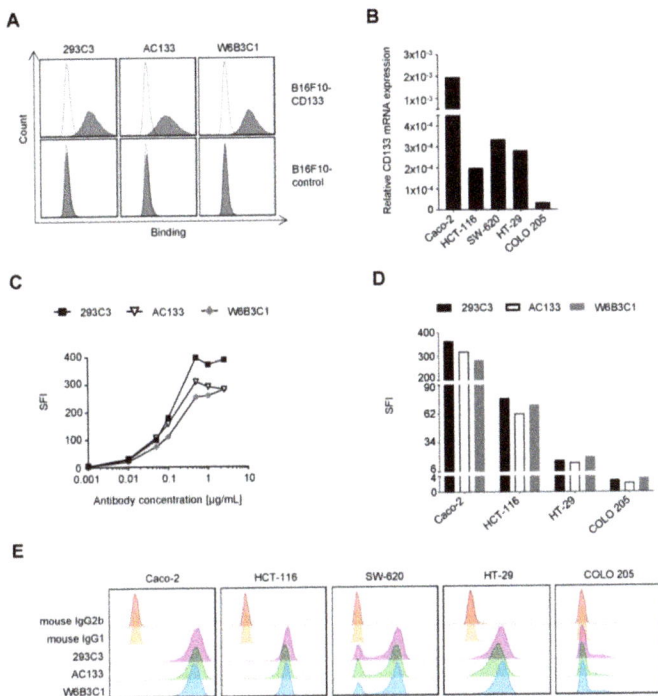

Figure 1. Comparative binding analysis of different CD133 monoclonal antibodies (mAbs) to colorectal cancer (CRC) cells. (**A**) Specific binding of three different commercially available CD133 mAbs (293C3, AC133, and W6B3C1) was determined by flow cytometry using B16F10-CD133 and B16F10-control transfectants. Cells were incubated with 5 µg/mL CD133 mAb followed by a goat anti-mouse phycoerythrin (PE) conjugate. Shaded peaks: CD133 mAbs; open peaks: controls. (**B**) Relative CD133 mRNA expression in five CRC cell lines—which were used as a model for mAb binding analyses—was determined by quantitative PCR as described in the method section. (**C**) The CD133 mAb surface binding was comparatively analyzed in flow cytometry experiments by incubating CD133 mRNA^{high} Caco-2 cells with increasing mAb concentrations of the different CD133 mAbs or isotype controls followed by a goat anti-mouse PE conjugate. Specific fluorescence intensity (SFI) levels were calculated as described in the method section. (**D,E**) The CD133 mAb binding to the panel of five CRC cell lines was comparatively analyzed by flow cytometry. Cells were incubated with 1 µg/mL CD133 mAb or isotype controls followed by a goat anti-mouse PE conjugate. Specific fluorescence intensity (SFI) levels (not applicable for SW-620 cells due to bimodal CD133 expression) and histograms are depicted in (**D,E**), respectively. Representative data of one experiment from a total of at least two with similar results is shown.

Table 1. Biological characteristics of the employed CRC cell lines.

Cell Line	Origin [1]	MSI Status [1]	KRAS [1]	Relative CD133 mRNA [2]	SFI 293C3 [2]	SFI AC133 [2]	SFI W6B3C1 [2]
Caco-2	Primary tumor	MSS	wt	1.96×10^{-3}	364.2	319.1	284.4
HCT-116	Primary tumor	MSI	G13D	1.99×10^{-4}	76.9	62.1	70.7
HT-29	Primary tumor	MSS	wt	2.82×10^{-4}	16.8	14.7	20.3
COLO 205	Metastasis	MSS	wt	3.33×10^{-5}	3.0	2.3	3.5
SW-620	Metastasis	MSS	G12V	3.34×10^{-4}	n.a.	n.a.	n.a.

[1] Information on cell lines' biological characteristics were derived from [24,25]. [2] Data were derived from Figure 1B,D. KRAS: Kirsten rat sarcoma viral oncogene; MSS/MSI: microsatellite stability/instability; n.a.: not applicable; SFI: specific fluorescence intensity.

2.2. Generation and Characterization of 293C3-SDIE in CRC

As previously described [14], mAb clone 293C3 was chimerized (backbone: human immunoglobulin G1/K constant region) and Fc-optimized by introducing the S239D/I332E modification in the constant heavy chain domain 2 (CH2) which is illustrated in Figure 2A. An Fc-optimized control protein with irrelevant target specificity termed Iso-SDIE served as control. Upon production as described in the method section, 293C3-SDIE was obtained with good yields, and analysis by sodium dodecyl sulfate–polyacrylamide gel electrophoresis (SDS-PAGE) and gel filtration revealed the expected molecular weights of ~24, ~50, and ~148 kDa for light chain (LC), heavy chain (HC), and full mAb, respectively, and confirmed the lack of aggregates (Figure 2B). Flow cytometric analyses including dose titrations with B16F10 transfectants confirmed that the chimerization and Fc-optimization process had not affected the specificity and affinity of 293C3-SDIE as compared to the parental murine mAb (Figure 2C,D). Next we performed dose titration experiments using three CRC cell lines with high, intermediate, and low CD133 surface antigen densities (Caco-2, CD133^{high}; HCT-116, CD133^{int}; HT-29, CD133^{low}). Flow cytometry revealed that saturating doses positively correlated with CD133 surface levels, but in all cases 1 μg/mL was sufficient to achieve saturating binding (Figure 2E).

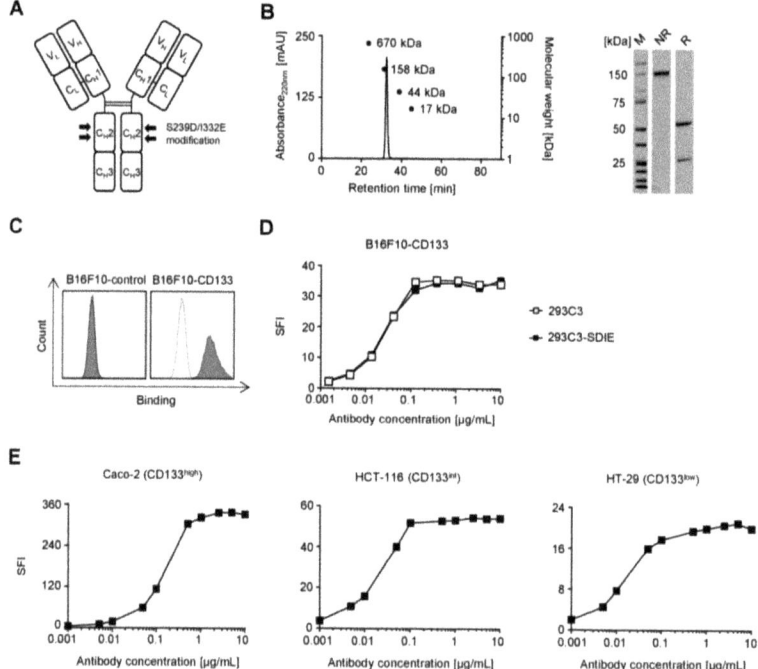

Figure 2. Generation and characterization of 293C3-SDIE in colorectal cancer (CRC). (**A**) Schematic illustration of 293C3-SDIE. (**B**) Purified 293C3-SDIE was analyzed by size exclusion chromatography (left) and SDS-PAGE (right). mAU: milli absorption unit; R: reduced; NR: non-reduced; M: marker. (**C**) B16F10-CD133 and B16F10-control transfectants were incubated with 10 μg/mL 293C3-SDIE or Iso-SDIE followed by an anti-human phycoerythrin (PE) conjugate. Shaded peaks: 293C3-SDIE; open peaks: Iso-SDIE. (**D**) B16F10-CD133 transfectants were incubated with the indicated concentrations of 293C3 or 293C3-SDIE and their respective isotype controls followed by an anti-mouse or anti-human PE conjugate. (**E**) The colorectal cancer (CRC) cell lines Caco-2 (CD133^{high}: left), HCT-116 (CD133^{int}: middle), and HT-29 (CD133^{low}: right) were incubated with the indicated concentrations of 293C3-SDIE or Iso-SDIE followed by an anti-human PE conjugate. Int: intermediate; SFI: specific fluorescence intensity.

2.3. Direct Effects of 293C3-SDIE on CRC Cell Viability

As CD133 was previously suggested to be involved in tumor cell survival and proliferation and CD133 mAb binding could have an influence in this context [16,26], we next determined whether 293C3-SDIE directly affected tumor cell viability. To this end, the CRC cell lines Caco-2, HCT-116, and HT-29 with high, intermediate, and low CD133 antigen densities, respectively, were incubated with 293C3-SDIE in the absence of immune effector cells. Notably, all these cell lines also express EGFR, which is therapeutically targeted by cetuximab and panitumumab (Figure 3A), and these two mAbs were included in the analysis. Analysis of ATP levels as surrogate marker for the amount of viable cells revealed that 293C3-SDIE had no effect (Figure 3B). While two of the CRC cell lines were not responsive to the EGFR blockade, the viability of Caco-2 cells was clearly reduced by the anti-EGFR mAbs. This differential reactivity is in line with data previously published by other investigators [27]. Since CD133 can interact with EGFR and has been hypothesized to contribute to resistance to EGFR-targeting drugs [16], we also determined whether simultaneous targeting of CD133 by 293C3-SDIE would sensitize CRC cells to anti-EGFR mAb treatment. To this end, CRC cells were incubated with either cetuximab or panitumumab alone or in combination with 293C3-SDIE, but anti-EGFR mAbs treatment effects were not further increased by 293C3-SDIE.

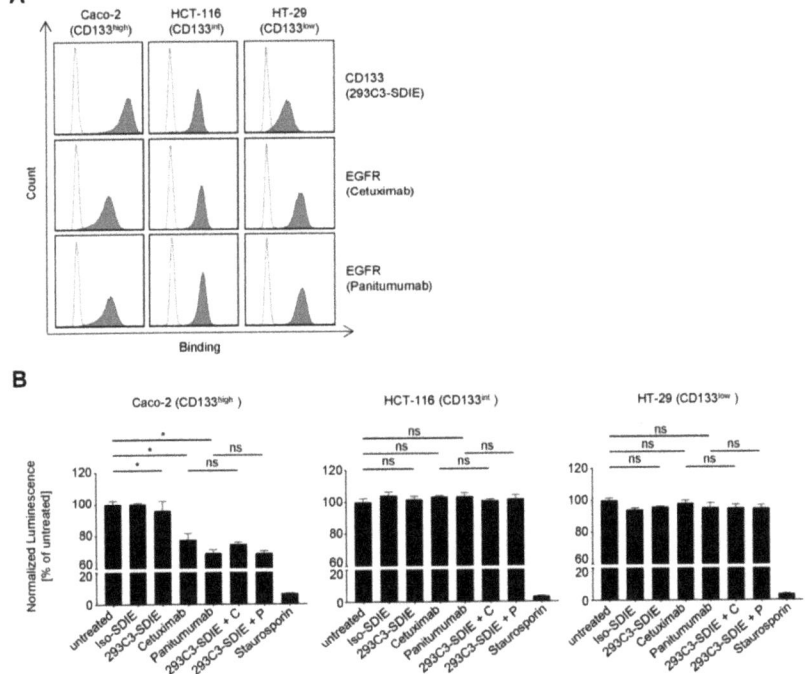

Figure 3. Direct effects of 293C3-SDIE on colorectal cancer (CRC) cell viability. (**A**) CD133 and epidermal growth factor receptor (EGFR) expression on CRC cell lines were comparatively analyzed by flow cytometry using 293C3-SDIE, cetuximab and panitumumab and their respective isotype controls (all at 1 µg/mL) followed by an anti-human phycoerythrin (PE) conjugate. Shaded peaks: specific mAbs; open peaks: isotype controls. (**B**) Caco-2 (left), HCT-116 (middle), and HT-29 (right) cells were incubated with 1 µg/mL of the indicated mAbs for three days. ATP levels were then determined by CellTiterGlo assays. Representative data of one experiment from a total of at least two with similar results are shown. C: cetuximab; int: intermediate; ns: not significant; P: panitumumab; *: significant (p-value < 0.05).

2.4. Induction of NK Cell Reactivity Against CRC Cells by 293C3-SDIE

Next we determined how 293C3-SDIE induced NK cell mediated anti-tumor immunity against CRC cells. To this end, peripheral blood mononuclear cells (PBMCs) of healthy donors containing NK cells as effector cells were cultured with the CRC cell lines Caco-2, HCT-116, and HT-29 with their high, intermediate, and low CD133 antigen densities, respectively, in the presence or absence of 293C3-SDIE or isotype control. Flow cytometric analysis of CD69 on NK cells revealed that 293C3-SDIE profoundly induced NK cell activation, while the control mAb with irrelevant target specificity had no effect (Figure 4A). In line, 293C3-SDIE specifically induced NK cell degranulation as revealed by flow cytometric detection of CD107a (Figure 4B). Additionally, the NK cell release of Interferon (IFN)-γ, an immunomodulatory cytokine that elicits direct anti-tumor effects and by which NK cells shape subsequent adaptive immune responses, was specifically induced by 293C3-SDIE (Figure 4C). Notably, in all cases the observed 293C3-SDIE effects positively correlated with antigen density.

Finally we examined whether the above-described effects on NK cell activity were mirrored by ADCC and a resulting tumor cell lysis. Europium based cytotoxicity assays revealed that treatment with 293C3-SDIE induced a clearly target-antigen restricted lysis, and this was observed with all tested cell lines (Figure 5). In line with the results observed for NK cell activity, lysis rates again positively correlated with CD133 antigen density on CRC target cells. Thus, 293C3-SDIE is capable to potently stimulate NK cell immunity against CRC cells. Furthermore, it is of particular interest that 293C3-SDIE was able to induce anti-tumor immunity against microsatellite stabile (Caco-2, HT-29) and RAS-mutated (HCT-116) CRC forms, where checkpoint blockade and anti-EGFR mAbs were found to lack efficiency in patients, respectively.

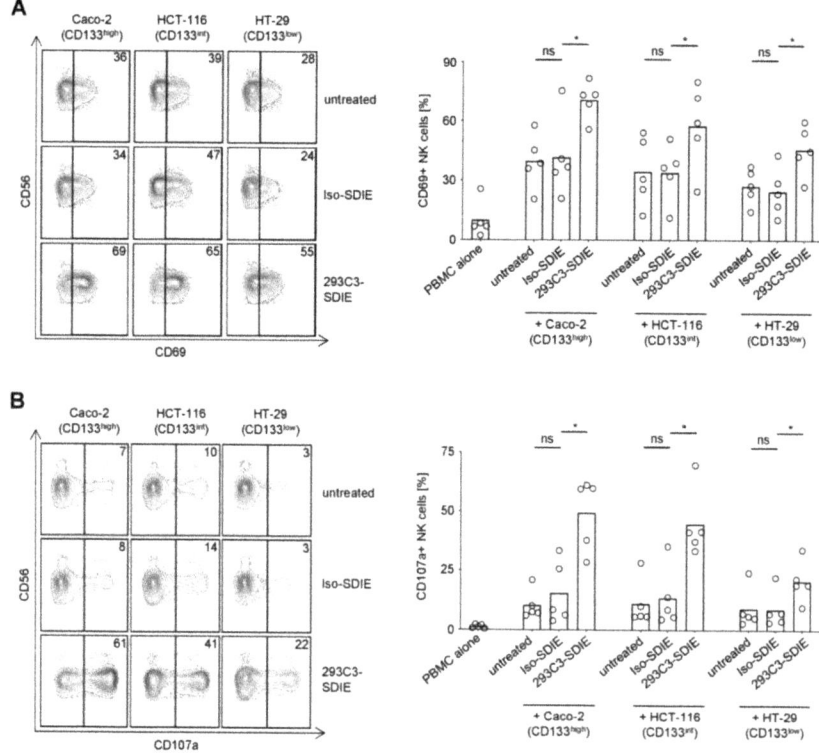

Figure 4. *Cont.*

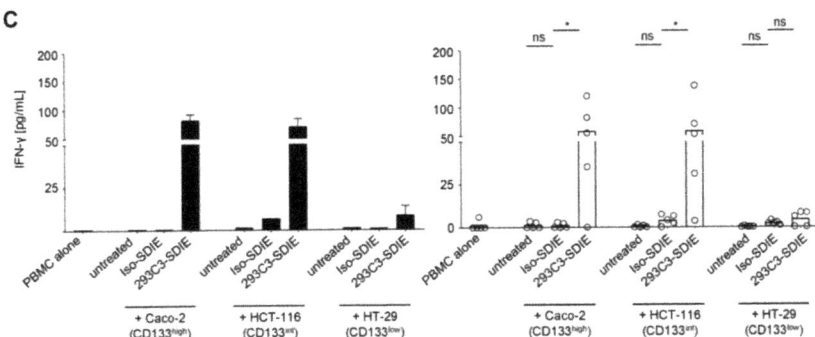

Figure 4. Induction of natural killer (NK) cell activity by 293C3-SDIE in the presence of colorectal cancer (CRC) cells. Peripheral blood mononuclear cells (PBMC) of healthy donors were cultured with or without the indicated CRC cell lines at an effector to target ratio of 2.5:1 in the presence or absence of 293C3-SDIE/Iso-SDIE (1 µg/mL). On the left, exemplary results obtained in a single experiment with PBMC of a single donor are shown; right panels depict combined analyses of data obtained with PBMC from five independent donors (bars represent respective means). (**A**) Activation of NK cells identified as CD14-CD56+CD3- cells within PBMC was determined after 24 h by flow cytometry for CD69. (**B**) Cells were cultured for 4 h in the presence of anti-human CD107a-PE/GolgiStop/GolgiPlug and NK cells subsequently analyzed by flow cytometry for CD107a as surrogate marker for degranulation. (**C**) Cells were cultured for 6 h before supernatants were analyzed for Interferon (IFN)-γ by an enzyme-linked immunosorbent assay. Int: intermediate; ns: not significant; *: significant (p-value < 0.05).

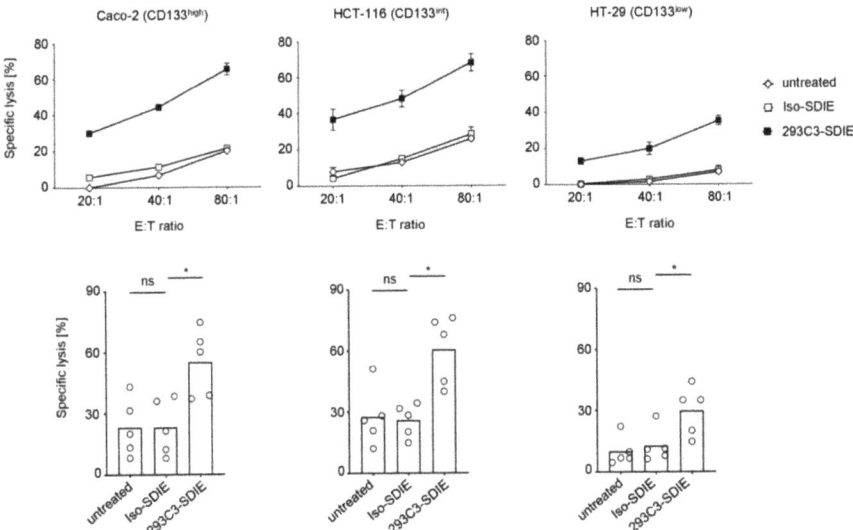

Figure 5. Induction of natural killer (NK) cell mediated colorectal cancer (CRC) cell lysis by 293C3-SDIE. Peripheral blood mononuclear cells (PBMC) of healthy donors were cultured with Caco-2 (left), HCT-116 (middle), and HT-29 cells (right) in the presence or absence of 293C3-SDIE/Iso-SDIE (1 µg/mL). Tumor cell lysis was measured after 2 h by Europium based cytotoxicity assays. In the top exemplary data over a broad range of effector to target (E:T) ratios with PBMC of one donor and in the bottom pooled data (bars represent respective means) at an E:T ratio of 80:1 with PBMC of five different donors are shown. Int: intermediate; ns: not significant; *: significant (p-value < 0.05).

3. Discussion

In the present study, we report on the preclinical characterization of 293C3-SDIE for treatment of CRC. 293C3-SDIE is a chimerized and Fc-optimized CD133 mAb recently introduced for induction of NK cell ADCC against leukemia. Evaluation in CRC appeared rational since CD133 is highly expressed in solid tumors, particularly in CRC, where it constitutes a negative prognostic marker, and immunotherapeutic options so far are rather limited. Our analyses revealed that 293C3-SDIE is well suited to target CD133 expressing CRC cells for NK cell ADCC because 293C3-SDIE showed convincing binding characteristics in CRC and potently induced anti-tumor immunity as determined in multiple experimental settings using CRC cell lines and NK cells contained in PBMC from healthy donors as effector cells.

NK cells belong to the group of cytotoxic lymphocytes and not only exert functions in innate immunity, but also influence adaptive immune responses [28]. They largely contribute to cancer immunosurveillance; thus, multiple efforts presently aim to engraft NK cells in cancer treatment [29]. A well established approach to achieve this goal is the application of antitumor antibodies to induce ADCC, as highlighted by the success, e.g., of rituximab, which is established for the treatment of B cell malignancies and the efficacy of which is largely based on ADCC [8]. While other immune cells, e.g., monocytes, also express CD16, it is firmly established that in humans it is NK cells that mediate this important antibody function [6,7]. At present, multiple strategies aim to further increase ADCC by generating Fc-optimized antitumor mAbs with enhanced affinity to CD16. Besides by modifications of the glycosylation pattern, this can be achieved by amino acid modifications such as the substitutions S239D/I332E (SDIE modification) in the Fc part's CH2 domain contained in 293C3-SDIE. Notably, many other Fc-optimized mAbs that currently undergo clinical evaluation, e.g., MOR00208 (anti-CD19; ClinicalTrials.gov ID: NCT01685021), margetuximab (anti-HER2; NCT01828021), FLYSYN (anti-FLT3; NCT02789254), MEN1112 (anti-CD157; NCT02353143) and BI 836858 (anti-CD33; NCT02240706, NCT03013998), comprise the SDIE modification.

After evaluating 293C3-SDIE for treatment of leukemia, we reasoned that CD133 would also constitute a promising target antigen for an Fc-optimized antibody in CRC. So far, established antibody-based approaches in CRC are restricted to a minority of patients only. Cetuximab and panitumumab are approved for treatment of patients with metastatic disease and only for patients with wildtype RAS accounting for 44% of metastatic CRC patients [30]. Immune checkpoint blockade is only available for CRC patients with metastasized disease and microsatellite instability-high/DNA mismatch repair deficiency, which accounts for ~5% of metastatic CRC patients [31]. CD133 has been suggested to be involved, amongst others, in chemotherapy resistance and metastasis, and was found to constitute a negative prognostic marker in CRC as shown in two meta-analyses [16,18,19]. CD133 is further expressed in a high number of CRC cases [17,18], which constitutes an important prerequisite for a therapeutic target antigen. It is thus not surprising that presently various CD133 targeting immunotherapeutics are under development, which, beyond 293C3-SDIE, comprises immunotoxins, CAR-T cells, bi-/tri-/tetraspecific mAbs, nanoparticles, adaptamers, and dendritic cell (DC)-based vaccination strategies. While most of these approaches aim to stimulate antitumor immunity against CD133-expressing target cells, they differ largely in many aspects, including, among others, the efforts required for production and the associated "costs of goods" and, importantly, efficacy and potential side effects.

While substantial further preclinical work and results of clinical studies are required to decide on the finally optimal CD133-targeting strategy, our findings demonstrate that 293C3-SDIE is produced well and with only minor aggregation tendency. This is in contrast to more artificial constructs such as the bispecific T cell engager (BiTE) format, where aggregates can cause unspecific T cell activation. In addition, 293C3-SDIE would constitute a "ready-to-use," off the shelf product, which would avoid the delay of treatment (about three weeks) that is required for the production of CAR-T cells and contributes to their vast costs upon clinical application. Furthermore, the concentration of 1 µg/mL 293C3-SDIE that was found to be sufficient to saturate CD133 binding and to potently induce ADCC appears easily achievable in humans, since other anti-tumor mAbs such as cetuximab and panitumumab achieve about 100-fold higher mean plasma peak levels in CRC patients upon recommended dosing [32,33]. With regard to potential toxicity/side effects, it must be considered that CD133 is not a tumor-exclusive antigen and, amongst others, expressed on healthy hematopoietic progenitor cells [34,35]. However, in our previous in vitro studies with 293C3-SDIE, no toxicity against healthy hematopoietic progenitor cells was observed, likely due to their profoundly lower CD133 antigen levels [14]. In addition, the first two clinical phase I studies evaluating CD133 targeting therapeutics—anti-CD133 CAR-T cells and DC-based CD133 vaccination—did not reveal any unbearable toxicity against healthy CD133 expressing cells [36,37]. Nevertheless, this issue and the question whether and how it is effective to target the CD133 positive cell fraction—potentially representing CSCs as reported in previous studies for CRC [38–40]—requires further elucidation. In any case, the results presented in this study demonstrate that 293C3-SDIE constitutes a promising novel option for CRC treatment, which we particularly envisage for elimination of residual disease after cytoreductive therapy.

4. Materials and Methods

4.1. Production, Purification, and Quality Control of Fc-Optimized Antibodies

293C3-SDIE and Iso-SDIE were produced as described previously [14]. In brief, plasmids for HC and LC were generated using the EndoFree Plasmid Maxi kit from Qiagen (Hilden, Germany) according to the manufacturer's protocol. Antibodies were expressed in ExpiCHO cells (Gibco, Carlsbad, CA, USA) according to the manufacturer's recommendations and purified by affinity (Mabselect; GE Healthcare, Chicago, IL, USA) and subsequent preparative size exclusion chromatography (HiLoad 16/60 Superdex 200; GE Healthcare, Chicago, IL, USA). Prior to use in functional experiments, mAbs were cleared from endotoxins using the Endotrap HD kit from Hyglos (Bernried, Germany). Ultimately, antibodies were run on analytical size exclusion columns (Superdex 200 Increase 10/300 GL; GE Healthcare; Chicago, IL, USA) and 4–12% gradient SDS-PAGE gels (Invitrogen; Carlsbad, CA, USA) using the gel filtration and Precision Plus standard from Bio-Rad (Hercules, CA, USA), respectively.

4.2. Cells

B16F10-CD133 and B16F10-control cells were generated by transfecting B16F10 cells with pcDNA™3.1 based vectors coding for human CD133 (accession no. BC012089.1) or FLT3 (accession no. NM_004119.2) as control. Cells were cultivated in selection medium, i.e., Dulbecco's Modified Eagle Medium (DMEM) containing 1 µg/mL G418 (Biochrom; Berlin, Germany).

The CRC cell lines Caco-2 and HCT-116 were from the German Collection of Microorganisms and Cell Cultures (Braunschweig, Germany) and HT-29 from the American Type Culture Collection (Manassas, VA, USA). The CRC cell lines SW-620 and COLO 205 were obtained internally at the University of Tuebingen. Authenticity was routinely determined by validating the respective immunophenotype described by the provider using flow cytometry after thawing, and cell lines were cultured for a maximum of 2 months prior to use in experiments. Contamination with mycoplasma was excluded by routine testing of all cultures every 3 months. All CRC cell lines were maintained in DMEM.

PBMC were isolated by density gradient centrifugation (Biocoll; Biochrom, Berlin, Germany) from thrombopheresis products of healthy volunteers and viably stored in liquid nitrogen. Prior to functional experiments, PBMC were cultured overnight in RPMI1640 for 18–24 h.

All above-mentioned media contained Glutamax, 10% heat-inactivated fetal calf serum (Biochrom; Berlin, Germany), and 1% Penicillin/Streptomycin (Lonza; Verviers, Belgium). All cells were kept in a humidified atmosphere at 37 °C and 5% CO_2.

4.3. Flow Cytometry

Flow cytometric analyses were performed using either fluorescently labeled or unlabeled mAbs followed by species-specific PE conjugates. Murine anti-human CD133 mAbs 293C3, AC133 and W6B3C1 were purchased from Miltenyi Biotec (Bergisch Gladbach, Germany). CD69-PE and CD107a-PE were from BD Pharmingen (San Diego, CA, USA), CD56-APC and CD14-PE/Cy7 from BioLegend (San Diego, CA, USA) and CD3-eFluor450 from eBioscience (San Diego, CA, USA). The goat anti-mouse PE conjugate was obtained from Dako (Glostrup, Denmark), the donkey anti-human PE conjugate was from Jackson ImmunoResearch (West Grove, PA, USA). The corresponding isotype controls were from BD Pharmingen (San Diego, CA, USA). Dead cells were excluded from analysis by 7-AAD (BioLegend; San Diego, CA, USA). Analysis was conducted using a FACS Canto II or FACS Fortessa (both BD Biosciences; Heidelberg, Germany). Specific fluorescence intensity (SFI) levels were calculated by dividing mean fluorescences obtained with a specific mAb by mean fluorescences obtained with the respective isotype control.

4.4. PCR Analysis

PCR analysis was performed as described previously [41]. In brief, total RNA was isolated using the High Pure RNA Isolation Kit (Roche, Mannheim, Germany) and transcribed into cDNA using FastGene Scriptase II (NIPPON Genetics Europe; Düren, Germany) according to the manufacturer's instructions. CD133 primers were 5'-TGGGGCTGCTGTTTATTATTCT-3' and 5'- TGCCACAAAACCATAGAAGATG-3' [42]. Primer assays (QuantiTect Primer Assay) for 18S ribosomal RNA were from Qiagen (Hilden, Germany). Amplification of cDNA was performed using PerfeCTa SYBR Green FastMix (Quanta Biosciences; Beverly, MA, USA) on a LightCycler 480 (Roche, Basel, Switzerland) instrument. Relative CD133 mRNA expression—normalized to 18S rRNA—was calculated by the $\Delta\Delta$ cycle-threshold (Ct) method.

4.5. Analysis of Direct mAb Effects on CRC Cell Viability

For analysis of direct mAb effects on CRC cell viability, CRC cell lines were seeded in white 96-well plates and treated with the indicated antibodies for 3 days. Subsequently, ATP levels as surrogate marker for live cells were determined using the CellTiterGlo assay from Promega (Madison, WI, USA) according to the manufacturer's protocol. Cetuximab (Erbitux©) and panitumumab (Vectibix©) were from Eli Lilly (Indianapolis, IN, USA) and Amgen (Thousand Oaks, CA, USA). Staurosporin (Abcam; Cambridge, UK) was used as a positive control. Values depict means of technical triplicates with standard deviation.

4.6. Analysis of NK Cell Activation, Degranulation and Cytokine Secretion

PBMC of healthy donors were cultured with or without the indicated CRC cell lines at an effector/target (E:T) ratio of 2.5:1 in the presence or absence of 293C3-SDIE/Iso-SDIE (1 µg/mL). CD69 upregulation on NK cells (CD14-/CD56+/CD3- within PBMC fraction) after 24 h was analyzed by flow cytometry. For studies on NK cell degranulation, cells were cultured for 4 h in the presence of anti-CD107a-PE, BD GolgiStop and BD GolgiPlug (both BD Biosciences; Heidelberg, Germany). Subsequently, CD107a upregulation on NK cells was determined by flow cytometry. IFN-γ secretion into the supernatants was measured after 6 h by an enzyme-linked immunosorbent assay (ELISA) using the ELISA mAb set from Thermo Scientific (Rockford, USA) according to the manufacturer's instructions. The KPL TMB Microwell Peroxidase Substrate System was from SeraCare Life Science (Milford, CT, USA) and the Streptavidin-Poly-HRP20 Conjugate from Fitzgerald Industries International (North Acton, MA, USA). If not indicated otherwise, IFN-γ values depict means of technical replicates with standard deviation.

4.7. Analysis of NK Cell Cytotoxicity

Lysis of CRC cells by PBMC of healthy donors in the presence or absence of 293C3-SDIE/Iso-SDIE (1 µg/mL) was assessed by 2 h Europium based cytotoxicity assays as previously described [13]. Specific lysis was calculated as follows: 100× (experimental release—spontaneous release)/(maximum release—spontaneous release). If not indicated otherwise, values depict means of technical triplicates with standard deviation.

4.8. Statistics

Statistical analysis was performed with GraphPad Prism 8 (GraphPad Software, San Diego, CA, USA). The 95% confidence level was used, and p-values were calculated by one-way ANOVA and subsequent Tukey's multiple comparison tests. Where indicated, statistically significantly different results ($p < 0.05$) between two groups are marked by "*", and results not statistically different are marked by "ns".

Author Contributions: Conceptualization: H.R.S. and B.J.S.; methodology: B.J.S., F.R., L.Z., L.G.H., and H.J.B.; validation: H.R.S., B.J.S., and F.R.; formal analysis: B.J.S. and F.R.; investigation, F.R. and B.J.S.; resources: H.R.S., L.G.H., H.J.B., L.Z., and G.J.; data curation: B.J.S. and F.R.; writing—original draft preparation: B.J.S.; writing—review and editing: H.R.S. and G.J.; visualization: B.J.S. and F.R.; supervision: H.R.S.; project administration: B.J.S.; funding acquisition: H.R.S.

Funding: This study was supported by grants from Deutsche Forschungsgemeinschaft (SA1360/9-1 and SA1360/7-3), Wilhelm Sander-Stiftung (2007.115.3), Deutsche Krebshilfe (111828 and 70112914), and Germany's Excellence Strategy (EXC 2180/1).

Acknowledgments: The authors thank Martin Pflügler and Stefanie Müller for support in mAb purification and PCR analysis, respectively. Flow cytometry sample acquisition was performed on shared instruments of the Flow Cytometry Core Facility Tuebingen. We acknowledge support by Deutsche Forschungsgemeinschaft and Open Access Publishing Fund of University of Tübingen.

Conflicts of Interest: The authors declare no conflict of interest.

References

1. Rothschilds, A.M.; Wittrup, K.D. What, Why, Where, and When: Bringing Timing to Immuno-Oncology. *Trends Immunol.* **2019**, *40*, 12–21. [CrossRef] [PubMed]
2. Keating, G.M. Rituximab: A review of its use in chronic lymphocytic leukaemia, low-grade or follicular lymphoma and diffuse large B-cell lymphoma. *Drugs* **2010**, *70*, 1445–1476. [CrossRef] [PubMed]
3. Arteaga, C.L.; Sliwkowski, M.X.; Osborne, C.K.; Perez, E.A.; Puglisi, F.; Gianni, L. Treatment of HER2-positive breast cancer: Current status and future perspectives. *Nat. Rev. Clin. Oncol.* **2012**, *9*, 16–32. [CrossRef] [PubMed]
4. Cruz, E.; Kayser, V. Monoclonal antibody therapy of solid tumors: Clinical limitations and novel strategies to enhance treatment efficacy. *Biologics* **2019**, *13*, 33–51. [CrossRef] [PubMed]
5. Kellner, C.; Otte, A.; Cappuzzello, E.; Klausz, K.; Peipp, M. Modulating Cytotoxic Effector Functions by Fc Engineering to Improve Cancer Therapy. *Transfus. Med. Hemother.* **2017**, *44*, 327–336. [CrossRef] [PubMed]
6. Vivier, E.; Tomasello, E.; Baratin, M.; Walzer, T.; Ugolini, S. Functions of natural killer cells. *Nat. Immunol.* **2008**, *9*, 503–510. [CrossRef] [PubMed]
7. Seidel, U.J.; Schlegel, P.; Lang, P. Natural killer cell mediated antibody-dependent cellular cytotoxicity in tumor immunotherapy with therapeutic antibodies. *Front. Immunol.* **2013**, *4*, 76. [CrossRef] [PubMed]
8. Weiner, G.J. Rituximab: Mechanism of action. *Semin. Hematol.* **2010**, *47*, 115–123. [CrossRef]
9. Lazar, G.A.; Dang, W.; Karki, S.; Vafa, O.; Peng, J.S.; Hyun, L.; Chan, C.; Chung, H.S.; Eivazi, A.; Yoder, S.C.; et al. Engineered antibody Fc variants with enhanced effector function. *Proc. Natl. Acad. Sci. USA* **2006**, *103*, 4005–4010. [CrossRef]
10. Hofmann, M.; Grosse-Hovest, L.; Nubling, T.; Pyz, E.; Bamberg, M.L.; Aulwurm, S.; Buhring, H.J.; Schwartz, K.; Haen, S.P.; Schilbach, K.; et al. Generation, selection and preclinical characterization of an Fc-optimized FLT3 antibody for the treatment of myeloid leukemia. *Leukemia* **2012**, *26*, 1228–1237. [CrossRef]

11. Schmiedel, B.J.; Scheible, C.A.; Nuebling, T.; Kopp, H.G.; Wirths, S.; Azuma, M.; Schneider, P.; Jung, G.; Grosse-Hovest, L.; Salih, H.R. RANKL Expression, Function, and Therapeutic Targeting in Multiple Myeloma and Chronic Lymphocytic Leukemia. *Cancer Res.* **2013**, *73*, 683–694. [CrossRef] [PubMed]
12. Schmiedel, B.J.; Werner, A.; Steinbacher, J.; Nuebling, T.; Buechele, C.; Grosse-Hovest, L.; Salih, H.R. Generation and Preclinical Characterization of a Fc-optimized GITR-Ig Fusion Protein for Induction of NK Cell Reactivity Against Leukemia. *Mol. Ther.* **2013**, *21*, 877–886. [CrossRef] [PubMed]
13. Steinbacher, J.; Baltz-Ghahremanpour, K.; Schmiedel, B.J.; Steinle, A.; Jung, G.; Kubler, A.; Andre, M.C.; Grosse-Hovest, L.; Salih, H.R. An Fc-optimized NKG2D-immunoglobulin G fusion protein for induction of natural killer cell reactivity against leukemia. *Int. J. Cancer* **2015**, *136*, 1073–1084. [CrossRef] [PubMed]
14. Koerner, S.P.; Andre, M.C.; Leibold, J.S.; Kousis, P.C.; Kubler, A.; Pal, M.; Haen, S.P.; Buhring, H.J.; Grosse-Hovest, L.; Jung, G.; et al. An Fc-optimized CD133 antibody for induction of NK cell reactivity against myeloid leukemia. *Leukemia* **2017**, *31*, 459–469. [CrossRef] [PubMed]
15. Grosse-Gehling, P.; Fargeas, C.A.; Dittfeld, C.; Garbe, Y.; Alison, M.R.; Corbeil, D.; Kunz-Schughart, L.A. CD133 as a biomarker for putative cancer stem cells in solid tumours: Limitations, problems and challenges. *J. Pathol.* **2013**, *229*, 355–378. [CrossRef] [PubMed]
16. Jang, J.W.; Song, Y.; Kim, S.H.; Kim, J.; Seo, H.R. Potential mechanisms of CD133 in cancer stem cells. *Life Sci.* **2017**, *184*, 25–29. [CrossRef]
17. PROM1. Available online: https://www.proteinatlas.org/ENSG00000007062-PROM1/pathology (accessed on 25 April 2019).
18. Chen, S.; Song, X.; Chen, Z.; Li, X.; Li, M.; Liu, H.; Li, J. CD133 expression and the prognosis of colorectal cancer: A systematic review and meta-analysis. *PLoS ONE* **2013**, *8*, e56380. [CrossRef]
19. Huang, R.; Mo, D.; Wu, J.; Ai, H.; Lu, Y. CD133 expression correlates with clinicopathologic features and poor prognosis of colorectal cancer patients: An updated meta-analysis of 37 studies. *Medicine* **2018**, *97*, e10446. [CrossRef]
20. Glumac, P.M.; LeBeau, A.M. The role of CD133 in cancer: A concise review. *Clin. Transl. Med.* **2018**, *7*, 18. [CrossRef]
21. Feng, H.L.; Liu, Y.Q.; Yang, L.J.; Bian, X.C.; Yang, Z.L.; Gu, B.; Zhang, H.; Wang, C.J.; Su, X.L.; Zhao, X.M. Expression of CD133 correlates with differentiation of human colon cancer cells. *Cancer Biol. Ther.* **2010**, *9*, 216–223. [CrossRef]
22. Feng, J.M.; Miao, Z.H.; Jiang, Y.; Chen, Y.; Li, J.X.; Tong, L.J.; Zhang, J.; Huang, Y.R.; Ding, J. Characterization of the conversion between CD133+ and CD133- cells in colon cancer SW620 cell line. *Cancer Biol. Ther.* **2012**, *13*, 1396–1406. [CrossRef] [PubMed]
23. Wang, C.; Xie, J.; Guo, J.; Manning, H.C.; Gore, J.C.; Guo, N. Evaluation of CD44 and CD133 as cancer stem cell markers for colorectal cancer. *Oncol. Rep.* **2012**, *28*, 1301–1308. [CrossRef] [PubMed]
24. Ahmed, D.; Eide, P.W.; Eilertsen, I.A.; Danielsen, S.A.; Eknaes, M.; Hektoen, M.; Lind, G.E.; Lothe, R.A. Epigenetic and genetic features of 24 colon cancer cell lines. *Oncogenesis* **2013**, *2*, e71. [CrossRef] [PubMed]
25. Berg, K.C.G.; Eide, P.W.; Eilertsen, I.A.; Johannessen, B.; Bruun, J.; Danielsen, S.A.; Bjornslett, M.; Meza-Zepeda, L.A.; Eknaes, M.; Lind, G.E.; et al. Multi-omics of 34 colorectal cancer cell lines-a resource for biomedical studies. *Mol. Cancer* **2017**, *16*, 116. [CrossRef] [PubMed]
26. Chen, W.; Li, F.; Xue, Z.M.; Wu, H.R. Anti-human CD133 monoclonal antibody that could inhibit the proliferation of colorectal cancer cells. *Hybridoma* **2010**, *29*, 305–310. [CrossRef] [PubMed]
27. Song, N.; Liu, S.; Zhang, J.; Liu, J.; Xu, L.; Liu, Y.; Qu, X. Cetuximab-induced MET activation acts as a novel resistance mechanism in colon cancer cells. *Int. J. Mol. Sci.* **2014**, *15*, 5838–5851. [CrossRef] [PubMed]
28. Vivier, E.; Raulet, D.H.; Moretta, A.; Caligiuri, M.A.; Zitvogel, L.; Lanier, L.L.; Yokoyama, W.M.; Ugolini, S. Innate or adaptive immunity? The example of natural killer cells. *Science* **2011**, *331*, 44–49. [CrossRef]
29. Ljunggren, H.G.; Malmberg, K.J. Prospects for the use of NK cells in immunotherapy of human cancer. *Nat. Rev. Immunol.* **2007**, *7*, 329–339. [CrossRef]
30. Peeters, M.; Kafatos, G.; Taylor, A.; Gastanaga, V.M.; Oliner, K.S.; Hechmati, G.; Terwey, J.H.; van Krieken, J.H. Prevalence of RAS mutations and individual variation patterns among patients with metastatic colorectal cancer: A pooled analysis of randomised controlled trials. *Eur. J. Cancer* **2015**, *51*, 1704–1713. [CrossRef]

31. Venderbosch, S.; Nagtegaal, I.D.; Maughan, T.S.; Smith, C.G.; Cheadle, J.P.; Fisher, D.; Kaplan, R.; Quirke, P.; Seymour, M.T.; Richman, S.D.; et al. Mismatch repair status and BRAF mutation status in metastatic colorectal cancer patients: A pooled analysis of the CAIRO, CAIRO2, COIN, and FOCUS studies. *Clin. Cancer Res.* **2014**, *20*, 5322–5330. [CrossRef]
32. Erbitux EMA. Available online: https://www.ema.europa.eu/en/documents/product-information/erbitux-epar-product-information_de.pdf (accessed on 3 May 2019).
33. Vectibix EMA. Available online: https://www.ema.europa.eu/en/documents/product-information/vectibix-epar-product-information_de.pdf (accessed on 3 May 2019).
34. Yin, A.H.; Miraglia, S.; Zanjani, E.D.; Almeida-Porada, G.; Ogawa, M.; Leary, A.G.; Olweus, J.; Kearney, J.; Buck, D.W. AC133, a novel marker for human hematopoietic stem and progenitor cells. *Blood* **1997**, *90*, 5002–5012. [PubMed]
35. Handgretinger, R.; Gordon, P.R.; Leimig, T.; Chen, X.; Buhring, H.J.; Niethammer, D.; Kuci, S. Biology and plasticity of CD133+ hematopoietic stem cells. *Ann. N. Y. Acad. Sci.* **2003**, *996*, 141–151. [CrossRef] [PubMed]
36. Wang, Y.; Chen, M.; Wu, Z.; Tong, C.; Dai, H.; Guo, Y.; Liu, Y.; Huang, J.; Lv, H.; Luo, C.; et al. CD133-directed CAR T cells for advanced metastasis malignancies: A phase I trial. *Oncoimmunology* **2018**, *7*, e1440169. [CrossRef] [PubMed]
37. Rudnick, J.D.; Fink, K.L.; Landolfi, J.C.; Markert, J.; Piccioni, D.E.; Glantz, M.J.; Swanson, S.J.; Gringeri, A.; Yu, J. Immunological targeting of CD133 in recurrent glioblastoma: A multi-center phase I translational and clinical study of autologous CD133 dendritic cell immunotherapy. *J. Clin. Oncol.* **2017**, *35*, 2059. [CrossRef]
38. O'Brien, C.A.; Pollett, A.; Gallinger, S.; Dick, J.E. A human colon cancer cell capable of initiating tumour growth in immunodeficient mice. *Nature* **2007**, *445*, 106–110. [CrossRef] [PubMed]
39. Ricci-Vitiani, L.; Lombardi, D.G.; Pilozzi, E.; Biffoni, M.; Todaro, M.; Peschle, C.; De Maria, R. Identification and expansion of human colon-cancer-initiating cells. *Nature* **2007**, *445*, 111–115. [CrossRef] [PubMed]
40. Abbasian, M.; Mousavi, E.; Arab-Bafrani, Z.; Sahebkar, A. The most reliable surface marker for the identification of colorectal cancer stem-like cells: A systematic review and meta-analysis. *J. Cell. Physiol.* **2019**, *234*, 8192–8202. [CrossRef] [PubMed]
41. Nuebling, T.; Schumacher, C.E.; Hofmann, M.; Hagelstein, I.; Schmiedel, B.J.; Maurer, S.; Federmann, B.; Rothfelder, K.; Roerden, M.; Dorfel, D.; et al. The Immune Checkpoint Modulator OX40 and Its Ligand OX40L in NK-Cell Immunosurveillance and Acute Myeloid Leukemia. *Cancer Immunol. Res.* **2018**, *6*, 209–221. [CrossRef]
42. Hirashima, K.; Yue, F.; Kobayashi, M.; Uchida, Y.; Nakamura, S.; Tomotsune, D.; Matsumoto, K.; Takizawa-Shirasawa, S.; Yokoyama, T.; Kanno, H.; et al. Cell biological profiling of reprogrammed cancer stem cell-like colon cancer cells maintained in culture. *Cell Tissue Res.* **2019**, *375*, 697–707. [CrossRef]

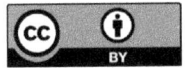

© 2019 by the authors. Licensee MDPI, Basel, Switzerland. This article is an open access article distributed under the terms and conditions of the Creative Commons Attribution (CC BY) license (http://creativecommons.org/licenses/by/4.0/).

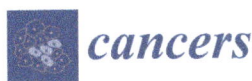

Article

Differential Effects of Ang-2/VEGF-A Inhibiting Antibodies in Combination with Radio- or Chemotherapy in Glioma

Gergely Solecki [1,2,3], Matthias Osswald [1,2], Daniel Weber [2], Malte Glock [2], Miriam Ratliff [1,4], Hans-Joachim Müller [5], Oliver Krieter [5], Yvonne Kienast [5], Wolfgang Wick [1,2] and Frank Winkler [1,2,*]

1. Neurology Clinic and Neurooncology Program at the National Center for Tumor Disease, University Hospital Heidelberg, Im Neuenheimer Feld 400, 69120 Heidelberg, Germany; gergely.solecki@web.de (G.S.); matthias.osswald@med.uni-heidelberg.de (M.O.); Miriam.Ratliff@umm.de (M.R.); wolfgang.wick@med.uni-heidelberg.de (W.W.)
2. German Cancer Consortium (DKTK), Clinical Cooperation Unit Neurooncology, German Cancer Research Center (DKFZ), 69120 Heidelberg, Germany; daniel.weber97@gmx.de (D.W.); malte.glock@web.de (M.G.)
3. Business Unit Service and Customer Care, Carl Zeiss Microscopy GmbH, 07745 Jena, Germany
4. Neurosurgery Department, University Medical Center Mannheim, 68167 Mannheim, Germany
5. Pharmaceutical Research and Early Development (pRED), Roche Innovation Center Munich, 82377 Munich, Germany; hans-joachim.mueller@mnet-mail.de (H.-J.M.); Oliver.Krieter@roche.com (O.K.); yvonne.kienast@roche.com (Y.K.)
* Correspondence: frank.winkler@med.uni-heidelberg.de; Tel.: +49-0-6221/56-7396

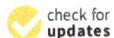

Received: 31 December 2018; Accepted: 28 February 2019; Published: 6 March 2019

Abstract: Antiangiogenic strategies have not shown striking antitumor activities in the majority of glioma patients so far. It is unclear which antiangiogenic combination regimen with standard therapy is most effective. Therefore, we compared anti-VEGF-A, anti-Ang2, and bispecific anti-Ang-2/VEGF-A antibody treatments, alone and in combination with radio- or temozolomide (TMZ) chemotherapy, in a malignant glioma model using multiparameter two-photon in vivo microscopy in mice. We demonstrate that anti-Ang-2/VEGF-A lead to the strongest vascular changes, including vascular normalization, both as monotherapy and when combined with chemotherapy. The latter was accompanied by the most effective chemotherapy-induced death of cancer cells and diminished tumor growth. This was most probably due to a better tumor distribution of the drug, decreased tumor cell motility, and decreased formation of resistance-associated tumor microtubes. Remarkably, all these parameters where reverted when radiotherapy was chosen as combination partner for anti-Ang-2/VEGF-A. In contrast, the best combination partner for radiotherapy was anti-VEGF-A. In conclusion, while TMZ chemotherapy benefits most from combination with anti-Ang-2/VEGF-A, radiotherapy does from anti-VEGF-A. The findings imply that uninformed combination regimens of antiangiogenic and cytotoxic therapies should be avoided.

Keywords: Ang-2; antiangiogenic therapy; in vivo imaging; radio- and chemotherapy; VEGF-A

1. Introduction

Glioblastoma (GB) is the most common and most malignant adult primary brain tumor [1]. It is associated with a poor prognosis and a high burden for the patient. The standard treatment is maximum safe resection, followed by radiotherapy and concomitant and adjuvant temozolomide (TMZ) chemotherapy. Despite this intensive treatment, overall survival (OS) remains under two years [2], largely because of inherent tumor resistance mechanisms [3–5]. Therefore, better therapeutic strategies are urgently needed, which includes those that make standard radio- and chemotherapy more efficient.

GBs are characterized by dense but structurally and functionally abnormal blood vessels, which are driven by a high level of proangiogenic factors, particularly VEGF-A [6–8] and Angiopoietin 2 (Ang-2) [9–12]. Ang-2 inhibition has previously been described to increase the effectiveness of anti-VEGF-A therapy in glioma [9–11,13].

The aberrant glioma blood supply is likely to compromise the effects of radio- and chemotherapy in malignant gliomas: due to high levels of tumor hypoxia [6] and potentially also by reduced delivery of TMZ to the glioma cells [14]. Thus, reestablishment of a more physiological microvascular function by antiangiogenic therapies, called vascular normalization, might increase the effectiveness of radio- and/or chemotherapy in gliomas [6,15–18]. This concept is supported from clinical data outside the brain, where combination of anti-VEGF-A therapies with chemotherapy showed the best antitumor effectivities [19,20]. However, in two phase III clinical trials in frontline GB (AVAglio and RTOG 0825) where standard radiochemotherapy was combined with the anti-VEGF-A antibody bevacizumab (Avastin®, Genentech Inc., South San Francisco, CA, USA), progression free survival (PFS), was improved by 4.4 months, while OS was unchanged [21,22]. Similar results were obtained in the EORTC 26101 study where bevacizumab was combined with lomustine chemotherapy vs. lomustine alone in patients with progressive GB [23]. Together these results unequivocally confirm that bevacizumab activity in controlled clinical trials remains far below expectations in newly diagnosed and relapsed GB.

The reason for that is not clear. Next to the possibility that only subgroups of GB patients benefit [4,24,25], other explanations for the so far disappointing overall benefits of anti-VEGF-A therapy include: (1) suboptimal vascular normalization of single VEGF-A inhibition, which is insufficient to increase the effectiveness of cytotoxic therapy and (2) lack of synergy or even detrimental effects for the combination with cytotoxic therapy. For chemotherapy, for example, vascular normalization with partial re-erection of the blood-brain barrier might compromise tumor penetration of the drug.

Therefore, to increase the benefit from antiangiogenic treatment strategies in glioma, it appears necessary to test these two possibilities: by directly comparing how inhibitors of VEGF-A, Ang-2, and both affect multiple critical parameters of tumor biology, and, most importantly, whether that benefits concomitant chemotherapy, radiotherapy, or both. Therefore, in this study we provide such a comprehensive comparison, making use of a newly developed multi-parameter longitudinal in vivo multi-photon microscopy technology. The results speak for a complex and dynamic system of interactions between the treatment modalities, and finally suggest that anti-Ang-2/VEGF-A is the best combination partner for chemotherapy, but anti-VEGF-A for radiotherapy.

2. Results

2.1. A Dynamic Multi-Parameter Microscopy Model to Study Therapeutic Interactions

To achieve parallel inhibition of both human and mouse VEGF-A and Ang-2, a bispecific antibody was used that employed the CrossMab technology [10,11,26–28] (the humanized antibody is vanucizumab [29,30]), combining the anti-Ang-2 specific IgG1 antibody LC06 with the anti-VEGF-A antibody B20.4.1 [31]. To directly compare the effects of VEGF-A, Ang-2, and dual inhibition on glioma biology, we tested the effects of these three antibodies vs. control antibody in an identical, clinically relevant dose (5 mg/kg BW every third day) (for treatment groups, see Figure S1A). To follow both morphology and pathophysiological features of glioma cells and tumor blood vessels alike, which would allow deeper insights into the complex world of interactions during the different combination therapies, we established a novel in vivo two-photon microscopy technology. This experimental setup made it possible to determine multiple parameters in the same tumor over multiple time points (Figure S1B).

2.2. Differential Vascular Effects of Antiangiogenic Combination Regimens

Dynamic angiograms of the same glioma region over time revealed striking morphological changes indicative of vascular normalization with anti-Ang-2/VEGF-A: blood vessels became thinner, much more ordered, and a clearer hierarchy developed, better resembling blood microvessels of the normal brain (Figure 1A). In contrast, both anti-VEGF-A and anti-Ang-2 monotherapy caused antiangiogenic changes of the tumor vasculature, reducing the number of newly built blood vessels over time when compared to tumors treated with the control antibody, but a clear morphological normalization of the existing tumor vasculature was not evident (Figure 1A). In line with this finding, the microvascular blood flow velocity, a good integrative parameter to measure tumor hemodynamics [32] and a particular robust one to determine functional vascular normalization [7] was decreasing in control tumors over time, while only dual Ang-2/VEGF-A inhibition rescuing levels to those seen in normal brain (Figure 1B). Remarkably, this was different when the antiangiogenic antibodies were combined with radiotherapy, where only anti-VEGF-A achieved a significant normalization of blood flow velocities compared to controls (Figure 1C), while in combination with chemotherapy it was again anti-Ang-2/VEGF-A that stood out as vascular normalization strategy (Figure 1D). Functional vascular normalization was paralleled by morphological vascular normalization in these distinct combination regimens (anti-VEGF-A plus RT, Suppl. Figure 2A; anti-Ang-2/VEGF-A plus chemotherapy, Figure S2B).

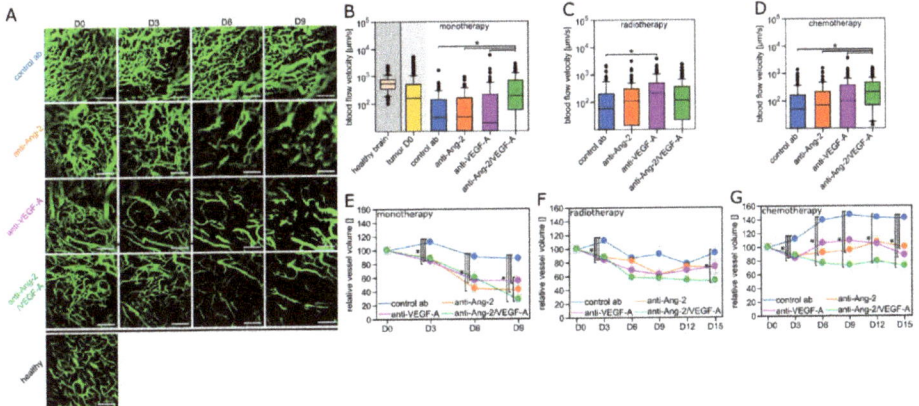

Figure 1. Vascular parameters for antiangiogenic treatment groups in monotherapy, and in combination with radio- or chemotherapy. (**A**) Representative angiograms for control, anti-Ang-2, anti-VEGF-A, and anti-Ang-2/VEGF-A monotherapy in comparison to healthy brain vasculature. Note that morphological vascular normalization occurs preferentially on days three and six under anti-Ang-2/VEGF-A dual inhibition. Scale bars: 150 µm. (**B–D**) Microvascular blood flow velocity in the healthy brain, in tumor blood vessels at the beginning of therapy (tumor D0), and on D6 in all four treatment groups. (**B**) Without cytotoxic combination partner; (**C**) in combination with radiotherapy; (**D**) in combination with TMZ chemotherapy. A total of 68–112 vessels from 5–11 animals per group were quantified. Box plots representing median values with 10th, 25th, 75th, and 90th percentiles. * $p < 0.05$ one-way ANOVA on ranks and post hoc Dunn's test. (**E–G**) Vessel volume over time for the different antiangiogenic antibodies given without cytotoxic therapy (**E**) or in combination with radiotherapy (**F**) or chemotherapy (**G**). Overall, 11–23 regions from 6–12 animals per group. Data are expressed as mean ± SD. * $p < 0.05$ one-way ANOVA and post hoc Tukey test.

As a point of caution, it has been a long matter of debate whether the effects of vascular normalization can actually help the tumor cells gain better access to oxygen and nutrients, thereby creating unwanted effects. Indeed, when quantifying the occurrence of mitotic figures in glioma cells in vivo, we found that antiangiogenic treatments lead to a short-time "burst" of glioma cell proliferation that ceased at later time points and was not present when antiangiogenic agents where combined with chemo- or radiotherapy (Figure S3A–D).

The total microvascular volume was reduced by all three antiangiogenic agents, as monotherapies and in all combinations with chemo- or radiotherapy; consistently, the strongest long-term reductions were seen with anti-Ang-2/VEGF-A (Figure 1E–G; compare also Figure 1A and Figure S2A,B). Of note, this effect was most evident in combination with chemotherapy (Figure 1G).

Together, this data speaks for differential activities of the three antiangiogenic antibodies on important parameters of tumor vascularization and, unexpectedly, for partially divergent effects when they are combined with radio- or chemotherapy.

2.3. Tumor Growth Inhibition is Limited to Regimens Where Vascular Normalization Occurs

Tumor growth over time was determined through the cranial window by measuring the area occupied by RFP-positive glioma cells, ensuring that real anti-tumor and not mere anti-edema effects were assessed. Furthermore, we ruled out that anti-edema effects of antiangiogenic therapies influence measurements of gross tumor size by demonstrating that density of tumor cell nuclei in a given tumor volume does not change during all three antiangiogenic treatments (Figure S3E,F).

All three antiangiogenic therapies did not significantly slow down tumor growth when given without a cytotoxic combination partner (Figure 2A). When combined with radiotherapy, anti-VEGF-A showed strongest tumor growth inhibition, significantly better than with anti-Ang-2/VEGF-A (Figure 2B). This reflects the superiority of this combination regimen regarding vascular normalization (Figure 1C, Figure S1A). In contrast, TMZ chemotherapy was most effective when combined with anti-Ang-2/VEGF-A (Figure 2C), again matching the strongest vascular normalization seen with this combination regimen (Figure 1D, Figure S2B).

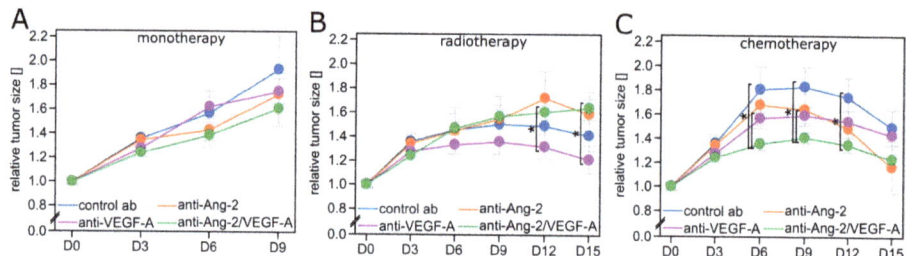

Figure 2. Tumor size over time. Brain tumor size as measured through the cranial window over time in 6–7 animals per group. Antiangiogenic therapy without cytotoxic therapy (**A**) or in combination with radiotherapy (**B**) or temozolomide (TMZ) chemotherapy (**C**). Data are expressed as mean ± SEM. * $p < 0.05$ two-tailed Student's t-test.

2.4. Tumor Cell Death Patterns Suggest Improved TMZ Penetration

We have demonstrated before that VEGF pathway inhibition improves the antitumor effects of radiotherapy in glioma due to increased tumor oxygenation during vascular normalization [6]. To get indications whether vascular normalization also helps TMZ chemotherapy by improving tumor penetration of the drug, we analyzed the occurrence of nuclear changes indicative of cell death with respect to blood vessel proximity in all combination regimens in vivo over time. For that we exploited that in addition to cytoplasmatic RFP, glioma cells stably expressed both RFP in the cytoplasm, and GFP in the nucleus.

Added to radiotherapy, anti-VEGF-A, the strongest vascular normalization regimen in this combination, did not significantly modify the distance of pathological events in relation to perfused blood vessels (Figure 3A,B). In contrast, when combined with chemotherapy, anti-Ang-2/VEGF-A, but also anti-VEGF-A, did significantly increase the median distance of pathological nuclei to the nearest blood vessel, compared to the control antibody (Figure 3A,B). Together, this data supports the concept that vascular normalization can increase the effectivity of chemotherapy by allowing better drug penetration to the glioma cells.

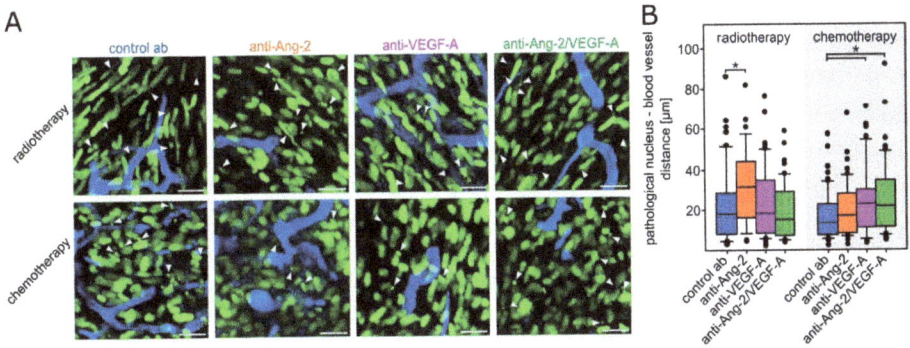

Figure 3. Dynamic changes of tumor cell nuclear parameters. (**A**) Representative images of pathological nuclei in dependence from the vessel distance. Green fluorescent protein (GFP) expressing nuclei are shown in green and the tumor vasculature is visualized in blue. The small arrows are only highlighting typically pathological nuclei. Scale bars: 20 μm. (**B**) Distance of the pathological nuclei from the proximal vessel on D9. A total of 35–68 cells from 4–7 animals per group were quantified. Box plots representing median values with 10th, 25th, 75th, and 90th percentiles. * $p < 0.05$ one-way ANOVA on ranks and post hoc Dunn's test.

2.5. Tumor Microtube Formation and Cellular Motility Closely Reflect Divergent Responses to Combination Regimens

We have recently discovered that glioma cells extend ultra-long cellular extensions, called tumor microtubes (TMs), to interconnect with each other to a multicellular network in which tumor cells resists the harmful effects of radiotherapy. TMs even increase in response to radiotherapy [3]. Therefore, the occurrence and length of TMs under different therapy strategies was determined on D0, D9, and D28 after the start of the antiangiogenic treatment (Figure 4A–D). In combination with radiotherapy, anti-Ang-2 and anti-Ang-2/VEGF-A both increased TM formation, while anti-VEGF-A (the optimum combination partner) did not. Likewise, in combination with chemotherapy, the ideal combination partner anti-Ang-2/VEGF-A, and also anti-VEGF-A, reduced TM length over time, compared to control and anti-Ang-2 antibodies.

One possible unwanted effect of antiangiogenic therapy is increased tumor cell invasiveness (Figure 4E) [33–36]. Anti-Ang-2/VEGF-A monotherapy slightly reduced nuclear motility, compared to control and the two other antiangiogenic antibodies (Figure 4F). While anti-Ang-2 and anti-Ang-2/VEGF-A increased motility compared to control when combined with radiotherapy, anti-VEGF-A did not (Figure 4G). In contrast, in combination with chemotherapy, anti-VEGF-A failed to reduce nuclear motility, but anti-Ang-2/VEGF-A and anti-Ang-2 did (Figure 4H).

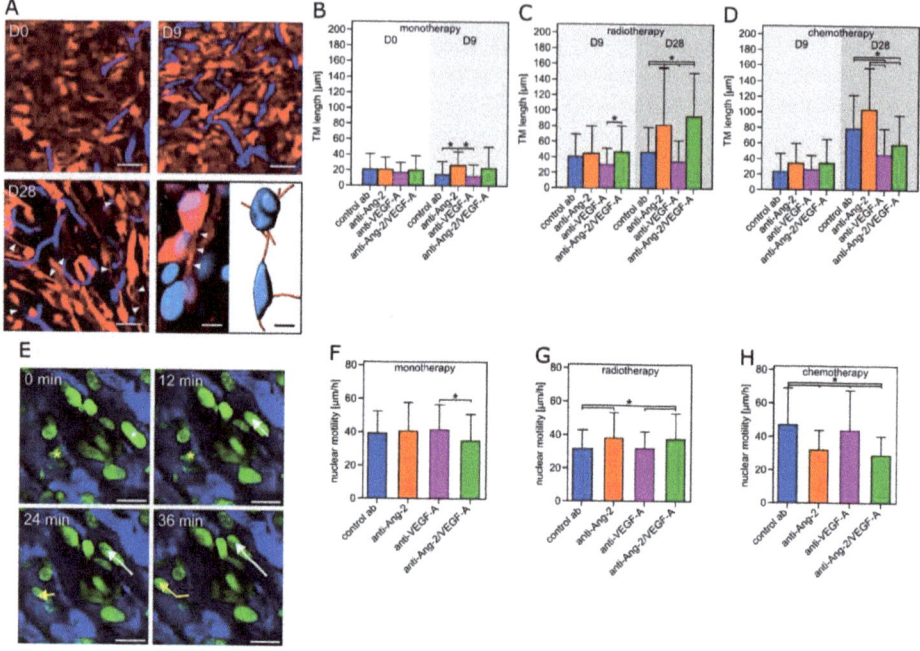

Figure 4. Tumor microtubes (TM) development and tumor cell motility. (**A**) Representative images of cellular morphology including TM development for the control antibody plus TMZ chemotherapy group. Note development of long cellular protrusions of 1–2 µm diameter, which is consistent with the criteria of TMs. Lower right panel: 3D reconstruction of TM-mediated glioma cell connections. Scale bars: 50 µm and 10 µm (right lower corner). (**B**–**D**) TM length for antiangiogenic monotherapy, and combinations with radiotherapy or chemotherapy. $n = 60$ cells from 3 animals per group. (**E**) Representative tracks of the movement of two nuclei over 36 min. Scale bars: 25 µm. (**F**–**H**) Velocity of tumor cell nuclei for the monotherapy and the combined treatment with irradiation or TMZ. $n = 60$–140 nuclei from 3–7 animals per group. Data are expressed as mean ± SD. * $p < 0.05$ one-way ANOVA on ranks and post hoc Dunn's test.

3. Discussion

In this study, we conducted a characterization of different antiangiogenic strategies in combinations with radio- and chemotherapy in glioblastoma. We found that anti-VEGF-A was the optimal combination partner for radiotherapy, while a bispecific antibody inhibiting both Ang-2 and VEGF-A was the best for chemotherapy throughout multiple parameters of tumor progression and therapy resistance. Importantly, there was an excellent correlation with morphological and functional vascular normalization [6,14,18], supporting that this concept has therapeutic relevance for primary brain tumors. Unexpectedly, the cytotoxic combination partner (chemo- vs. radiotherapy) had profound influence on how the antiangiogenic treatments influenced the different parameters of tumor biology, frequently even producing opposite effects (Figure 5).

It has been demonstrated before that the VEGF and angiopoietin pathways are interrelated in glioma, making dual inhibition a plausible strategy. In patients with recurrent GB treated with bevacizumab, plasma Ang-2 concentrations were significantly increased at the time of relapse, pointing towards a potential role of Ang-2 in the development of resistance against VEGF-A targeting treatments [37]. This supports previous preclinical reports that Ang-2 upregulation is typically found during VEGF pathway inhibition [6,9,38]. Furthermore, a particular strong vascular normalization during co-inhibition of the VEGF-A and Ang-2 pathways is also supported by recent preclinical findings [9,11]. Moreover, dose-dependent effects of antiangiogenics need to be taken into account, which can reach from merely normalization effects in lower doses to frank vascular pruning in higher doses, including differential effects on cancer cells [7,14]. The dose selected for this study was a lower dose, which is however still in the range of doses given to patients, were a maximum effect on vascular normalization could be expected, and less vascular regression.

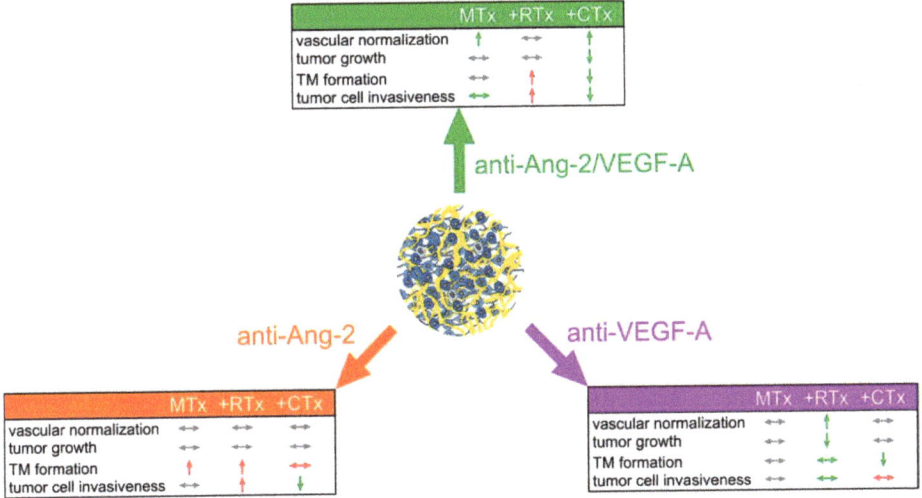

Figure 5. Summary of results. Schematic summary of the different experimental groups: antiangiogenic treatments as monotherapy or in combination with radiotherapy or chemotherapy for the most important parameters. Arrows down: parameter is decreased; arrows up: parameter is increased; sideways arrows: parameter is not affected; green arrows: beneficial effect compared to the other treatment groups; red arrows: unwanted effect compared to the other treatment groups; grey arrows: no effect compared to the other treatment groups.

However, dual inhibition of VEGF-A and Ang-2 did only improve the effects of TMZ chemotherapy, which included multiple favorable effects on parameters of glioma progression and therapy resistance. We demonstrate that nuclear changes indicative of glioma cell regression are not limited to the direct perivascular region in this combination anymore, supporting improved tumor penetration of TMZ by anti-Ang-2/VEGF-A co-inhibition. One can wonder why vascular normalization with re-erection of the blood-brain barrier is helping chemotherapy at all. In fact, contradictory findings have been reported whether antiangiogenic therapy improves chemotherapy penetration into the tumor or even hinders it [39–44]. However, TMZ is well known to effectively cross the blood-brain barrier (BBB) [45], which is the likely reason why it had similar clinical effects when compared to standard radiotherapy in a recent phase III study of low-grade glioma, where relevant BBB breakdown is normally not present [46]. With such a chemotherapeutic agent, BBB re-erection of any antiangiogenic treatment should be of minor relevance, and better drug delivery to the tumor by increase of its normally low blood flow velocity, but also by decrease of its high interstitial fluid pressure and other pathophysiological tumor features [14] during vascular normalization are likely to improve cytotoxic drug effectiveness. This view is supported by the findings of our study, where anti-Ang-2/VEGF-A was the only antiangiogenic treatment that normalized tumor blood vessels when combined with TMZ chemotherapy, and also significantly reduced tumor growth. Limitations remain. The tumor growth delay detected here might not translate into improved patient survival and the anti-edema effects of antiangiogenics may have clinical benefit even if the tumor load is increasing [47].

VEGF-A is responsible for the stimulation of proliferation and migration of endothelial cells and the enhancement of the vascular permeability [48]. Gliomas and other tumors often show highly elevated expression levels. For this reason, the therapeutic inhibition of this pathway was an important advance and is now targeted for a broad range of cancer entities [26,49]. However, further studies demonstrated that the efficacy of VEGF-A inhibition could be compromised by up-regulation of other angiogenic pathways [50]. One important component of this resistance is Ang-2, which is promoting neovascularization and tumor growth by Tie2 signaling in a VEGF-A independent manner [51–53]. While the single inhibition of Ang-2 led to a modest (if at all) beneficial effect on tumor growth and vascular normalization, which is in line with our results, the dual inhibition of both VEGF-A and Ang-2 proved beneficial for the therapy of CNS [9–11] and non-CNS [26,29,54–59] tumors.

In this study, we provide additional data in which opposite effects of anti-VEGF-A vs. anti-Ang-2 vs. dual inhibition on glioma growth are evident, depending on whether standard chemotherapy or standard radiotherapy is used as the combination partner. This might be best explained by three observations. First, chemotherapy and radiotherapy by themselves (without an active antiangiogenic combination partner) modulate blood vessel morphology, with antiangiogenic, anti-vascular, and partially also vascular normalization effects (control antibody groups: Figure S2, compared to Figure 1A) [60–62]. This can explain that the overall change of vascular morphology and function is somewhat unpredictable when an antiangiogenic agent is added. Second, the resulting differential vascular normalization effects observed with the various combination regimens can lead to various levels of tumor hypoxia, which is known to increase resistance to radiotherapy and TMZ [6,14–18]. Lastly, an additional or alternative explanation can be sought in our finding that relevant parameters of tumor resistance (e.g., TM formation, cellular invasiveness) are divergently increased or decreased. It has been described that radiotherapy can increase glioma cell invasiveness [63,64] as one potential mechanism. Importantly, both radio- and chemotherapy can increase the number of TMs and their interconnections and the multicellular networks formed by TMs in gliomas are prime factors of primary and adaptive resistance against radiotherapy and TMZ chemotherapy [3,65,66]. Moreover, TMs drive glioma cell invasion in the brain. An increased glioma cell invasiveness that can occur during inhibition of angiogenesis has been proposed as one major mechanism of resistance against antiangiogenics [33–36], although this could not be clearly demonstrated in patients yet [67]. Finally, it is very well possible that other well-described effects of antiangiogenics and/or cytotoxic therapies, like modulation of the immune tumor microenvironment and DNA damage response, play a role here. Our study provides the first evidence that antiangiogenic agents can even decrease cellular resistance mechanisms of glioma cells, but only if the right cytotoxic combination partner is selected.

In summary, we provide evidence that inhibition of VEGF-A might be the best combination strategy for radiotherapy, but inhibition of both Ang-2 and VEGF-A for chemotherapy. This provides interesting cues how to best develop dual anti-Ang-2/VEGF-A inhibitors in the clinic: combination with chemotherapy (either adjuvant TMZ in newly diagnosed glioblastoma or lomustine in recurrent glioblastoma) appears the most promising clinical trial strategy, while combination with radiotherapy might even be avoided. Since all phase III studies in primary or recurrent glioblastoma did not find unexpected CNS toxicities or other toxicities when the anti-VEGF-A antibody bevacizumab was combined with chemo-/radiotherapy (Chinot et al. 2014; Gilbert et al. 2014; Wick et al. 2017 [21–23]), at least safety and tolerability seem to not be a major issue with these treatment strategies. The most important consequence of the surprisingly complex interactions between antiangiogenic and cytotoxic treatments reported here is to better study them in preclinical and early clinical settings in the future to avoid testing uninformed combination regimens in controlled clinical trials.

4. Materials and Methods

4.1. Cell Culture

Cell culture was done under adherent conditions with Dulbeccos's Modified Eagle's Medium (DMEM, Sigma-Aldrich, Munich, Germany), which was supplemented with 10% fetal bovine serum (FBS, Sigma-Aldrich, Munich, Germany) and 1% penicillin-streptomycin (PS, Sigma-Aldrich, Munich,

Germany). For the cultured cells a contamination and authentification test was done by Multiplexion (Heidelberg, Germany). U-87MG, a human glioblastoma cell line obtained from the American Type Culture Collection (LGC Standards, Wesel, Germany), which is growing angiogenic in the mouse brain was used. O^6-methylguanine-DNA methyltransferase (MGMT) promotor methylation of this cell line was already confirmed in former publications [68]. Furthermore, when 24 brain tumor cell lines were analyzed for VEGF-A and Ang-2 mRNA expression, the U-87MG cell line showed both, being considerably representative with respect to expression levels. The cells were stably co-transduced with the red cytoplasmic construct LeGO-T2 (plasmid #27342 Addgene, Cambridge, MA, USA) and the green nuclear fluorescent plasmid LV-GFP (plasmid #25999 Addgene, Cambridge, MA, USA). The co-transduced cells were selected by fluorescence-associated cell sorting (FACSAria™ Special Order System, BD Biosciences, Heidelberg, Germany). To distinguish between single and double transduced cells, compensation was used. To separate dead and alive cells, propidium iodide (Sigma-Aldrich, Munich, Germany) staining was used.

4.2. Animals and Surgical Procedures

Naval Medical Research Institute (NMRI) nude male mice, between 8 and 10 weeks old (Charles River, Sulzfeld, Germany) were used to study the angiogenesis of human brain tumor cells within the mouse brain. All efforts were made to minimize animal suffering and to reduce the number of animals used. The operation of the chronic cranial window was done as previously described [3,69]. One week after window implantation a 1 µL cell suspension, containing 50,000 tumor cells, was injected cortically 500 µm deep with a stereotactical injector (Hamilton, Bonaduz, Switzerland and Stoelting, Wood Dale, IL, USA). When the tumor reached a mean diameter of 2 mm in vivo imaging and therapy was started. The animals were sacrificed when they got moribund and/or developed a weight loss of over 20%, which was particularly important in light of the frequent intravital imaging sessions that were an additional burden for tumor-bearing mice. The animals were treated every third day with the control (MOPC21), the anti-Ang-2 (LC06, RO6872894), the anti-VEGF-A (B20.4.1, RO6872895), or the anti-Ang-2/VEGF-A antibodies (LC06/B20.4.1, RO6872840) (F. Hoffmann-La Roche, Penzberg, Germany). All antibodies were administered in the same concentration of 5 mg/kg body weight (bw). For the radiotherapy group, tumors were irradiated with 7 Gy on D4, D5, and D6 (three consecutive days; total dose 21 Gy) after the start of the antiangiogenic treatment. The radiation was done with a 6 MV linear accelerator with a 6 mm collimator (adjusted to the window size) at a dose rate of 3 Gy min^{-1} (Artiste, Siemens, Erlangen, Germany). The administered radiation dose is in the range of the commonly used 60 Gy in 2 Gy fractions for glioma patients, assuming an α/β of ~10 in the linear quadratic model, and taking into account a radiation time of three days (Osswald et al. 2015; Winkler et al. 2004 [3,6]). For the chemotherapy group, animals were orally administered with TMZ (Schering-Plough, Kenilworth, NJ, USA) using a feeding needle on the three consecutive days during D4–D6 of therapy. TMZ concentration was 20 mg/kg bw per day (Figure S3A,B). This dose was selected because it was shown to exert measurable anti-tumor effects as single agent in preliminary studies on U87 and other glioma models (Weil et al. 2017 [65]) in our laboratory, but still low enough to be comparable to bioavailable doses given to patients. All animal procedures were performed in accordance with the institutional laboratory animal research guidelines after approval of the Regierungspräsidium Karlsruhe, Germany (governmental authority).

4.3. In Vivo Multiphoton Laser Scanning Microscopy (MPLSM)

In vivo imaging was performed with a LSM 7MP microscope (Carl Zeiss Microscopy, Jena, Germany) provided with a Coherent Chameleon UltraII laser (Coherent, Glasgow, UK) with a 500–550 nm and a 575–610 nm band pass filter. With the following wavelengths fluorophores were detected: 750 nm (FITC-dextrane, tdTomato) and 850 nm (GFP, TRITC-dextrane). To prevent phototoxic effects laser power was always kept as low as possible. During the imaging process animals were anaesthetized with a low gas narcosis including 1.5% isoflurane (Baxter, Unterschleißheim,

Germany) and 98.5% oxygen (Guttroff, Heidelberg, Germany). During imaging body temperature was kept constantly at 37 °C by a heating pad. To acquire angiographies of brain blood vessel, 0.1 mL high molecular dextrans were injected intravenously: tetramethylrhodamine isothiocyanate (TRITC, 500 kDa, 10 mg mL^{-1}, Sigma-Aldrich, Munich, Germany), and fluorescein isothiocyanate (FITC, 2 MDa, 10 mg mL^{-1}, Sigma-Aldrich, Munich, Germany). The angiographic image (size: 607.28 × 607.28 × 123 µm) allowed longitudinal tracking of two consecutive regions in the center of the brain tumor, which was done every third day from D0 to D15 after beginning with antiangiogenic treatment.

The large cranial window also allowed to study the entire tumor up to a depth of up to 1000 µm that sufficiently allowed to assess the tumor diameter. Verification experiments were performed, comparing the diameter measured by in vivo two-photon microscopy with the maximum diameter measured by standard histology and fluorescence microscopy of tumor-bearing brain sections. Here, a strong correlation was detected [7]. The mean tumor diameter under the cranial window was measured by a tile scan in a depth of 400 µm.

On D0 and D6, microvascular blood flow velocity was measured by a line scan as described before [7]. The cellular morphology and the length of the TMs were determined in a depth of 51 µm on D0, D9, and D28. On D3, D9, and D15 the nuclei were detected with a higher magnification (size: 151.82 × 151.82 × 48 µm) to quantify the nuclear density and the nuclear morphology. Additionally, the nuclear motility of the cells of the same region (size: 151.82 × 151.82 × 99 µm) was measured over 1.5 h.

4.4. Quantification and Visualization of MPLSM Data

In vivo images were recorded with the ZEN Software (Carl Zeiss Microscopy, Jena, Germany). Images were analyzed with the ImageJ 1.51f software (Wayne Rasband, National Institutes of Health, Bethesda, MD, USA). The diameter was determined by a tile scan in a depth of about 400 µm, where the tumor bulk reached its major dimensions. The diameter was calculated as the average of the minor and major axis of an ellipse. For quantification the diameters were normalized to the mean diameter on D0.

The blood flow velocity was measured by a line scan with a minimum length of 10 µm, detecting 2000 events in microvessels. Moreover, 16 randomly chosen vessels were measured per animal. The resulting scan identifies single erythrocytes as angular black lines, where the x-axis is according to the length of the detected distance and the y-axis is the elapsed time of the measurement. The angle is converging more and more to 90° when the cells are static. By knowing the resolution of both parameters and by the measurement of the slope of 30 randomly chosen red blood cells, a calculation of the mean velocity is possible, by inversion of the result.

For the nuclear density and the quantification of mitotic cells, stacks cropped to thickness of 67 µm (151.82 × 151.82 µm) in a depth of 35–102 µm were analyzed. The nuclear density was calculated by dividing the manually counted cell number with the volume of the stack. For the quantification of the mitotic activity, the percentage of mitotic cells was detected. Due to distances up to 100 µm between vessels and pathological nuclei, the whole and not the cropped stacks were analyzed manually. In control animals, nuclear size and shape was very homogenous. In distinct treatment groups, nuclear morphological changes of apoptosis or necrosis where evident. Tortuous, abnormally flexed, strongly condensed or swollen nuclei were evaluated as pathological (see Figure 3A). The distance between the center of the pathological nucleus and the exterior of the wall of the blood vessels was measured manually.

TMs were identified as thin and long cytoplasmatic protrusions, which often interconnect tumor cells [3]. For the measurement of the TM length single slices in a depth of 51 µm were quantified for two regions per animal. For every region 30 random cells were picked, where the length of the longest and most prominent TM of the cell was determined.

Cellular invasiveness was detected for 3D stacks in a depth of 51–150 µm, which were recorded in 40 cycles long (over 1.5 h lasting) time series. For 20 randomly chosen nuclei, x, y, and z coordinates were identified for 10 different time points. Since the expansion of the tissue by laser irradiation and breathing artefacts also modifies coordinates, striking blood vessel bifurcations were used as an inertial system.

3D representative pictures for the angiograms, nuclear morphologies, nuclear densities, nuclear motilities and the 3D rendering of the TMs were acquired with Imaris 7.5.1 (Bitplane, Zürich, Switzerland). Finally, the pictures were edited with Inkscape 0.91 (GNU General Public License) and GIMP 2.8.14 (GNU General Public License).

4.5. Statistical Analysis

The measured results were arranged in Excel 2016 (Microsoft Corporation, Redmond, WA, USA) and tested for outliers by a Nalimov test. The outlier-cleared datasets were transferred to the statistic software SigmaPlot 13.0 (Systat Software, San Jose, CA, USA). Equal variance and normal distribution were tested (Kolmogorov-Smirnov or Shapiro-Wilk). For results with normal distribution and equal variance, the two-sided Student's *t*-test was used. Otherwise, the Mann-Whitney U statistic was applied. For measurements with more than two groups, ANOVA on ranks or ANOVA was used in combination with the suitable post-hoc test (Dunn's method for the non-parametric and the Tukey test for the parametric). Results were significant from the corresponding control at a critical p-value below 0.05. Results were plotted in a line diagram by presenting the mean ± standard error of mean (SEM). In a bar chart the results were displayed as mean ± standard deviation (SD). Box plots depicted the median values with the percentiles and error bars. Results shown in a line diagram and in a bar chart have a linear scale; results in a box plot had a common logarithm scale for the ordinate. Finally, the pictures were finished with the graphic editors Inkscape 0.91 (GNU General Public License) and GIMP 2.8.14 (GNU General Public License).

5. Conclusions

Despite very high angiogenic activity of malignant gliomas, the current clinical effectiveness of antiangiogenic drugs and their combination regimens falls short of expectations. Here we show that inhibition of VEGF-A might be the best combination strategy for radiotherapy, but dual inhibition of Ang-2 plus VEGF-A for chemotherapy. This provides interesting cues how to best develop dual anti-Ang-2/VEGF-A inhibitors in the clinic. Combination with chemotherapy (either with adjuvant TMZ in primary glioblastoma, or lomustine in recurrent glioblastoma) appears most promising. Remarkably, the VEGF-A blocking antibody bevacizumab has never been tested with radiotherapy alone in a controlled clinical trial, which might be its optimal combination partner according to the results of this study. The most important consequence of the surprisingly complex interactions between antiangiogenic and cytotoxic treatments is to better study them in preclinical and early clinical settings in the future - to avoid testing uninformed combination regimens in controlled clinical trials.

Supplementary Materials: The following are available online at http://www.mdpi.com/2072-6694/11/3/314/s1, Figure S1: Experimental design, Figure S2: Differential changes of tumor blood vessel angiograms during combination of antiangiogenic treatment with radio- or chemotherapy, Figure S3: Transient pro-mitotic effects, and nuclear densities.

Author Contributions: G.S., M.O., H.-J.M., O.K., Y.K., W.W. and F.W. were responsible for experimental design, data interpretation, and writing of the manuscript. G.S. performed cell culture, surgical procedures, and MPLSM experiments. D.W. and M.G. performed cell culture experiments and surgical procedures. M.R. performed cell culture and was responsible for writing the manuscript.

Funding: Research grant from F. Hoffmann-La Roche AG to F.W.; research funding from Apogenix, Boehringer Ingelheim, MSD, Roche and Pfizer to W.W.

Acknowledgments: We would like to thank Christiane Stahl-Arnsberger, Peter Häring, Clemens Lang, Vanessa Mendes, and Mona Splinter for the irradiation of the mice; Felix Bestvater, Gaby Blaser, Manuela Brom, and Damir Krunic for assistance with the confocal microscope; Miriam Gömmel for the preparation of cranial windows; Mostafa Jarahian for FACS sorting of transduced cells; Anna S. Berghoff, Sara Ciprut, and Tobias Kessler for proofreading of the publication.

Conflicts of Interest: G.S. is an employee of Carl Zeiss Microscopy GmbH. H.-J.M., O.K. and Y.K. are employees of F. Hoffmann-La Roche AG. W.W. has participated in a speaker's bureau for BMS, Genentech/Roche and MSD, he received research funding from Apogenix, Boehringer Ingelheim, Merck, Sharp, and Dohme (MSD), Roche and Pfizer and has a consultant relationship with BMS, Genentech/Roche and MSD. F.W. received research grants from F. Hoffmann-La Roche AG, Boehringer, Glaxo Smith Kline, and Genentech.

References

1. Louis, D.N.; Perry, A.; Reifenberger, G.; von Deimling, A.; Figarella-Branger, D.; Cavenee, W.K.; Ohgaki, H.; Wiestler, O.D.; Kleihues, P.; Ellison, D.W. The 2016 World Health Organization Classification of Tumors of the Central Nervous System: A summary. *Acta Neuropathol.* **2016**, *131*, 803–820. [CrossRef] [PubMed]
2. Stupp, R.; Mason, W.P.; van den Bent, M.J.; Weller, M.; Fisher, B.; Taphoorn, M.J.; Belanger, K.; Brandes, A.A.; Marosi, C.; Bogdahn, U.; et al. Radiotherapy plus concomitant and adjuvant temozolomide for glioblastoma. *N. Engl. J. Med.* **2005**, *352*, 987–996. [CrossRef] [PubMed]
3. Osswald, M.; Jung, E.; Sahm, F.; Solecki, G.; Venkataramani, V.; Blaes, J.; Weil, S.; Horstmann, H.; Wiestler, B.; Syed, M.; et al. Brain tumour cells interconnect to a functional and resistant network. *Nature* **2015**, *528*, 93–98. [CrossRef] [PubMed]
4. Wick, W.; Platten, M.; Wick, A.; Hertenstein, A.; Radbruch, A.; Bendszus, M.; Winkler, F. Current status and future directions of anti-angiogenic therapy for gliomas. *Neuro Oncol.* **2016**, *18*, 315–328. [CrossRef] [PubMed]
5. Osswald, M.; Solecki, G.; Wick, W.; Winkler, F. A malignant cellular network in gliomas: Potential clinical implications. *Neuro Oncol.* **2016**, *18*, 479–485. [CrossRef] [PubMed]
6. Winkler, F.; Kozin, S.V.; Tong, R.T.; Chae, S.S.; Booth, M.F.; Garkavtsev, I.; Xu, L.; Hicklin, D.J.; Fukumura, D.; di Tomaso, E.; et al. Kinetics of vascular normalization by VEGFR2 blockade governs brain tumor response to radiation: Role of oxygenation, angiopoietin-1, and matrix metalloproteinases. *Cancer Cell* **2004**, *6*, 553–563. [CrossRef] [PubMed]
7. Von Baumgarten, L.; Brucker, D.; Tirniceru, A.; Kienast, Y.; Grau, S.; Burgold, S.; Herms, J.; Winkler, F. Bevacizumab has differential and dose-dependent effects on glioma blood vessels and tumor cells. *Clin. Cancer Res.* **2011**, *17*, 6192–6205. [CrossRef] [PubMed]
8. Plate, K.H.; Breier, G.; Weich, H.A.; Mennel, H.D.; Risau, W. Vascular endothelial growth factor and glioma angiogenesis: Coordinate induction of VEGF receptors, distribution of VEGF protein and possible in vivo regulatory mechanisms. *Int. J. Cancer* **1994**, *59*, 520–529. [CrossRef] [PubMed]
9. Scholz, A.; Harter, P.N.; Cremer, S.; Yalcin, B.H.; Gurnik, S.; Yamaji, M.; Di Tacchio, M.; Sommer, K.; Baumgarten, P.; Bahr, O.; et al. Endothelial cell-derived angiopoietin-2 is a therapeutic target in treatment-naive and bevacizumab-resistant glioblastoma. *EMBO Mol. Med.* **2016**, *8*, 39–57. [CrossRef] [PubMed]
10. Kloepper, J.; Riedemann, L.; Amoozgar, Z.; Seano, G.; Susek, K.; Yu, V.; Dalvie, N.; Amelung, R.L.; Datta, M.; Song, J.W.; et al. Ang-2/VEGF bispecific antibody reprograms macrophages and resident microglia to anti-tumor phenotype and prolongs glioblastoma survival. *Proc. Natl. Acad. Sci. USA* **2016**, *113*, 4476–4481. [CrossRef] [PubMed]
11. Peterson, T.E.; Kirkpatrick, N.D.; Huang, Y.; Farrar, C.T.; Marijt, K.A.; Kloepper, J.; Datta, M.; Amoozgar, Z.; Seano, G.; Jung, K.; et al. Dual inhibition of Ang-2 and VEGF receptors normalizes tumor vasculature and prolongs survival in glioblastoma by altering macrophages. *Proc. Natl. Acad. Sci. USA* **2016**, *113*, 4470–4475. [CrossRef] [PubMed]
12. Stratmann, A.; Risau, W.; Plate, K.H. Cell type-specific expression of angiopoietin-1 and angiopoietin-2 suggests a role in glioblastoma angiogenesis. *Am. J. Pathol.* **1998**, *153*, 1459–1466. [CrossRef]
13. Chae, S.S.; Kamoun, W.S.; Farrar, C.T.; Kirkpatrick, N.D.; Niemeyer, E.; de Graaf, A.M.; Sorensen, A.G.; Munn, L.L.; Jain, R.K.; Fukumura, D. Angiopoietin-2 interferes with anti-VEGFR2-induced vessel normalization and survival benefit in mice bearing gliomas. *Clin. Cancer Res.* **2010**, *16*, 3618–3627. [CrossRef] [PubMed]
14. Jain, R.K. Normalization of tumor vasculature: An emerging concept in antiangiogenic therapy. *Science* **2005**, *307*, 58–62. [CrossRef] [PubMed]

15. Huber, P.E.; Bischof, M.; Jenne, J.; Heiland, S.; Peschke, P.; Saffrich, R.; Grone, H.J.; Debus, J.; Lipson, K.E.; Abdollahi, A. Trimodal cancer treatment: Beneficial effects of combined antiangiogenesis, radiation, and chemotherapy. *Cancer Res.* **2005**, *65*, 3643–3655. [CrossRef] [PubMed]
16. Sorensen, A.G.; Batchelor, T.T.; Zhang, W.T.; Chen, P.J.; Yeo, P.; Wang, M.; Jennings, D.; Wen, P.Y.; Lahdenranta, J.; Ancukiewicz, M.; et al. A "vascular normalization index" as potential mechanistic biomarker to predict survival after a single dose of cediranib in recurrent glioblastoma patients. *Cancer Res.* **2009**, *69*, 5296–5300. [CrossRef] [PubMed]
17. McGee, M.C.; Hamner, J.B.; Williams, R.F.; Rosati, S.F.; Sims, T.L.; Ng, C.Y.; Gaber, M.W.; Calabrese, C.; Wu, J.; Nathwani, A.C.; et al. Improved intratumoral oxygenation through vascular normalization increases glioma sensitivity to ionizing radiation. *Int. J. Radiat. Oncol. Biol. Phys.* **2010**, *76*, 1537–1545. [CrossRef] [PubMed]
18. Jain, R.K. Normalizing tumor vasculature with anti-angiogenic therapy: A new paradigm for combination therapy. *Nat. Med.* **2001**, *7*, 987–989. [CrossRef] [PubMed]
19. Jain, R.K.; Martin, J.D.; Stylianopoulos, T. The role of mechanical forces in tumor growth and therapy. *Annu. Rev. Biomed. Eng.* **2014**, *16*, 321–346. [CrossRef] [PubMed]
20. Batchelor, T.T.; Gerstner, E.R.; Emblem, K.E.; Duda, D.G.; Kalpathy-Cramer, J.; Snuderl, M.; Ancukiewicz, M.; Polaskova, P.; Pinho, M.C.; Jennings, D.; et al. Improved tumor oxygenation and survival in glioblastoma patients who show increased blood perfusion after cediranib and chemoradiation. *Proc. Natl. Acad. Sci. USA* **2013**, *110*, 19059–19064. [CrossRef] [PubMed]
21. Gilbert, M.R.; Dignam, J.J.; Armstrong, T.S.; Wefel, J.S.; Blumenthal, D.T.; Vogelbaum, M.A.; Colman, H.; Chakravarti, A.; Pugh, S.; Won, M.; et al. A randomized trial of bevacizumab for newly diagnosed glioblastoma. *N. Engl. J. Med.* **2014**, *370*, 699–708. [CrossRef] [PubMed]
22. Chinot, O.L.; Wick, W.; Mason, W.; Henriksson, R.; Saran, F.; Nishikawa, R.; Carpentier, A.F.; Hoang-Xuan, K.; Kavan, P.; Cernea, D.; et al. Bevacizumab plus radiotherapy-temozolomide for newly diagnosed glioblastoma. *N. Engl. J. Med.* **2014**, *370*, 709–722. [CrossRef] [PubMed]
23. Wick, W.; Gorlia, T.; Bendszus, M.; Taphoorn, M.; Sahm, F.; Harting, I.; Brandes, A.A.; Taal, W.; Domont, J.; Idbaih, A.; et al. Lomustine and Bevacizumab in Progressive Glioblastoma. *N. Engl. J. Med.* **2017**, *377*, 1954–1963. [CrossRef] [PubMed]
24. Sandmann, T.; Bourgon, R.; Garcia, J.; Li, C.; Cloughesy, T.; Chinot, O.L.; Wick, W.; Nishikawa, R.; Mason, W.; Henriksson, R.; et al. Patients With Proneural Glioblastoma May Derive Overall Survival Benefit From the Addition of Bevacizumab to First-Line Radiotherapy and Temozolomide: Retrospective Analysis of the AVAglio Trial. *J. Clin. Oncol.* **2015**, *33*, 2735–2744. [CrossRef] [PubMed]
25. Kessler, T.; Sahm, F.; Blaes, J.; Osswald, M.; Rubmann, P.; Milford, D.; Urban, S.; Jestaedt, L.; Heiland, S.; Bendszus, M.; et al. Glioma cell VEGFR-2 confers resistance to chemotherapeutic and antiangiogenic treatments in PTEN-deficient glioblastoma. *Oncotarget* **2015**, *6*, 31050–31068. [CrossRef] [PubMed]
26. Kienast, Y.; Klein, C.; Scheuer, W.; Raemsch, R.; Lorenzon, E.; Bernicke, D.; Herting, F.; Yu, S.; The, H.H.; Martarello, L.; et al. Ang-2-VEGF-A CrossMab, a novel bispecific human IgG1 antibody blocking VEGF-A and Ang-2 functions simultaneously, mediates potent antitumor, antiangiogenic, and antimetastatic efficacy. *Clin. Cancer Res.* **2013**, *19*, 6730–6740. [CrossRef] [PubMed]
27. Thomas, M.; Kienast, Y.; Scheuer, W.; Bahner, M.; Kaluza, K.; Gassner, C.; Herting, F.; Brinkmann, U.; Seeber, S.; Kavlie, A.; et al. A novel angiopoietin-2 selective fully human antibody with potent anti-tumoral and anti-angiogenic efficacy and superior side effect profile compared to Pan-Angiopoietin-1/-2 inhibitors. *PLoS ONE* **2013**, *8*, e54923. [CrossRef] [PubMed]
28. Liang, W.C.; Wu, X.; Peale, F.V.; Lee, C.V.; Meng, Y.G.; Gutierrez, J.; Fu, L.; Malik, A.K.; Gerber, H.P.; Ferrara, N.; et al. Cross-species vascular endothelial growth factor (VEGF)-blocking antibodies completely inhibit the growth of human tumor xenografts and measure the contribution of stromal VEGF. *J. Biol. Chem.* **2006**, *281*, 951–961. [CrossRef] [PubMed]
29. Baker, L.C.; Boult, J.K.; Thomas, M.; Koehler, A.; Nayak, T.; Tessier, J.; Ooi, C.H.; Birzele, F.; Belousov, A.; Zajac, M.; et al. Acute tumour response to a bispecific Ang-2-VEGF-A antibody: Insights from multiparametric MRI and gene expression profiling. *Br. J. Cancer* **2016**, *115*, 691–702. [CrossRef] [PubMed]
30. Klein, C.; Schaefer, W.; Regula, J.T. The use of CrossMAb technology for the generation of bi- and multispecific antibodies. *mAbs* **2016**, *8*, 1010–1020. [CrossRef] [PubMed]

31. Schaefer, W.; Regula, J.T.; Bahner, M.; Schanzer, J.; Croasdale, R.; Durr, H.; Gassner, C.; Georges, G.; Kettenberger, H.; Imhof-Jung, S.; et al. Immunoglobulin domain crossover as a generic approach for the production of bispecific IgG antibodies. *Proc. Natl. Acad. Sci. USA* **2011**, *108*, 11187–11192. [CrossRef] [PubMed]
32. Kamoun, W.S.; Chae, S.S.; Lacorre, D.A.; Tyrrell, J.A.; Mitre, M.; Gillissen, M.A.; Fukumura, D.; Jain, R.K.; Munn, L.L. Simultaneous measurement of RBC velocity, flux, hematocrit and shear rate in vascular networks. *Nat. Methods* **2010**, *7*, 655–660. [CrossRef] [PubMed]
33. Lu, K.V.; Chang, J.P.; Parachoniak, C.A.; Pandika, M.M.; Aghi, M.K.; Meyronet, D.; Isachenko, N.; Fouse, S.D.; Phillips, J.J.; Cheresh, D.A.; et al. VEGF inhibits tumor cell invasion and mesenchymal transition through a MET/VEGFR2 complex. *Cancer Cell* **2012**, *22*, 21–35. [CrossRef] [PubMed]
34. Fischer, I.; Cunliffe, C.H.; Bollo, R.J.; Raza, S.; Monoky, D.; Chiriboga, L.; Parker, E.C.; Golfinos, J.G.; Kelly, P.J.; Knopp, E.A.; et al. High-grade glioma before and after treatment with radiation and Avastin: Initial observations. *Neuro Oncol.* **2008**, *10*, 700–708. [CrossRef] [PubMed]
35. Paez-Ribes, M.; Allen, E.; Hudock, J.; Takeda, T.; Okuyama, H.; Vinals, F.; Inoue, M.; Bergers, G.; Hanahan, D.; Casanovas, O. Antiangiogenic therapy elicits malignant progression of tumors to increased local invasion and distant metastasis. *Cancer Cell* **2009**, *15*, 220–231. [CrossRef] [PubMed]
36. Keunen, O.; Johansson, M.; Oudin, A.; Sanzey, M.; Rahim, S.A.; Fack, F.; Thorsen, F.; Taxt, T.; Bartos, M.; Jirik, R.; et al. Anti-VEGF treatment reduces blood supply and increases tumor cell invasion in glioblastoma. *Proc. Natl. Acad. Sci. USA* **2011**, *108*, 3749–3754. [CrossRef] [PubMed]
37. Labussiere, M.; Cheneau, C.; Prahst, C.; Gallego Perez-Larraya, J.; Farina, P.; Lombardi, G.; Mokhtari, K.; Rahimian, A.; Delattre, J.Y.; Eichmann, A.; et al. Angiopoietin-2 May Be Involved in the Resistance to Bevacizumab in Recurrent Glioblastoma. *Cancer Investig.* **2016**, *34*, 39–44. [CrossRef] [PubMed]
38. Cortes-Santiago, N.; Hossain, M.B.; Gabrusiewicz, K.; Fan, X.; Gumin, J.; Marini, F.C.; Alonso, M.M.; Lang, F.; Yung, W.K.; Fueyo, J.; et al. Soluble Tie2 overrides the heightened invasion induced by anti-angiogenesis therapies in gliomas. *Oncotarget* **2016**, *7*, 16146–16157. [CrossRef] [PubMed]
39. Tong, R.T.; Boucher, Y.; Kozin, S.V.; Winkler, F.; Hicklin, D.J.; Jain, R.K. Vascular normalization by vascular endothelial growth factor receptor 2 blockade induces a pressure gradient across the vasculature and improves drug penetration in tumors. *Cancer Res.* **2004**, *64*, 3731–3736. [CrossRef] [PubMed]
40. Grossman, R.; Brastianos, H.; Blakeley, J.O.; Mangraviti, A.; Lal, B.; Zadnik, P.; Hwang, L.; Wicks, R.T.; Goodwin, R.C.; Brem, H.; et al. Combination of anti-VEGF therapy and temozolomide in two experimental human glioma models. *J. Neuro Oncol.* **2014**, *116*, 59–65. [CrossRef] [PubMed]
41. Van der Veldt, A.A.; Lubberink, M.; Bahce, I.; Walraven, M.; de Boer, M.P.; Greuter, H.N.; Hendrikse, N.H.; Eriksson, J.; Windhorst, A.D.; Postmus, P.E.; et al. Rapid decrease in delivery of chemotherapy to tumors after anti-VEGF therapy: Implications for scheduling of anti-angiogenic drugs. *Cancer Cell* **2012**, *21*, 82–91. [CrossRef] [PubMed]
42. Rohrig, F.; Vorlova, S.; Hoffmann, H.; Wartenberg, M.; Escorcia, F.E.; Keller, S.; Tenspolde, M.; Weigand, I.; Gatzner, S.; Manova, K.; et al. VEGF-ablation therapy reduces drug delivery and therapeutic response in ECM-dense tumors. *Oncogene* **2016**, *36*. [CrossRef] [PubMed]
43. Ma, J.; Waxman, D.J. Modulation of the antitumor activity of metronomic cyclophosphamide by the angiogenesis inhibitor axitinib. *Mol. Cancer Ther.* **2008**, *7*, 79–89. [CrossRef] [PubMed]
44. Arjaans, M.; Schroder, C.P.; Oosting, S.F.; Dafni, U.; Kleibeuker, J.E.; de Vries, E.G. VEGF pathway targeting agents, vessel normalization and tumor drug uptake: From bench to bedside. *Oncotarget* **2016**, *7*, 21247–21258. [CrossRef] [PubMed]
45. Agarwala, S.S.; Kirkwood, J.M. Temozolomide, a novel alkylating agent with activity in the central nervous system, may improve the treatment of advanced metastatic melanoma. *Oncologist* **2000**, *5*, 144–151. [CrossRef] [PubMed]
46. Baumert, B.G.; Hegi, M.E.; van den Bent, M.J.; von Deimling, A.; Gorlia, T.; Hoang-Xuan, K.; Brandes, A.A.; Kantor, G.; Taphoorn, M.J.; Hassel, M.B.; et al. Temozolomide chemotherapy versus radiotherapy in high-risk low-grade glioma (EORTC 22033-26033): A randomised, open-label, phase 3 intergroup study. *Lancet Oncol.* **2016**, *17*, 1521–1532. [CrossRef]
47. Winkler, F.; Osswald, M.; Wick, W. Anti-Angiogenics: Their Role in the Treatment of Glioblastoma. *Oncol. Res. Treat.* **2018**, *41*, 181–186. [CrossRef] [PubMed]

48. Lange, C.; Storkebaum, E.; de Almodovar, C.R.; Dewerchin, M.; Carmeliet, P. Vascular endothelial growth factor: A neurovascular target in neurological diseases. *Nat. Rev. Neurol.* **2016**, *12*, 439–454. [CrossRef] [PubMed]
49. Jayson, G.C.; Kerbel, R.; Ellis, L.M.; Harris, A.L. Antiangiogenic therapy in oncology: Current status and future directions. *Lancet* **2016**, *388*, 518–529. [CrossRef]
50. Bergers, G.; Hanahan, D. Modes of resistance to anti-angiogenic therapy. *Nat. Rev. Cancer* **2008**, *8*, 592–603. [CrossRef] [PubMed]
51. Thomas, M.; Felcht, M.; Kruse, K.; Kretschmer, S.; Deppermann, C.; Biesdorf, A.; Rohr, K.; Benest, A.V.; Fiedler, U.; Augustin, H.G. Angiopoietin-2 stimulation of endothelial cells induces alphavbeta3 integrin internalization and degradation. *J. Biol. Chem.* **2010**, *285*, 23842–23849. [CrossRef] [PubMed]
52. Scharpfenecker, M.; Fiedler, U.; Reiss, Y.; Augustin, H.G. The Tie-2 ligand angiopoietin-2 destabilizes quiescent endothelium through an internal autocrine loop mechanism. *J. Cell Sci.* **2005**, *118*, 771–780. [CrossRef] [PubMed]
53. Felcht, M.; Luck, R.; Schering, A.; Seidel, P.; Srivastava, K.; Hu, J.; Bartol, A.; Kienast, Y.; Vettel, C.; Loos, E.K.; et al. Angiopoietin-2 differentially regulates angiogenesis through TIE2 and integrin signaling. *J. Clin. Investig.* **2012**, *122*, 1991–2005. [CrossRef] [PubMed]
54. Bessho, H.; Wong, B.; Huang, D.; Tan, J.; Ong, C.K.; Iwamura, M.; Hart, S.; Dangl, M.; Thomas, M.; Teh, B.T. Effect of Ang-2-VEGF-A Bispecific Antibody in Renal Cell Carcinoma. *Cancer Investig.* **2015**, *33*, 378–386. [CrossRef] [PubMed]
55. Brown, J.L.; Cao, Z.A.; Pinzon-Ortiz, M.; Kendrew, J.; Reimer, C.; Wen, S.; Zhou, J.Q.; Tabrizi, M.; Emery, S.; McDermott, B.; et al. A human monoclonal anti-ANG2 antibody leads to broad antitumor activity in combination with VEGF inhibitors and chemotherapy agents in preclinical models. *Mol. Cancer Ther.* **2010**, *9*, 145–156. [CrossRef] [PubMed]
56. Daly, C.; Eichten, A.; Castanaro, C.; Pasnikowski, E.; Adler, A.; Lalani, A.S.; Papadopoulos, N.; Kyle, A.H.; Minchinton, A.I.; Yancopoulos, G.D.; et al. Angiopoietin-2 functions as a Tie2 agonist in tumor models, where it limits the effects of VEGF inhibition. *Cancer Res.* **2013**, *73*, 108–118. [CrossRef] [PubMed]
57. Hashizume, H.; Falcon, B.L.; Kuroda, T.; Baluk, P.; Coxon, A.; Yu, D.; Bready, J.V.; Oliner, J.D.; McDonald, D.M. Complementary actions of inhibitors of angiopoietin-2 and VEGF on tumor angiogenesis and growth. *Cancer Res.* **2010**, *70*, 2213–2223. [CrossRef] [PubMed]
58. Koh, Y.J.; Kim, H.Z.; Hwang, S.I.; Lee, J.E.; Oh, N.; Jung, K.; Kim, M.; Kim, K.E.; Kim, H.; Lim, N.K.; et al. Double antiangiogenic protein, DAAP, targeting VEGF-A and angiopoietins in tumor angiogenesis, metastasis, and vascular leakage. *Cancer Cell* **2010**, *18*, 171–184. [CrossRef] [PubMed]
59. Myers, A.L.; Williams, R.F.; Ng, C.Y.; Hartwich, J.E.; Davidoff, A.M. Bevacizumab-induced tumor vessel remodeling in rhabdomyosarcoma xenografts increases the effectiveness of adjuvant ionizing radiation. *J. Pediatr. Surg.* **2010**, *45*, 1080–1085. [CrossRef] [PubMed]
60. Browder, T.; Butterfield, C.E.; Kraling, B.M.; Shi, B.; Marshall, B.; O'Reilly, M.S.; Folkman, J. Antiangiogenic scheduling of chemotherapy improves efficacy against experimental drug-resistant cancer. *Cancer Res.* **2000**, *60*, 1878–1886. [PubMed]
61. Kerbel, R.S.; Kamen, B.A. The anti-angiogenic basis of metronomic chemotherapy. *Nat. Rev. Cancer* **2004**, *4*, 423–436. [CrossRef] [PubMed]
62. Goel, S.; Duda, D.G.; Xu, L.; Munn, L.L.; Boucher, Y.; Fukumura, D.; Jain, R.K. Normalization of the vasculature for treatment of cancer and other diseases. *Physiol. Rev.* **2011**, *91*, 1071–1121. [CrossRef] [PubMed]
63. Wild-Bode, C.; Weller, M.; Rimner, A.; Dichgans, J.; Wick, W. Sublethal irradiation promotes migration and invasiveness of glioma cells: Implications for radiotherapy of human glioblastoma. *Cancer Res.* **2001**, *61*, 2744–2750. [PubMed]
64. Pei, J.; Park, I.H.; Ryu, H.H.; Li, S.Y.; Li, C.H.; Lim, S.H.; Wen, M.; Jang, W.Y.; Jung, S. Sublethal dose of irradiation enhances invasion of malignant glioma cells through p53-MMP 2 pathway in U87MG mouse brain tumor model. *Radiat. Oncol.* **2015**, *10*, 164. [CrossRef] [PubMed]
65. Weil, S.; Osswald, M.; Solecki, G.; Grosch, J.; Jung, E.; Lemke, D.; Ratliff, M.; Hanggi, D.; Wick, W.; Winkler, F. Tumor microtubes convey resistance to surgical lesions and chemotherapy in gliomas. *Neuro Oncol.* **2017**, *19*, 1316–1326. [CrossRef] [PubMed]

66. Lou, E. Can you hear them now? Tumor microtubes form cellular communication networks that protect gliomas from surgical lesions and chemotherapy treatments. *Neuro Oncol.* **2017**, *19*, 1289–1291. [CrossRef] [PubMed]
67. Wick, A.; Dorner, N.; Schafer, N.; Hofer, S.; Heiland, S.; Schemmer, D.; Platten, M.; Weller, M.; Bendszus, M.; Wick, W. Bevacizumab does not increase the risk of remote relapse in malignant glioma. *Ann. Neurol.* **2011**, *69*, 586–592. [CrossRef] [PubMed]
68. Pyko, I.V.; Nakada, M.; Sabit, H.; Teng, L.; Furuyama, N.; Hayashi, Y.; Kawakami, K.; Minamoto, T.; Fedulau, A.S.; Hamada, J. Glycogen synthase kinase 3beta inhibition sensitizes human glioblastoma cells to temozolomide by affecting O6-methylguanine DNA methyltransferase promoter methylation via c-Myc signaling. *Carcinogenesis* **2013**, *34*, 2206–2217. [CrossRef] [PubMed]
69. Yuan, F.; Salehi, H.A.; Boucher, Y.; Vasthare, U.S.; Tuma, R.F.; Jain, R.K. Vascular permeability and microcirculation of gliomas and mammary carcinomas transplanted in rat and mouse cranial windows. *Cancer Res.* **1994**, *54*, 4564–4568. [PubMed]

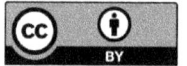

© 2019 by the authors. Licensee MDPI, Basel, Switzerland. This article is an open access article distributed under the terms and conditions of the Creative Commons Attribution (CC BY) license (http://creativecommons.org/licenses/by/4.0/).

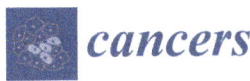

Article

Influence of Vitamin D in Advanced Non-Small Cell Lung Cancer Patients Treated with Nivolumab

Jessica Cusato [1], Carlo Genova [2], Cristina Tomasello [3], Paolo Carrega [4,5], Selene Ottonello [6,7], Gabriella Pietra [6,8], Maria Cristina Mingari [6,7,8], Irene Cossu [9], Erika Rijavec [10], Anna Leggieri [3], Giovanni Di Perri [1], Maria Giovanna Dal Bello [10], Simona Coco [10], Simona Boccardo [10], Guido Ferlazzo [4,5,11], Francesco Grossi [2,*,†] and Antonio D'Avolio [1,12,†]

1. Department of Medical Sciences, University of Turin, Amedeo di Savoia Hospital, 10149 Turin, Italy; jessica.cusato@unito.it (J.C.); giovanni.diperri@unito.it (G.D.P.); antonio.davolio@unito.it (A.D.)
2. Medical Oncology Unit, Fondazione IRCCS Ca' Granda Ospedale Maggiore Policlinico, 20122 Milan, Italy; carlo.genova1985@gmail.com
3. S.C. Farmacie Ospedaliere-Ospedale M.Vittoria-ASL Città di Torino, 10143 Turin, Italy; cristina.tomasello@aslcittaditorino.it (C.T.); anna.leggieri@aslcittaditorino.it (A.L.)
4. Laboratory of Immunology and Biotherapy, Department of Human Pathology, University of Messina, 98125 Messina, Italy; paolo.carrega@unime.it (P.C.); guido.ferlazzo@unime.it (G.F.)
5. Cell Factory Center, University of Messina, 98125 Messina, Italy
6. Department of Experimental Medicine (DiMES), University of Genoa, 16132 Genoa, Italy; sele_8@hotmail.it (S.O.); gabriella.pietra68@gmail.com (G.P.); mariacristina.mingari@hsanmartino.it (M.C.M.)
7. Center of Excellence for Biomedical Research (CEBR), University of Genoa, 16132 Genoa, Italy
8. Immunology Unit, IRCCS Ospedale Policlinico San Martino, 16132 Genoa, Italy
9. Giannina Gaslini Institute, Via Gerolamo Gaslini, 5, 16147 Genova, Italy; ire-ne@hotmail.it
10. Lung Cancer Unit, IRCCS Ospedale Policlinico San Martino, 16132 Genoa, Italy; erika.rijavec@hsanmartino.it (E.R.); mariagiovanna.dalbello@hsanmartino.it (M.G.D.B.); simona.coco@hsanmartino.it (S.C.); simona.boccardo@hsanmartino.it (S.B.)
11. Division of Clinical Pathology, University Hospital Policlinico G. Martino, 98125 Messina, Italy
12. Interdepartmental Center for Clinical and Experimental Pharmacology (CIFACS), University of Turin, 10149 Turin, Italy
* Correspondence: francesco.grossi@policlinico.mi.it; Tel.: +39-025-503-2556
† These authors contributed equally to this work.

Received: 11 December 2018; Accepted: 16 January 2019; Published: 21 January 2019

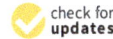

Abstract: Nivolumab is one of the most commonly used monoclonal antibodies for advanced non-small cell lung cancer treatment, to the extent that the presence of its anti-antibody is considered a negative prognostic factor. Vitamin D (VD) modulates expression of the genes involved in drug metabolism and elimination. Immune system regulation and immunodeficiency is frequent in non-small cell lung cancer patients. To date, no data have been reported about the relationship between nivolumab and VD. The aim of this study was to quantify plasma 25-hydroxyVD (25-VD) and 1,25-VD, nivolumab, and its anti-antibody before starting treatment (baseline) and at 15, 45 and 60 days of therapy. VD-pathway-associated gene single nucleotide polymorphisms (SNPs) were also evaluated. Molecules were quantified through enzyme-linked immunosorbent assay, and SNPs through real-time PCR. Forty-five patients were enrolled. Median nivolumab concentrations were 12.5 µg/mL, 22.3 µg/mL and 27.1 µg/mL at 15, 45 and 60 days respectively. No anti-nivolumab antibodies were found. Correlations were observed between nivolumab concentrations and 25-VD levels. Nivolumab concentrations were affected by VD-pathway-related gene SNPs. *VDBP* AC/CC genotype and baseline 25-VD < 10 ng/mL predicted a nivolumab concentration cut-off value of <18.7 µg/mL at 15 days, which was associated with tumor progression. This is the first study showing VD marker predictors of nivolumab concentrations in a real-life context of non-small cell lung cancer treatment.

Keywords: monoclonal antibody; NSCLC; immunotherapy; ELISA; pharmacokinetics; pharmacogenetics

1. Introduction

Immunotherapy represents the most revolutionary treatment for solid cancers nowadays. To date, several types of immunotherapy are available, including monoclonal antibodies, non-specific immunotherapies, oncolytic virus therapy, T-cell therapy and cancer vaccines. The evolution of immune checkpoint inhibitors as anticancer treatment options represents one of the most successful approaches in cancer drug research in the past few years [1]. Checkpoint inhibitor antibodies, such as anti-programmed cell death protein 1 (PD-1) and its ligand (PD-L1), are new drugs acting as tumor suppressing factors since they are able to modulate the interaction between the immune cell and the tumor cell [2]. These therapies proved to be a safe and effective option in advanced non-small cell lung cancer (NSCLC) and can be recommended selectively [3].

Nivolumab, a monoclonal antibody, binds to the immunomodulating PD-1, blocking ligand interaction and downstream signaling pathways. The result is a positive regulation of T-cell function resulting in an antitumor effect [4]. In 2015, this drug was approved by the FDA for the treatment of patients with advanced squamous and non-squamous NSCLC with progression, or after platinum-based chemotherapy (second-line therapy) [5]. In a randomized trial, 272 patients treated with nivolumab had an overall survival of 3.2 months longer than those on docetaxel [2].

In a conference abstract, authors measured nivolumab plasma concentrations in patients and suggested that partial responders had higher nivolumab mean trough concentrations (27.4 µg/mL) compared to subjects with tumor progression (18.7 µg/mL) [6].

PD-1 inhibitors typically cause fewer and less severe treatment-related adverse events (AEs) compared with conventional chemotherapy compounds, although immunorelated AEs can occur requiring monitoring and specialized management to prevent serious complications [7]. Moreover, immunogenicity in terms of the presence of nivolumab's anti-antibodies is considered a negative prognostic factor [8]. Immunogenicity and immune checkpoints in general are regulated by different factors such as vitamin D (VD) [9]. Reported studies show that VD controls different pathways related to innate and adaptive immunity regulating the expression of many genes involved in drug metabolism/elimination through its receptor (VDR). Moreover, in another study, single nucleotide polymorphisms (SNPs) in genes involved in the VD pathway could affect VD kinetics and, consequently, its action. Polymorphisms present near genes involved in cholesterol production, hydroxylation, and VD transport are able to predict who could have risk of VD insufficiency, as suggested by Wang et al. [10]. Genetic variations near DHCR7 (4p12 (overall $p = 1.9 \times 10(-109)$ for rs2282679, in GC); 11q12 ($p = 2.1 \times 10(-27)$ for rs12785878), near CYP2R1 (11p15 ($p = 3.3 \times 10(-20)$ for rs10741657) and near CYP24A1 (20q13)) have genome-wide significance in that population. Furthermore, participants with a score obtained combining the three variants in the highest quartile are at increased risk of 25-VD levels lower than 75 nmol/L or than 50 nmol/L, compared with those in the lowest quartile.

Since VD deficiency is frequent in lung cancer patients [11] and no data on nivolumab and its relationship with VD are currently available, the aim of this study was to quantify 25-hydroxyVD (25-VD), 1,25-hydroxyVD (1,25-VD), nivolumab, and its anti-antibody levels in patients' plasma at different timings, also considering their influence in predicting the cut-off value (18.7 µg/mL) associated with tumor progression.

2. Results

2.1. Patient Characteristics

Baseline (BL) characteristics for the 45 included patients are reported in Table 1. Thirty-one (69) were male, the median age was 73 years and the median body mass index (BMI) was 23.4 Kg/m^2.

Table 1. Baseline characteristics of study population.

Characteristics		n (%), Median (IQR)
n		45
Age (years)		73 (65–79.5)
Male sex		31 (69)
BMI (Kg/m^2)		23.4 (20.1–26.4)
Caucasian		45 (100)
NSCLC type	Adenocarcinoma	34 (52.3)
	Squamous cell carcinoma	9 (13.8)
	Poorly differentiated carcinoma	1 (1.5)
	Large-cell neuroendocrine carcinoma	1 (1.5)
Concomitant drugs	Cardiovascular	24 (36.9)
	Diabetes	4 (6.2)
	Opioids	9 (13.8)
	Protease inhibitors	20 (30.8)
	Corticosteroid	12 (18.5)
	Vitamin D	2 (3.1)
Pre-treatment drugs	Cisplatine	24 (53.3)
	Docetaxel	10 (22.2)
	Carboplatine	24 (53.3)
	Gemcitabine	12 (26.7)
	Gefitinib	2 (4.4)
	Pemetrexed	30 (66.7)
	Afatinib	1 (2.2)
	Osimertinib	1 (2.2)
	Erlotinib	20 (44.4)
	Vinorelbine	10 (22.2)
	Paclitaxel	3 (6.7)
	Bevacizumab	3 (6.7)
	Etoposide	4 (8.9)
	Zoledronic acid	1 (2.2)
	Bavicizumab	1 (2.2)
	Farletuzumab	1 (2.2)
	Radiotherapy	1 (2.2)

2.2. Nivolumab and Vitamin D Concentrations

Median nivolumab concentrations were 12.5 µg/mL (9.5–17.1 µg/mL), 22.3 µg/mL (IQR:18.30–34.88 µg/mL) and 27.1 µg/mL (IQR:17.4–39.4 µg/mL), respectively, at 15, 45, and 60 days (Figure 1). No anti-nivolumab antibodies were detected.

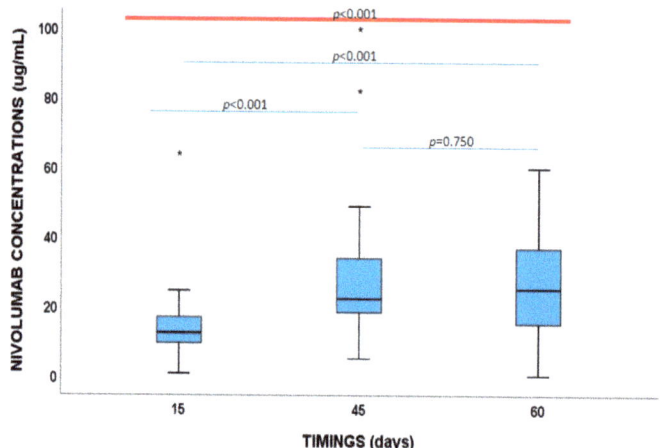

Figure 1. Nivolumab plasma concentrations at 15, 45 and 60 days.

The 25-VD concentration was 12.8 ng/mL (10.1–16.6 ng/mL), 13.6 ng/mL (10.9–16.1 ng/mL), 11.8 ng/mL (10.1–18.9 ng/mL), and 12.9 ng/mL (10.8–17.0 ng/mL) at BL, 15, 45, and 60 days, respectively.

The 1,25-VD value was 33.7 pg/mL (23.4–40.6 ng/mL), 34.7 ng/mL (22.3–45.4 ng/mL), 28.5 ng/mL (20.7–41.5 ng/mL), and 35.7 ng/mL (IQR:19.2–49.0 ng/mL), respectively, at BL, 15, 45, and 60 days.

Correlations (see Figure 2) were observed between nivolumab concentrations at 15 days and BL 25-VD levels ($p = 0.024$, Pearson's coefficient (PC) 0.451) and at 15 days ($p = 0.017$, PC = 0.542). Nivolumab exposure at 60 days was correlated with 25-VD at BL ($p = 0.001$, PC = 0.730), at 15 ($p < 0.001$, PC = 0.858), 45 ($p = 0.001$, PC = 0.779), and 60 days ($p < 0.001$, PC = 0.900). Furthermore, in a sub-group, patients were stratified according to 25-VD deficiency. BL 25-VD levels < 10 ng/mL were associated with lower nivolumab concentrations at 15 days ($p = 0.103$, a trend without statistical significance), 45 days ($p = 0.018$), and 60 days ($p = 0.021$). Fifteen days of 25-VD < 10 ng/mL levels were associated with lower nivolumab concentrations at 15 days ($p = 0.019$), 45 days ($p = 0.019$), and 60 days ($p = 0.028$). Finally, 60 days of 25-VD < 10 ng/mL was associated with lower nivolumab levels at 60 days ($p = 0.030$). No correlation was observed for 1,25-VD or toxicities and nivolumab exposure.

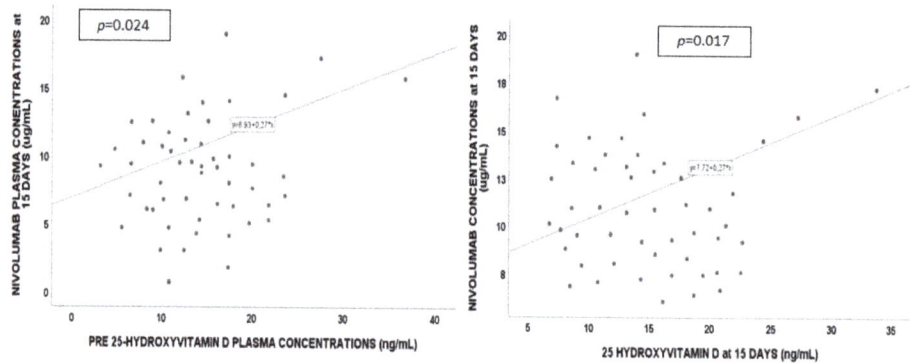

Figure 2. *Cont.*

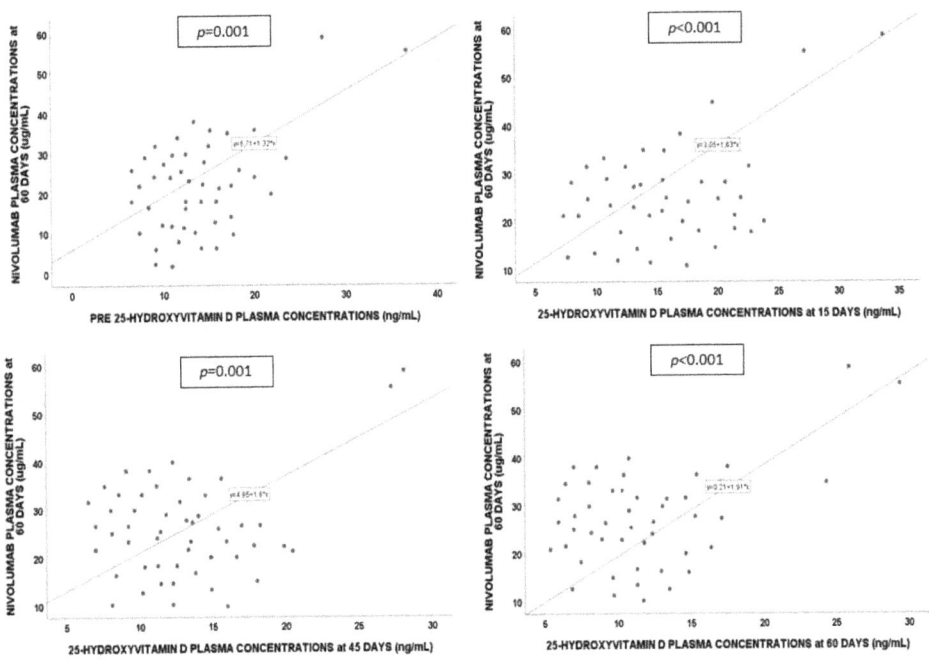

Figure 2. Nivolumab and 25-hydroxyvitamin D correlations at different timings.

2.3. Pharmacogenetics

Variant genotype frequencies (%) were calculated and are reported in Table 2.

Table 2. Variant allele frequencies.

Single Nucleotide Polymorphism (SNP)	% Homozygous Wild Type	% Heterozygous	% Homozygous Mutant
CYP27B1 +2838 C > T	20 CC	2.2 CT	77.8 TT
CYP27B1 −1260 G > T	73.3 CC	15.6 CT	11.1 TT
CYP24A1 rs2248359 T > C	42.2 TT	40 TC	17.8 CC
CYP24A1 rs927650 C > T	33.3 CC	22.2 CT	44.5 TT
CYP24A1 rs2585428 A > G	31.1 AA	28.9 AC	40 CC
VDR Cdx2 A > G	17.8 AA	13.3 AG	68.9 GG
VDR TaqI T > C	33.3 TT	26.7 TC	40 CC
VDR FokI T > C	11.1 TT	42.2 TC	46.7 CC
VDR BsmI G > A	42.2 GG	57.8 GA	-
VDR ApaI C > A	26.7 CC	28.9 CA	44.4 AA
VDBP rs7041 T > G	6.7 TT	62.2 TG	31.1 GG

No genetic variants showed to affect VD concentrations. Nivolumab plasma concentrations at 15 days (Figure 3) were associated with *VDR* TaqI CC ($p = 0.042$), ApaI CA/AA ($p = 0.030$) and *CYP27B1*-1260 TT ($p = 0.014$). Nivolumab exposure at 45 days (Figure 4) were influenced by *VDR* Cdx2 AG/GG ($p = 0.019$), *VDBP* rs7041 AC/CC ($p = 0.035$), and *CYP27B1*-1260 TT ($p = 0.028$); nivolumab exposure at 60 days (Figure 5) was affected by *VDR* Cdx2 AG/GG ($p = 0.022$) and TaqI TC/CC ($p = 0.021$). VDR: vitamin D receptor.

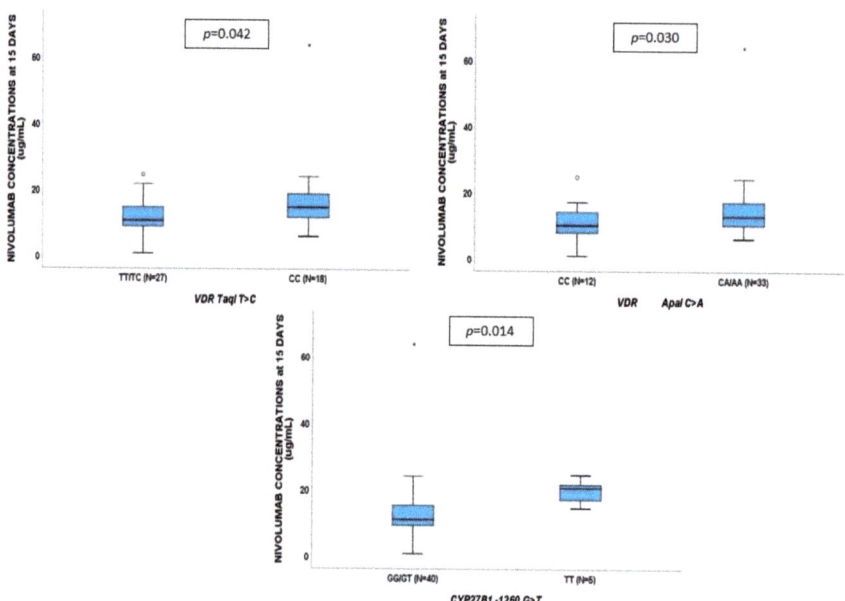

Figure 3. Influence of gene variants on nivolumab plasma concentrations at 15 days.

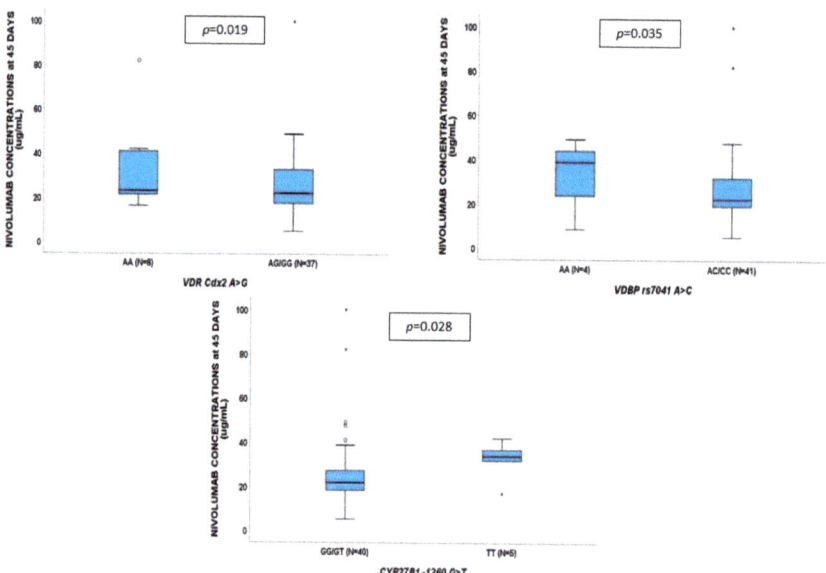

Figure 4. Influence of gene variants on nivolumab plasma concentrations at 45 days.

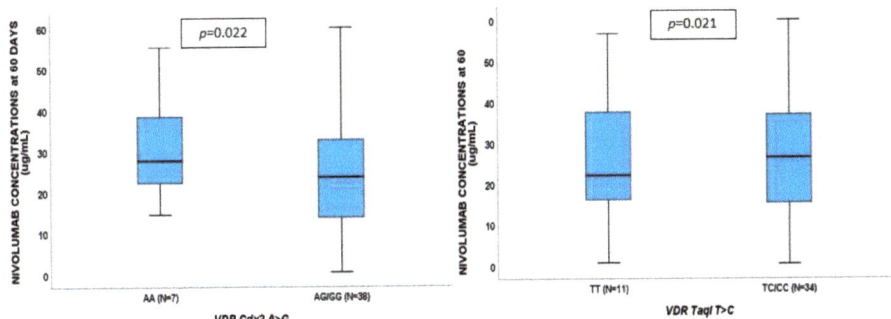

Figure 5. Influence of gene variants on nivolumab plasma concentrations at 60 days.

2.4. Regression Analysis

A logistical regression analysis was performed to evaluate whether factors (demographic, clinical, pharmacological or genetic) were able to predict nivolumab concentrations <18.7 µg/mL at 15 days (see Table 3). According to a Bonferroni test, $p < 0.003$ was considered to be the adjusted p-value, but no factors reached this value in the univariate analysis. In the multivariate model, *VDBP* (GC) AC/CC genotype and BL 25-VD were predictors of this cut-off value, associated with tumor progression (Figure 6).

Table 3. Logistic regression analyses: Factors able to predict nivolumab concentrations <18.7 µg/mL at 15 days of therapy. Bold represents statistically significant values. NC: not comparable, all the factors belong to a single group. Thus, statistics could show p-values and *odd-ratio* (OR).

Variables	Nivolumab Concentrations ≤ 18.7 µg/mL			
	Univariate		Multivariate	
	p-Value	OR (95% IC)	p-Value	OR (95% IC)
BMI < 25 Kg/m^2	0.766	1.270 (0.392–6.112)		
Age > 60 years	0.939	0.970 (0.091–9.145)		
Gender (male)	0.213	2.260 (0.692–12.419)		
Drug dosage < 200 mg	0.945	1.056 (0.099–4.867)		
VDBP (GC) AC/CC	0.059	11.667 (0.909–149.700)	**0.049**	**10.667 (0.830–137.145)**
CYP24A1 3999 CC	NC			
VDR TaqI TC/CC	0.164	3.077 (0.632–14.976)		
CYP27B1 -1260 GG	0.148	3.250 (0.658–16.040)		
Pre 25-hydroxyvitamin D levels	NC		NC	
Pre 1,25-hydroxyvitamin D levels	0.124	3.840 (0.692–21.312)		
Adenocarcinoma NSCLC type	NC			
Squamous cell carcinoma	NC			
Cisplatine pre-treatment	0.093	4.442 (0.852–24.853)		
Carboplatine pre-treatment	0.190	0.300 (0.051–1.854)		
Pemetrexed pre-treatment	NC			

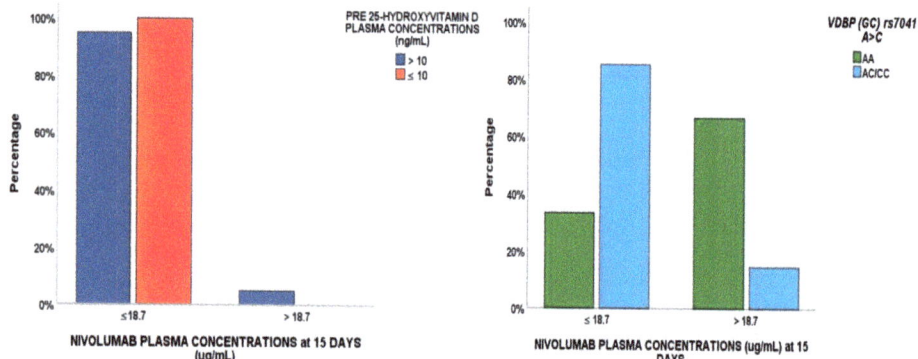

Figure 6. *VDBP* rs7041 SNP and pre-25 hydroxyvitamin D levels predictors of the nivolumab cut-off value of 18.7 µg/mL at 15 days, associated with tumor progression.

3. Discussion

Nivolumab represents an active treatment strategy with the potential of long-term disease control [12]. Unfortunately, biomarkers of reliable efficacy are lacking, thus nivolumab has not been considered to be cost-effective in several national health systems [13,14].

However, a meta-analysis [3] on immune checkpoint inhibitors and chemotherapy in the treatment of advanced NSCLC showed significant advantages in terms of overall survival, progression-free survival, and overall response rate, compared with conventional chemotherapy in patients with advanced disease.

VD is able to regulate the immune system. Its synthesis begins by the action of ultraviolet light in the context of skin tissue. Cholecalciferol is hydroxylated to calcifediol (25-VD) in the liver through cytochrome P-450 (CYP, 27A1, 2R1). In the kidney, calcitriol (1,25-VD, the active form) is synthesized through CYP27B1 and transported in the bloodstream through vitamin D binding protein (VDBP). The inactivation of 25-VD to calcitroic acid (24,25-VD) is carried on by CYP24A1. VD deficiency is frequently observed in cancer patients. Bochen et al. suggested that VD serum levels were significantly lower in head and neck cancer patients compared to controls, particularly in patients with lymphatic metastasis [15]. Different studies show that a lower 25-VD serum level is associated with several negative outcomes in lung cancer. Feng et al. analyzed seventeen studies in a meta-analysis and found a statistically significant relationship between 25-VD, lung cancer risk, and mortality, but a relationship with overall lung cancer survival was not observed [16]. In addition, they suggested differences between males and females and in Caucasian and Asian populations in terms of cancer risk.

In the current study, 25-VD influenced nivolumab concentrations, but not 1,25-VD. Here, we only evaluate nivolumab and VD concentrations and not the effect on the immune cells. VD deficiency could have a relapse due to the immune system, which is directly related to this treatment. In fact, in another study, a relationship between immune cells and 25-VD and not with 1,25-VD was found, as shown for regulatory T cell function in multiple sclerosis patients [17]. Information about the influence of VD on the immune system is lacking in this study. This limitation will be the aim of further studies by our group.

Furthermore, 1,25-VD is present with a concentration 1000 times lower than 25-VD in the blood. Such low 1,25-VD concentrations could be more difficult to measure compared to 25-VD levels. Finally, the absence of statistical significance could be due to the small sample size.

In the current study, the nivolumab plasma levels in a real-life context of NSCLC are described at different timings and, in addition, the role of 25-VD concentrations and *VDBP* rs7041 A > C SNP in predicting concentrations lower than 18.7 µg/mL (the cut-off value associated with tumor progression as shown by Stijn et al. [6]) is suggested.

Various *VDBP* genetic variants are known. The two most common polymorphisms, 1296 A > C (rs7041, Glu432Asp) and 1307 C > A (rs4588, Thr436Lys), are localized in exon 11 and they are in complete linkage disequilibrium [18]. Circulating VDBP seems not to be influenced by rs7041 SNP, however, considering the 1296/1307 diplotype, there is a slight transport increase in AC/CA, compared to AA/CA. It is probable that lysine to threonine substitution at position 436 eliminates an O-glycosylation site from the molecule and the loss of glycosylation influences the half-life of VDBP. Moreover, glutamine to asparagine changes in the 432 position affect the extent of O-glycosylation at the 436. It is not known how changes in the VDBP molecule modify its serum concentration, but the described substitutions could result in altered rates of transcription, changes in mRNA stability, or in a self-clearance of the protein [19]. In a recent study of Caucasian women, the AA genotype was related to higher breast cancer risk, compared to healthy controls [20].

Controversial studies are present in the literature concerning the influence of VDBP rs7041 on VD levels. Lafi et al. show that genotypes containing the variant allele of rs7041 (TT, TG) are associated with lower 25-VD concentrations than the GG genotype, whereas Daffara et al. did not find an association in coronary heart disease patients and suggest that 25-VD levels, but not VDBP genetic status, independently predicted the presence of coronary lesions at angiography [21,22]. Also, in the current study, an association between the *VDBP* genetic variant and VD levels has been evidenced, although a borderline influence ($p = 0.049$) is present with the nivolumab cut-off value. However, the best predicting factor remains 25-VD < 10 ng/mL, as showed in the regression. It is important to understand the nature of the relationship between these variables: is the VD associated with poorer outcomes, or it could be an underlying condition? In our opinion, VD deficiency could be able to affect the outcome, since it is involved in the regulation of the immune system. Furthermore, in deficient individuals before starting therapy, the situation could be more difficult to manage and complications could be more severe (for example, concerning cachexia).

Schmid et al. showed that immunotherapy efficacy was dependent on the metastatic location [23]. For these reasons, it is very important to understand which biomarkers could predict patients with a higher probability of tumor progression.

Our study would recommend to clinicians to evaluate 25-VD levels and the *VDBP* rs7041 genotype, before starting therapy, and to quantify nivolumab concentrations at 15 days, to eventually consider a drug dosage modification or VD supplementation, reducing the risk of tumor progression. It is important to highlight that these analyses are preliminary and have several limitations: They are conducted on few individuals (only 45 patients), only one cohort is analyzed, and *VDBP* SNP has a borderline influence ($p = 0.049$).

4. Materials and Methods

Patients were treated with nivolumab, affected by advanced NSCLC, treated within the Italian Nivolumab Expanded Access Program (NCT02475382), and enrolled in a mono-institutional translational research study at the Lung Cancer Unit of the Ospedale San Martino (Genova, Italy). This study was approved by the Local Ethics Committee (registry number: P.R. 191REG2015). Patients were eligible if they met the following criteria: (i) cytologically or histologically confirmed advanced/metastatic NSCLC, (ii) progression after at least one line of platinum-based chemotherapy, (iii) Eastern Cooperative Oncology Group Performance Status (ECOG-PS) = 0–2, (iv) no previous treatment with immune checkpoint inhibitors, (v) any brain metastasis had to be treated and clinically stable for at least 14 days before starting nivolumab, (vi) no treatment with corticosteroids at a dose higher than 10 mg/day of prednisone or equivalent. Eligible patients received nivolumab at 3 mg/kg every 14 days, with assessment by computed tomography scan (CT-scan) every 8 weeks. Nivolumab was administered until the onset of unacceptable toxicities, patient refusal, death, or up to 96 weeks from the start of treatment. Treatment beyond tumor progression was allowed based on the investigators' judgment, as long as clinical benefit was perceived.

Values of 25-VD and 1,25-VD were evaluated at BL and at 15, 45, and 60 days after starting therapy, with enzyme-linked immunosorbent assay technique (DRG DIAGNOSTIC, Marburg, Germany) and with LIAISON® XL (DiaSorin, Saluggia, Italy), respectively. Nivolumab and its anti-antibody were quantified with validated ELISA kits (Matrix Biotek, Ankara, Turkey).

Whole blood was drawn in EDTA tubes, genomic DNA was isolated from blood samples (MagnaPure Compact, Roche, Monza, Italy), and genotypes were assessed through a real-time polymerase chain reaction allelic discrimination system (LightCycler 480, Roche, Monza, Italy). The investigated gene SNPs were: *CYP27B1* (encoding cytochrome 27B1 enzyme responsible for VD active metabolite 1,25-VD production) rs4646536 (+2838) C > T and rs10877012 (−1260) G > T, *VDR* (encoding VD receptor) rs7975232 (ApaI) C > A, rs731236 (TaqI) T > C, rs10735810 (FokI) T > C, rs11568820 (Cdx2) A > G and rs1544410 (BsmI) G > A, *CYP24A1* (encoding cytochrome 27B1 enzyme responsible for VD inactive metabolite 24,25-dyhydroxyvitamin D (24,25-VD) production) rs2248359 (3999) T > C, rs927650 (22776) C > T and rs2585428 (8620) A > G and finally *GC* (encoding VD transporter, VDBP) rs7041 A > C.

The analysis of PD-L1 was performed in 29 out of 45 patients with available tumor tissue at diagnosis using Immunohistochemistry. In particular, the PD-L1 expression was assessed manually using the rabbit monoclonal anti-human PD-L1 antibody clone 28-8 (Pharm DX DAKO, CA, USA), according to the FDA approved auto-stainer link 48 protocol. The tumor samples were defined as positive when at least 1% of tumor cells showed a strong staining according to their membrane location. All variables were tested for normality through the Shapiro–Wilk test. Normal variables were described as average and standard deviation, non-normal variables as median values and interquartile range (IQR), and categorical variables as numbers and percentages. Allele frequencies were tested for Hardy–Weinberg equilibrium. Kruskal–Wallis and Mann–Whitney tests were adopted for differences in continuous variables between genetic groups, considering statistical significance with a two-sided p-value < 0.05. Stepwise multivariate logistic regression analysis was performed including variables with a p-value below 0.2 at univariate analysis to evaluate whether factors were able to predict nivolumab levels <18.7 µg/mL at 15 days. A Bonferroni correction was performed, since an adjustment made to p-values is needed when several dependent or independent statistical tests are being performed simultaneously on a single data set [24].

Tests were performed using IBM SPSS Statistics 25.0 for Windows (Chicago, IL, USA).

5. Conclusions

In conclusion, this is the first study showing an association between VD-related biomarkers and nivolumab plasma concentrations.

In the current study, for the first time, VD deficiency seems to result in altered nivolumab clearance, as shown by different associations. It is interesting to highlight that, according to these analyses, the reduction in VD concentration was not through antibodies.

Future studies will aim to analyze the effect of VD deficiency on the immune system, for example, evaluating the immunologic profile according to VD-related biomarkers or PD-1 or PD-L1 levels and their genetic variants.

These are preliminary and limited analyses, and further studies in larger and different cohorts are needed to clarify these aspects, and to improve the knowledge in the field of the monoclonal antibody treatment used in NSCLC.

Author Contributions: J.C. conceived and directed the project, performed vitamin D and nivolumab quantification, the statistical analyses and wrote the article; C.G. enrolled patients, follwed up during treatment, recovered all clinical data and contributed to the writing of the article; C.T. performed vitamin D and nivolumab quantification and wrote the article; P.C. organized the sample collection, processed the serum at the diffent timepoints, contributed to data obtainment and the writing of the article; S.O. processed sample at the different timepoints, G.P. processed the serum at the diffent timepoints; M.C.M. contributed to the data collection; I.C. processed the serum at the diffent timepoints; E.R. contributed to the data collection; A.L. evaluated the pharmacoeconomical impact of this study; G.D.P. contributed to the acquisition of the fundings; M.G.D.B. and S.C.

coordinateed the sample collection and recorded the clinical information in database for analyses; S.B. performed the immunohistochemistry and data interpretation for PD-L1 expression; G.F. contributed to the organization of the study; F.G. supervised the project, contributed to the design of the research, to the analysis of the results and to the writing of the manuscript; A.D. supervised the project, contributed to the acquisition of the fundings, to the design of the research, to the analysis of the results and to the writing of the manuscript. All authors discussed the results, rviewed and approved the manuscript.

Funding: C.G. received honoraria from Astra Zeneca, Boehringer Ingelheim, Bristol-Myers Squibb, Merck Sharp and Dohme, Roche; E.R. received honoraria from Astra Zeneca, Boehringer Ingelheim, Bristol-Myers Squibb, Roche; F.G. received honoraria from AMGEN, Astra Zeneca, Bristol-Myers Squibb, Boehringer Ingelheim, Celgene, Merck Sharp and Dohme, Pfizer, Pierre Fabre, Roche.The PD-L1 analysis was supported by a grant from Compagnia San Paolo (SC: 2017-0529).

Acknowledgments: We thank CoQua Lab (www.coqualab.it) for its methodological support and assistance in the preparation and execution of the study and analysis.

Conflicts of Interest: The authors declare no conflict of interest.

References

1. Couzin-Frankel, J. Breakthrough of the year 2013. Cancer immunotherapy. *Science* **2013**, *342*, 1432–1433. [CrossRef] [PubMed]
2. Alsaab, H.O.; Sau, S.; Alzhrani, R.; Tatiparti, K.; Bhise, K.; Kashaw, S.K.; Iyer, A.K. PD-1 and PD-L1 checkpoint signaling inhibition for cancer immunotherapy: Mechanism, combinations, and clinical outcome. *Front. Pharm.* **2017**, *8*, 561. [CrossRef] [PubMed]
3. Khan, M.; Lin, J.; Liao, G.; Tian, Y.; Liang, Y.; Li, R.; Liu, M.; Yuan, Y. Comparative analysis of immune checkpoint inhibitors and chemotherapy in the treatment of advanced non-small cell lung cancer: A meta-analysis of randomized controlled trials. *Medicine (Baltimore)* **2018**, *97*, e11936. [CrossRef] [PubMed]
4. Tykodi, S.S.; Schadendorf, D.; Cella, D.; Reck, M.; Harrington, K.; Wagner, S.; Shaw, J.W. Patient-reported outcomes with nivolumab in advanced solid cancers. *Cancer Treat. Rev.* **2018**, *70*, 75–87. [CrossRef] [PubMed]
5. (FDA) FaDA. *FDA Grants Nivolumab Accelerated Approval for Third-Line Treatment of Metastatic Small Cell Lung Cancer*; Food and Drug Administration: Silver Spring, MD, USA, 2015.
6. Koolen, S.L.W.; Basak, E.A.; Hurkmans, D.; Schreurs, M.W.J.; Bins, S.; Oomen De Hoop, E.; Wijkhuis, A.J.M.; Den Besten, I.; Sleijfer, S.; Debets, R.; et al. Correlation between nivolumab exposure and treatment outcome in NSCLC. In Proceedings of the 2018 ASCO Annual Meeting, Chicago, IL, USA, 1–5 June 2018.
7. Michot, J.M.; Bigenwald, C.; Champiat, S.; Collins, M.; Carbonnel, F.; Postel-Vinay, S.; Berdelou, A.; Varga, A.; Bahleda, R.; Hollebecque, A.; et al. Immune-related adverse events with immune checkpoint blockade: A comprehensive review. *Eur. J. Cancer* **2016**, *54*, 139–148. [CrossRef] [PubMed]
8. Agrawal, S.; Statkevich, P.; Bajaj, G.; Feng, Y.; Saeger, S.; Desai, D.D.; Park, J.S.; Waxman, I.M.; Roy, A.; Gupta, M. Evaluation of immunogenicity of nivolumab monotherapy and its clinical relevance in patients with metastatic solid tumors. *J. Clin. Pharmacol.* **2017**, *57*, 394–400. [CrossRef] [PubMed]
9. Bersanelli, M.; Leonetti, A.; Buti, S. The link between calcitriol and anticancer immunotherapy: Vitamin D as the possible balance between inflammation and autoimmunity in the immune-checkpoint blockade. *Immunotherapy* **2017**, *9*, 1127–1131. [CrossRef]
10. Wang, T.J.; Zhang, F.; Richards, J.B.; Kestenbaum, B.; Van Meurs, J.B.; Berry, D.; Kiel, D.P.; Streeten, E.A.; Ohlsson, C.; Koller, D.L.; et al. Common genetic determinants of vitamin D insufficiency: A genome-wide association study. *Lancet* **2010**, *376*, 180–188. [CrossRef]
11. Ma, K.; Xu, W.; Wang, C.; Li, B.; Su, K.; Li, W. Vitamin D deficiency is associated with a poor prognosis in advanced non-small cell lung cancer patients treated with platinum-based first-line chemotherapy. *Cancer Biomark.* **2017**, *18*, 297–303. [CrossRef]
12. Horn, L.; Spigel, D.R.; Vokes, E.E.; Holgado, E.; Ready, N.; Steins, M.; Poddubskaya, E.; Borghaei, H.; Felip, E.; Paz-Ares, L.; et al. Nivolumab versus docetaxel in previously treated patients with advanced non-small-cell lung cancer: Two-year outcomes from two randomized, open-label, phase III trials (CheckMate 017 and CheckMate 057). *J. Clin. Oncol.* **2017**, *35*, 3924–3933. [CrossRef]
13. Aguiar, P.N., Jr.; Perry, L.A.; Penny-Dimri, J.; Babiker, H.; Tadokoro, H.; De Mello, R.A.; Lopes, G.L., Jr. The effect of PD-L1 testing on the cost-effectiveness and economic impact of immune checkpoint inhibitors for the second-line treatment of NSCLC. *Ann. Oncol.* **2017**, *28*, 2256–2263. [CrossRef] [PubMed]

14. Matter-Walstra, K.; Schwenkglenks, M.; Aebi, S.; Dedes, K.; Diebold, J.; Pietrini, M.; Klingbiel, D.; Von Moos, R.; Gautschi, O. A cost-effectiveness analysis of nivolumab versus docetaxel for advanced nonsquamous NSCLC including PD-L1 testing. *J. Thorac. Oncol.* **2016**, *11*, 1846–1855. [CrossRef] [PubMed]
15. Bochen, F.; Balensiefer, B.; Korner, S.; Bittenbring, J.T.; Neumann, F.; Koch, A.; Bumm, K.; Marx, A.; Wemmert, S.; Papaspyrou, G.; et al. Vitamin D deficiency in head and neck cancer patients-prevalence, prognostic value and impact on immune function. *Oncoimmunology* **2018**, *7*, e1476817. [CrossRef]
16. Feng, Q.; Zhang, H.; Dong, Z.; Zhou, Y.; Ma, J. Circulating 25-hydroxyvitamin D and lung cancer risk and survival: A dose-response meta-analysis of prospective cohort studies. *Medicine (Baltimore)* **2017**, *96*, e8613. [CrossRef] [PubMed]
17. Smolders, J.; Menheere, P.; Thewissen, M.; Peelen, E.; Tervaert, J.W.; Hupperts, R.; Damoiseaux, J. Regulatory T cell function correlates with serum 25-hydroxyvitamin D, but not with 1,25-dihydroxyvitamin D, parathyroid hormone and calcium levels in patients with relapsing remitting multiple sclerosis. *J. Steroid Biochem. Mol. Biol.* **2010**, *121*, 243–246. [CrossRef] [PubMed]
18. Malik, S.; Fu, L.; Juras, D.J.; Karmali, M.; Wong, B.Y.; Gozdzik, A.; Cole, D.E. Common variants of the vitamin D binding protein gene and adverse health outcomes. *Crit. Rev. Clin. Lab. Sci.* **2013**, *50*, 1–22. [CrossRef] [PubMed]
19. Carpenter, T.O.; Zhang, J.H.; Parra, E.; Ellis, B.K.; Simpson, C.; Lee, W.M.; Balko, J.; Fu, L.; Wong, B.Y.; Cole, D.E. Vitamin D binding protein is a key determinant of 25-hydroxyvitamin D levels in infants and toddlers. *J. Bone Miner. Res.* **2013**, *28*, 213–221. [CrossRef] [PubMed]
20. Anderson, L.N.; Cotterchio, M.; Cole, D.E.; Knight, J.A. Vitamin D-related genetic variants, interactions with vitamin D exposure, and breast cancer risk among Caucasian women in Ontario. *Cancer Epidemiol. Biomark. Prev.* **2011**, *20*, 1708–1717. [CrossRef]
21. Lafi, Z.M.; Irshaid, Y.M.; El-Khateeb, M.; Ajlouni, K.M.; Hyassat, D. Association of rs7041 and rs4588 polymorphisms of the vitamin D binding protein and the rs10741657 polymorphism of CYP2R1 with vitamin D status among Jordanian patients. *Genet. Test Mol. Biomar.* **2015**, *19*, 629–636. [CrossRef]
22. Daffara, V.; Verdoia, M.; Rolla, R.; Nardin, M.; Marino, P.; Bellomo, G.; Carriero, A.; De Luca, G. Impact of polymorphism rs7041 and rs4588 of Vitamin D Binding Protein on the extent of coronary artery disease. *Nutr. Metab. Cardiovasc. Dis.* **2017**, *27*, 775–783. [CrossRef]
23. Schmid, S.; Diem, S.; Li, Q.; Krapf, M.; Flatz, L.; Leschka, S.; Desbiolles, L.; Klingbiel, D.; Jochum, W.; Fruh, M. Organ-specific response to nivolumab in patients with non-small cell lung cancer (NSCLC). *Cancer Immunol. Immunother.* **2018**, *67*, 1825–1832. [CrossRef] [PubMed]
24. Du Prel, J.B.; Rohrig, B.; Hommel, G.; Blettner, M. Choosing statistical tests: Part 12 of a series on evaluation of scientific publications. *Dtsch. Arztebl. Int.* **2010**, *107*, 343–348. [PubMed]

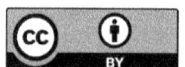

© 2019 by the authors. Licensee MDPI, Basel, Switzerland. This article is an open access article distributed under the terms and conditions of the Creative Commons Attribution (CC BY) license (http://creativecommons.org/licenses/by/4.0/).

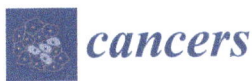

Review

Tumor Neovascularization and Developments in Therapeutics

Yuki Katayama, Junji Uchino *, Yusuke Chihara, Nobuyo Tamiya, Yoshiko Kaneko, Tadaaki Yamada and Koichi Takayama

Department of Pulmonary Medicine, Kyoto Prefectural University of Medicine, 465 Kajiicho, Kawaramachi-Hirokoji, Kamigyo-ku, Kyoto 602-8566, Japan; ktym2487@koto.kpu-m.ac.jp (Y.K.); c1981311@koto.kpu-m.ac.jp (Y.C.); koma@koto.kpu-m.ac.jp (N.T.); kaneko-y@koto.kpu-m.ac.jp (Y.K.); tayamada@koto.kpu-m.ac.jp (T.Y.); takayama@koto.kpu-m.ac.jp (K.T.)
* Correspondence: uchino@koto.kpu-m.ac.jp; Tel.: +81-75-251-5513

Received: 28 December 2018; Accepted: 4 March 2019; Published: 6 March 2019

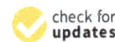

Abstract: Tumors undergo fast neovascularization to support the rapid proliferation of cancer cells. Vasculature in tumors, unlike that in wound healing, is immature and affects the tumor microenvironment, resulting in hypoxia, acidosis, glucose starvation, immune cell infiltration, and decreased activity, all of which promote cancer progression, metastasis, and drug resistance. This innate defect of tumor vasculature can however represent a useful therapeutic target. Angiogenesis inhibitors targeting tumor vascular endothelial cells important for angiogenesis have attracted attention as cancer therapy agents that utilize features of the tumor microenvironment. While angiogenesis inhibitors have the advantage of targeting neovascularization factors common to all cancer types, some limitations to their deployment have emerged. Further understanding of the mechanism of tumor angiogenesis may contribute to the development of new antiangiogenic therapeutic approaches to control tumor invasion and metastasis. This review discusses the mechanism of tumor angiogenesis as well as angiogenesis inhibition therapy with antiangiogenic agents.

Keywords: cancer therapy; neovascularization; angiogenesis; tumor microenvironment

1. Introduction

Vasculogenesis refers to the process by which vascular endothelial cells differentiate from endothelial precursor cells to form the lumen. Neovascularization refers to the process, whereby new blood vessels are formed from existing ones following endothelial cell proliferation and migration [1]. This process is essential during physiological angiogenesis, such as systemic blood supply in the fetal stage, luteinization related to postpartum menstrual cycle, and wound healing [2]. During tumor proliferation, oxygen and nutrients required for solid tumor growth are supplied from neighboring blood capillaries. However, because the diffusion distance of oxygen is 100–200 µm, for tumors to grow to ≥1–2 mm, generation of new blood vessels towards the tumor (i.e., neovascularization) is required [3,4]. Tumors located >100–200 µm from capillaries often encounter hypoxic conditions, which promote the expression of hypoxia-inducible factor-1 (HIF-1). HIF-1 induces the expression of angiogenic proteins, such as vascular endothelial growth factor (VEGF), epidermal growth factor, fibroblast growth factor (FGF), hepatocyte growth factor (HGF), and platelet-derived growth factor (PDGF), which then stimulate hypervascularization [5,6]. The sustained expression of these angiogenic factors results in abnormally structured angiogenic tumor vessels. Tortuous and dilated tumor vessels show increased vascular permeability and high interstitial pressure, further reducing blood perfusion and increasing hypoxic conditions in the tumor microenvironment [7–9]. Administration of angiogenesis inhibitors leads to tumor vascular normalization, a reduction in vascular permeability and interstitial fluid pressure, and an improvement in tumor perfusion. A normalized tumor vascular system with reduced hypoxic conditions not only augments the effects of radiotherapy and chemotherapy but also enhances antitumor immunity [10–12]. The findings can contribute to a new approach (i.e., the combination of angiogenesis inhibitors and immunotherapy) to further improve the overall survival of cancer patients. This review discusses the molecular mechanisms of tumor angiogenesis and outlines options for cancer therapy with antiangiogenic agents including combined immunotherapy.

2. Molecules Involved in Neovascularization

Neovascularization is regulated by a balance between angiogenesis-inducing factors and angiogenesis-inhibiting factors such as those outlined in Table 1. Here, we describe the molecules that induce angiogenesis and their mechanisms. Among angiogenesis-inducing factors, VEGF plays an important role in the initiation of angiogenesis. The VEGF family consists of five members, namely VEGFA, VEGFB, VEGFC, VEGFD, and placental growth factor (P1GF). VEGF signals are transmitted through three VEGF receptor tyrosine kinases: VEGFR1, VEGFR2, and VEGFR3 [8,13]. The VEGF family of proteins is the most critical factor for the induction of neovascularization. VEGF induces proliferation of endothelial cells, promotes cell migration, and decreases the rate of apoptosis. It also increases vascular permeability and promotes migration and circulation of other cells [13,14]. VEGFA and its receptor, VEGFR2, have major angiogenic effects [15]. Upon binding to the VEGF receptor on the vascular endothelial cell membrane, VEGF induces dimerization and autophosphorylation of the receptor and initiates a signaling cascade that activates a variety of downstream pathways. Phosphorylation of phospholipase C (PLC) γ activates the RAS/mitogen-activated protein kinase (MAPK) cascade via protein kinase C (PKC) activation and regulates gene expression and cell proliferation [16–18]. In addition, activation of the phosphoinositide-3-kinase (PI3K)/protein kinase B (AKT) pathway produces NO via AKT, suppresses apoptosis, and activates endothelial cell NO synthase, thereby enhancing vascular permeability [19–22]. VEGFR1 has a weak kinase activity and limits VEGFR2-induced angiogenic effects by regulating the amount of VEGFA that can be bound by VEGFR2 [23]. The following has been reported: (i) VEGFR3 and its ligand, VEGFC, are responsible for lymphangiogenesis; (ii) VEGFC and VEGFD contribute to tumor angiogenesis by binding to VEGFR2 and VEGFR3; (iii) VEGFR3 is expressed in the tip cells of tumor vessels [15,24].

Table 1. Endogenous regulators of angiogenesis.

Activators	Functions	Inhibitors	Functions
Vascular endothelial growth factor family	Induction of angiogenesis, enhancement of vascular permeability	Angiopoietin-2	Antagonist of Ang1
Epidermal growth factor	Promotes growth of vascular endothelial cells	Thrombospondin-1,2	Inhibits endothelial migration, growth, adhesion and survival
Fibroblast growth factor	Induction of angiogenesis	collagen	Substrate for MMPs
Platelet-derived growth factor	Involved in migration of vascular endothelial cells	Endostatin	Inhibits endothelial survival and migration
Angiopoietin-1	Stabilization of vascular endothelium	Angiostatin	Suppresses tumor angiogenesis
Transforming growth factor	Production of extracellular matrix	TIMPs	Suppresses pathological angiogenesis
Ephrin	Control of blood vessel and lymph duct formation	Platelet Factor-4	Inhibits binding of bFGF and VEGF
Matrix metalloproteinase	Degradation of extracellular matrix, activation of angiogenesis inducing factor	Vasostatin	Inhibits endothelial growth

Angiopoietins play a critical role in the maturation of blood vessels. Human angiopoietins consist of three ligands, Ang-1, Ang-2, and Ang-4. Ang-1 and Ang-2 are of critical importance in angiogenesis and are outlined hereafter. The Tie family of receptors includes receptor tyrosine kinases specifically expressed in the vascular endothelium. They include Tie1 and Tie2. Tie2 is activated by Ang-1, which is secreted by platelets and peri-endothelial cells; whereas Tie1 is an orphan receptor homolog of Tie2, whose expression enhances Tie2 activation [25]. The Ang-1/Tie-2 signaling pathway is specific for endothelial cells. Ang-1 binds to the Tie-2 tyrosine kinase receptor of endothelial cells, whose downstream phosphorylation activity stimulates cell survival by activating the PI3K-AKT pathway [26–28]. Furthermore, it contributes to the maturation of blood vessels by inhibiting the proinflammatory pathway initiated by nuclear factor-kappa B (NF-κβ) [26–28]. In contrast, in the absence of cell-cell adhesion, extracellular matrix-anchored Tie2 regulates angiogenesis via extracellular signal-regulated kinase (ERK) 1/2 signaling [29]. Ang-2 antagonizes Ang-1 activity and, in the presence of low levels of VEGF, leads to detachment of pericytes and regression of blood vessels. However, in the presence of high levels of VEGF, Ang-2 elicits an inflammatory response and destabilizes existing vessels. This, in turn, promotes angiogenesis and lymphangiogenesis by weakening the interaction between endothelial cells and pericytes and increasing endothelial cell migration [1,30,31].

3. Characteristics of Angiogenic Tumor Vessels

Angiogenesis-promoting factors such as VEGF induced by the tumor microenvironment (e.g., hypoxia), stimulate sustained and abnormal neovascularization [32,33]. The vessels formed during neovascularization are unlike those formed during wound healing and exhibit unusual morphological characteristics. In normal vessels, the distribution of arteries, capillaries, and veins is stable, and the vessels have an ordered hierarchical structure. In comparison, angiogenic tumor vessels are dilated and tortuous. Furthermore, vascular density and blood vessel diameter are not uniform [34,35]. A simple squamous epithelium, known as vascular endothelial cells, covers the lumen of capillaries, which is lined with pericytes and covered by the basement membrane. Angiogenesis promoting factors induce weakening and migration of vascular endothelial cell junctions and change the vascular wall structure [36,37]. Pericytes and vascular endothelial cell junctions between pericytes and vascular smooth muscle cells are also weakened, and the number of pericytes is reduced [38,39]. The basement membranes are multilayered and collagen IV thickness is uneven. Weakened cell junctions between endothelial cells and pericytes result in their infiltration into the tumor stroma [38,39]. The morphological abnormalities observed in tumor blood vessels raise the question of whether there are phenotypic differences at the molecular and functional levels between tumor endothelial cells (TECs) that line tumor blood vessels and normal endothelial cells. TECs express higher levels of proangiogenic genes such as VEGFR, VEGF, and EGFR. The Hu antigen, a neuronal protein identified in the serum of patients with small cell lung cancer and paraneoplastic encephalomyelitis/sensory neuronopathy, promotes TECs survival by stabilizing VEGF mRNA. TECs also up-regulates integrin αVβ3 and cause cytogenetic abnormalities [40]. Moreover, in comparison with normal endothelial cells, TECs have a high proliferative capacity, migratory ability, and angiogenic potential [41]. Additionally, cells showing stem cell/precursor cell-like properties have been reported in the TECs population, together with those originating from bone marrow-derived vascular endothelial progenitor cells and tissues derived from tissue stem cells [42]. Furthermore, a population expressing stem cell markers such as aldehyde dehydrogenase and having high angiogenic potential has also been reported [43]. ATP-binding cassette sub-family B member 1 (ABCB1) is the most well-known drug efflux transporter and TECs strongly expressing ABCB1 are resistant to drugs [44]. Importantly, cancer microenvironment factors such as hypoxia, are also thought to be involved in tumor vascular endothelial cell abnormalities, together with humoral factors derived from cancer cells and exosomes [45,46]. Tumor vascular endothelial markers are expressed in cancer cells when cultured under hypoxia or in a low-serum medium. Furthermore, Kubota et al. reported that an ataxia telangiectasia mutated kinase was strongly activated in immature vessels in response to the accumulation of reactive oxygen species, where it provided a defensive function [47]. More recently, Maishi et al. demonstrated that biglycan secreted by TECs induced intravascular invasion and metastasis of cancer cells and reported a new mechanism of cancer metastasis induction from tumor vessels [48]. As can be seen, various factors typical of the cancer microenvironment exert complex and diverse properties in tumor vascular endothelial cells.

4. Regulatory Mechanisms of Neovascularization

4.1. HIF-1α

Hypoxic conditions in the tumor microenvironment up-regulate angiogenesis inducing factors such as VEGF, PDGF, P1GF, and HGF. However, reactions activated by such a hypoxic environment are thought to be elicited primarily by HIF-1α [49,50]. HIF is a transcription factor heterodimer consisting of subunits HIF-1α and HIF-1β [51,52]. When oxygen tension is normal, HIF-1α is quickly degraded [53]. Under normal oxygen concentration, HIF-1α is modified by prolyl 4 hydroxylase (PHD), which acts as a direct oxygen sensor by catalyzing the binding of molecular oxygen to a specific proline on HIF-1α [52]. The Von Hippel-Lindau cancer suppression protein binds to hydroxylated HIF-1α to activate the protein complex and targets HIF-1α for proteasome-dependent degradation following its ubiquitination [54]. Under normal oxygen conditions, asparagine residues near the C-terminus are hydroxylated by factor inhibiting HIF-1 (FIH-1), which also requires oxygen for its activity. FIH-1 reduces HIF-1α transcriptional activity by preventing the binding of p300 and cAMP response element binding protein (CREB) to HIF-α [55,56]. As PHD is inactive and HIF-1α is not hydroxylated in a low-oxygen environment, the Von Hippel-Lindau factor cannot bind and direct HIF-1α for proteasome-mediated proteolysis. Instead, HIF-1α can bind to p300 and CREB. The HIF-1α-conjugated protein is also believed to be transferred to the nucleus, heterodimerized by HIF-1β, and immediately involved in initiating transcription of target genes. With a binding site corresponding to 5′-RCGTG-3′, the HIF heterodimer transcription factor activates target genes via a hypoxia response sequence (HRE) [57]. HIF-1α binds to the HRE of VEGFA, PDGF, and transforming growth factor-alpha, inducing their expression (Figure 1) [58].

In addition to angiogenesis, HIF-1α activates glucose metabolism, thereby leading to acidosis in the tumor microenvironment. HIF-1α enhances the expression of glucose transporter 1, 3 and increases the uptake of glucose into cells [59]. Additionally, it cleaves glycolytic enzymes (phosphofructokinase L, hexokinase, aldolase A, and lactate dehydrogenase A) by activating ATP production and promoting glycolysis [60,61]. HIF-1α activates pyruvate dehydrogenase kinase 1, which then inactivates pyruvate dehydrogenase, resulting in suppression of the TCA cycle [62]. Thus, overexpression of HIF-1α under hypoxic conditions accelerates lactic acid production by promoting glycolysis and suppressing the TCA cycle, leading to an acidic tumor microenvironment. The latter contributes to tumor survival by conferring apoptosis resistance [63], increasing invasion and metastatic potential [64], and providing immune tolerance through T cell suppression [65].

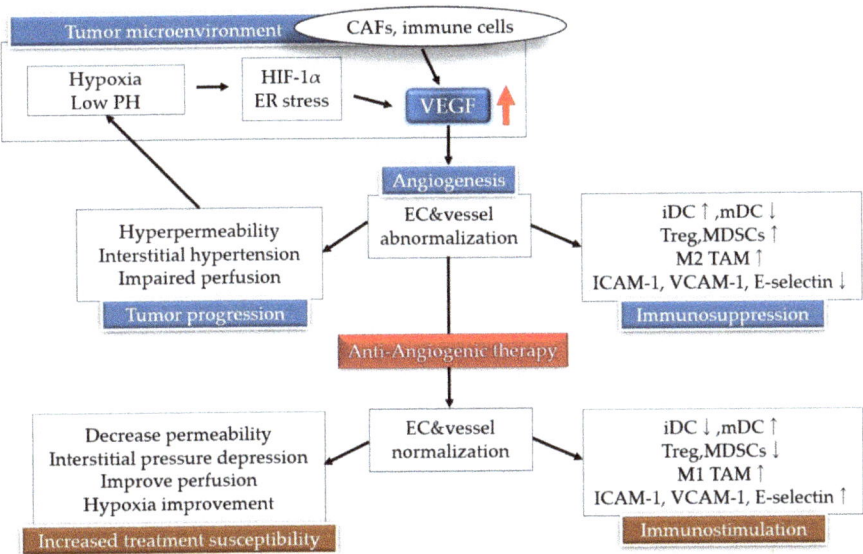

Figure 1. Hypoxia inducible factor (HIF) and vascular endothelial growth factor (VEGF) link the angiogenesis signaling pathways. Low oxygen tension (hypoxia) results in constitutive activation of the HIF pathway and VEGF. The tumor hypoxic environment leads to an immunosuppressive tumor microenvironment by inducing regulatory T cells (Tregs), myeloid-derived suppressor cells (MDSCs), and M2 tumor-associated macrophages (TAMs). Antiangiogenic therapy results in blood vessel regression by suppression of neovascularization, leading to tumor starvation and tumors falling into dormant states. CAFs, cancer-associated fibroblasts; iDCs, immature dendritic cells; mDCs, mature dendritic cells; ICAM-1, intercellular adhesion molecule 1; VCAM-1, vascular cell adhesion molecule 1.

4.2. Endoplasmic Reticulum Stress Signals

The endoplasmic reticulum is a protein folding and maturation site within the cell, where membrane proteins are glycosylated and secreted. Failure to mature results in the accumulation of proteins with an abnormal higher-order structure. Accumulation of such abnormal proteins causes endoplasmic reticulum stress, and the cellular responses elicited to deal with it are collectively referred to as the endoplasmic reticulum stress response. Tumor microenvironment characteristics such as hypoxia, acidosis, and glucose deprivation contribute to the activation of the endoplasmic reticulum stress pathway and promote cancer cell survival. Up-regulation of the endoplasmic reticulum molecular chaperone, BiP/GRP78 has been observed in multiple cancer cells, indicating that it is involved in their proliferation and metastasis [66]. VEGF expression is induced in the protein kinase R like endoplasmic reticulum kinase (PERK)-activating transcription factor 4 (ATF4) pathway in the endoplasmic reticulum stress environment [67]. The inositol-requiring kinase enzyme 1 alpha (IRE1α) signal also promotes cell growth in certain cancer cell types due to up-regulation of cyclin A1 via X-box binding protein 1 (XBP-1) downstream of IRE1α [68]. Expression of XBP-1 is elevated in breast cancer cells and hepatocellular carcinoma. Therefore, XBP-1 expression is believed to contribute to the survival of cancer cells by inducing BiP/GRP78 expression [69]. As in the case of PERK and IRE1α signals, ATF6 is thought to be involved in neovascularization by controlling the expression of VEGF [70]. In addition to cancer cells, tumor tissues and their microenvironments include fibroblasts, mesenchymal stem cells, and immune cells including macrophages and T cells. Cells that build these tumor microenvironments can induce angiogenesis by producing multiple growth factors, cytokines, and chemokines. Fibroblasts in tumor tissue are the major constituents of tumor stromal tissue and are said to play a vital role in cancer development. Known as cancer-associated fibroblasts (CAFs) they secrete stromal cell-derived factor 1 (SDF1). CAF-derived SDF1 not only directly stimulates cancer cell proliferation via C-X-C chemokine receptor type 4 on tumor cells, but also recruits endothelial progenitor cells towards the tumor and induces angiogenesis [71]. In colorectal cancer, angiogenesis is promoted by CAF-induced secretion of interleukin 6 and a concomitant increase in VEGF production [72]. Macrophages involved in carcinogenesis and malignancy are called tumor-associated macrophages (TAMs). Most TAMs are composed of M2 macrophages, which affect tumor development through increased immunosuppression and angiogenesis. TAMs stimulate angiogenesis directly by facilitating the production of angiogenesis promoting factors such as VEGF, and indirectly by localizing matrix metallopeptidase 9 to the tumor microenvironment. There, metallopeptidase 9 induces angiogenesis by cleaving and releasing VEGF from the matrix [73,74]. In addition, vascular endothelial cells produce Ang-2c and TAMs express its receptor, Tie2, further stimulating angiogenesis in tumor tissues [75].

5. Antiangiogenic Therapy

Clinical treatment approaches targeting tumor angiogenesis include the anti-VEGF monoclonal antibody bevacizumab, anti-VEGFR2 monoclonal antibody ramucirumab, VEGFR ligand traps (e.g., aflibercept, VEGFR, PDGFR, c-KIT), and multi-target tyrosine kinase inhibitors (e.g., sunitinib and sorafenib) [76,77] (Table 2, Figure 2). Bevacizumab, a humanized monoclonal immunoglobulin G1 antibody, is the most widely studied antiangiogenic agent that prevents VEGFA from binding to receptors, thus hindering neovascularization and the activation of signal transduction cascades [78]. After bevacizumab combined with chemotherapy was first approved by the U.S. Food and Drug Administration (FDA) in 2004, the drug was also approved by the FDA for use in non-small cell lung cancer, metastatic colorectal cancer, renal cell carcinoma (RCC), ovarian cancer, glioblastoma multiforme, cervical cancer, fallopian tube cancer, and primary peritoneal cancer [79].

Table 2. Angiogenesis inhibitors approved by FDA.

Drug	Target Molecule	Approved Disease
Bevacizumab	Anti-VEGF monoclonal antibody	mCRC, NSCLC, mRCC, ovarian cancer, malignant glioma, advanced cervical cancer, fallopian tube cancer, primary peritoneal cancer
Ramucirumab	Anti-VEGFR2 monoclonal antibody	Advanced gastric or gastroesophageal junction adenocarcinoma, NSCLC, advanced colorectal cancer
Ziv-aflibercept	Soluble decoy of VEGFR	Metastatic colorectal cancer
Sunitinib	TKI: VEGFR, PDGFR, FLT3, KIT	RCC, Gastrointestinal stromal tumor, pancreatic neuroendocrine tumor
Sorafenib	TKI: VEGFR, PDGFR, FLT3, KIT, Raf	RCC, unresectable hepatocellular carcinoma, metastatic or recurrent thyroid carcinoma
Axitinib	TKI: VEGFR, PDGFR, KIT	Advanced RCC
Pazopanib	Multiple targeted receptor TKI	RCC, Advanced soft tissue sarcoma
Vandetanib	TKI: VEGFR, EGFR, RET	Unresectable or metastatic medullary thyroid cancer

Ramucirumab combined with chemotherapy has been shown to extend overall survival of gastric cancer, non-small cell lung cancer, and rectal cancer patients. In 2012, aflibercept (i.e., a peptide-antibody fusion targeting the VEGF ligand) combined with fluorouracil, irinotecan, and folinic acid was also approved by the FDA for use in colorectal cancer [80]. Sunitinib and sorafenib, which are multi-target tyrosine kinase inhibitors, have been approved as monotherapy agents based on improvement in overall survival and progression-free survival in phase III studies in metastatic-differentiated thyroid cancer, unresectable hepatocellular carcinoma, and advanced RCC [81–83].

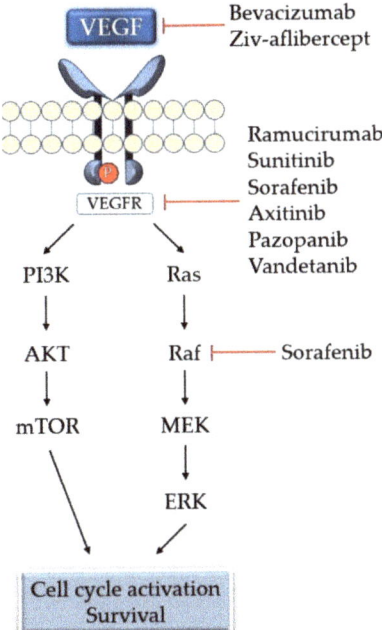

Figure 2. Vascular endothelial growth factor (VEGF) binds to the VEGF receptor, a receptor tyrosine kinase, leading to receptor dimerization and subsequent auto phosphorylation of the receptor complex. The phosphorylated receptor then interacts with a variety of cytoplasmic signaling molecules, leading to signal transduction and eventually angiogenesis. Examples of clinical drugs (Table 2) that inhibit the pathway are shown. PI3K, phosphoinositide-3-kinase; AKT, protein kinase B; mTOR, mechanistic target of rapamycin; MEK, MAPK/ERK kinase; ERK, extracellular signal-regulated kinase.

6. Resistance Mechanism of Angiogenesis Inhibitors

Resistance to angiogenesis inhibitors develops through a variety of mechanisms such as activation of an alternate angiogenic pathway that promotes tumor angiogenesis. When VEGF and VEGFR are inhibited, other angiogenic factors such as P1GF, SDF1, Ang-1, FGF, HGF, and cytokines, are induced [84]. In preclinical models, FGF1, FGF2, Ang-1, Ephrin-A1, and Ephrin-A2 have been induced in pancreatic tumors treated with anti-VEGFR2 antibody [85]. HGF, bFGF, and P1GF levels were increased in patients with metastatic colorectal cancer before disease progression when treated with a combination of fluorouracil, irinotecan, and bevacizumab [86]. Cancers such as colorectal cancer, RCC, and neuroendocrine tumors are often highly dependent on the induction of angiogenesis by VEGF. On the opposite end, cancers that are less susceptible to anti-VEGF antibodies, such as breast cancer, pancreatic cancer, malignant melanoma or prostate cancer, use different angiogenesis mechanisms and angiogenic factors [87]. Long-term administration of angiogenesis inhibitors induces hypoxia in the tumor microenvironment by over-pruning blood vessels and up-regulates HIF-1α [88]. Angiogenesis promoting factors, such as P1GF, VEGF, Ang-1, and FGF, which are induced by HIF-1α, recruit bone marrow-derived dendritic cells (BMDCs) that mediate the growth of new blood vessels to support tumors. The presence of BMDCs in the tumor environment induces resistance to angiogenesis inhibition [89,90]. In addition to BMDCs, the hypoxic environment within the tumor promotes recruitment of regulatory T cells (Tregs), bone marrow-derived repression cells (MDSCs), and M2 TAMs.

Immune cell populations in tumors promote angiogenesis, tumor growth, epithelial-mesenchymal transition, metastasis, and immunosuppression of the tumor microenvironment [91,92]. Besides acquiring resistance to angiogenesis inhibition by inducing other cells, tumor cells have also been reported to escape the effect of angiogenesis inhibitors by adopting different neovascularization modalities, including vascular co-option and vasculogenic mimicry [93]. Vessel co-option refers to the process whereby cancer cells incorporate pre-existing vessels from surrounding tissue instead of inducing new vessel growth [94]. The main factors regulating vessel co-option are VEGF and angiopoietins. Moreover, several studies have reported an increase in vessel co-option after inhibition of angiogenesis [95]. Anti-VEGF antibody treatment in glioblastoma promotes an increase in vessel co-option, and similar phenomena have been reported in other solid tumors [96]. Vasculogenic mimicry refers to a situation, whereby tumor cells function like endothelial cells and form a blood vessel-like structure [97]. This phenomenon has been reported in malignant melanoma, sarcoma, glioma, breast cancer, and many other cancer types [98–100]. Preclinical studies have reported increased vasculogenic mimicry by angiogenesis inhibition therapy with bevacizumab, and the effectiveness of combining angiogenesis inhibitors with chemotherapy has been suggested.

7. Neovascularization and Immunity

Tumor angiogenesis and tumor immunity share a complex relationship. When exposed to hypoperfusion/vascular hyperpermeability by immature tumor neovasculature, the tumor microenvironments becomes hypoxic and VEGF is up-regulated. This induces a decrease in T cell activation by dendritic cells (DCs), a reduction in the number of intratumorally infiltrating lymphocytes, and an increase in immunosuppressive cells, all of which affect immune function [101]. Steady-state immature dendritic cells (iDCs) in vivo are superior in antigen uptake ability, but have weak T cell stimulating ability and induce immune tolerance through Treg activity. iDCs that phagocytose and process the antigen, migrate to regional lymph nodes where they convert to mature dendritic cells (mDCs) that present the antigen to T cells and activate them [102]. Although DC maturation is activated by the NF-κB pathway, the increase in VEGF due to the hypoxic environment of the tumor reduces the number of mDCs by inhibiting DC maturation through inhibition of the NF-κB pathway and suppresses immunity [103–105]. Furthermore, VEGF binds to VEGFR2, inhibits the T cell activation function of mDCs, up-regulates the expression of programmed cell death ligand 1 (PD-L1) (B7-H1/CD274), and suppresses the function of DCs [106]. The migration and adhesion of vascular adhesion molecules to vascular endothelial cells plays an important role in the activation of immunity by causing the accumulation of immune cells, such as macrophages, NK cells, granulocytes, B cells, and T cells [107]. VEGF promotes abnormal neovascularization and affects immune cell migration, which reduces the expression of cell adhesion molecules, such as intercellular adhesion molecule 1, vascular cell adhesion molecule 1, and E-selectin. The down-regulation of cell adhesion molecules inhibits tumor invasion by immune cells and reduces the immune response [108–110]. A tumor immune response is induced by tilting the quantitative and functional balance of tumor-attacking effector T cells and immunosuppressive cells to the former dominant state. The tumor hypoxic environment enhances the expression of SDF1-α and C-C motif chemokine 28, thereby inducing immunosuppressive cells such as Tregs, MDSCs, and M2 TAMs, and suppresses tumor immunity [91,92,111]. When VEGF binds to VEGFR on MDSCs, signal transducer and activator of transcription 3 signaling is activated and induces MDSC proliferation [112], VEGF also promotes an increase in Tregs in the tumor microenvironment [113,114]. Increasing the recruitment of T cells and promoting tumor invasion by angiogenesis inhibitors have shown the effect of tilting the tumor microenvironment towards immunity promotion. Bevacizumab and sorafenib induce DC maturation and improve T cell activation [115]. Inhibition of VEGF increases E-selectin expression on the tumor vascular endothelium and promotes an increase in T cell tumor invasion [116]. In the laboratory, administration of bevacizumab led to a decrease in MDSCs in the RCC mouse model, as well as a decrease in Tregs in vitro and in vivo [114,117]. A similar decrease in Tregs has been observed in RCC patients treated with sunitinib, where it correlated with overall survival [118].

8. Angiogenesis Inhibitors and Immunotherapy

Although the immune system is very effective in inducing an immune response against foreign antigens, malignant tumors can avoid immune surveillance via multiple mechanisms of immune tolerance. Overexpression of immune checkpoint molecules inducing immune tolerance has been demonstrated in some solid tumors, and correlates with poor prognosis [119]. Programmed-cell death-1 (PD-1 is a checkpoint molecule expressed on the outer surface of NK cells, B cells, DCs, monocytes, and CD4 + and CD8 + T cells [120]. When PD-1 is expressed by T cell stimulation and binds to PD-L1 and PD-L2 on antigen-presenting cells and some cancer cells, the Ras/MAPK/ERK kinase/ERK pathway and PI3K/AKT pathway are inhibited and inactivate T cells [120]. PD-L1 is expressed in cancers of tissues such as the lung, colon, ovaries, as well as in malignant melanoma and its expression is enhanced by the inflammatory cytokine interferon gamma [121]. Additionally, activation of HIF-1 in a hypoxic environment within a tumor leads to elevated expression of PD-L1 in cancer tissue [122]. In other words, cancer cells escape immune surveillance by inactivating locally accumulated T cells through the PD-1/PD-L1 pathway. Immunological checkpoint inhibitors such as nivolumab and pembrolizumab, which are PD-1 inhibitors, and atezolizumab, which is a PD-L1 inhibitor, promote the antitumor activity of T cells by blocking these pathways, and are clinically effective in several cancer types [122]. As mentioned in the previous section, angiogenesis inhibitors and immunological checkpoint inhibitors are expected to have a combined immunostimulatory effect. Increased infiltration of CD4 + and CD8 + T cells, in addition to macrophages, into the tumor space and increased expression of PD-L1 in the tumor by co-administration of bevacizumab and sunitinib have been shown in the RCC mouse model [123]. Additionally, a decrease in MDSCs in tumor tissue and an increase in PD-1 expression in tumor infiltrating lymphocytes have been observed in RCC patients treated with sunitinib [124]. Combination therapy with atezolizumab and bevacizumab resulted in an increase in CD8 + T cells and major histocompatibility complex 1 in the tumor, as well as up-regulation of chemokines and down-regulation of genes associated with neovascularization in patients with metastatic RCC [125]. Several phase III studies on the combined treatment of angiogenesis inhibitors and immunity checkpoint inhibitors are in progress, and the results of these preclinical and clinical trials are listed in Table 3. Two phase III trials have shown that a combination therapy of atezolizumab and bevacizumab is effective and tolerable. Comparisons of combination chemotherapies (carboplatin and paclitaxel) and atezolizumab + bevacizumab in untreated non-small cell lung cancer have shown better survival (response rate, progression-free survival, and overall survival) in the atezolizumab + bevacizumab group than in the chemotherapy + bevacizumab group. Subgroup analysis of the low PD-L1 expression group, the group with low effector T cell gene expression, and the liver metastases group also shows similar results [126]. In a study of patients with metastatic RCC characterized by ≥1% PD-L1 expression, the combination therapy (bevacizumab and atezolizumab) group had a longer progression-free survival than the sunitinib monotherapy group [127].

Table 3. Selected ongoing phase III clinical trials involving anti-angiogenic inhibitors combined with cancer immunotherapy.

Tumor Type	Combination Drugs	Study Status	NCT ID
Stage IV NSCLC	Atezolizumab+Carboplatin+paclitaxel+Bevacizumab	Active, not recruiting	NCT02366143
Advanced RCC	Bevacizumab+Atezolizumab	Active, not recruiting	NCT02420821
Advanced RCC	Avelumab+Axitinib	Active, not recruiting	NCT02684006
Advanced RCC	Lenvatinib/Everolimus or Lenvatinib/Pembrolizumab	Recruiting	NCT02811861
Recurrent OC, FTC, or PPC	Pegylated Liposomal Doxorubicin+Atezolizumab+Bevacizumab	Recruiting	NCT02839707
RCC	Pembrolizumab+Axitinib	Active, not recruiting	NCT02853331
Late relapse OC	Atezolizumab+Chemotherapy+Bevacizumab	Recruiting	NCT02891824
OC,FTC,or PPC	Atezolizumab+Carboplatin+paclitaxel+Bevacizumab	Recruiting	NCT03038100
Early relapse OC	Atezolizumab+Bevacizumab+Chemotherapy	Recruiting	NCT03353831
Locally Advanced or Metasatatic HCC	Atezolizumab+Bevacizumab	Recruiting	NCT03434379

9. Conclusions

In this review, we have discussed the mechanism of tumor angiogenesis as well as antiangiogenic therapy from the perspective of the tumor microenvironment. Although angiogenesis inhibitors have been used in combination with chemotherapy for more than 10 years, resulting overall survival has increased by only a few months and resistance to treatment has often developed rapidly. Angiogenesis inhibitors have failed to improve overall survival in some cancers such as breast cancer. These findings highlight the complexity of the pathways involved in tumor neovascularization and raise questions about the effective use of antiangiogenic therapy in cancer treatment. Therefore, we need to better understand the role of neovascularization in different cancers and how they avoid the effects of antiangiogenic therapy. A combination therapy with angiogenesis inhibitors and immunotherapy effectively enhances the benefits of angiogenesis inhibitors and represents the most promising path ahead.

Author Contributions: Y.K. (Yuki Katayama): Writing—Original draft preparation, J.U.: Writing—review & editing; Y.C., N.T., Y.K. (Yoshiko Kaneko) and T.Y.: Editing review; K.T.: Supervision.

Acknowledgments: We would like to thank Editage (www.editage.jp) for English language editing.

Conflicts of Interest: The authors declare no conflict of interest.

References

1. Folkman, J. Angiogenesis: An organizing principle for drug discovery? *Nat. Rev. Drug Discov.* **2007**, *6*, 273–286. [CrossRef] [PubMed]
2. Tepper, O.M.; Capla, J.M.; Galiano, R.D.; Ceradini, D.J.; Callaghan, M.J.; Kleinman, M.E.; Gurtner, G.C. Adult vasculogenesis occurs through in situ recruitment, proliferation, and tubulization of circulating bone marrow-derived cells. *Blood* **2005**, *105*, 1068–1077. [CrossRef] [PubMed]
3. Carmeliet, P.; Jain, R.K. Angiogenesis in cancer and other diseases. *Nature* **2000**, *407*, 249–257. [CrossRef] [PubMed]
4. Folkman, J.; Kalluri, R. Cancer with disease. *Nature* **2004**, *427*, 787. [CrossRef] [PubMed]
5. Itatani, Y.; Kawada, K.; Yamamoto, T.; Sakai, Y. Molecular Sciences Resistance to Anti-Angiogenic Therapy in Cancer-Alterations to Anti-VEGF Pathway. *Int. J. Mol. Sci.* **2018**, *19*, 1232. [CrossRef] [PubMed]
6. Bergers, G.; Benjamin, L.E.; Francisco, S. Tumorigenesis and the angiogenic switch. *Nat. Rev. Cancer* **2003**, *6*, 401–410. [CrossRef] [PubMed]
7. Maeda, H.; Wu, J. Tumor vascular permeability and the EPR effect in macromolecular therapeutics: A review. *J. Control. Release* **2000**, *65*, 271–284. [CrossRef]
8. Snuderl, M.; Batista, A.; Kirkpatrick, N.D.; De Almodovar, C.R.; Riedemann, L.; Walsh, E.C.; Anolik, R.; Huang, Y.; Martin, J.D.; Kamoun, W.; et al. Targeting placental growth factor/neuropilin 1 pathway inhibits growth and spread of medulloblastoma. *Cell* **2013**, *152*, 1065–1076. [CrossRef] [PubMed]
9. Dvorak, H.F. Vascular permeability factor/vascular endothelial growth factor: A critical cytokine in tumor angiogenesis and a potential target for diagnosis and therapy. *J. Clin. Oncol.* **2002**, *20*, 4368–4380. [CrossRef] [PubMed]
10. Klein, D. The Tumor Vascular Endothelium as Decision Maker in Cancer Therapy. *Front. Oncol.* **2018**, *8*, 367. [CrossRef] [PubMed]
11. Huang, Y.; Goel, S.; Duda, D.G.; Fukumura, D.; Jain, R.K. Vascular normalization as an emerging strategy to enhance cancer immunotherapy. *Cancer Res.* **2013**, *73*, 2943–2948. [CrossRef] [PubMed]
12. Jain, R.K. Normalizing Tumor Microenvironment to Treat Cancer: Bench to Bedside to Biomarkers. *J. Clin. Oncol.* **2013**, *31*, 2205–2218. [CrossRef] [PubMed]
13. Karaman, S.; Leppänen, V.-M.; Alitalo, K. Vascular endothelial growth factor signaling in development and disease. *Development* **2018**, *145*, dev151019. [CrossRef] [PubMed]
14. Neufeld, G.; Cohen, T.; Gengrinovitch, S.; Poltorak, Z. Vascular endothelial growth factor (VEGF) and its receptors. *FASEB J.* **1999**, *13*, 9–22. [CrossRef] [PubMed]

15. Tammela, T.; Zarkada, G.; Wallgard, E.; Murtomäki, A.; Suchting, S.; Wirzenius, M.; Waltari, M.; Hellström, M.; Schomber, T.; Peltonen, R.; et al. Blocking VEGFR-3 suppresses angiogenic sprouting and vascular network formation. *Nature* **2008**, *454*, 656–660. [CrossRef] [PubMed]
16. Meadows, K.N.; Bryant, P.; Pumiglia, K. Vascular Endothelial Growth Factor Induction of the Angiogenic Phenotype Requires Ras Activation. *J. Biol. Chem.* **2001**, *276*, 49289–49298. [CrossRef] [PubMed]
17. Shu, X.; Wu, W.; Mosteller, R.D.; Broek, D. Sphingosine kinase mediates vascular endothelial growth factor-induced activation of ras and mitogen-activated protein kinases. *Mol. Cell. Biol.* **2002**, *22*, 7758–7768. [CrossRef] [PubMed]
18. Takahashi, T.; Yamaguchi, S.; Chida, K.; Shibuya, M. A single autophosphorylation site on KDR/Flk-1 is essential for VEGF-A-dependent activation of PLC-gamma and DNA synthesis in vascular endothelial cells. *EMBO J.* **2001**, *20*, 2768–2778. [CrossRef] [PubMed]
19. Gerber, H.P.; McMurtrey, A.; Kowalski, J.; Yan, M.; Keyt, B.A.; Dixit, V.; Ferrara, N. Vascular endothelial growth factor regulates endothelial cell survival through the phosphatidylinositol 3'-kinase/Akt signal transduction pathway. Requirement for Flk-1/KDR activation. *J. Biol. Chem.* **1998**, *273*, 30336–30343. [CrossRef] [PubMed]
20. Fujio, Y.; Walsh, K. Akt mediates cytoprotection of endothelial cells by vascular endothelial growth factor in an anchorage-dependent manner. *J. Biol. Chem.* **1999**, *274*, 16349–16354. [CrossRef] [PubMed]
21. Michell, B.J.; Griffiths, J.E.; Mitchelhill, K.I.; Rodriguez-Crespo, I.; Tiganis, T.; Bozinovski, S.; de Montellano, P.R.; Kemp, B.E.; Pearson, R.B. The Akt kinase signals directly to endothelial nitric oxide synthase. *Curr. Biol.* **1999**, *9*, 845–848. [CrossRef]
22. Murohara, T.; Horowitz, J.R.; Silver, M.; Tsurumi, Y.; Chen, D.; Sullivan, A.; Isner, J.M. Vascular endothelial growth factor/vascular permeability factor enhances vascular permeability via nitric oxide and prostacyclin. *Circulation* **1998**, *97*, 99–107. [CrossRef] [PubMed]
23. Shibuya, M. Vascular endothelial growth factor receptor-1 (VEGFR-1/Flt-1): A dual regulator for angiogenesis. *Angiogenesis* **2006**, *9*, 225–230. [CrossRef] [PubMed]
24. Kubo, H.; Fujiwara, T. Involvement of vascular endothelial growth factor receptor-3 in maintenance of integrity of endothelial cell lining during tumor angiogenesis. *Blood* **2000**, *96*, 546–553. [PubMed]
25. Parikh, S.M. The Angiopoietin-Tie2 Signaling Axis in Systemic Inflammation. *J. Am. Soc. Nephrol.* **2017**, *28*, 1973–1982. [CrossRef] [PubMed]
26. Fujikawa, K.; de Aos Scherpenseel, I.; Jain, S.K.; Presman, E.; Varticovski, L.; Varticovski, L. Role of PI 3-Kinase in Angiopoietin-1-Mediated Migration and Attachment-Dependent Survival of Endothelial Cells. *Exp. Cell Res.* **1999**, *253*, 663–672. [CrossRef] [PubMed]
27. Kim, I.; Kim, H.G.; So, J.N.; Kim, J.H.; Kwak, H.J.; Koh, G.Y. Angiopoietin-1 regulates endothelial cell survival through the phosphatidylinositol 3'-Kinase/Akt signal transduction pathway. *Circ. Res.* **2000**, *86*, 24–29. [CrossRef] [PubMed]
28. Hughes, D.P.; Marron, M.B.; Brindle, N.P.J. The Antiinflammatory Endothelial Tyrosine Kinase Tie2 Interacts With a Novel Nuclear Factor-κB Inhibitor ABIN-2. *Circ. Res.* **2003**, *92*, 630–636. [CrossRef] [PubMed]
29. Fukuhara, S.; Sako, K.; Minami, T.; Noda, K.; Kim, H.Z.; Kodama, T.; Shibuya, M.; Takakura, N.; Koh, G.Y.; Mochizuki, N. Differential function of Tie2 at cell-cell contacts and cell-substratum contacts regulated by angiopoietin-1. *Nat. Cell Biol.* **2008**, *10*, 513–526. [CrossRef] [PubMed]
30. Adams, R.H.; Alitalo, K. Molecular regulation of angiogenesis and lymphangiogenesis. *Nat. Rev. Mol. Cell Biol.* **2007**, *8*, 464–478. [CrossRef] [PubMed]
31. Holash, J.; Wiegand, S.J.; Yancopoulos, G.D. New model of tumor angiogenesis: Dynamic balance between vessel regression and growth mediated by angiopoietins and VEGF. *Oncogene* **1999**, *18*, 5356–5362. [CrossRef] [PubMed]
32. Nagy, N. Endothelial cells promote migration and proliferation of enteric neural crest cells via β1 integrin signaling. *Dev. Biol.* **2009**, *330*, 263–272. [CrossRef] [PubMed]
33. Kalinski, P. *Tumor Immune Microenvironment in Cancer Progression and Cancer Therapy*; Springer International Publishing: New York, NY, USA, 2017; ISBN 331967577X.
34. Tong, R.T.; Boucher, Y.; Kozin, S.V.; Winkler, F.; Hicklin, D.J.; Jain, R.K. Vascular Normalization by Vascular Endothelial Growth Factor Receptor 2 Blockade Induces a Pressure Gradient Across the Vasculature and Improves Drug Penetration in Tumors. *Cancer Res.* **2004**, *64*, 3731–3736. [CrossRef] [PubMed]

35. Streit, M.; Riccardi, L.; Velasco, P.; Brown, L.F.; Hawighorst, T.; Bornstein, P.; Detmar, M. Thrombospondin-2: A potent endogenous inhibitor of tumor growth and angiogenesis. *Proc. Natl. Acad. Sci. USA* **1999**, *Dec 21*, 14888–14893. [CrossRef]
36. Hashizume, H.; Baluk, P.; Morikawa, S.; McLean, J.W.; Thurston, G.; Roberge, S.; Jain, R.K.; McDonald, D.M. Openings between defective endothelial cells explain tumor vessel leakiness. *Am. J. Pathol.* **2000**, *156*, 1363–1380. [CrossRef]
37. Fitzgerald, G.; Soro-Arnaiz, I.; De Bock, K. The Warburg Effect in Endothelial Cells and its Potential as an Anti-angiogenic Target in Cancer. *Front. Cell Dev. Biol.* **2018**, *6*, 100. [CrossRef] [PubMed]
38. Inai, T.; Mancuso, M.; Hashizume, H.; Baffert, F.; Haskell, A.; Baluk, P.; Hu-lowe, D.D.; Shalinsky, D.R.; Thurston, G.; Yancopoulos, G.D.; et al. Inhibition of Vascular Endothelial Growth Factor (VEGF) Signaling in Cancer Causes Loss of Endothelial Fenestrations, Regression of Tumor Vessels, and Appearance of Basement Membrane Ghosts. *Am. J. Pathol.* **2004**, *165*, 35–52. [CrossRef]
39. Ferland-McCollough, D.; Slater, S.; Richard, J.; Reni, C.; Mangialardi, G. Pericytes, an overlooked player in vascular pathobiology. *Pharmacol. Ther.* **2017**, *171*, 30–42. [CrossRef] [PubMed]
40. Hida, K.; Kawamoto, T.; Ohga, N.; Akiyama, K.; Hida, Y.; Shindoh, M. Altered angiogenesis in the tumor microenvironment. *Pathol. Int.* **2011**, *61*, 630–637. [CrossRef] [PubMed]
41. Matsuda, K.; Ohga, N.; Hida, Y.; Muraki, C.; Tsuchiya, K.; Kurosu, T.; Akino, T.; Shih, S.-C.; Totsuka, Y.; Klagsbrun, M.; et al. Isolated tumor endothelial cells maintain specific character during long-term culture. *Biochem. Biophys. Res. Commun.* **2010**, *394*, 947–954. [CrossRef] [PubMed]
42. Naito, H.; Kidoya, H.; Sakimoto, S.; Wakabayashi, T.; Takakura, N. Identification and characterization of a resident vascular stem/progenitor cell population in preexisting blood vessels. *EMBO J.* **2012**, *31*, 842–855. [CrossRef] [PubMed]
43. Ohmura-Kakutani, H.; Akiyama, K.; Maishi, N.; Ohga, N.; Hida, Y.; Kawamoto, T.; Iida, J.; Shindoh, M.; Tsuchiya, K.; Shinohara, N.; et al. Identification of tumor endothelial cells with high aldehyde dehydrogenase activity and a highly angiogenic phenotype. *PLoS ONE* **2014**, *9*, e113910. [CrossRef] [PubMed]
44. Naito, H.; Wakabayashi, T.; Kidoya, H.; Muramatsu, F.; Takara, K.; Eino, D.; Yamane, K.; Iba, T.; Takakura, N. Endothelial side population cells contribute to tumor angiogenesis and antiangiogenic drug resistance. *Cancer Res.* **2016**, *76*, 3200–3210. [CrossRef] [PubMed]
45. Akiyama, K.; Ohga, N.; Hida, Y.; Kawamoto, T.; Sadamoto, Y.; Ishikawa, S.; Maishi, N.; Akino, T.; Kondoh, M.; Matsuda, A.; et al. Tumor endothelial cells acquire drug resistance by MDR1 up-regulation via VEGF signaling in tumor microenvironment. *Am. J. Pathol.* **2012**, *180*, 1283–1293. [CrossRef] [PubMed]
46. Kondoh, M.; Ohga, N.; Akiyama, K.; Hida, Y.; Maishi, N.; Towfik, A.M.; Inoue, N.; Shindoh, M.; Hida, K. Hypoxia-induced reactive oxygen species cause chromosomal abnormalities in endothelial cells in the tumor microenvironment. *PLoS ONE* **2013**, *8*, e80349. [CrossRef] [PubMed]
47. Okuno, Y.; Nakamura-Ishizu, A.; Otsu, K.; Suda, T.; Kubota, Y. Pathological neoangiogenesis depends on oxidative stress regulation by ATM. *Nat. Med.* **2012**, *18*, 1208–1216. [CrossRef] [PubMed]
48. Maishi, N.; Ohba, Y.; Akiyama, K.; Ohga, N.; Hamada, J.-I.; Nagao-Kitamoto, H.; Alam, M.T.; Yamamoto, K.; Kawamoto, T.; Inoue, N.; et al. Tumour endothelial cells in high metastatic tumours promote metastasis via epigenetic dysregulation of biglycan. *Sci. Rep.* **2016**, *6*, 28039. [CrossRef] [PubMed]
49. Fukumura, D.; Jain, R.K. Tumor microvasculature and microenvironment: Targets for anti- angiogenesis and normalization. *Microvasc. Res.* **2007**, *74*, 72–84. [CrossRef] [PubMed]
50. Ramakrishnan, S.; Anand, V.; Roy, S. Vascular endothelial growth factor signaling in hypoxia and inflammation. *J. Neuroimmune Pharmacol.* **2014**, *9*, 142–160. [CrossRef] [PubMed]
51. Wang, G.L.; Jiang, B.-H.; Rue, E.A.; Semenza, G.L. Hypoxia-inducible factor 1 is a basic-helix-loop-helix-PAS heterodimer regulated by cellular O2 tension (dioxin receptor/erythropoietin/hypoxia/transcription). *Proc. Natl. Acad. Sci. USA* **1995**, *92*, 5510–5514. [CrossRef] [PubMed]
52. Masoud, G.N.; Li, W. HIF-1α pathway: Role, regulation and intervention for cancer therapy. *Acta Pharm. Sin. B* **2015**, *5*, 378–389. [CrossRef] [PubMed]
53. dos Santos, S.A.; de Andrade Júnior, D.R. HIF-1alpha and infectious diseases: A new frontier for the development of new therapies. *Rev. Inst. Med. Trop. Sao Paulo* **2017**, *59*. [CrossRef] [PubMed]
54. Zhang, J.; Zhang, Q. VHL and Hypoxia Signaling: Beyond HIF in Cancer. *Biomedicines* **2018**, *6*, 35. [CrossRef] [PubMed]

55. Lando, D.; Peet, D.J.; Whelan, D.A.; Gorman, J.J.; Whitelaw, M.L. Asparagine hydroxylation of the HIF transactivation domain: A hypoxic switch. *Science (80-)* **2002**, *295*, 858–861. [CrossRef] [PubMed]
56. Taylor, C.T.; Doherty, G.; Fallon, P.G.; Cummins, E.P. Hypoxia-dependent regulation of inflammatory pathways in immune cells. *J. Clin. Investig.* **2016**, *126*, 3716–3724. [CrossRef] [PubMed]
57. Salceda, S.; Caro, J. Hypoxia-inducible factor 1alpha (HIF-1alpha) protein is rapidly degraded by the ubiquitin-proteasome system under normoxic conditions. *J. Biol. Chem.* **1997**, *14*, 3470–3481.
58. Zimna, A.; Kurpisz, M. Hypoxia-Inducible Factor-1 in Physiological and Pathophysiological Angiogenesis: Applications and Therapies. *BioMed Res. Int.* **2015**, *2015*, 549412. [CrossRef] [PubMed]
59. Maxwell, P.H.; Dachs, G.U.; Gleadle, J.M.; Nicholls, L.G.; Harris, A.L.; Stratford, I.J.; Hankinson, O.; Pugh, C.W.; Ratcliffe, P.J. Hypoxia-inducible factor-1 modulates gene expression in solid tumors and influences both angiogenesis and tumor growth. *Proc. Natl. Acad. Sci. USA* **1997**, *94*, 8104–8109. [CrossRef] [PubMed]
60. Hu, C.-J.; Wang, L.-Y.; Chodosh, L.A.; Keith, B.; Simon, M.C. Differential roles of hypoxia-inducible factor 1alpha (HIF-1alpha) and HIF-2alpha in hypoxic gene regulation. *Mol. Cell. Biol.* **2003**, *23*, 9361–9374. [CrossRef] [PubMed]
61. Bacon, A.; Harris, A. Hypoxia-inducible factors and hypoxic cell death in tumour physiology. *Ann. Med.* **2004**, *36*, 530–539. [CrossRef] [PubMed]
62. Kirito, K.; Hu, Y.; Komatsu, N. HIF-1 prevents the overproduction of mitochondrial ROS after cytokine stimulation through induction of PDK-1. *Cell Cycle* **2009**, *8*, 2844–2849. [CrossRef] [PubMed]
63. Wu, H.; Ding, Z.; Hu, D.; Sun, F.; Dai, C.; Xie, J.; Hu, X. Central role of lactic acidosis in cancer cell resistance to glucose deprivation-induced cell death. *J. Pathol.* **2012**, *227*, 189–199. [CrossRef] [PubMed]
64. Estrella, V.; Chen, T.; Lloyd, M.; Wojtkowiak, J.; Cornnell, H.H.; Ibrahim-Hashim, A.; Bailey, K.; Balagurunathan, Y.; Rothberg, J.M.; Sloane, B.F.; et al. Acidity Generated by the Tumor Microenvironment Drives Local Invasion. *Cancer Res.* **2013**, *73*, 1524–1535. [CrossRef] [PubMed]
65. Mendler, A.N.; Hu, B.; Prinz, P.U.; Kreutz, M.; Gottfried, E.; Noessner, E. Tumor lactic acidosis suppresses CTL function by inhibition of p38 and JNK/c-Jun activation. *Int. J. Cancer* **2012**, *131*, 633–640. [CrossRef] [PubMed]
66. Miao, Y.R.; Eckhardt, B.L.; Cao, Y.; Pasqualini, R.; Argani, P.; Arap, W.; Ramsay, R.G.; Anderson, R.L. Inhibition of established micrometastases by targeted drug delivery via cell surface-associated GRP78. *Clin. Cancer Res.* **2013**, *19*, 2107–2116. [CrossRef] [PubMed]
67. Pereira, E.R.; Frudd, K.; Awad, W.; Hendershot, L.M. Endoplasmic Reticulum (ER) stress and Hypoxia response pathways interact to Potentiate Hypoxia-inducible Factor 1 (HIF-1) Transcriptional activity on targets like Vascular Endothelial Growth Factor (VEGF). *J. Biol. Chem.* **2014**, *289*, 3352–3364. [CrossRef] [PubMed]
68. Giampietri, C.; Petrungaro, S.; Conti, S.; Facchiano, A.; Filippini, A.; Ziparo, E. Cancer Microenvironment and Endoplasmic Reticulum Stress Response. *Mediators Inflamm.* **2015**, *2015*, 417281. [CrossRef] [PubMed]
69. Han, J.; Kaufman, R.J. Physiological/pathological ramifications of transcription factors in the unfolded protein response. *Genes Dev.* **2017**, *31*, 1417–1438. [CrossRef] [PubMed]
70. Karali, E.; Bellou, S.; Stellas, D.; Klinakis, A.; Murphy, C.; Fotsis, T. VEGF Signals through ATF6 and PERK to Promote Endothelial Cell Survival and Angiogenesis in the Absence of ER Stress. *Mol. Cell* **2014**, *54*, 559–572. [CrossRef] [PubMed]
71. Orimo, A.; Gupta, P.B.; Sgroi, D.C.; Arenzana-Seisdedos, F.; Delaunay, T.; Naeem, R.; Carey, V.J.; Richardson, A.L.; Weinberg, R.A. Stromal Fibroblasts Present in Invasive Human Breast Carcinomas Promote Tumor Growth and Angiogenesis through Elevated SDF-1/CXCL12 Secretion. *Cell* **2005**, *121*, 335–348. [CrossRef] [PubMed]
72. Nagasaki, T.; Hara, M.; Nakanishi, H.; Takahashi, H.; Sato, M.; Takeyama, H. Interleukin-6 released by colon cancer-associated fibroblasts is critical for tumour angiogenesis: Anti-interleukin-6 receptor antibody suppressed angiogenesis and inhibited tumour–stroma interaction. *Br. J. Cancer* **2014**, *110*, 469–478. [CrossRef] [PubMed]
73. Riabov, V.; Gudima, A.; Wang, N.; Mickley, A.; Orekhov, A.; Kzhyshkowska, J. Role of tumor associated macrophages in tumor angiogenesis and lymphangiogenesis. *Front. Physiol.* **2014**, *5*, 75. [CrossRef] [PubMed]
74. Deryugina, E.I.; Quigley, J.P. Tumor angiogenesis: MMP-mediated induction of intravasation- and metastasis-sustaining neovasculature. *Matrix Biol.* **2015**, *44–46*, 94–112. [CrossRef] [PubMed]

75. De Palma, M.; Venneri, M.A.; Galli, R.; Sergi, L.S.; Politi, L.S.; Sampaolesi, M.; Naldini, L. Tie2 identifies a hematopoietic lineage of proangiogenic monocytes required for tumor vessel formation and a mesenchymal population of pericyte progenitors. *Cancer Cell* **2005**, *8*, 211–226. [CrossRef] [PubMed]
76. He, Y.-C.; Halford, M.M.; Achen, M.G.; Stacker, S.A. Exploring the role of endothelium in the tumour response to anti-angiogenic therapy. *Biochem. Soc. Trans.* **2014**, *42*, 1569–1575. [CrossRef] [PubMed]
77. Fontanella, C.; Ongaro, E.; Bolzonello, S.; Guardascione, M.; Fasola, G.; Aprile, G. Clinical advances in the development of novel VEGFR2 inhibitors. *Ann. Transl. Med.* **2014**, *2*, 123. [PubMed]
78. Amadio, M.; Govoni, S.; Pascale, A. Targeting VEGF in eye neovascularization: What's new?: A comprehensive review on current therapies and oligonucleotide-based interventions under development. *Pharmacol. Res.* **2016**, *103*, 253–269. [CrossRef] [PubMed]
79. Tewari, K.S.; Sill, M.W.; Long, H.J., III; Penson, R.T.; Huang, H.; Ramondetta, L.M.; Landrum, L.M.; Oaknin, A.; Reid, T.J.; Leitao, M.M.; et al. Improved Survival with Bevacizumab in Advanced Cervical Cancer. *N. Engl. J. Med.* **2014**, *370*, 734–743. [CrossRef] [PubMed]
80. Scartozzi, M.; Vincent, L.; Chiron, M.; Cascinu, S. Aflibercept, a New Way to Target Angiogenesis in the Second Line Treatment of Metastatic Colorectal Cancer (mCRC). *Target. Oncol.* **2016**, *11*, 489–500. [CrossRef] [PubMed]
81. Motzer, R.J.; Hutson, T.E. Overall Survival in Renal-Cell Carcinoma with Pazopanib versus Sunitinib. *N. Engl. J. Med.* **2014**, *370*, 1769–1770. [CrossRef] [PubMed]
82. Rini, B.I.; Escudier, B.; Tomczak, P.; Kaprin, A.; Szczylik, C.; Hutson, T.E.; Michaelson, M.D.; Gorbunova, V.A.; Gore, M.E.; Rusakov, I.G.; et al. Comparative effectiveness of axitinib versus sorafenib in advanced renal cell carcinoma (AXIS): A randomised phase 3 trial. *Lancet* **2011**, *378*, 1931–1939. [CrossRef]
83. Brose, M.S.; Nutting, C.M.; Jarzab, B.; Elisei, R.; Siena, S.; Bastholt, L.; de la Fouchardiere, C.; Pacini, F.; Paschke, R.; Shong, Y.K.; et al. Sorafenib in radioactive iodine-refractory, locally advanced or metastatic differentiated thyroid cancer: A randomised, double-blind, phase 3 trial. *Lancet (London, England)* **2014**, *384*, 319–328. [CrossRef]
84. van Beijnum, J.R.; Nowak-Sliwinska, P.; Huijbers, E.J.M.; Thijssen, V.L.; Griffioen, A.W. The Great Escape; the Hallmarks of Resistance to Antiangiogenic Therapy. *Pharmacol. Rev.* **2015**, *67*, 441–461. [CrossRef] [PubMed]
85. Casanovas, O.; Hicklin, D.J.; Bergers, G.; Hanahan, D. Drug resistance by evasion of antiangiogenic targeting of VEGF signaling in late-stage pancreatic islet tumors. *Cancer Cell* **2005**, *8*, 299–309. [CrossRef] [PubMed]
86. Kopetz, S.; Hoff, P.M.; Morris, J.S.; Wolff, R.A.; Eng, C.; Glover, K.Y.; Adinin, R.; Overman, M.J.; Valero, V.; Wen, S.; et al. Phase II Trial of Infusional Fluorouracil, Irinotecan, and Bevacizumab for Metastatic Colorectal Cancer: Efficacy and Circulating Angiogenic Biomarkers Associated With Therapeutic Resistance. *J. Clin. Oncol.* **2010**, *28*, 453–459. [CrossRef] [PubMed]
87. Vasudev, N.S.; Reynolds, A.R. Anti-angiogenic therapy for cancer: Current progress, unresolved questions and future directions. *Angiogenesis* **2014**, *17*, 471–494. [CrossRef] [PubMed]
88. Goel, S.; Duda, D.G.; Xu, L.; Munn, L.L.; Boucher, Y.; Fukumura, D.; Jain, R.K. Normalization of the Vasculature for Treatment of Cancer and Other Diseases. *Physiol. Rev.* **2011**, *91*, 1071–1121. [CrossRef] [PubMed]
89. Zhao, Y.; Adjei, A.A. New Drug Development and Clinical Pharmacology Targeting Angiogenesis in Cancer Therapy: Moving Beyond Vascular Endothelial Growth Factor. *Oncologist* **2015**, *20*, 660–673. [CrossRef] [PubMed]
90. Yang, L.; DeBusk, L.M.; Fukuda, K.; Fingleton, B.; Green-Jarvis, B.; Shyr, Y.; Matrisian, L.M.; Carbone, D.P.; Lin, P.C. Expansion of myeloid immune suppressor Gr+CD11b+ cells in tumor-bearing host directly promotes tumor angiogenesis. *Cancer Cell* **2004**, *6*, 409–421. [CrossRef] [PubMed]
91. Petit, I.; Jin, D.; Rafii, S. The SDF-1-CXCR4 signaling pathway: A molecular hub modulating neo-angiogenesis. *Trends Immunol.* **2007**, *28*, 299–307. [CrossRef] [PubMed]
92. Ceradini, D.J.; Kulkarni, A.R.; Callaghan, M.J.; Tepper, O.M.; Bastidas, N.; Kleinman, M.E.; Capla, J.M.; Galiano, R.D.; Levine, J.P.; Gurtner, G.C. Progenitor cell trafficking is regulated by hypoxic gradients through HIF-1 induction of SDF-1. *Nat. Med.* **2004**, *10*, 858–865. [CrossRef] [PubMed]
93. Hillen, F.; Griffioen, A.W. Tumour vascularization: Sprouting angiogenesis and beyond. *Cancer Metastasis Rev.* **2007**, *26*, 489–502. [CrossRef] [PubMed]

94. Coelho, A.L.; Gomes, M.P.; Catarino, R.J.; Rolfo, C.; Lopes, A.M.; Medeiros, R.M.; Araújo, A.M.; Coelho, A.L.; Gomes, M.P.; Catarino, R.J.; et al. Angiogenesis in NSCLC: Is vessel co-option the trunk that sustains the branches? *Oncotarget* **2017**, *8*, 39795–39804. [CrossRef] [PubMed]
95. Frentzas, S.; Simoneau, E.; Bridgeman, V.L.; Vermeulen, P.B.; Foo, S.; Kostaras, E.; Nathan, M.; Wotherspoon, A.; Gao, Z.-H.; Shi, Y.; et al. Vessel co-option mediates resistance to anti-angiogenic therapy in liver metastases. *Nat. Med.* **2016**, *22*, 1294–1302. [CrossRef] [PubMed]
96. Qian, C.-N.; Tan, M.-H.; Yang, J.-P.; Cao, Y. Revisiting tumor angiogenesis: Vessel co-option, vessel remodeling, and cancer cell-derived vasculature formation. *Chin. J. Cancer* **2016**, *35*, 10. [CrossRef] [PubMed]
97. Ge, H.; Luo, H. Overview of advances in vasculogenic mimicry—A potential target for tumor therapy. *Cancer Manag. Res.* **2018**, *10*, 2429–2437. [CrossRef] [PubMed]
98. Sood, A.K.; Seftor, E.A.; Fletcher, M.S.; Gardner, L.M.; Heidger, P.M.; Buller, R.E.; Seftor, R.E.; Hendrix, M.J. Molecular determinants of ovarian cancer plasticity. *Am. J. Pathol.* **2001**, *158*, 1279–1288. [CrossRef]
99. Van Der Schaft, D.W.J.; Hillen, F.; Pauwels, P.; Kirschmann, D.A.; Castermans, K.; Egbrink, M.G.A.; Tran, M.G.B.; Sciot, R.; Hauben, E.; Hogendoorn, P.C.W.; et al. Tumor Cell Plasticity in Ewing Sarcoma, an Alternative Circulatory System Stimulated by Hypoxia. *Cancer Res.* **2005**, *65*, 11520–11529. [CrossRef] [PubMed]
100. Hillen, F.; Baeten, C.I.M.; van de Winkel, A.; Creytens, D.; van der Schaft, D.W.J.; Winnepenninckx, V.; Griffioen, A.W. Leukocyte infiltration and tumor cell plasticity are parameters of aggressiveness in primary cutaneous melanoma. *Cancer Immunol. Immunother.* **2008**, *57*, 97–106. [CrossRef] [PubMed]
101. Hawiger, D.; Inaba, K.; Dorsett, Y.; Guo, M.; Mahnke, K.; Rivera, M.; Ravetch, J.V.; Steinman, R.M.; Nussenzweig, M.C. Dendritic cells induce peripheral T cell unresponsiveness under steady state conditions in vivo. *J. Exp. Med.* **2001**, *194*, 769–779. [CrossRef] [PubMed]
102. Reis e Sousa, C. Dendritic cells in a mature age. *Nat. Rev. Immunol.* **2006**, *6*, 476–483. [CrossRef] [PubMed]
103. Gabrilovich, D.I.; Chen, H.L.; Girgis, K.R.; Cunningham, H.T.; Meny, G.M.; Nadaf, S.; Kavanaugh, D.; Carbone, D.P. Production of vascular endothelial growth factor by human tumors inhibits the functional maturation of dendritic cells. *Nat. Med.* **1996**, *2*, 1096–1103. [CrossRef] [PubMed]
104. Gabrilovich, D.; Ishida, T.; Oyama, T.; Ran, S.; Kravtsov, V.; Nadaf, S.; Carbone, D.P. Vascular endothelial growth factor inhibits the development of dendritic cells and dramatically affects the differentiation of multiple hematopoietic lineages in vivo. *Blood* **1998**, *92*, 4150–4166. [PubMed]
105. Oyama, T.; Ran, S.; Ishida, T.; Nadaf, S.; Kerr, L.; Carbone, D.P.; Gabrilovich, D.I. Vascular endothelial growth factor affects dendritic cell maturation through the inhibition of nuclear factor-kappa B activation in hemopoietic progenitor cells. *J. Immunol.* **1998**, *160*, 1224–1232. [PubMed]
106. Mimura, K.; Kono, K.; Takahashi, A.; Kawaguchi, Y.; Fujii, H. Vascular endothelial growth factor inhibits the function of human mature dendritic cells mediated by VEGF receptor-2. *Cancer Immunol. Immunother.* **2007**, *56*, 761–770. [CrossRef] [PubMed]
107. Kinashi, T. Intracellular signalling controlling integrin activation in lymphocytes. *Nat. Rev. Immunol.* **2005**, *5*, 546–559. [CrossRef] [PubMed]
108. Clark, R.A.; Huang, S.J.; Murphy, G.F.; Mollet, I.G.; Hijnen, D.; Muthukuru, M.; Schanbacher, C.F.; Edwards, V.; Miller, D.M.; Kim, J.E.; et al. Human squamous cell carcinomas evade the immune response by down-regulation of vascular E-selectin and recruitment of regulatory T cells. *J. Exp. Med.* **2008**, *205*, 2221–2234. [CrossRef] [PubMed]
109. Afanasiev, O.K.; Nagase, K.; Simonson, W.; Vandeven, N.; Koelle, D.M.; Clark, R.; Nghiem, P. Vascular E-selectin expression correlates with CD8 lymphocyte infiltration and improved outcome in Merkel cell carcinoma. *J. Investig. Dermatol.* **2013**, *133*, 206–221. [CrossRef] [PubMed]
110. Griffioen, A.W.; Damen, C.A.; Martinotti, S.; Blijham, G.H.; Groenewegen, G. Endothelial Intercellular Adhesion Molecule-i Expression Is Suppressed in Human. *Cancer Res.* **1996**, *1*, 1111–1117.
111. Facciabene, A.; Peng, X.; Hagemann, I.S.; Balint, K.; Barchetti, A.; Wang, L.; Gimotty, P.A.; Gilks, C.B.; Lal, P.; Zhang, L.; et al. Tumour hypoxia promotes tolerance and. *Nature* **2011**, *475*, 226–230. [CrossRef] [PubMed]
112. Gabrilovich, D.I.; Nagaraj, S. Myeloid-derived suppressor cells as regulators of the immune system. *Nat. Rev. Immunol.* **2009**, *9*, 162–174. [CrossRef] [PubMed]
113. Li, B.; Lalani, A.S.; Harding, T.C.; Luan, B.; Koprivnikar, K.; Huan Tu, G.; Prell, R.; VanRoey, M.J.; Simmons, A.D.; Jooss, K. Vascular Endothelial Growth Factor Blockade Reduces Intratumoral Regulatory T

Cells and Enhances the Efficacy of a GM-CSF-Secreting Cancer Immunotherapy. *Clin. Cancer Res.* **2006**, *12*, 6808–6816. [CrossRef] [PubMed]
114. Wada, J.; Suzuki, H.; Fuchino, R.; Yamasaki, A.; Nagai, S.; Yanai, K.; Koga, K.; Nakamura, M.; Tanaka, M.; Morisaki, T.; et al. The contribution of vascular endothelial growth factor to the induction of regulatory T-cells in malignant effusions. *Anticancer Res.* **2009**, *29*, 881–888. [PubMed]
115. Alfaro, C.; Suarez, N.; Gonzalez, A.; Solano, S.; Erro, L.; Dubrot, J.; Palazon, A.; Hervas-Stubbs, S.; Gurpide, A.; Lopez-Picazo, J.M.; et al. Influence of bevacizumab, sunitinib and sorafenib as single agents or in combination on the inhibitory effects of VEGF on human dendritic cell differentiation from monocytes. *Br. J. Cancer* **2009**, *100*, 1111–1119. [CrossRef] [PubMed]
116. Borgström, P.; Hughes, G.K.; Hansell, P.; Wolitsky, B.A.; Sriramarao, P. Leukocyte adhesion in angiogenic blood vessels. Role of E-selectin, P-selectin, and beta2 integrin in lymphotoxin-mediated leukocyte recruitment in tumor microvessels. *J. Clin. Investig.* **1997**, *99*, 2246–2253. [CrossRef] [PubMed]
117. Kusmartsev, S.; Eruslanov, E.; Kübler, H.; Tseng, T.; Sakai, Y.; Su, Z.; Kaliberov, S.; Heiser, A.; Rosser, C.; Dahm, P.; et al. Oxidative stress regulates expression of VEGFR1 in myeloid cells: Link to tumor-induced immune suppression in renal cell carcinoma. *J. Immunol.* **2008**, *181*, 346–353. [CrossRef] [PubMed]
118. Adotevi, O.; Pere, H.; Ravel, P.; Haicheur, N.; Badoual, C.; Merillon, N.; Medioni, J.; Peyrard, S.; Roncelin, S.; Verkarre, V.; et al. A Decrease of Regulatory T Cells Correlates With Overall Survival After Sunitinib-based Antiangiogenic Therapy in Metastatic Renal Cancer Patients. *J. Immunother.* **2010**, *33*, 991–998. [CrossRef] [PubMed]
119. Keir, M.E.; Butte, M.J.; Freeman, G.J.; Sharpe, A.H. PD-1 and Its Ligands in Tolerance and Immunity. *Annu. Rev. Immunol.* **2008**, *26*, 677–704. [CrossRef] [PubMed]
120. Okazaki, T.; Chikuma, S.; Iwai, Y.; Fagarasan, S.; Honjo, T. A rheostat for immune responses: The unique properties of PD-1 and their advantages for clinical application. *Nat. Immunol.* **2013**, *14*, 1212–1218. [CrossRef] [PubMed]
121. Bai, J.; Gao, Z.; Li, X.; Dong, L.; Han, W.; Nie, J. Regulation of PD-1/PD-L1 pathway and resistance to PD-1/PDL1 blockade. *Oncotarget* **2017**, *8*, 110693–110707. [CrossRef] [PubMed]
122. Ribas, A.; Wolchok, J.D. Cancer immunotherapy using checkpoint blockade. *Science* **2018**, *359*, 1350–1355. [CrossRef] [PubMed]
123. Liu, X.-D.; Hoang, A. Resistance to anti-angiogenic therapy is associated with an immunosuppressive tumor microenvironment in metastatic renal cell carcinoma. *Cancer Immunol. Res.* **2015**, *3*, 1017–1029. [CrossRef] [PubMed]
124. Guislain, A.; Gadiot, J.; Kaiser, A.; Jordanova, E.S.; Broeks, A.; Sanders, J.; van Boven, H.; de Gruijl, T.D.; Haanen, J.B.A.G.; Bex, A.; et al. Sunitinib pretreatment improves tumor-infiltrating lymphocyte expansion by reduction in intratumoral content of myeloid-derived suppressor cells in human renal cell carcinoma. *Cancer Immunol. Immunother.* **2015**, *64*, 1241–1250. [CrossRef] [PubMed]
125. Wallin, J.J.; Bendell, J.C.; Funke, R.; Sznol, M.; Korski, K.; Jones, S.; Hernandez, G.; Mier, J.; He, X.; Hodi, F.S.; et al. Atezolizumab in combination with bevacizumab enhances antigen-specific T-cell migration in metastatic renal cell carcinoma. *Nat. Commun.* **2016**, *7*, 12624. [CrossRef] [PubMed]
126. Socinski, M.A.; Jotte, R.M.; Cappuzzo, F.; Orlandi, F.; Stroyakovskiy, D.; Nogami, N.; Rodríguez-Abreu, D.; Moro-Sibilot, D.; Thomas, C.A.; Barlesi, F.; et al. Atezolizumab for First-Line Treatment of Metastatic Nonsquamous NSCLC. *N. Engl. J. Med.* **2018**, *378*, 2288–2301. [CrossRef] [PubMed]
127. Motzer, R.J.; Powles, T.; Atkins, M.B.; Escudier, B.; McDermott, D.F.; Suarez, C.; Bracarda, S.; Stadler, W.M.; Donskov, F.; Lee, J.-L.; et al. IMmotion151: A Randomized Phase III Study of Atezolizumab Plus Bevacizumab vs. Sunitinib in Untreated Metastatic Renal Cell Carcinoma (mRCC). *J. Clin. Oncol.* **2018**, *36*, 578. [CrossRef]

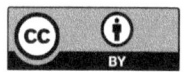

© 2019 by the authors. Licensee MDPI, Basel, Switzerland. This article is an open access article distributed under the terms and conditions of the Creative Commons Attribution (CC BY) license (http://creativecommons.org/licenses/by/4.0/).

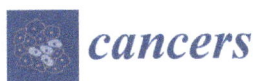

Review

Therapeutic Monoclonal Antibodies and Antibody Products: Current Practices and Development in Multiple Myeloma

Francesca Bonello, Roberto Mina, Mario Boccadoro and Francesca Gay *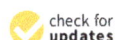

Myeloma Unit, Division of Hematology, University of Torino, Azienda Ospedaliero-Universitaria Città della Salute e della Scienza di Torino, 10126 Torino, Italy; francesca.bonello@edu.unito.it (F.B.); roberto.mina.rm@gmail.com (R.M.); mario.boccadoro@unito.it (M.B.)
* Correspondence: fgay@cittadellasalute.to.it; Tel.: +39-011-6333-4279/4301; Fax: +39-011-6333-4187

Received: 8 November 2019; Accepted: 16 December 2019; Published: 19 December 2019

Abstract: Immunotherapy is the latest innovation for the treatment of multiple myeloma (MM). Monoclonal antibodies (mAbs) entered the clinical practice and are under evaluation in clinical trials. MAbs can target highly selective and specific antigens on the cell surface of MM cells causing cell death (CD38 and CS1), convey specific cytotoxic drugs (antibody-drug conjugates), remove the breaks of the immune system (programmed death 1 (PD-1) and PD-ligand 1/2 (L1/L2) axis), or boost it against myeloma cells (bi-specific mAbs and T cell engagers). Two mAbs have been approved for the treatment of MM: the anti-CD38 daratumumab for newly-diagnosed and relapsed/refractory patients and the anti-CS1 elotuzumab in the relapse setting. These compounds are under investigation in clinical trials to explore their synergy with other anti-MM regimens, both in the front-line and relapse settings. Other antibodies targeting various antigens are under evaluation. B cell maturation antigens (BCMAs), selectively expressed on plasma cells, emerged as a promising target and several compounds targeting it have been developed. Encouraging results have been reported with antibody drug conjugates (e.g., GSK2857916) and bispecific T cell engagers (BiTEs®), including AMG420, which re-directs T cell-mediated cytotoxicity against MM cells. Here, we present an overview on mAbs currently approved for the treatment of MM and promising compounds under investigation.

Keywords: multiple myeloma (MM); immunotherapy; monoclonal antibodies (mAbs); antibody products; B cell maturation antigens (BCMAs); bispecific T cell engagers (BiTEs®)

1. Introduction

Multiple myeloma (MM) is a hematologic malignancy characterized by a clonal expansion of aberrant plasma cells in the bone marrow inducing bone lesions, anemia, renal insufficiency and hypercalcemia. In the last two decades, the treatment armamentarium of effective anti-myeloma drugs, used both at diagnosis and at relapse, has been significantly expanded with various compounds of different drug-classes. However, despite the availability of several treatment options, MM still remains an incurable disease whose natural history is characterized by phases of disease remission followed by relapses. The remission duration tends to progressively decrease at every subsequent relapse and MM inevitably becomes refractory to all available agents. Therefore, even if the survival of MM patients, both young and elderly, has steadily increased over time, to date, roughly 50% of patients are alive at 5 years after diagnosis [1–3].

With the introduction of effective novel agent combinations, based on immunomodulatory agents (IMiDs) and proteasome inhibitors (PIs), the treatment goal for first-line therapies is now the achievement of minimal residual disease (MRD) negativity [4], which is currently reported in

50–80% of transplant-eligible [5–8] and in 15–30% of transplant-ineligible patients [9–11]. A large meta-analysis demonstrated that reaching MRD negativity (though with some variability in terms of methods and cut-offs adopted) significantly prolonged progression-free survival (PFS) and overall survival (OS) as compared to a MRD-positive status [12]. For this reason, efforts should be made to improve the effectiveness of first-line therapies in inducing deep and durable responses. Regardless of the effectiveness of newer combinations available at diagnosis, the prognosis of high-risk patients (e.g., patients with unfavorable genetics or molecular abnormalities, International Staging System (ISS) stage III, extramedullary disease, or those who experience an early relapse after first-line therapies) is dismal compared to that of standard-risk patients. This evidence prompts the development of different strategies and the adoption of newer drugs in this population, currently representing an unmet medical need.

Furthermore, despite the depth of response obtained with first-line therapies and the duration of the remission, relapse is inevitable in almost all patients with MM, who progressively become refractory to all approved drugs, particularly to IMiDs and PIs. The development of compounds with different mechanisms of action, aiming at synergizing with currently used agents and overcoming drug-induced resistance, is therefore a priority.

Immunotherapy, either passive—with monoclonal antibodies (mAbs) or cellular products directed against neoplastic cells—or active—when the patient's immune system is stimulated to mount an immune response against tumor cells—represents a pivotal strategy for the treatment of both solid and hematologic malignancies.

MAbs have entered the clinical practice for the treatment of MM [13]. They are selective compounds targeting surface antigens that are highly expressed on aberrant plasma cells and not (or at low density) on normal tissues, thus promoting on-target activity while limiting off-target toxicity. MAbs elicit their therapeutic actions through different mechanisms, including a direct cytotoxicity on the neoplastic cell and immune-mediated mechanisms such as antibody-dependent cell-mediated cytotoxicity (ADCC), antibody-dependent cell-mediated phagocytosis (ADCP) and complement-dependent cytotoxicity (CDC). Monoclonal antibodies can also be exploited to directly target the myeloma cell while conveying a cytotoxic agent, as in the case of antibody-drug conjugates (ADCs), or to engage and activate T cells against the myeloma cell as with bispecific T cell engagers.

Several potential targets have been identified on the myeloma cells and likewise constructs have been designed and tested in MM patients, some of them having already entered the clinical practice.

This review focuses on the strength and controversies of the current treatment strategies exploiting mAbs in MM, as well as on newer experimental immunotherapeutic approaches such as ADCs and bispecific T-cell engagers (BiTEs®).

2. Monoclonal Antibodies

2.1. Anti-CD38 Monoclonal Antibodies

2.1.1. Rationale

CD38 is a transmembrane type II glycoprotein that is highly expressed on normal plasma cells as well as on MM cells [14]. CD38 is also present at lower levels on normal lymphoid and myeloid cells, on red blood cells, as well as on solid tissues such as muscle cells (especially in the airway system), epithelial cells in the prostate and pancreatic beta cells. CD38 acts as a receptor, as an adhesion molecule, and as an ectoenzyme [15–17].

Anti-CD38 mAbs elicit their action targeting CD38+ MM cells and inducing effector mechanisms such as ADCC (which relies mainly on natural killer [NK] cells), ADCP, and CDC [18–21]. An in vitro comparison between the different anti-CD38 molecules showed that ADCC was equally induced by all of them, whereas daratumumab induced the highest CDC at low concentration and ADCP [22]. Alongside immune-mediated cytotoxicity, anti-CD38 mAbs have an immunomodulatory activity that relies on the modulation of immune cells. Myeloid-derived suppressor cells (MDSC), regulatory B cells

(Bregs, which promote tumor growth and immune escape), as well as a subset of regulatory T cells (Tregs) express CD38, and their levels are reduced after daratumumab exposure. Conversely, daratumumab results in significant expansion of CD8+ cytotoxic and CD4+ helper T cells, likely following the depletion of regulatory cells. Remarkably, expanded effector T cells also show increased killing capacity due to augmented levels of granzyme B, which activates caspases and triggers cell apoptosis [23–25]. In addition, among the activities promoted by CD38, there is a nicotinamide adenine dinucleotide (NAD)-ase activity, which results in reduced levels of NAD+ in T cells, responsible for the loss of their effector functions (exhausted T cells). In murine models, anti-CD38 mAbs administration induced higher levels of NAD+ in T effector cells, thus enhancing their antitumor activity [23]. The main mechanisms of action of anti-CD38 monoclonal antibodies are summarized in Figure 1.

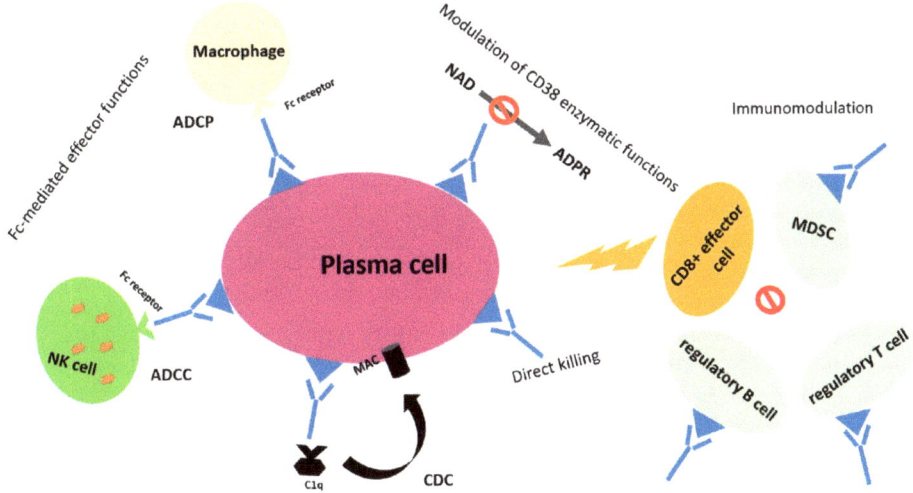

Figure 1. Main mechanisms of action of anti-CD38 monoclonal antibodies. Abbreviations: MDSC, myeloid-derived suppressor cell; ADCC, antibody-dependent cell-mediated cytotoxicity; CDC, complement-dependent cytotoxicity; NAD, nicotinamide adenine dinucleotide; ADPR, adenosine ribose; MAC, membrane attack complex.

In vitro studies showed a marked synergism between anti-CD38 mAbs (daratumumab, isatuximab and MOR202) and IMiDs (lenalidomide and pomalidomide), mainly owing to an enhanced NK activity elicited by IMiDs that increases both number and activity of NK cells and consequently ADCC, as well as the cytotoxic activity of macrophages, thus stimulating ADCP [26]. This evidence prompted the investigation of the in vivo effect of the addition of anti-CD38 mAbs to IMiD-based combinations. Anti-CD38 mAbs also show an additive effect with PIs [27], although the exact mechanisms are less clear.

2.1.2. Clinical Development

Daratumumab

Daratumumab was the first fully human anti-CD38 mAb to be tested in clinical trials. Results of the main clinical trials are summarized in Table 1.

Table 1. Results of the main clinical trials with anti-CD38 monoclonal antibodies daratumumab and isatuximab.

Study	Phase	Number of Patients	Median Previous Line	Regimen	ORR	Median PFS (Months)	Median OS (Months)
RELAPSED PATIENTS							
GEN501 + SIRIUS POOLED [28]	II	148	5	Daratumumab single agent	31.1%	4	20.1
POLLUX [29]	III	569	1	Dara-Rd vs. Rd	92.9% vs. 76.4%	NR vs. 17.5	1-year OS 92.1% vs. 86.8%
CASTOR [30,31]	III	498	2	Dara-Vd vs. Vd	83.8% vs. 63.2%	16.7 vs. 7.1	NA
NCT01998971 [32]	II	103	4	Dara-Poma-dex	60%	8.8	17.5
NCT01998971 [33]	Ib	85	2	Dara-Kd	84%	1-year PFS 74%	1-year OS 82%
NCT01749969 [34]	Ib	57	5	Isa-Rd	56%	8.5	NR
NCT02283775 [35]	Ib	45	3	Isa-Pd	62%	17.6	NR
NCT02332850 [36]	Ib	33	3	Isa-Kd	66%	NR	NR
ICARIA [37]	III	307	3	Isa-Pd vs. Pd	60% vs. 35%	11.5 vs. 6.5	NA
NEWLY DIAGNOSED PATIENTS							
ALCYONE [11]	III	706 TNE	–	Dara-VMP vs. VMP	90.9% vs. 73.9%	NR vs. 18.1	NA
MAIA [38]	III	737 TNE	–	Dara-Rd vs. Rd	92.9% vs. 81.3%	NR vs. 31.9	NA
CASSIOPEIA [39]	III	1085 TE	–	Dara-VTd vs. VTd	≥CR 39% vs. 26%	NA	NA
GRIFFIN [40]	II	207 TE	–	Dara-VRd vs. VRd	51.5% vs. 42.3%	NA	NA

Abbreviations: ORR, overall response rate; PFS, progression-free survival; OS, overall survival; Dara, daratumumab; Isa, isatuximab; V, bortezomib; C, cyclophosphamide; d, dex, dexamethasone; T, thalidomide; R, lenalidomide; K, carfilzomib; Poma, pomalidomide; M, melphalan; P, prednisone; NR, not reached; NA, not yet available; TNE, transplant ineligible; TE, transplant eligible; CR, complete response.

In the phase I GEN501 study, which investigated different doses of daratumumab in relapsed/refractory (RR)MM patients, the greatest activity was reported at the dose of 16 mg/kg, at which 36% of patients achieved a partial response (PR) or better. These results were confirmed by the phase II SIRIUS trial, which reported a 29% overall response rate (ORR) in heavily pretreated patients, resulting into median PFS and OS of 3.7 and 17.5 months, respectively [41]. These results led to the approval, by both the Food and Drug Administration (FDA) and the European Medicines Agency (EMA), of daratumumab as single agent for RRMM patients with 3 prior lines of therapy including a PI and an IMiD.

The synergism showed in vitro by daratumumab and lenalidomide was first translated into a marked in vivo activity of the 3-drug combination daratumumab-lenalidomide-dexamethasone (Dara-Rd) observed in RRMM patients enrolled in the phase II GEN503 study and then confirmed by the phase III POLLUX study. In the POLLUX trial, 569 RRMM patients were randomized to receive standard lenalidomide-dexamethasone (Rd) versus Dara-Rd until disease progression or intolerance [29]. ORR was higher in the triplet arm (93% vs. 76%) as well as the rate of patients achieving minimal residual disease (MRD) negativity (26% vs. 6% of patients, threshold 10^{-5}). Median PFS was not reached (NR) versus

17.5 months (hazard ratio [HR] 0.41, $p < 0.001$) in the Dara-Rd versus Rd arms; this benefit was also consistent in patients with high-risk cytogenetics (HR 0.53, $p = 0.09$) [42]. Of notice, the addition of daratumumab to Rd did not significantly increase the rates of grade 3–4 toxicities, with the exception of neutropenia (54% vs. 39%) and infections (28.3% vs. 22.8%). These data supported the approval of Dara-Rd for the treatment of MM patients who had previously received at least 1 line of therapy.

Daratumumab was then evaluated with pomalidomide and dexamethasone (Dara-Pd). In a preliminary phase II trial, this 3-drug regimen showed, in a heavily pretreated population (the median number of prior therapies was 4), ORR (60%) and median PFS (8.8 months) that compared favorably with those of Pd alone (ORR 31%, median PFS 3.8 months) despite the limitations of a cross-trial comparison [32,43]. Following the results of this study, the triplet Dara-Pd received accelerated approval by the FDA for RRMM patients who previously received both an IMiD and a PI. This combination is appealing considering that, in the near future, the majority of newly diagnosed (ND)MM patients will become refractory to continuous lenalidomide after their first line of therapy. Definitive results will come from the phase III trial APOLLO (NCT03180736) comparing Dara-Pd vs. Pd in RRMM patients.

Daratumumab has also been associated with PIs. The phase III CASTOR trial compared bortezomib-dexamethasone (Vd) administered for 8 cycles to daratumumab-Vd (Dara-Vd) for 8 cycles, followed by monthly daratumumab until progression in RRMM patients [30]. The addition of daratumumab resulted in higher ORR (83% vs. 63%) and MRD negativity rate (12% vs. 2%, threshold 10^{-5}), and in prolonged PFS (median, 16.7 vs. 7.1 months; HR 0.31; $p < 0.0001$) [31]. Importantly, the MRD negativity rate continued to increase over time for patients receiving Dara-Vd as compared to those receiving Vd, thus highlighting the benefit of continuous treatment with daratumumab. The PFS advantage was also consistent for patients previously exposed to bortezomib (HR 0.35, $p < 0.001$) and for patients with high-risk cytogenetic features detected by fluorescence in situ hybridization (FISH, HR 0.45, $p = 0.05$). The triplet Dara-Vd is currently approved by the FDA and EMA for RRMM patients.

A phase Ib study with carfilzomib-dexamethasone-daratumumab (KdD) induced an objective response in 84% of RRMM patients after both lenalidomide and bortezomib [33]. It was recently announced that the phase III CANDOR study (NCT03158688) comparing Kd to KdD met its primary endpoint, with a 37% reduction in the risk of progression or death (HR 0.63, 95% CI 0.464–0.854, $p = 0.0014$) in patients receiving daratumumab [44].

Because CD38 expression is higher in the early stages of the disease, and mAbs greatly rely on the immune system to exploit their anti-MM activity, it seems reasonable to expect that moving daratumumab to the first-line setting, when the immune-system of a treatment-naïve patient is less compromised, could increase its efficacy. In older patients with newly diagnosed (ND)MM, daratumumab plus bortezomib-melphalan-prednisone (Dara-VMP), followed by daratumumab maintenance, significantly increased the MRD negativity rate as compared to the standard of care VMP (22% vs. 6%, $p < 0.001$, threshold 10^{-5}), ultimately prolonging the median PFS (NR after a median follow-up of 17 months vs. 18.1 months, HR 0.50, $p < 0.001$) [11]. Highlighting the role of continuous treatment, a substantial benefit in PFS was detected during the maintenance phase when a lower rate of relapses was observed in patients receiving daratumumab compared with observation (sustained response after 18 months: 77% vs. 60%). This evidence supports the benefit of continuous therapy with daratumumab, which allows better disease control over time compared to fixed duration treatment. A longer follow-up is needed to detect an OS benefit. Dara-VMP has recently been approved by both the FDA and EMA, thus becoming one of the standards of care for transplant-ineligible patients. Impressive results in terms of higher MRD negativity rates (24.2% vs. 7.3%, respectively; $p < 0.001$, threshold 10^{-5}) and reduced risk of progression or death (median NR vs. 32 months after a median follow-up of 28 months, HR 0.56, $p < 0.001$) were observed when Dara-Rd was compared to Rd in NDMM patients not suitable for autologous stem-cell transplantation (ASCT; MAIA study [38]). In both Dara-VMP and Dara-Rd regimens, the addition of daratumumab did not negatively affect the safety profiles of VMP and Rd, despite a higher rate of grade 3–4 infections being reported in both studies in patients receiving daratumumab (Dara-VMP 23.1% vs. VMP 14.7%; Dara-Rd 32% vs. Rd

23%); also, the frequency of grade 3–4 neutropenia was higher in patients receiving daratumumab in the MAIA study (50% vs. 35%).

Daratumumab has also been incorporated in the induction, consolidation, and maintenance approach in combination with standard triplets such as bortezomib-thalidomide-dexamethasone (VTd) and bortezomib-lenalidomide-dexamethasone (VRd) as initial treatment for NDMM patients eligible for high-dose melphalan and ASCT.

The phase III CASSIOPEIA trial randomized 1085 transplant-eligible patients to VTd with or without daratumumab as induction and consolidation, followed by daratumumab maintenance or no maintenance. After the consolidation phase, the proportion of MRD-negative patients was higher in the Dara-VTd group than in the VTd group (64% vs. 44%, $p < 0.001$, threshold 10^{-5}). This translated into a significantly reduced risk of progression or death in the Dara-VTd arm as compared to the control group (HR for PFS 0.47, $p < 0.001$) [39]. The higher MRD negativity rate reported with daratumumab was also confirmed in ISS-III and high-risk FISH patients (64% vs. 46%, $p = 0.01$; 60% vs. 40%, $p = 0.06$, respectively), with a trend towards PFS improvement with daratumumab (HR 0.66, 95% CI 0.31–1.39; HR 0.67, 95% CI 0.35–1.30, respectively) in these subsets of patients that traditionally represent unmet clinical needs [45]. Mobilization and stem collection after a more intensified induction including daratumumab were adequate. Although patients in the Dara-VTd arm required the use of plerixafor more frequently (22% vs. 8%) and collected less CD34+ cells (median 6.3×10^6/kg vs. 8×10^6/kg), successful ASCT and hematopoietic reconstitution were not affected. Data on maintenance are eagerly awaited. Following the results of the CASSIOPEIA trial, in September 2019, the FDA has approved frontline Dara-VTd as induction for transplant-eligible patients. VRd ± daratumumab as induction and post-ASCT consolidation followed by lenalidomide ± daratumumab maintenance is being compared in the ongoing phase II GRIFFIN trial [40]. The quadruplet significantly improved the MRD negativity rate (threshold 10^{-5}) at the end of consolidation, as compared to VRd (47.9% vs. 17.9%, HR 0.23, $p < 0.001$). In both trials, patients treated with daratumumab experienced no significant increase in grade 3–4 non-hematologic adverse events (AEs). Data on maintenance will shed light on the role of daratumumab maintenance, either alone or in combination with lenalidomide.

Other ongoing phase II/III trials evaluating front-line daratumumab in ASCT-eligible patients include the EMN17/PERSEUS trial, which explores the addition of daratumumab to VRd as induction and consolidation and to lenalidomide as maintenance treatment, and the EMN18 study, which compares induction and consolidation with daratumumab-bortezomib-cyclophosphamide-dexamethasone (Dara-VCd) to standard VTd followed by ASCT and maintenance with ixazomib ± daratumumab [46]. The main ongoing trials are summarized in Table 2.

Table 2. Main ongoing trials involving daratumumab and isatuximab in multiple myeloma patients.

Study	Setting	Phase	Study Design
DARATUMUMAB			
NCT03710603 [46]	NDMM TE (690 pts)	III	Dara-VRd + ASCT + Dara-VRd consolidation + Dara-R maintenance vs. VRd + ASCT + VRd consolidation + R maintenance

Table 2. Cont.

NCT03896737	NDMM TE (≈400 pts)	II	Dara-VCd + double ASCT + Dara-VCd consolidation vs. VTd + double ASCT + VTd consolidation Second randomization: Ixa maintenance vs. Ixa-Dara
NCT03180736	RRMM (302 pts)	III	Dara-Poma-dex vs. Poma-dex
NCT03158688	RRMM (466 pts)	III	Dara-Kd vs. Kd
ISATUXIMAB			
NCT02513186 [47,48]	NDMM NTE (88 pts)	I/II	Isa-VCd vs. Isa-VRd
NCT03319667 [49]	NDMM, NTE (475 pts)	III	Isa-VRd vs. VRd
NCT03275285	RRMM (302 pts)	III	Isa-Kd vs. Kd
NCT02990338 [50]	RRMM (300 pts)	III	Isa-Poma-dex vs. Poma-dex

Abbreviations: pts, patients; NDMM, newly diagnosed multiple myeloma; RRMM, relapsed/refractory MM; Dara, daratumumab; Isa, isatuximab; ASCT, autologous stem-cell transplantation; TE, transplant eligible; NTE, transplant ineligible; Ixa, ixazomib; V, bortezomib; C, cyclophosphamide; d, dex, dexamethasone; T, thalidomide; R, lenalidomide; K, carfilzomib; Poma, pomalidomide.

It is currently a matter of debate whether patients with smoldering (S)MM should receive therapy with the aim of preventing the progression to symptomatic MM and the associated morbidity. Two randomized trials demonstrated the benefit of lenalidomide, with or without dexamethasone, in delaying the time to progression to active MM versus observation; importantly, the longer follow-up of the Spanish trial allowed for the detection of an OS advantage for lenalidomide-treated patients [51]. In this setting, a highly targeted therapy with a good safety profile stands out as an ideal option. In the phase II CENTAURUS trial, single-agent daratumumab resulted in an ORR of 56% in high-risk SMM patients, and median PFS was NR after a median follow-up of 26 months [52,53]. The randomized phase III AQUILA study is currently comparing daratumumab administered for 3 years versus standard observation in high-risk SMM (NCT03301220).

One of the limitations to the use of daratumumab is its long infusion time (3.5 h). To deal with this issue, a shorter infusion schedule was tested—daratumumab was administered over a 90 min infusion at the usual dose (16 mg/kg) from the third infusion onward, without increasing the risk for infusion-related reactions (IRRs) or further short-term AEs [54]. A game changer in this setting will be the possibility of delivering daratumumab subcutaneously over a short period of time. The PAVO study explored subcutaneous daratumumab in combination with the recombinant human hyaluronidase PH20 enzyme (rHuPH20), which allowed for the reaching and maintaining of a high-serum concentration of the mAb [55]. At the end of phase Ib of the study, a flat dose of 1800 mg was recommended on the basis of pharmacokinetics, safety (all-grade IRRs 25%), and efficacy data (ORR 42%).

Isatuximab

Isatuximab (SAR 650984) is an anti-CD38 immunoglobulin G (IgG)-k chimeric monoclonal antibody that, besides having the same mechanisms of action of daratumumab, holds a unique direct proapoptotic effect independent from the Fc cross-linking [56,57]. Results of the main clinical trials are summarized in Table 1.

Similarly to daratumumab, isatuximab showed a promising activity when administered as a single agent in heavily pre-treated MM patients [58] and has therefore been combined with different anti-MM compounds. A phase Ib trial combined isatuximab at different dose levels with Rd in heavily pretreated MM patients (5 median prior lines of therapy), of whom 68% had already received carfilzomib or pomalidomide and 82% were refractory to lenalidomide. ORR was 51% (and 52% in lenalidomide-refractory patients) and median PFS was 8.5 months. IRRs were the most common AEs related to isatuximab (56% of patients, mainly of grades 1–2 and limited to first infusions) [34]. Another phase Ib trial combined isatuximab with Pd in relapsed patients (3 median prior lines of therapy)—the ORR was 62% and the median PFS was 17.6 months [35]. For both combinations, the selected dose of isatuximab was 10 mg/kg for 4 weekly doses and every 2 weeks thereafter. Of notice, preliminary results of a phase Ib trial in which isatuximab was combined to Kd showed a promising 66% ORR [36].

The ongoing phase III ICARIA trial (NCT02990338) is comparing the triplet isatuximab-pomalidomide-dexamethasone (Isa-Pd) to Pd in 307 RRMM patients who had received at least 2 previous lines of therapy (median lines: 3 in both groups). After a median follow-up of 11.6 months, a consistent benefit in terms of ORR (60% vs. 35%, $p < 0.001$) and PFS (median PFS 11.5 vs. 6.5, HR 0.59, $p = 0.001$) for the triplet arm compared to the control group was shown. Subgroup analysis revealed that PFS benefit was also maintained in high-risk patients (median PFS 7.5 vs. 3.7 months, HR 0.66, 95% CI 0.30–1.28). The median OS was NR in either group, although a trend to improved OS was observed in the triplet arm (HR 0.687, 95% CI 0.461–1.023; $p = 0.06$) [37]. Regarding the safety profile, Isa-Pd induced a slightly higher rate of grade 3–4 infections (42.8% vs. 30.2%) and neutropenia (84.9% vs. 70.1%) [50]. The ongoing phase III IKEMA trial is evaluating the combination of isatuximab with Kd in RRMM patients (NCT03275285).

In transplant-ineligible NDMM patients, isatuximab (10 mg/kg) is being evaluated in a phase Ib trial in combination with VRd as induction (4 cycles) followed by maintenance with Isa-Rd. Preliminary results showed an ORR of 93%, with 38.5% of patients achieving MRD negativity [47]. Another phase Ib trial is evaluating induction with 12 cycles of isatuximab (10/20 mg/kg) plus bortezomib-cyclophosphamide-dexamethasone (VCd), followed by maintenance with single-agent isatuximab in a similar patient population. The ORR was 87%, whereas data on MRD status and PFS are not yet available [48].

In order to improve the poor prognosis of high-risk patients, a phase Ib trial that was specifically designed for high-risk NDMM patients is currently testing a quadruplet regimen combining isatuximab-carfilzomib-lenalidomide-dexamethasone (GMMG-CONCEPT trial [59]).

Finally, the phase III IMROZ study is currently comparing the quadruplet isatuximab-VRd (Isa-VRd) to VRd as upfront treatment for transplant-ineligible patients (NCT03319667). Another ongoing trial is comparing the quadruplet Isa-VRd to isatuximab-VCd (Isa-VCd) in transplant-ineligible patients at diagnosis (NCT02513186).

MOR202 and TAK-079

MOR202 and TAK-079 are two anti-CD38 mAbs under development. In preliminary trials, MOR202 proved to be effective in combination with IMiDs; as expected, as this agent does not seem to induce CDC, a low rate of IRRs was observed (10%) [60,61]. In detail, the ORR was 28% in patients receiving MOR202 plus dexamethasone, which increased up to 65% in those receiving MOR202 plus

Rd and to 43% in those receiving MOR202 with Pd. However, further development of MOR202 has been discontinued in the United States and Europe. Subcutaneous TAK-079 is currently being tested in preliminary clinical trials on RRMM patients as monotherapy (NCT03439280) and in combination with standard regimens Rd or VRd (NCT03984097). We still need to further define the role of newer anti-CD38 mAbs in the treatment scenario for MM, where daratumumab and isatuximab have proven high efficacy and manageability.

2.2. Anti-Signaling Lymphocytic Activation Molecule Family 7 (SLAMF7) Monoclonal Antibodies

2.2.1. Rationale

Signaling lymphocytic activation molecule family 7 (SLAMF7 or CS1) is a cell surface glycoprotein whose expression is essentially restricted to NK cells and both normal and abnormal plasma cells, with 95% of myeloma plasma cells being SLAMF7-positive [62]. In plasma cells and MM cells, the SLAMF7 pathway promotes cell growth and survival, as well as the interaction with the bone marrow micro-environment. Its highly selective expression on plasma cells makes SLAMF7 an optimal target for mAbs.

2.2.2. Clinical Development

Elotuzumab is a humanized IgG-1 monoclonal antibody targeting SLAMF7 that promotes NK-mediated ADCC, directly activates NK cells and interferes with the MM cell adhesion to the bone marrow stromal cells [63–65]. Elotuzumab showed no clinically meaningful activity when administered as a single agent—in a phase I dose-escalating study, the best response achieved by RRMM patients treated at different doses of elotuzumab was stable disease (SD, 26%) [66] (Table 3).

Table 3. Results of the main clinical trials with anti-signaling lymphocytic activation molecule family 7 (SLAMF7) monoclonal antibody elotuzumab.

Study	Phase	Number of Patients	Median Previous Line	Regimen	ORR	Median PFS (Months)	Median OS (Months)
NCT00425347 [66]	I	35	5	Elo (0.5–20 mg/kg)	0	NA	NA
ELOQUENT-2 [67,68]	III	321	2	Elo-Rd vs. Rd	79% vs. 66%	19.4 vs.14.9	48 vs. 40
ELOQUENT-3 [69]	II	117	3	Elo-Poma-dex vs. Pd	53%vs.26%	10.3 vs. 4.7	NA
NCT00726869 [70]	I	28	2	Elo-V	48%	9.5	NA
NCT01478048 [71]	II	152	NA	Elo-Vd vs. Vd	66% vs. 63%	9.7 vs. 6.9	2-year OS 73% vs. 66%

Abbreviations: Elo, elotuzumab; ORR, overall response rate; PFS, progression-free survival; OS, overall survival; d, dex, dexamethasone; R, lenalidomide; Poma, pomalidomide; V, bortezomib; NR, not reached; NA, not yet available.

Preclinical data showed a synergistic activity of elotuzumab with IMiDs, the latter altering cytokine production and enhancing the activity of NK cells, the main target of elotuzumab immune activity. Promising results in terms of efficacy and tolerability were observed combining elotuzumab with Rd in phase I and II studies, thus providing the rationale for the phase III study ELOQUENT-2, which compared elotuzumab-Rd (Elo-Rd) to Rd in RRMM patients that were not refractory to lenalidomide [67,68,72]. In this study, elotuzumab was administered at the dose of 10 mg/kg and treatment was continued until progression or intolerance [66]. The triplet regimen containing elotuzumab proved to be more effective than Rd in terms of both PFS (19.4 vs. 14.9 months, HR 0.70, $p < 0.001$) and OS (48 vs. 40 months), without adding significant toxicity [73,74]. Patients at first relapse after a remission duration >3.5 years obtained the greater PFS advantage with Elo-Rd [75], showing that the greatest benefit with Elo-Rd could be obtained in patients with a slow and indolent progression. Elo-Rd is currently approved by both the FDA and EMA for the treatment of RRMM patients after 1 line of therapy.

The synergistic activity between elotuzumab and IMiDs prompted the investigators to test elotuzumab both in the upfront setting in combination with lenalidomide and at relapse with the third-generation IMiD pomalidomide [76]. The ongoing phase III study ELOQUENT-1, whose results are not yet available, enrolled NDMM patients ineligible for high-dose melphalan and ASCT in order to investigate the benefit of the addition of elotuzumab to the standard doublet Rd, possibly establishing a new standard of care in this setting.

In the randomized phase II ELOQUENT-3 trial, the addition of elotuzumab to Pd in RRMM patients significantly increased the ORR (53% vs. 26%) and prolonged median PFS (10.3 vs. 4.7 months, HR 0.54, $p = 0.008$), as compared to Pd alone. Again, the safety profiles of the two arms of the study were overlapping, meaning that elotuzumab did not add significant toxicity to Pd [69]. On this basis, in 2018 the FDA approved the triplet elotuzumab-Pd for the treatment of RRMM patients who had received at least 2 prior regimens including lenalidomide and a PI.

In preclinical models, elotuzumab activity was potentiated by bortezomib, which makes myeloma cells more vulnerable to NK-mediated lysis [77]. This combination was subsequently tested in clinical trials. In a phase I study on RRMM patients, elotuzumab was combined with bortezomib, showing an ORR of 48% and a median time to progression of 9.5 months [70]. The triplet elotuzumab-Vd (Elo-Vd, with elotuzumab administered at 10 mg/kg) was subsequently compared to Vd in a phase II trial on 152 RRMM patients, half of which had already received bortezomib in previous lines of therapy. ORR was similar between the two groups (66% vs. 63%), and a slight PFS advantage was observed in the triplet arm that nonetheless did not reach statistical significance (median, 9.7 vs. 6.9 months, HR 0.72, $p = 0.09$) [71]. The most common grade ≥3 AEs were infections (Elo-Vd 21% vs. Vd 13%) and thrombocytopenia (Elo-Vd 9% vs. Vd 17%). Because elotuzumab elicits its action by binding its Fc portion to the Fc gamma receptor III on NK cells, different allelic variants of the receptor were analyzed to evaluate possible predictors of elotuzumab efficacy. In this study, patients homozygous for the high-affinity Fc gamma receptor IIIa (FcγRIIIa) V allele showed longer PFS as compared to patients homozygous for the low-affinity allele. Considering the number of treatment options currently approved, the availability of a predictor of response could help clinicians in the choice of the most appropriate treatment.

Elotuzumab-Rd has also been investigated as a prevention strategy in high-risk SMM. In a phase II study (NCT02279394), patients received 8 cycles of elotuzumab-Rd and were subsequently allowed to continue with elotuzumab and lenalidomide maintenance until progression to symptomatic MM [78]. Preliminary data showed an ORR of 84% with no patients progressing at MM at the present follow-up of 29 months. Grade 3–4 toxicities included neutropenia (16%) and infections (12%), mainly related to lenalidomide. Again, single-agent elotuzumab did not show any clinical activity when in the setting of SMM [79].

Of interest, the rate of IRRs observed with elotuzumab—which were mostly mild in nature (grades 1–2) and rarely leading to treatment discontinuation—was definitely lower (10%) than that observed with other mAbs, making elotuzumab-based combinations appealing options for the treatment of frail patients [80].

Numerous studies are currently ongoing with elotuzumab-based combinations, such as elotuzumab-VRd (Elo-VRd, NCT02375555), elotuzumab-KRd (Elo-KRd, NCT02969837) and elotuzumab plus pomalidomide-bortezomib-dexamethasone (NCT02718833).

2.3. Anti-Programmed Death 1 (PD-1) Monoclonal Antibodies

2.3.1. Rationale

The programmed death 1 (PD-1) receptor is a transmembrane glycoprotein expressed on antigen-activated T cells and B cells. The binding of PD-1 ligands (PD-1-L1 and PD-1-L2) on PD-1 receptor results in the downregulation of immune T cell functions [81]. Preclinical data showed that PD-1/L1 is highly expressed on myeloma cells and, at variable levels, on normal plasma cells. It is also expressed at high levels on dendritic cells in the myeloma microenvironment [82,83]. Moreover, T cells derived from myeloma patients showed higher rates of PD-1 expression as compared to T cells from healthy donors, suggesting that the PD-1/PD-L1 pathway plays an important role in the immune escape of myeloma cells. Given these premises, targeting PD-1 and PD-L1 with monoclonal antibodies seems to be a promising strategy for the treatment of MM.

2.3.2. Clinical Development

Monoclonal antibodies directed against the PD-1/PD-L1 pathway can be divided into molecules targeting PD-1 (e.g., pembrolizumab and cemiplimab) and molecules targeting PD-L1 (e.g., durvalumab). Pembrolizumab monotherapy did not show efficacy as a single agent in 30 heavily pretreated myeloma patients (4 median prior lines of therapy) [84]. Pembrolizumab was subsequently combined with immunomodulatory agents, as preclinical data suggested that IMiDs could contribute to the downregulation of the PD-1/PD-L1 pathway [85]. In phase II trials, ORR was 50% in RRMM patients receiving pembrolizumab plus Rd and 60% in patients receiving pembrolizumab plus Pd [86]. However, in 2017, following the preliminary results of the two randomized phase III trials KEYNOTE 185 (pembrolizumab-Rd vs. Rd) and KEYNOTE 183 (pembrolizumab-Pd vs. Pd), the FDA prompted the discontinuation of any further investigations of these combinations, in light of the increased risk of death for patients in the pembrolizumab group versus the control group (HR for OS in pembrolizumab-Pd vs. Pd 1.61; HR for OS in pembrolizumab-Rd vs. Rd 2.06) [87,88]. The main concern with this combination is indeed the increased risk of enhancing immune-mediated toxicity, resulting in various AEs, such as dermatologic, pulmonary, cardiac, gastrointestinal and hepatic toxicities. These results questioned the utility of anti-PD-1 mAbs in MM, at least in combination with IMiDs. Different molecules are currently under evaluation in combination with other agents. The anti-PD-1 cemiplimab is being evaluated in a phase I/II trial in combination with isatuximab (NCT03194867), whereas durvalumab is being tested in combination with daratumumab (NCT03000452). However, the future role of this class of molecules in the treatment of MM remains debated.

3. Antibody Drug Conjugates

3.1. Rationale

Antibody drug conjugates (ADCs) are monoclonal antibodies bound by a chemical linker to a cytotoxic compound directed against surface antigens of the targeted cells. ADCs selectively target cells expressing their target antigen and are then internalized releasing the cytotoxic component through lysosome degradation, causing cell death. This targeted delivery limits the systemic exposure to the cytotoxic compound, sparing the non-malignant cells and tissues that do not express the target antigen, consequently limiting its off-target toxic effects [89,90]. In the past few years, interest has been raised around ADCs for the treatment of lymphoid malignancies, with brentuximab vedotin being the first agent of this class to receive FDA and EMA approval for the treatment of relapsed/refractory Hodgkin lymphoma and anaplastic large cell lymphoma in 2011–2012 [91,92]. In MM, ADCs showed preclinical activity in in vitro and in xenograft models and are currently under evaluation in clinical trials for relapsed MM patients [93–95]. One of the main challenges with ADCs is the choice of the most appropriate surface antigens to be targeted, which should be highly expressed only on malignant cells and not on normal tissues. Several target antigens have been identified on plasma cells: CD56, CD138, CD74, Fc receptor-like 5 and B cell maturation antigen (BCMA) [96]; of these, CD56 is expressed only on MM cells, with no expression on normal plasma cells, whereas other antigens are expressed on both malignant and non-malignant plasma cells, although at different levels [97]. The cytotoxic compound is typically a small molecular weight toxin with potent activity at low concentrations. Such molecules, usually not employed for systemic chemotherapy due to their excessive toxicity, can cause cell death due to two different mechanisms: cell cycle interference through microtubules inhibitions and DNA damage. Maytansinoid derivatives are microtubule inhibitors, including DM1 (emtansine and mertansine), DM4 (soravtansine and ravtansine) and auristatin derivatives (including monomethyl-auristatin E (MMAE, vedotin) and monomethyl auristatin F (MMAF, mafodotin)) [98–101]. Calicheamicins, duocarymycins and pyrrolobenzodiazepine dimmers are DNA-damaging agents [102,103].

3.2. Clinical Development

Table 4 summarizes the results of the main studies with ADCs in MM.

Table 4. Results of preliminary clinical trials with antibody-drug conjugates (ADCs).

Study	Phase	ADC	Target	Cytotoxic Agent	Respinse	Key Toxicities (G3–4)
NCT02064387 [104–106]	I	GSK2857916	BCMA	MMAF	ORR 60% PFS 12 m	Thrombocyotpenia 35% Corneal events 14%
NCT01001442 [107]	I	Indatuximab-ravtansine	CD138	DM4	ORR 6% PFS 3 m OS 26 m	Fatigue (7%) Anemia (7%) Diarrhea (4%)
NCT01638936 [108]		Indatuximab-ravtansine + Rd or + Poma-dex	CD138	DM4	ORR 77% PFS 16.4 m ORR 79% PFS NR	Diarrhea Fatigue Nausea
NCT00991562 [109]	I	Lorvotuzumab-mertansine	CD56	DM1	ORR 6% PFS 6.5 m	Peripheral neuropathy (5.3%)
NCT01101594 [110]	I	Milatuzumab-doxorubicin	CD74	Doxorubicin	ORR 0%	Anemia (4%) Back pain (4%) CRS (4%)

Abbreviations: R, lenalidomide; d, dex, dexamethasone; ORR, overall response rate; PFS, progression-free survival; OS, overall survival; NR, not reached; CRS, cytokine release syndrome; G, grade; MMAF, monomethyl auristatin F; BCMA, B cell maturation antigen.

In 2018, the results of a first in-human phase I study investigating GSK2857916, a BCMA-targeting mAb conjugated to the antimitotic agent monomethyl auristatin F (MMAF), in 73 RRMM patients were published. BCMA, a transmembrane receptor required for B cell maturation, was chosen as an optimal target, as it is expressed almost exclusively on MM cells and plasma cells [104–106]. In the dose-escalation phase of the study, 38 patients received escalating doses of IV GSK2857916 (0.03–4.6 mg/kg) every 3 weeks. In the dose-expansion phase of the study, 35 patients received the recommended phase II dose of GSK2857916 (3.4 mg/kg) every 3 weeks until progression. Among heavily pre-treated patients, GSK2857916 induced an objective response in 60% of them, with 15% of patients achieving a CR or a stringent CR (sCR). Remarkably, the ORR in patients previously treated with anti-CD38 mAbs and refractory to both IMiDs and PIs was 38%. Responses were rapid (median time to response 1.2 months) and durable (median duration of response 14.3 months). Overall, median PFS was 12 months; median PFS was 7.9 months in double-refractory patients (to IMiDs and PIs) and 6.2 months in double-refractory patients with prior daratumumab. The most common treatment-related toxicities were thrombocytopenia (63%; grades 3–4: 26%) and corneal events in terms of blurred vision and photophobia (51%; grades 3–4: 3%). Ocular toxicity was mainly limited to grades 1–2 and was reversible and easily manageable with dose reductions (51% of patients) [104,106]. Because GSK285791 showed high ORR in patients previously treated with anti-CD38 mAbs, a phase I/II clinical trial exploring its efficacy as monotherapy in patients with previous exposure to daratumumab/isatuximab has recently completed enrollment and results will soon be available (NCT03525678). Ongoing trials are evaluating its safety and efficacy in combination with pembrolizumab (NCT03848845), pomalidomide (NCT03715478), and lenalidomide versus bortezomib (NCT03544281).

Indatuximab-ravtansine (BT062) is an anti-CD138 IgG4 monoclonal antibody that delivers the microtubule inhibitor maytansinoid ravtansine to CD138-positive cells. CD138 is a transmembrane protein receptor upregulated by myeloma cells. BT062 monotherapy was evaluated in 67 heavily pretreated RRMM patients (median previous therapies 7, range 1–15). The most common grade 3–4 toxicities were fatigue (7%), anemia (7%), and diarrhea (4%). At the maximum tolerated dose (MTD) of BT062 (140 mg/m^2), 62% of patients achieved SD, whereas an objective response was observed in 5% of patients only. Median PFS and OS were 3 and 26 months, respectively [107]. BT062 is currently under evaluation in combination with lenalidomide or pomalidomide plus dexamethasone in RRMM patients. In patients receiving BT062 + lenalidomide (n = 47), ORR was 77% and median PFS was 16.4 months, whereas in those receiving the ADC in combination with pomalidomide (n = 17) ORR was 79% and median PFS was NR after 7 months of follow-up. These triplets were well tolerated, with main AEs being fatigue and diarrhea [108].

Lorvotuzumab-mertansine (IMGN901) is an anti-CD56 mAb linked to the maytansinoid mertansine, which inhibits microtubules assembly interfering with cell cycle and therefore causing cell death. A phase I trial enrolling 37 heavily pre-treated patients (78% had ≥3 lines of therapy) with CD56+ RRMM explored the safety and efficacy of single-agent IMGN901. The MTD was established at 112 mg/m^2. Forty-three percent of patients experienced SD, 6% PR, and no patient reached a very good (VG)PR or better, with a median PFS of 6.5 months. The toxicity profile was manageable and drug discontinuation due to AEs was observed in 24% of patients, with peripheral neuropathy (grades 3–4: 5.3%) being the most common toxicity leading to discontinuation [109]. IMGN901 is also being evaluated in combination with Rd. Preliminary reports showed an ORR of 56%, including 2 CRs and 8 VGPRs. The most common toxicity was peripheral neuropathy, although no grade 3–4 events occurred at the MTD of 75 mg/m^2 [111].

ADCs, particularly GSK285791, displayed a promising efficacy among heavily pre-treated patients. Their unique mechanism of action and preliminary efficacy data make these drugs an appealing treatment option in patients who have become refractory to IMiDs, PIs, and anti-CD38. Furthermore, the lack of cross-resistance with currently approved agents also prompts their investigation in the earlier phase of the disease, such as in the context of a consolidation strategy in high-risk patients or those MRD-positive after the induction/transplant phases.

Other compounds are under preliminary evaluation in MM. CD74, a transmembrane glycoprotein expressed in more than 90% of B cell malignancies, is the target of the ADC milatuzumab-doxorubicin (of hLL1-DOX) [110]. In a preliminary study, the ADC proved to be well tolerated, with SD being the best response achieved (26% patients) with this agent used as monotherapy for RRMM patients [112]. Preclinical results showing synergistic activity of hLL1-DOX with PIs and IMiDs provide the biological rationale for the evaluation of this ADC in combination with other agents.

4. Bispecific T Cell Engagers

Bispecific monoclonal antibodies are engineered molecules meant to redirect immune effector cells, mainly T and NK cells, to tumor cells, thus restoring the immune suppressor activity of the immune system against neoplastic cells. Bispecific T cell engager molecules are a class of bispecific antibodies combining the minimal binding domains (variable fragments (Fv), single chains) of two different monoclonal antibodies on one polypeptide chain [113]. They are characterized by a small size, allowing optimal proximity between the engaged T cell and the target tumor cell; for this very reason, they are active at low concentrations, as compared to bispecific antibodies. Bispecific antibodies usually link the invariant part of CD3 of the T cell receptor (TCR) on T cells and a tumor-specific antigen, thus leading to T cell activation and proliferation and tumor cell apoptosis [114]. The first approved bispecific T cell engager was the anti-CD19 blinatumomab for the treatment of RR B cell acute lymphoblastic leukemia [115].

Among potential targets on plasma cells, BCMA, CD38 and SLAMF7 have been chosen to design anti-MM bispecific antibodies [23,116], with BCMA representing the most promising target. Another potential target due to its high expression on PC is G-protein coupled receptor C family 5D (GPRC5D), whose function is still unclear [117,118].

Clinical Development

AMG420 is an anti-BCMA bispecific T cell engager that is currently being evaluated in the first in-human dose escalation trial enrolling RRMM patients (4 median prior lines of therapy). AMG420 was administered as a continuous intravenous infusion due to its short half-life at doses ranging from 0.2 to 800 mcg/die. At the MTD of 400 mcg/day, the ORR was 70%, with 5/10 patients obtaining MRD-negative sCRs (10^{-4}) [119]. Dose-limiting toxicities were cytokine release syndrome (CRS, 1 patient) and peripheral neuropathy (2 patients). Only 1 grade 3 CRS was observed, and no grade 3–4 AEs related to the central nervous system were registered at the MTD. Another anti-BCMA BiTE®, AMG 701, has a longer half-life (112 h), thus allowing weekly short-term infusion. AMG 701 is currently being investigated in the first phase I trial [120].

BiTEs® currently under investigation are listed in Table 5.

Table 5. Bispecific T cell-engaging agents (BiTEs®) for the treatment of multiple myeloma.

ClinicalTrials.Gov ID	Agent	Target
NCT02514239	AMG 420	BCMA
NCT03287908	AMG 701	BCMA
NCT03486067	CC-93269	BCMA
NCT03145181	JNJ-64007957	BCMA
NCT03269136	PF-06863135	BCMA
NCT03761108	REGN5458	BCMA
NCT03399799	JNJ-64407564	GPRC5D
NCT03309111	GBR 1342	CD38

Abbreviations: BCMA, B cell maturation antigen; CPRC5D, G-protein coupled receptor C family 5D.

5. Conclusions and Future Directions

Immunotherapy, and in particular mAbs, is no longer an appealing future perspective, but rather a valuable present therapeutic option for MM patients—having demonstrated to induce a response where conventional agents had failed—to increase the depth of response obtained with standard regimens acting in synergy with them and, ultimately, to prolong both PFS and OS. The 'guiding star' in this treatment landscape is definitely the anti-CD38 mAb, which rapidly turned from being a valid alternative for RRMM patients without further viable therapeutic options to being the backbone of virtually all present and future combinations adopted as frontline therapies. However, given the different combinations of both daratumumab and isatuximab with backbone therapies (available or under evaluation), we still need to define which anti-CD38 mAb should be used considering the unavailability of data on the superiority of one over the other. Another open issue is as to what could be the effectiveness of re-treatment with the same, or a different, CD38 mAb. Arguably, this last question will be answered in the near future, thanks to the increasing use of anti-CD38 mAb combinations in early lines. These issues are particularly challenging considering the wide heterogeneity of myeloma cell populations [121]. Immunotherapy seems to be a potential strategy for targeting virtually all tumor subclones, as effector mechanisms rely on the patient immune system. Ongoing studies are exploring the different potential mechanisms of resistance to anti-CD38 mAbs, as well as how to overcome them. Lower basal levels of the target antigen have been proposed as a possible mechanism of intrinsic resistance to mAbs [122,123]. Regarding daratumumab, the downregulation of CD38 on cell surfaces could partially explain the loss of response to mAb therapy [124]. Interestingly, myeloma cells exposed to isatuximab and MOR202 did not show such a downregulation [125,126]. An intriguing way to overcome the acquired resistance derived from antigen downregulation could be the addition of molecules able to re-induce CD38 expression on cell surface, such as all-trans retinoic acid (ATRA) or panobinostat [127,128]. Finally, other proposed mechanisms of resistance under evaluation include the modification of the expression of adhesion molecules and the overexpression of complement inhibitors. In the context of the currently available anti-CD38 combinations, the role of anti-SLAMF7 mAb-based combinations is unclear—both anti-CD38 and anti-SLAMF7 antibodies have been combined with the same backbones (Rd, Pd, Vd); both anti-CD38 and anti-SLAMF7 mAbs showed encouraging efficacy data even in high-risk patients, but not substantial enough to suggest an ability to completely overcome their adverse prognoses; and, finally, both mAbs have a very good safety profile. Studies showing the better efficacy of one mAb combination over the other are currently lacking. The role of both mAbs in the treatment of SMM also needs to be defined—their good safety profiles make them good candidates for the treatment of a still asymptomatic disease, but their efficacy and the possibility to improve OS still need to be shown. ADCs and BiTEs® are fascinating constructs potentially able to either carry toxic compounds or redirect T cells against MM cells in a very specific way, thus limiting off-target toxicities. The preliminary results obtained with single-agent ADCs or BiTEs® in heavily pre-treated patients are by far exceeding expectations, especially if compared to the results obtained with the currently available single-agent drugs. Future studies will shed light on their role in the treatment of MM patients and on their efficacy when used earlier in the course of the disease; they will also explore how to improve their feasibility and treatment compliance, especially in relation to the continuous intravenous infusion characteristic of the BiTEs® evaluated in MM thus far. In this field, the compounds showing the most encouraging preclinical results are bispecific antibodies with extended half-life such as the anti-BCMAs AMG701 and PF3135, which would allow a weekly administration [129,130]. Moreover, we still need to decipher the exact mechanisms of resistance and how to revert them, as well as the best drug-partners to enhance their efficacy in different settings. We have to devise the proper antigen selection and payload choice that will be critical for their success in the treatment of MM. MAbs can also be conjugated with radioisotopes in order to increase the antitumor effect of the molecules. Daratumumab has been combined with different radionuclides (e.g., actinium-225), resulting in an increased tumoricidal effect besides its Fc-effector functions in preclinical models [131]. Bispecific pretargeted radiolabeled antibodies showed an even greater biodistribution to tumor cells and, in future, can represent an appealing approach for the treatment of MM, especially for heavily pretreated patients who usually remain sensitive to radiation [132]. Regarding the use of mAbs, another field of interest is the use of radiolabeled antibodies for imaging assessment with immuno-positron emission tomography (immuno-PET) [133]. Indeed, surface antigens expressed on myeloma cells could be a target for radiolabeled mAbs, which would allow highly specific tumor detection and precise response assessment. Daratumumab has already been labeled to different positron emitters showing excellent targeting in preclinical models [134–136]. With these premises, immuno-PET could represent a useful tool for imaging assessment and also for guiding treatment strategies, as this technique could potentially be used to predict the effectiveness of mAb therapy.

Another issue is timing, that is to say, the most appropriate phase of treatment or disease in which these different classes of drugs should be used—if at diagnosis, at the evidence of MRD persistence in an effort to eradicate a resistant clone, or at relapse once conventional treatments have failed. In a highly competitive setting, with few validated targets (CS1, CD38, BCMA) and many different technologies (ADC, BiTEs®, chimeric antigen receptor [CAR] T cells), both preclinical and clinical studies are critical to identify the most promising compounds. Along with the refinement of the existing drug regimens and treatment strategies and the development of new ones, a better understanding of the role of the immune system in the pathogenesis of MM will certainly be necessary.

Author Contributions: Substantial contributions to the conception or design, F.B., R.M., M.B., and F.G.; acquisition, analysis, or interpretation of data, F.B., R.M., M.B., and F.G.; first draft, F.B., R.M., and F.G.; supervision, M.B. and F.G.; critical revision for important intellectual content, F.B., R.M., M.B., and F.G.; final approval of the version to be published, R.M., F.B., M.B., and F.G.; agreement to be accountable for all aspects of the work in ensuring that questions related to the accuracy or integrity of any part of the work are appropriately investigated and resolved, F.B., R.M., M.B., and F.G. All authors have read and agreed to the published version of the manuscript.

Funding: This research received no external funding.

Conflicts of Interest: F.B. declares no competing financial interests. R.M. has received honoraria from Amgen, Celgene, Takeda, and Janssen, and served on the advisory boards for Janssen. M.B. has received honoraria from Sanofi, Celgene, Amgen, Janssen, Novartis, Bristol-Myers Squibb, and AbbVie, and has received research funding from Sanofi, Celgene, Amgen, Janssen, Novartis, Bristol-Myers Squibb, and Mundipharma. F.G. has received honoraria from Amgen, Bristol-Myers Squibb, Celgene, Janssen, and Takeda, and served on the advisory boards for Amgen, Bristol-Myers Squibb, Celgene, Janssen, Roche, Takeda, and AbbVie.

References

1. Turesson, I.; Velez, R.; Kristinsson, S.Y.; Landgren, O. Patterns of Improved Survival in Patients with Multiple Myeloma in the Twenty-First Century: A Population-Based Study. *J. Clin. Oncol.* **2010**, *28*, 830–834. [CrossRef] [PubMed]
2. Kristinsson, S.Y.; Anderson, W.F.; Landgren, O. Improved long-term survival in multiple myeloma up to the age of 80 years. *Leukemia* **2014**, *28*, 1346–1348. [CrossRef] [PubMed]
3. Howlader, N.; Noone, A.; Krapcho, M.; Miller, D.; Brest, A.; Yu, M.; Ruhl, J.; Tatalovich, Z.; Mariotto, A.; Lewis, D.; et al. *SEER Cancer Statistics Review (CSR), 1975-2016*; Based on November 2018 SEER Data Submission, Posted to the SEER Web Site, April 2019; National Cancer Institute: Bethesda, MD, USA, 2019. Available online: https://seer.cancer.gov/csr/1975_2016/ (accessed on 19 December 2019).
4. Kumar, S.; Paiva, B.; Anderson, K.C.; Durie, B.; Landgren, O.; Moreau, P.; Munshi, N.; Lonial, S.; Bladé, J.; Mateos, M.-V.; et al. International Myeloma Working Group consensus criteria for response and minimal residual disease assessment in multiple myeloma. *Lancet. Oncol* **2016**, *17*, e328–e346. [CrossRef]
5. Attal, M.; Lauwers-Cances, V.; Hulin, C.; Leleu, X.; Caillot, D.; Escoffre, M.; Arnulf, B.; Macro, M.; Belhadj, K.; Garderet, L.; et al. Lenalidomide, Bortezomib, and Dexamethasone with Transplantation for Myeloma. *N. Engl. J. Med.* **2017**, *376*, 1311–1320. [CrossRef] [PubMed]
6. De Tute, R.M.; Rawstron, A.C.; Gregory, W.M.; Child, J.A.; Davies, F.E.; Bell, S.E.; Cook, G.; Szubert, A.J.; Drayson, M.T.; Jackson, G.H.; et al. Minimal residual disease following autologous stem cell transplant in myeloma: Impact on outcome is independent of induction regimen. *Haematologica* **2016**, *101*, e69–e71. [CrossRef]
7. Oliva, S.; Gambella, M.; Gilestro, M.; Muccio, V.E.; Gay, F.; Drandi, D.; Ferrero, S.; Passera, R.; Pautasso, C.; Bernardini, A.; et al. Minimal residual disease after transplantation or lenalidomidebased consolidation in myeloma patients: A prospective analysis. *Oncotarget* **2017**, *8*, 5924–5935. [CrossRef]
8. Gay, F.; Cerrato, C.; Petrucci, M.T.; Zambello, R.; Gamberi, B.; Ballanti, S.; Omedè, P.; Palmieri, S.; Troia, R.; Spada, S.; et al. Efficacy of carfilzomib lenalidomide dexamethasone (KRd) with or without transplantation in newly diagnosed myeloma according to risk status: Results from the forte trial. *J. Clin. Oncol.* **2019**, *37*, Abstract #8002 [ASCO 2019 Annual Meeting].
9. Paiva, B.; Cedena, M.T.; Puig, N.; Arana, P.; Vidriales, M.B.; Cordon, L.; Flores-Montero, J.; Gutierrez, N.C.; Martín-Ramos, M.L.; Martinez-Lopez, J.; et al. Minimal residual disease monitoring and immune profiling in multiple myeloma in elderly patients. *Blood* **2016**, *127*, 3165–3174. [CrossRef]
10. Rawstron, A.C.; Child, J.A.; de Tute, R.M.; Davies, F.E.; Gregory, W.M.; Bell, S.E.; Szubert, A.J.; Navarro-Coy, N.; Drayson, M.T.; Feyler, S.; et al. Minimal residual disease assessed by multiparameter flow cytometry in multiple myeloma: Impact on outcome in the Medical Research Council Myeloma IX Study. *J. Clin. Oncol.* **2013**, *31*, 2540–2547. [CrossRef]
11. Mateos, M.-V.; Dimopoulos, M.A.; Cavo, M.; Suzuki, K.; Jakubowiak, A.; Knop, S.; Doyen, C.; Lucio, P.; Nagy, Z.; Kaplan, P.; et al. Daratumumab plus Bortezomib, Melphalan, and Prednisone for Untreated Myeloma. *N. Engl. J. Med.* **2018**, *378*, 518–528. [CrossRef]
12. Munshi, N.C.; Avet-Loiseau, H.; Rawstron, A.C.; Owen, R.G.; Child, J.A.; Thakurta, A.; Sherrington, P.; Samur, M.K.; Georgieva, A.; Anderson, K.C.; et al. Association of Minimal Residual Disease With Superior Survival Outcomes in Patients With Multiple Myeloma: A Meta-analysis. *JAMA Oncol.* **2017**, *3*, 28–35. [CrossRef] [PubMed]
13. Giuliani, N.; Malavasi, F. Editorial: Immunotherapy in Multiple Myeloma. *Front. Immunol.* **2019**, *10*, 1945. [CrossRef] [PubMed]
14. Leo, R.; Boeker, M.; Peest, D.; Hein, R.; Bartl, R.; Gessner, J.E.; Seibach, J.; Wacker, G.; Deicher, H. Multiparameter analyses of normal and malignant human plasma cells: CD38++, CD56+, CD54+, cIg+ is the common phenotype of myeloma cells. *Ann. Hematol.* **1992**, *64*, 132–139. [CrossRef] [PubMed]

15. Malavasi, F.; Funaro, A.; Roggero, S.; Horenstein, A.; Calosso, L.; Mehta, K. Human CD38: A glycoprotein in search of a function. *Immunol. Today* **1994**, *15*, 95–97. [CrossRef]
16. Cagnetta, A.; Cea, M.; Calimeri, T.; Acharya, C.; Fulciniti, M.; Tai, Y.-T.; Hideshima, T.; Chauhan, D.; Zhong, M.Y.; Patrone, F.; et al. Intracellular NAD+ depletion enhances bortezomib-induced anti-myeloma activity. *Blood* **2013**, *122*, 1243–1255. [CrossRef] [PubMed]
17. Ausiello, C.M.; la Sala, A.; Ramoni, C.; Urbani, F.; Funaro, A.; Malavasi, F. Secretion of IFN-γ, IL-6, Granulocyte-Macrophage Colony-Stimulating Factor and IL-10 Cytokines after Activation of Human Purified T Lymphocytes upon CD38 Ligation. *Cell. Immunol.* **1996**, *173*, 192–197. [CrossRef]
18. Van de Donk, N.W.C.J. Immunomodulatory effects of CD38-targeting antibodies. *Immunol. Lett.* **2018**, *199*, 16–22. [CrossRef]
19. Casneuf, T.; Xu, X.S.; Adams, H.C.; Axel, A.E.; Chiu, C.; Khan, I.; Ahmadi, T.; Yan, X.; Lonial, S.; Plesner, T.; et al. Effects of daratumumab on natural killer cells and impact on clinical outcomes in relapsed or refractory multiple myeloma. *Blood Adv.* **2017**, *1*, 2105–2114. [CrossRef]
20. Wang, Y.; Zhang, Y.; Hughes, T.; Zhang, J.; Caligiuri, M.A.; Benson, D.M.; Yu, J. Fratricide of NK Cells in Daratumumab Therapy for Multiple Myeloma Overcome by Ex Vivo-Expanded Autologous NK Cells. *Clin. Cancer Res.* **2018**, *24*, 4006–4017. [CrossRef]
21. Overdijk, M.B.; Verploegen, S.; Bögels, M.; van Egmond, M.; van Bueren, J.J.L.; Mutis, T.; Groen, R.W.; Breij, E.; Martens, A.C.; Bleeker, W.K.; et al. Antibody-mediated phagocytosis contributes to the anti-tumor activity of the therapeutic antibody daratumumab in lymphoma and multiple myeloma. *MAbs* **2015**, *7*, 311–320. [CrossRef]
22. Lammerts van Bueren, J.; Jakobs, D.; Kaldenhoven, N.; Roza, M.; Hiddingh, S.; Meesters, J.; Voorhorst, M.; Gresnigt, E.; Wiegman, L.; Ortiz Buijsse, A.; et al. Direct in Vitro Comparison of Daratumumab with Surrogate Analogs of CD38 Antibodies MOR03087, SAR650984 and Ab79. *Blood* **2014**, *124*, Abstract #3474 [ASH 2014 56th Meeting].
23. Krejcik, J.; Casneuf, T.; Nijhof, I.S.; Verbist, B.; Bald, J.; Plesner, T.; Syed, K.; Liu, K.; van de Donk, N.W.C.J.; Weiss, B.M.; et al. Daratumumab depletes CD38+ immune regulatory cells, promotes T-cell expansion, and skews T-cell repertoire in multiple myeloma. *Blood* **2016**, *128*, 384–394. [CrossRef] [PubMed]
24. Chatterjee, S.; Daenthanasanmak, A.; Chakraborty, P.; Wyatt, M.W.; Dhar, P.; Selvam, S.P.; Fu, J.; Zhang, J.; Nguyen, H.; Kang, I.; et al. CD38-NAD+Axis Regulates Immunotherapeutic Anti-Tumor T Cell Response. *Cell Metab.* **2018**, *27*, 85–100. [CrossRef] [PubMed]
25. Van De Donk, N.W.; Adams, H.; Vanhoof, G.; Krejcik, J.; Van der Borght, K.; Casneuf, T.; Smets, T.; Axel, A.; Abraham, Y.; Ceulmans, H.; et al. Daratumumab in Combination with Lenalidomide Plus Dexamethasone Results in Persistent Natural Killer (NK) Cells with a Distinct Phenotype and Expansion of Effector Memory T-Cells in Pollux, a Phase 3 Randomized Study. *Blood* **2017**, *130*, Abstract #3124 [ASH 2017 58th Meeting].
26. Van de Donk, N.W.C.J.; Richardson, P.G.; Malavasi, F. CD38 antibodies in multiple myeloma: Back to the future. *Blood* **2018**, *131*, 13–29. [CrossRef] [PubMed]
27. Van Der Veer, M.S.; De Weers, M.; Van Kessel, B.; Bakker, J.M.; Wittebol, S.; Parren, P.W.H.I.; Lokhorst, H.M.; Mutis, T. The therapeutic human CD38 antibody daratumumab improves the anti-myeloma effect of newly emerging multi-drug therapies. *Blood Cancer J.* **2011**, *1*, e41. [CrossRef]
28. Usmani, S.Z.; Weiss, B.M.; Plesner, T.; Bahlis, N.J.; Belch, A.; Lonial, S.; Lokhorst, H.M.; Voorhees, P.M.; Richardson, P.G.; Chari, A.; et al. Clinical efficacy of daratumumab monotherapy in patients with heavily pretreated relapsed or refractory multiple myeloma. *Blood* **2016**, *128*, 37–44. [CrossRef]
29. Dimopoulos, M.A.; Oriol, A.; Nahi, H.; San-Miguel, J.; Bahlis, N.J.; Usmani, S.Z.; Rabin, N.; Orlowski, R.Z.; Komarnicki, M.; Suzuki, K.; et al. Daratumumab, Lenalidomide, and Dexamethasone for Multiple Myeloma. *N. Engl. J. Med.* **2016**, *375*, 1319–1331. [CrossRef]
30. Palumbo, A.; Chanan-Khan, A.; Weisel, K.; Nooka, A.K.; Masszi, T.; Beksac, M.; Spicka, I.; Hungria, V.; Munder, M.; Mateos, M.V.; et al. Daratumumab, Bortezomib, and Dexamethasone for Multiple Myeloma. *N. Engl. J. Med.* **2016**, *375*, 754–766. [CrossRef]
31. Spencer, A.; Lentzsch, S.; Weisel, K.; Avet-Loiseau, H.; Mark, T.M.; Spicka, I.; Masszi, T.; Lauri, B.; Levin, M.-D.; Bosi, A.; et al. Daratumumab plus bortezomib and dexamethasone versus bortezomib and dexamethasone in relapsed or refractory multiple myeloma: Updated analysis of CASTOR. *Haematologica* **2018**, *103*, 2079–2087. [CrossRef]

32. Chari, A.; Suvannasankha, A.; Fay, J.W.; Arnulf, B.; Kaufman, J.L.; Ifthikharuddin, J.J.; Weiss, B.M.; Krishnan, A.; Lentzsch, S.; Comenzo, R.; et al. Daratumumab plus pomalidomide and dexamethasone in relapsed and/or refractory multiple myeloma. *Blood* **2017**, *130*, 974–981. [CrossRef] [PubMed]
33. Chari, A.; Martinez-Lopez, J.; Mateos, M.-V.; Bladé, J.; Benboubker, L.; Oriol, A.; Arnulf, B.; Rodriguez-Otero, P.; Pineiro, L.; Jakubowiak, A.; et al. Daratumumab plus carfilzomib and dexamethasone in patients with relapsed or refractory multiple myeloma. *Blood* **2019**, *134*, 421–431. [CrossRef] [PubMed]
34. Martin, T.; Baz, R.; Benson, D.M.; Lendvai, N.; Wolf, J.; Munster, P.; Lesokhin, A.M.; Wack, C.; Charpentier, E.; Campana, F.; et al. A phase 1b study of isatuximab plus lenalidomide and dexamethasone for relapsed/refractory multiple myeloma. *Blood* **2017**, *129*, 3294–3303. [CrossRef] [PubMed]
35. Mikhael, J.; Richardson, P.; Usmani, S.Z.; Raje, N.; Bensinger, W.; Karanes, C.; Campana, F.; Kanagavel, D.; Dubin, F.; Liu, Q.; et al. A phase 1b study of isatuximab plus pomalidomide/dexamethasone in relapsed/refractory multiple myeloma. *Blood* **2019**, *134*, 123–133. [CrossRef] [PubMed]
36. Chari, A.; Richter, J.R.; Shah, N.; Wong, S.W.K.; Jagannath, S.; Cho, H.J.; Biran, N.; Wolf, J.; Parekh, S.S.; Munster, P.N.; et al. Phase I-b study of isatuximab + carfilzomib in relapsed and refractory multiple myeloma (RRMM). *J. Clin. Oncol.* **2018**, *36*, Abstract #8014 [ASCO 2018 Annual Meeting].
37. Attal, M.; Richardson, P.G.; Rajkumar, S.V.; San-Miguel, J.; Beksac, M.; Spicka, I.; Leleu, X.; Schjesvold, F.; Moreau, P.; Dimopoulos, M.A.; et al. Isatuximab plus pomalidomide and low-dose dexamethasone versus pomalidomide and low-dose dexamethasone in patients with relapsed and refractory multiple myeloma (ICARIA-MM): A randomised, multicentre, open-label, phase 3 study. *Lancet* **2019**, *394*, 2096–2107. [CrossRef]
38. Facon, T.; Kumar, S.; Plesner, T.; Orlowski, R.Z.; Moreau, P.; Bahlis, N.; Basu, S.; Nahi, H.; Hulin, C.; Quach, H.; et al. Daratumumab plus Lenalidomide and Dexamethasone for Untreated Myeloma. *N. Engl. J. Med.* **2019**, *380*, 2104–2115. [CrossRef]
39. Moreau, P.; Attal, M.; Hulin, C.; Arnulf, B.; Belhadj, K.; Benboubker, L.; Béné, M.C.; Broijl, A.; Caillon, H.; Caillot, D.; et al. Bortezomib, thalidomide, and dexamethasone with or without daratumumab before and after autologous stem-cell transplantation for newly diagnosed multiple myeloma (CASSIOPEIA): A randomised, open-label, phase 3 study. *Lancet* **2019**, *394*, 29–38. [CrossRef]
40. Voorhees, P.M.; Rodriguez, C.; Reeves, B.; Nathwani, N.; Costa, L.J.; Lutska, Y.; Hoehn, D.; Pei, H.; Ukropec, J.; Qi, M.; et al. Efficacy and Updated Safety Analysis of a Safety Run-in Cohort from Griffin, a Phase 2 Randomized Study of Daratumumab (Dara), Bortezomib (V), Lenalidomide (R), and Dexamethasone (D.; Dara-Vrd) Vs. Vrd in Patients (Pts) with Newly Diagnosed (ND) Multiple M. *Blood* **2018**, *132*, Abstract #151 [ASH 2018 59th Meeting].
41. Lonial, S.; Weiss, B.M.; Usmani, S.Z.; Singhal, S.; Chari, A.; Bahlis, N.J.; Belch, A.; Krishnan, A.; Vescio, R.A.; Mateos, M.V.; et al. Daratumumab monotherapy in patients with treatment-refractory multiple myeloma (SIRIUS): An open-label, randomised, phase 2 trial. *Lancet* **2016**, *387*, 1551–1560. [CrossRef]
42. Dimopoulos, M.A.; San-Miguel, J.; Belch, A.; White, D.; Benboubker, L.; Cook, G.; Leiba, M.; Morton, J.; Ho, P.J.; Kim, K.; et al. Daratumumab plus lenalidomide and dexamethasone versus lenalidomide and dexamethasone in relapsed or refractory multiple myeloma: Updated analysis of POLLUX. *Haematologica* **2018**, *103*, 2088–2096. [CrossRef] [PubMed]
43. San Miguel, J.; Weisel, K.; Moreau, P.; Lacy, M.; Song, K.; Delforge, M.; Karlin, L.; Goldschmidt, H.; Banos, A.; Oriol, A.; et al. Pomalidomide plus low-dose dexamethasone versus high-dose dexamethasone alone for patients with relapsed and refractory multiple myeloma (MM-003): A randomised, open-label, phase 3 trial. *Lancet Oncol.* **2013**, *14*, 1055–1066. [CrossRef]
44. Amgen Announces Phase 3 CANDOR Study Combining KYPROLIS®(carfilzomib) And DARZALEX®(daratumumab) Meets Primary Endpoint of Progression-Free Survival. Available online: https://www.amgen.com/media/news-releases/2019/09/amgen-announces-phase-3-candor-study-combining-kyprolis-carfilzomib-and-darzalex-daratumumab-meets-primary-endpoint-of-progressionfree-survival/ (accessed on 7 November 2019).
45. Sonneveld, P.; Attal, M.; Perrot, A.; Hulin, C.; Caillot, D.; Facon, T.; Leleu, X.; Belhadj-Merzoug, K.; Karlin, L.; Benboubker, L.; et al. Daratumumab Plus Bortezomib, Thalidomide, and Dexamethasone (D-VTd) in Transplant-eligible Newly Diagnosed Multiple Myeloma (NDMM): Subgroup Analysis of High-risk Patients (Pts) in CASSIOPEIA—International Myeloma Workshop (IMW) 2019 Abstract Book. 4 [Abstract #OAB–003]. Available online: http://imw2019boston.org/images/Abstracts/17th_IMW_Abstract_Book_FINAL_V2.pdf (accessed on 12 December 2019).

46. Sonneveld, P.; Broijl, A.; Gay, F.; Boccadoro, M.; Einsele, H.; Blade, J.; Dimopoulos, M.A.; Delforge, M.; Spencer, A.; Hajek, R.; et al. Bortezomib, lenalidomide, and dexamethasone (VRd) ± daratumumab (DARA) in patients (pts) with transplant-eligible (TE) newly diagnosed multiple myeloma (NDMM): A multicenter, randomized, phase III study (PERSEUS). *J. Clin. Oncol.* **2019**, *37*, Abstract #TPS8055 [ASCO 2019 Annual Meeting].
47. Ocio, E.M.; Otero, P.R.; Bringhen, S.; Oliva, S.; Nogai, A.; Attal, M.; Moreau, P.; Kanagavel, D.; Fitzmaurice, T.; Wu, J.; et al. Preliminary Results from a Phase I Study of Isatuximab (ISA) in Combination with Bortezomib, Lenalidomide, Dexamethasone (VRd) in Patients with Newly Diagnosed Multiple Myeloma (NDMM) Non-Eligible for Transplant. *Blood* **2018**, *132*, Abstract #595 [ASH 2018 60th Meeting].
48. Ocio, E.M.; Bringhen, S.; Oliva, S.; Rodriguez-Otero, P.; Kanagavel, D.; Oprea, C.; Wei, V.; Doroumian, S.; Martinez-Lopez, J. A Phase Ib Study of Isatuximab in Combination with Bortezomib, Cyclophosphamide, and Dexamethasone (VCDI) in Patients with Newly Diagnosed Multiple Myeloma Non-Eligible for Transplantation. *Blood* **2017**, *130*, Abstract #3160 [ASH 2017 59th Annual Meeting].
49. Orlowski, R.Z.; Goldschmidt, H.; Cavo, M.; Martin, T.G.; Paux, G.; Oprea, C.; Facon, T. Phase III (IMROZ) study design: Isatuximab plus bortezomib (V), lenalidomide (R), and dexamethasone (d) vs VRd in transplant-ineligible patients (pts) with newly diagnosed multiple myeloma (NDMM). *J. Clin. Oncol.* **2018**, *36*, Abstract #TPS8055 [ASCO 2018 Annual Meeting].
50. Richardson, P.G.; Attal, M.; Rajkumar, S.V.; San Miguel, J.; Beksac, M.; Spicka, I.; Leleu, X.; Schjesvold, F.; Moreau, P.; Dimopoulos, M.A.; et al. A phase III randomized, open label, multicenter study comparing isatuximab, pomalidomide, and low-dose dexamethasone versus pomalidomide and low-dose dexamethasone in patients with relapsed/refractory multiple myeloma (RRMM). *J. Clin. Oncol.* **2019**, *37*, Abstract #8004 [ASCO 2019 Annual Meeting].
51. Mateos, M.-V.; Hernández, M.-T.; Giraldo, P.; de la Rubia, J.; de Arriba, F.; López Corral, L.; Rosiñol, L.; Paiva, B.; Palomera, L.; Bargay, J.; et al. Lenalidomide plus dexamethasone for high-risk smoldering multiple myeloma. *N. Engl. J. Med.* **2013**, *369*, 438–447. [CrossRef] [PubMed]
52. Hofmeister, C.C.; Chari, A.; Cohen, Y.; Spencer, A.; Voorhees, P.M.; Estell, J.; Venner, C.P.; Sandhu, I.; Jenner, M.W.; Williams, C.; et al. Daratumumab Monotherapy for Patients with Intermediate or High-Risk Smoldering Multiple Myeloma (SMM): Centaurus, a Randomized, Open-Label, Multicenter Phase 2 Study. *Blood* **2017**, *130*, Abstract #510 [ASH 2017 59th Meeting].
53. Landgren, O.; Cavo, M.; Chari, A.; Cohen, Y.C.; Spencer, A.; Voorhees, P.M.; Estell, J.; Sandhu, I.; Jenner, M.; Williams, C.; et al. Updated Results from the Phase 2 Centaurus Study of Daratumumab (DARA) Monotherapy in Patients with Intermediate-Risk or High-Risk Smoldering Multiple Myeloma (SMM). *Blood* **2018**, *132*, Abstract #1994 [ASH 2018 60th Meeting].
54. Barr, H.; Dempsey, J.; Waller, A.; Huang, Y.; Williams, N.; Sharma, N.; Benson, D.M.; Rosko, A.E.; Efebera, Y.A.; Hofmeister, C.C. Ninety-minute daratumumab infusion is safe in multiple myeloma. *Leukemia* **2018**, *32*, 2495–2518. [CrossRef] [PubMed]
55. Chari, A.; Nahi, H.; Mateos, M.-V.; Lokhorst, H.M.; Kaufman, J.L.; Moreau, P.; Oriol, A.; Plesner, T.; Benboubker, L.; Hellemans, P.; et al. Subcutaneous Delivery of Daratumumab in Patients (pts) with Relapsed or Refractory Multiple Myeloma (RRMM): Pavo, an Open-Label, Multicenter, Dose Escalation Phase 1b Study. *Blood* **2017**, *130*, Abstract #838 [ASH 2017 59th Meeting].
56. Deckert, J.; Wetzel, M.-C.; Bartle, L.M.; Skaletskaya, A.; Goldmacher, V.S.; Vallee, F.; Zhou-Liu, Q.; Ferrari, P.; Pouzieux, S.; Lahoute, C.; et al. SAR650984, A Novel Humanized CD38-Targeting Antibody, Demonstrates Potent Antitumor Activity in Models of Multiple Myeloma and Other CD38+ Hematologic Malignancies. *Clin. Cancer Res.* **2014**, *20*, 4574–4583. [CrossRef]
57. Jiang, H.; Acharya, C.; An, G.; Zhong, M.; Feng, X.; Wang, L.; Dasilva, N.; Song, Z.; Yang, G.; Adrian, F.; et al. SAR650984 directly induces multiple myeloma cell death via lysosomal-associated and apoptotic pathways, which is further enhanced by pomalidomide. *Leukemia* **2016**, *30*, 399–408. [CrossRef] [PubMed]
58. Martin, T.; Strickland, S.; Glenn, M.; Charpentier, E.; Guillemin, H.; Hsu, K.; Mikhael, J. Phase I trial of isatuximab monotherapy in the treatment of refractory multiple myeloma. *Blood Cancer J.* **2019**, *9*, 41. [CrossRef] [PubMed]

59. Weisel, K.; Asemissen, A.M.; Schieferdecker, A.; Besemer, B.; Zago, M.; Mann, C.; Lutz, R.; Benner, A.; Tichy, D.; Bokemeyer, C.; et al. Isatuximab, Carfilzomib, Lenalidomide and Dexamethasone (I-KRd) in front-line treatment of high-risk Multiple Myeloma: Results of the Safety Run-In cohort in the phase II, multicenter GMMG-CONCEPT trial—International Myeloma Workshop (IMW), 2019 Abstract. 2019, 25–26 [Abstract #OAB–023]. Available online: http://imw2019boston.org/images/Abstracts/17th_IMW_Abstract_Book_FINAL_V2.pdf (accessed on 12 December 2019).
60. Raab, M.S.; Goldschmidt, H.; Agis, H.; Blau, I.W.; Einsele, H.; Engelhardt, M.; Ferstl, B.; Gramatzki, M.; Röllig, C.; Weisel, K.; et al. A phase I/IIa study of the human anti-CD38 antibody MOR202 (MOR03087) in relapsed or refractory multiple myeloma (rrMM). *J. Clin. Oncol.* **2015**, *33*, Abstract #8574 (ASCO 2015 Annual Meeting].
61. Raab, M.S.; Chatterjee, M.; Goldschmidt, H.; Agis, H.; Blau, I.; Einsele, H.; Engelhardt, M.; Ferstl, B.; Gramatzki, M.; Rollig, C.; et al. MOR202 with Low-Dose Dexamethasone (Dex) or Pomalidomide/Dex or Lenalidomide/Dex in Relapsed or Refractory Multiple Myeloma (RRMM): Primary Analysis of a Phase I/IIa, Multicenter, Dose-Escalation Study. *Blood* **2018**, *132*, Abstract #153 [ASH 2018 60th Meeting].
62. Hsi, E.D.; Steinle, R.; Balasa, B.; Szmania, S.; Draksharapu, A.; Shum, B.P.; Huseni, M.; Powers, D.; Nanisetti, A.; Zhang, Y.; et al. CS1, a potential new therapeutic antibody target for the treatment of multiple myeloma. *Clin. Cancer Res.* **2008**, *14*, 2775–2784. [CrossRef] [PubMed]
63. Pazina, T.; James, A.M.; MacFarlane, A.W.; Bezman, N.A.; Henning, K.A.; Bee, C.; Graziano, R.F.; Robbins, M.D.; Cohen, A.D.; Campbell, K.S. The anti-SLAMF7 antibody elotuzumab mediates NK cell activation through both CD16-dependent and –independent mechanisms. *Oncoimmunology* **2017**, *6*, e1339853. [CrossRef]
64. Collins, S.M.; Bakan, C.E.; Swartzel, G.D.; Hofmeister, C.C.; Efebera, Y.A.; Kwon, H.; Starling, G.C.; Ciarlariello, D.; Bhaskar, S.; Briercheck, E.L.; et al. Elotuzumab directly enhances NK cell cytotoxicity against myeloma via CS1 ligation: Evidence for augmented NK cell function complementing ADCC. *Cancer Immunol. Immunother.* **2013**, *62*, 1841–1849. [CrossRef]
65. Tai, Y.-T.; Dillon, M.; Song, W.; Leiba, M.; Li, X.-F.; Burger, P.; Lee, A.I.; Podar, K.; Hideshima, T.; Rice, A.G.; et al. Anti-CS1 humanized monoclonal antibody HuLuc63 inhibits myeloma cell adhesion and induces antibody-dependent cellular cytotoxicity in the bone marrow milieu. *Blood* **2008**, *112*, 1329–1337. [CrossRef]
66. Zonder, J.A.; Mohrbacher, A.F.; Singhal, S.; van Rhee, F.; Bensinger, W.I.; Ding, H.; Fry, J.; Afar, D.E.H.; Singhal, A.K. A phase 1, multicenter, open-label, dose escalation study of elotuzumab in patients with advanced multiple myeloma. *Blood* **2012**, *120*, 552–559. [CrossRef]
67. Lonial, S.; Vij, R.; Harousseau, J.-L.; Facon, T.; Moreau, P.; Mazumder, A.; Kaufman, J.L.; Leleu, X.; Tsao, L.C.; Westland, C.; et al. Elotuzumab in combination with lenalidomide and low-dose dexamethasone in relapsed or refractory multiple myeloma. *J. Clin. Oncol.* **2012**, *30*, 1953–1959. [CrossRef]
68. Richardson, P.G.; Jagannath, S.; Moreau, P.; Jakubowiak, A.J.; Raab, M.S.; Facon, T.; Vij, R.; White, D.; Reece, D.E.; Benboubker, L.; et al. Elotuzumab in combination with lenalidomide and dexamethasone in patients with relapsed multiple myeloma: Final phase 2 results from the randomised, open-label, phase 1b-2 dose-escalation study. *Lancet. Haematol.* **2015**, *2*, e516–e527. [CrossRef]
69. Dimopoulos, M.A.; Dytfeld, D.; Grosicki, S.; Moreau, P.; Takezako, N.; Hori, M.; Leleu, X.; LeBlanc, R.; Suzuki, K.; Raab, M.S.; et al. Elotuzumab plus Pomalidomide and Dexamethasone for Multiple Myeloma. *N. Engl. J. Med.* **2018**, *379*, 1811–1822. [CrossRef]
70. Jakubowiak, A.J.; Benson, D.M.; Bensinger, W.; Siegel, D.S.D.; Zimmerman, T.M.; Mohrbacher, A.; Richardson, P.G.; Afar, D.E.H.; Singhal, A.K.; Anderson, K.C. Phase I Trial of Anti-CS1 Monoclonal Antibody Elotuzumab in Combination With Bortezomib in the Treatment of Relapsed/Refractory Multiple Myeloma. *J. Clin. Oncol.* **2012**, *30*, 1960–1965. [CrossRef]
71. Jakubowiak, A.; Offidani, M.; Pégourie, B.; De La Rubia, J.; Garderet, L.; Laribi, K.; Bosi, A.; Marasca, R.; Laubach, J.; Mohrbacher, A.; et al. Randomized phase 2 study: Elotuzumab plus bortezomib/dexamethasone vs bortezomib/dexamethasone for relapsed/refractory MM. *Blood* **2016**, *127*, 2833–2840. [CrossRef]
72. Cives, M.; Simone, V.; Brunetti, O.; Longo, V.; Silvestris, F. Novel lenalidomide-based combinations for treatment of multiple myeloma. *Crit. Rev. Oncol. Hematol.* **2013**, *85*, 9–20. [CrossRef]
73. Lonial, S.; Dimopoulos, M.; Palumbo, A.; White, D.; Grosicki, S.; Spicka, I.; Walter-Croneck, A.; Moreau, P.; Mateos, M.-V.; Magen, H.; et al. Elotuzumab Therapy for Relapsed or Refractory Multiple Myeloma. *N. Engl. J. Med.* **2015**, *373*, 621–631. [CrossRef]

74. Dimopoulos, M.A.; Lonial, S.; Betts, K.A.; Chen, C.; Zichlin, M.L.; Brun, A.; Signorovitch, J.E.; Makenbaeva, D.; Mekan, S.; Sy, O.; et al. Elotuzumab plus lenalidomide and dexamethasone in relapsed/refractory multiple myeloma: Extended 4-year follow-up and analysis of relative progression-free survival from the randomized ELOQUENT-2 trial. *Cancer* **2018**, *124*, 4032–4043. [CrossRef]
75. Gavriatopoulou, M.; Terpos, E.; Dimopoulos, M.A. The extended 4-year follow-up results of the ELOQUENT-2 trial. *Oncotarget* **2019**, *10*, 82–83. [CrossRef]
76. Balasa, B.; Yun, R.; Belmar, N.A.; Fox, M.; Chao, D.T.; Robbins, M.D.; Starling, G.C.; Rice, A.G. Elotuzumab enhances natural killer cell activation and myeloma cell killing through interleukin-2 and TNF-α pathways. *Cancer Immunol. Immunother.* **2015**, *64*, 61–73. [CrossRef]
77. Van Rhee, F.; Szmania, S.M.; Dillon, M.; van Abbema, A.M.; Li, X.; Stone, M.K.; Garg, T.K.; Shi, J.; Moreno-Bost, A.M.; Yun, R.; et al. Combinatorial efficacy of anti-CS1 monoclonal antibody elotuzumab (HuLuc63) and bortezomib against multiple myeloma. *Mol. Cancer Ther.* **2009**, *8*, 2616–2624. [CrossRef]
78. Ghobrial, I.M.; Badros, A.Z.; Vredenburgh, J.J.; Matous, J.; Caola, A.M.; Savell, A.; Henrick, P.; Paba-Prada, C.E.; Schlossman, R.L.; Laubach, J.P.; et al. Phase II Trial of Combination of Elotuzumab, Lenalidomide, and Dexamethasone in High-Risk Smoldering Multiple Myeloma. *Blood* **2016**, *128*, Abstract #976 [ASH 2016 58th Meeting].
79. Jagannath, S.; Laubach, J.; Wong, E.; Stockerl-Goldstein, K.; Rosenbaum, C.; Dhodapkar, M.; Jou, Y.-M.; Lynch, M.; Robbins, M.; Shelat, S.; et al. Elotuzumab monotherapy in patients with smouldering multiple myeloma: A phase 2 study. *Br. J. Haematol.* **2018**, *182*, 495–503. [CrossRef]
80. Weisel, K.; Paner, A.; Engelhardt, M.; Taylor, F.; Cocks, K.; Espensen, A.; Popa-McKiver, M.; Chen, C.; Cavo, M. Quality-of-Life Outcomes in Patients with Relapsed/Refractory Multiple Myeloma Treated with Elotuzumab Plus Pomalidomide and Dexamethasone: Results from the Phase 2 Randomized Eloquent-3 Study. *Blood* **2018**, *132*, Abstract #2288 [ASH 2018 60th Meeting].
81. Parry, R.V.; Chemnitz, J.M.; Frauwirth, K.A.; Lanfranco, A.R.; Braunstein, I.; Kobayashi, S.V.; Linsley, P.S.; Thompson, C.B.; Riley, J.L. CTLA-4 and PD-1 receptors inhibit T-cell activation by distinct mechanisms. *Mol. Cell. Biol.* **2005**, *25*, 9543–9553. [CrossRef]
82. Paiva, B.; Azpilikueta, A.; Puig, N.; Ocio, E.M.; Sharma, R.; Oyajobi, B.O.; Labiano, S.; San-Segundo, L.; Rodriguez, A.; Aires-Mejia, I.; et al. PD-L1/PD-1 presence in the tumor microenvironment and activity of PD-1 blockade in multiple myeloma. *Leukemia* **2015**, *29*, 2110–2113. [CrossRef]
83. Ray, A.; Das, D.S.; Song, Y.; Richardson, P.; Munshi, N.C.; Chauhan, D.; Anderson, K.C. Targeting PD1–PDL1 immune checkpoint in plasmacytoid dendritic cell interactions with T cells, natural killer cells and multiple myeloma cells. *Leukemia* **2015**, *29*, 1441–1444. [CrossRef]
84. Ribrag, V.; Avigan, D.E.; Green, D.J.; Wise-Draper, T.; Posada, J.G.; Vij, R.; Zhu, Y.; Farooqui, M.Z.H.; Marinello, P.; Siegel, D.S. Phase 1b trial of pembrolizumab monotherapy for relapsed/refractory multiple myeloma: KEYNOTE-013. *Br. J. Haematol.* **2019**, *186*, e41–e44. [CrossRef]
85. Görgün, G.; Samur, M.K.; Cowens, K.B.; Paula, S.; Bianchi, G.; Anderson, J.E.; White, R.E.; Singh, A.; Ohguchi, H.; Suzuki, R.; et al. Lenalidomide enhances immune checkpoint blockade-induced immune response in multiple myeloma. *Clin. Cancer Res.* **2015**, *21*, 4607–4618. [CrossRef]
86. Badros, A.; Hyjek, E.; Ma, N.; Lesokhin, A.; Dogan, A.; Rapoport, A.P.; Kocoglu, M.; Lederer, E.; Philip, S.; Milliron, T.; et al. Pembrolizumab, pomalidomide, and low-dose dexamethasone for relapsed/refractory multiple myeloma. *Blood* **2017**, *130*, 1189–1197. [CrossRef]
87. Mateos, M.-V.; Blacklock, H.; Schjesvold, F.; Oriol, A.; Simpson, D.; George, A.; Goldschmidt, H.; Larocca, A.; Chanan-Khan, A.; Sherbenou, D.; et al. Pembrolizumab plus pomalidomide and dexamethasone for patients with relapsed or refractory multiple myeloma (KEYNOTE-183): A randomised, open-label, phase 3 trial. *Lancet Haematol.* **2019**, *6*, e459–e469. [CrossRef]
88. Usmani, S.Z.; Schjesvold, F.; Oriol, A.; Karlin, L.; Cavo, M.; Rifkin, R.M.; Yimer, H.A.; LeBlanc, R.; Takezako, N.; McCroskey, R.D.; et al. Pembrolizumab plus lenalidomide and dexamethasone for patients with treatment-naive multiple myeloma (KEYNOTE-185): A randomised, open-label, phase 3 trial. *Lancet Haematol.* **2019**, *6*, e448–e458. [CrossRef]
89. Tolcher, A.W. Antibody drug conjugates: Lessons from 20 years of clinical experience. *Ann. Oncol.* **2016**, *27*, 2168–2172. [CrossRef]
90. Wolska-Washer, A.; Robak, P.; Smolewski, P.; Robak, T. Emerging antibody-drug conjugates for treating lymphoid malignancies. *Expert Opin. Emerg. Drugs* **2017**, *22*, 259–273. [CrossRef]

91. Younes, A.; Gopal, A.K.; Smith, S.E.; Ansell, S.M.; Rosenblatt, J.D.; Savage, K.J.; Ramchandren, R.; Bartlett, N.L.; Cheson, B.D.; de Vos, S.; et al. Results of a Pivotal Phase II Study of Brentuximab Vedotin for Patients With Relapsed or Refractory Hodgkin's Lymphoma. *J. Clin. Oncol.* **2012**, *30*, 2183–2189. [CrossRef]
92. Pro, B.; Advani, R.; Brice, P.; Bartlett, N.L.; Rosenblatt, J.D.; Illidge, T.; Matous, J.; Ramchandren, R.; Fanale, M.; Connors, J.M.; et al. Brentuximab Vedotin (SGN-35) in Patients With Relapsed or Refractory Systemic Anaplastic Large-Cell Lymphoma: Results of a Phase II Study. *J. Clin. Oncol.* **2012**, *30*, 2190–2196. [CrossRef]
93. Tassone, P.; Gozzini, A.; Goldmacher, V.; Shammas, M.A.; Whiteman, K.R.; Carrasco, D.R.; Li, C.; Allam, C.K.; Venuta, S.; Anderson, K.C.; et al. In vitro and in vivo activity of the maytansinoid immunoconjugate huN901-N2'-deacetyl-N2'-(3-mercapto-1-oxopropyl)-maytansine against CD56+ multiple myeloma cells. *Cancer Res.* **2004**, *64*, 4629–4636. [CrossRef]
94. Tassone, P.; Goldmacher, V.S.; Neri, P.; Gozzini, A.; Shammas, M.A.; Whiteman, K.R.; Hylander-Gans, L.L.; Carrasco, D.R.; Hideshima, T.; Shringarpure, R.; et al. Cytotoxic activity of the maytansinoid immunoconjugate B-B4–DM1 against CD138+ multiple myeloma cells. *Blood* **2004**, *104*, 3688–3696. [CrossRef]
95. Stein, R.; Smith, M.R.; Chen, S.; Zalath, M.; Goldenberg, D.M. Combining Milatuzumab with Bortezomib, Doxorubicin, or Dexamethasone Improves Responses in Multiple Myeloma Cell Lines. *Clin. Cancer Res.* **2009**, *15*, 2808–2817. [CrossRef]
96. Robak, T.; Robak, E. Current Phase II antibody-drug conjugates for the treatment of lymphoid malignancies. *Expert Opin. Investig. Drugs* **2014**, *23*, 911–924.
97. Sherbenou, D.W.; Behrens, C.R.; Su, Y.; Wolf, J.L.; Martin, T.G.; Liu, B. The development of potential antibody-based therapies for myeloma. *Blood Rev.* **2015**, *29*, 81–91. [CrossRef]
98. Nittoli, T.; Kelly, M.P.; Delfino, F.; Rudge, J.; Kunz, A.; Markotan, T.; Spink, J.; Chen, Z.; Shan, J.; Navarro, E.; et al. Antibody drug conjugates of cleavable amino-alkyl and aryl maytansinoids. *Bioorganic Med. Chem.* **2018**, *26*, 2271–2279. [CrossRef]
99. Waight, A.B.; Bargsten, K.; Doronina, S.; Steinmetz, M.O.; Sussman, D.; Prota, A.E. Structural Basis of Microtubule Destabilization by Potent Auristatin Anti-Mitotics. *PLoS ONE* **2016**, *11*, e0160890. [CrossRef]
100. Gébleux, R.; Stringhini, M.; Casanova, R.; Soltermann, A.; Neri, D. Non-internalizing antibody-drug conjugates display potent anti-cancer activity upon proteolytic release of monomethyl auristatin E in the subendothelial extracellular matrix. *Int. J. Cancer* **2017**, *140*, 1670–1679. [CrossRef]
101. Yoshida, S.; Tuscano, E.; Duong, C.; Chung, J.; Li, Y.; Beckett, L.; Tuscano, J.M.; Satake, N. Efficacy of an anti-CD22 antibody-monomethyl auristatin E conjugate in a preclinical xenograft model of precursor B-cell acute lymphoblastic leukemia. *Leuk. Lymphoma* **2017**, *58*, 1254–1257. [CrossRef]
102. Peters, C.; Brown, S. Antibody-drug conjugates as novel anti-cancer chemotherapeutics. *Biosci. Rep.* **2015**, *35*, e00225. [CrossRef]
103. Jackson, P.J.M.; Kay, S.; Pysz, I.; Thurston, D.E. Use of pyrrolobenzodiazepines and related covalent-binding DNA-interactive molecules as ADC payloads: Is mechanism related to systemic toxicity? *Drug Discov. Today Technol.* **2018**, *30*, 71–83. [CrossRef]
104. Trudel, S.; Lendvai, N.; Popat, R.; Voorhees, P.M.; Reeves, B.; Libby, E.N.; Richardson, P.G.; Hoos, A.; Gupta, I.; Bragulat, V.; et al. Antibody–drug conjugate, GSK2857916, in relapsed/refractory multiple myeloma: An update on safety and efficacy from dose expansion phase I study. *Blood Cancer J.* **2019**, *9*, 37. [CrossRef]
105. Yong, K.L.; Germaschewski, F.M.; Rodriguez-Justo, M.; Bounds, D.; Lee, L.; Mayes, P.A.; Sully, K.; Seestaller-Wehr, L.M.; Fieles, W.E.; Tunstead, J.R.; et al. Evaluation Of Bcma As A Therapeutic Target In Multiple Myeloma Using An Antibody-Drug Conjugate. *Blood* **2013**, *122*, Abstract #4447 [ASH 2013 55th Meeting].
106. Trudel, S.; Lendvai, N.; Popat, R.; Voorhees, P.M.; Reeves, B.; Libby, E.N.; Richardson, P.G.; Anderson, L.D.; Sutherland, H.J.; Yong, K.; et al. Targeting B-cell maturation antigen with GSK2857916 antibody–drug conjugate in relapsed or refractory multiple myeloma (BMA117159): A dose escalation and expansion phase 1 trial. *Lancet Oncol.* **2018**, *19*, 1641–1653. [CrossRef]
107. Jagannath, S.; Heffner, L.T.; Ailawadhi, S.; Munshi, N.C.; Zimmerman, T.M.; Rosenblatt, J.; Lonial, S.; Chanan-Khan, A.; Ruehle, M.; Rharbaoui, F.; et al. Indatuximab Ravtansine (BT062) Monotherapy in Patients With Relapsed and/or Refractory Multiple Myeloma. *Clin. Lymphoma Myeloma Leuk.* **2019**, *19*, 372–380. [CrossRef] [PubMed]

108. Kelly, K.R.; Siegel, D.S.; Chanan-Khan, A.A.; Somlo, G.; Heffner, L.T.; Jagannath, S.; Zimmerman, T.; Munshi, N.C.; Madan, S.; Mohrbacher, A.; et al. Indatuximab Ravtansine (BT062) in Combination with Low-Dose Dexamethasone and Lenalidomide or Pomalidomide: Clinical Activity in Patients with Relapsed / Refractory Multiple Myeloma. *Blood* **2016**, *128*, Abstract #4486 [ASH 2016 58th Meeting].
109. Ailawadhi, S.; Kelly, K.R.; Vescio, R.A.; Jagannath, S.; Wolf, J.; Gharibo, M.; Sher, T.; Bojanini, L.; Kirby, M.; Chanan-Khan, A. A Phase I Study to Assess the Safety and Pharmacokinetics of Single-agent Lorvotuzumab Mertansine (IMGN901) in Patients with Relapsed and/or Refractory CD–56-positive Multiple Myeloma. *Clin. Lymphoma Myeloma Leuk.* **2019**, *19*, 29–34. [CrossRef] [PubMed]
110. Stein, R.; Mattes, M.J.; Cardillo, T.M.; Hansen, H.J.; Chang, C.-H.; Burton, J.; Govindan, S.; Goldenberg, D.M. CD74: A New Candidate Target for the Immunotherapy of B-Cell Neoplasms. *Clin. Cancer Res.* **2007**, *13*, 5556s–5563s. [CrossRef] [PubMed]
111. Berdeja, J.G.; Hernandez-Ilizaliturri, F.; Chanan-Khan, A.; Patel, M.; Kelly, K.R.; Running, K.L.; Murphy, M.; Guild, R.; Carrigan, C.; Ladd, S.; et al. Phase I Study of Lorvotuzumab Mertansine (LM, IMGN901) in Combination with Lenalidomide (Len) and Dexamethasone (Dex) in Patients with CD56-Positive Relapsed or Relapsed/Refractory Multiple Myeloma (MM). *Blood* **2012**, *120*, Abstract #728 [ASH 2012 54th Meeting].
112. Kaufman, J.L.; Niesvizky, R.; Stadtmauer, E.A.; Chanan-Khan, A.; Siegel, D.; Horne, H.; Wegener, W.A.; Goldenberg, D.M. Phase I, multicentre, dose-escalation trial of monotherapy with milatuzumab (humanized anti-CD74 monoclonal antibody) in relapsed or refractory multiple myeloma. *Br. J. Haematol.* **2013**, *163*, 478–486. [CrossRef]
113. Wolf, E.; Hofmeister, R.; Kufer, P.; Schlereth, B.; Baeuerle, P.A. BiTEs: Bispecific antibody constructs with unique anti-tumor activity. *Drug Discov. Today* **2005**, *10*, 1237–1244. [CrossRef]
114. Madduri, D.; Dhodapkar, M.V.; Lonial, S.; Jagannath, S.; Cho, H.J. SOHO State of the Art Updates and Next Questions: T-Cell–Directed Immune Therapies for Multiple Myeloma: Chimeric Antigen Receptor–Modified T Cells and Bispecific T-Cell–Engaging Agents. *Clin. Lymphoma Myeloma Leuk.* **2019**, *19*, 537–544. [CrossRef]
115. Topp, M.S.; Gökbuget, N.; Stein, A.S.; Zugmaier, G.; O'Brien, S.; Bargou, R.C.; Dombret, H.; Fielding, A.K.; Heffner, L.; Larson, R.A.; et al. Safety and activity of blinatumomab for adult patients with relapsed or refractory B-precursor acute lymphoblastic leukaemia: A multicentre, single-arm, phase 2 study. *Lancet Oncol.* **2015**, *16*, 57–66. [CrossRef]
116. Bonello, F.; D'Agostino, M.; Moscvin, M.; Cerrato, C.; Boccadoro, M.; Gay, F. CD38 as an immunotherapeutic target in multiple myeloma. *Expert Opin. Biol. Ther.* **2018**, *18*, 1209–1221. [CrossRef] [PubMed]
117. Atamaniuk, J.; Gleiss, A.; Porpaczy, E.; Kainz, B.; Grunt, T.W.; Raderer, M.; Hilgarth, B.; Drach, J.; Ludwig, H.; Gisslinger, H.; et al. Overexpression of G protein-coupled receptor 5D in the bone marrow is associated with poor prognosis in patients with multiple myeloma. *Eur. J. Clin. Invest.* **2012**, *42*, 953–960. [CrossRef] [PubMed]
118. Kodama, T.; Kochi, Y.; Nakai, W.; Mizuno, H.; Baba, T.; Habu, K.; Sawada, N.; Tsunoda, H.; Shima, T.; Miyawaki, K.; et al. Anti-GPRC5D/CD3 Bispecific T-Cell–Redirecting Antibody for the Treatment of Multiple Myeloma. *Mol. Cancer Ther.* **2019**, *18*, 1555–1564. [CrossRef] [PubMed]
119. Topp, M.S.; Duell, J.; Zugmaier, G.; Attal, M.; Moreau, P.; Langer, C.; Kroenke, J.; Facon, T.; Salnikov, A.; Lesley, R.; et al. Evaluation of AMG 420, an anti-BCMA bispecific T-cell engager (BiTE) immunotherapy, in R/R multiple myeloma (MM) patients: Updated results of a first-in-human (FIH) phase I dose escalation study. *J. Clin. Oncol.* **2019**, *37*, Abstract #8007 [ASCO 2019 Annual Meeting].
120. Cho, S.-F.; Lin, L.; Xing, L.; Liu, J.; Yu, T.; Wen, K.; Hsieh, P.; Munshi, N.; Anderson, K.; Tai, Y.-T. Anti-Bcma BiTE® AMG 701 Potently Induces Specific T Cell Lysis of Human Multiple Myeloma (MM) Cells and Immunomodulation in the Bone Marrow Microenvironment. *Blood* **2018**, *132*, Abstract #592 [ASH 2018 60th Meeting]. [CrossRef]
121. Rasche, L.; Kortüm, K.M.; Raab, M.S.; Weinhold, N. The impact of tumor heterogeneity on diagnostics and novel therapeutic strategies in multiple myeloma. *Int. J. Mol. Sci.* **2019**, *20*, 1248. [CrossRef]
122. Nijhof, I.S.; Casneuf, T.; van Velzen, J.; van Kessel, B.; Axel, A.E.; Syed, K.; Groen, R.W.J.; van Duin, M.; Sonneveld, P.; Minnema, M.C.; et al. CD38 expression and complement inhibitors affect response and resistance to daratumumab therapy in myeloma. *Blood* **2016**, *128*, 959–970. [CrossRef]
123. Danhof, S.; Strifler, S.; Hose, D.; Kortüm, M.; Bittrich, M.; Hefner, J.; Einsele, H.; Knop, S.; Schreder, M. Clinical and biological characteristics of myeloma patients influence response to elotuzumab combination therapy. *J. Cancer Res. Clin. Oncol.* **2019**, *145*, 561–571. [CrossRef]

124. Ghose, J.; Viola, D.; Terrazas, C.; Caserta, E.; Troadec, E.; Khalife, J.; Gunes, E.G.; Sanchez, J.; McDonald, T.; Marcucci, G.; et al. Daratumumab induces CD38 internalization and impairs myeloma cell adhesion. *Oncoimmunology* **2018**, *7*, e1486948. [CrossRef]
125. Moreno, L.; Perez, C.; Zabaleta, A.; Manrique, I.; Alignani, D.; Ajona, D.; Blanco, L.; Lasa, M.; Maiso, P.; Rodriguez, I.; et al. The Mechanism of Action of the Anti-CD38 Monoclonal Antibody Isatuximab in Multiple Myeloma. *Clin. Cancer Res.* **2019**, *25*, 3176–3187. [CrossRef] [PubMed]
126. Raab, M.S.; Chatterjee, M.; Goldschmidt, H.; Agis, H.; Blau, I.; Einsele, H.; Engelhardt, M.; Ferstl, B.; Gramatzki, M.; Röllig, C.; et al. A Phase I/IIa Study of the CD38 Antibody MOR202 Alone and in Combination with Pomalidomide or Lenalidomide in Patients with Relapsed or Refractory Multiple Myeloma. *Blood* **2016**, *128*, Abstract #1152 [ASH 2016 58th Meeting].
127. Nijhof, I.S.; Groen, R.W.J.; Lokhorst, H.M.; Van Kessel, B.; Bloem, A.C.; Van Velzen, J.; De Jong-Korlaar, R.; Yuan, H.; Noort, W.A.; Klein, S.K.; et al. Upregulation of CD38 expression on multiple myeloma cells by all-trans retinoic acid improves the efficacy of daratumumab. *Leukemia* **2015**, *29*, 2039–2049. [CrossRef] [PubMed]
128. García-Guerrero, E.; Gogishvili, T.; Danhof, S.; Schreder, M.; Pallaud, C.; Pérez-Simón, J.A.; Einsele, H.; Hudecek, M. Panobinostat induces CD38 upregulation and augments the antimyeloma efficacy of daratumumab. *Blood* **2017**, *129*, 3386–3388. [CrossRef] [PubMed]
129. Cho, S.-F.; Lin, L.; Xing, L.; Wen, K.; Yu, T.; Hsieh, P.A.; Li, Y.; Munshi, N.C.; Wahl, J.; Matthes, K.; et al. AMG 701 Potently Induces Anti-Multiple Myeloma (MM) Functions of T Cells and IMiDs Further Enhance Its Efficacy to Prevent MM Relapse In Vivo. Abstract #135, ASH 2019 61st Meeting. Available online: https://ash.confex.com/ash/2019/webprogram/Paper128528.html (accessed on 13 December 2019).
130. Raje, N.; Jakubowiak, A.; Gasparetto, C.; Cornell, R.F.; Krupka, H.I.; Navarro, D.; Forgie, A.J.; Udata, C.; Basu, C.; Chou, J.; et al. Safety, Clinical Activity, Pharmacokinetics, and Pharmacodynamics from a Phase I Study of PF-06863135, a B-Cell Maturation Antigen (BCMA)–CD3 Bispecific Antibody, in Patients with Relapsed/Refractory Multiple Myeloma (RRMM). Abstract #1869, ASH 2019 61st. Available online: https://ash.confex.com/ash/2019/webprogram/Paper121805.html (accessed on 13 December 2019).
131. Dawicki, W.; Allen, K.J.H.; Jiao, R.; Malo, M.E.; Helal, M.; Berger, M.S.; Ludwig, D.L.; Dadachova, E. Daratumumab-225Actinium conjugate demonstrates greatly enhanced antitumor activity against experimental multiple myeloma tumors. *Oncoimmunology* **2019**, *8*, 1607673. [CrossRef]
132. Teiluf, K.; Seidl, C.; Blechert, B.; Gaertner, F.C.; Gilbertz, K.P.; Fernandez, V.; Bassermann, F.; Endell, J.; Boxhammer, R.; Leclair, S.; et al. α-radioimmunotherapy with 213Bi-anti-CD38 immunoconjugates is effective in a mouse model of human multiple myeloma. *Oncotarget* **2015**, *6*, 4692–4703. [CrossRef]
133. Pandit-Taskar, N. Functional Imaging Methods for Assessment of Minimal Residual Disease in Multiple Myeloma: Current Status and Novel ImmunoPET Based Methods. *Semin. Hematol.* **2018**, *55*, 22–32. [CrossRef]
134. Ghai, A.; Maji, D.; Cho, N.; Chanswangphuwana, C.; Rettig, M.; Shen, D.; DiPersio, J.; Akers, W.; Dehdashti, F.; Achilefu, S.; et al. Preclinical development of CD38-Targeted [89 Zr]Zr-DFO-Daratumumab for Imaging Multiple Myeloma. *J. Nucl. Med.* **2018**, *59*, 216–222. [CrossRef]
135. Caserta, E.; Chea, J.; Minnix, M.; Viola, D.; Vonderfecht, S.; Yazaki, P.; Crow, D.; Khalife, J.; Sanchez, J.F.; Palmer, J.M.; et al. Copper 64-labeled daratumumab as a PET/CT imaging tracer for multiple myeloma. *Blood* **2018**, *131*, 741–745. [CrossRef]
136. Ulaner, G.; Sobol, N.; O'Donoghue, J.; Burnazi, E.; Staton, K.; Weber, W.; Lyashchenko, S.; Lewis, J.; Landgren1, C.O. Preclinical development and First-in-human imaging of 89Zr-Daratumumab for CD38 targeted imaging of myeloma. *J. Nucl. Med.* **2019**, *60*, Abstract #203.

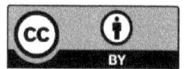

© 2019 by the authors. Licensee MDPI, Basel, Switzerland. This article is an open access article distributed under the terms and conditions of the Creative Commons Attribution (CC BY) license (http://creativecommons.org/licenses/by/4.0/).

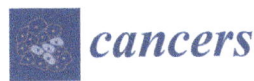

Review

Targeting the Tetraspanins with Monoclonal Antibodies in Oncology: Focus on Tspan8/Co-029

Mathilde Bonnet [1,†], Aurélie Maisonial-Besset [2,†], Yingying Zhu [3], Tiffany Witkowski [2], Gwenaëlle Roche [1], Claude Boucheix [3], Céline Greco [3,4] and Françoise Degoul [2,*]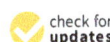

1. Université Clermont Auvergne, INSERM1071, Microbes, Intestins, Inflammation et Susceptibilité de l'hôte, 63001 Clermont-Ferrand CEDEX 1, France; mathilde.bonnet@uca.fr (M.B.); gwenaelle.roche@uca.fr (G.R.)
2. Université Clermont Auvergne, INSERM U1240, Imagerie Moléculaire et Stratégies Théranostiques, F-63000 Clermont Ferrand, France; aurelie.maisonial@uca.fr (A.M.-B.); tiffany.witkowski@inserm.fr (T.W.)
3. Université Paris-Sud, INSERM U935, Bâtiment Lavoisier, 14 Avenue Paul-Vaillant-Couturier, F-94800 Villejuif, France; julianzyy@hotmail.com (Y.Z.); claude.boucheix@inserm.fr (C.B.); celine.greco@inserm.fr (C.G.)
4. Department of Pain and Palliative Medicine AP HP, Hôpital Necker, 75015 Paris, France
* Correspondence: francoise.degoul@inserm.fr; Tel.: +33-(0)47-3150-1814
† These authors contributed equally to this work.

Received: 19 December 2018; Accepted: 30 January 2019; Published: 4 February 2019

Abstract: Tetraspanins are exposed at the surface of cellular membranes, which allows for the fixation of cognate antibodies. Developing specific antibodies in conjunction with genetic data would largely contribute to deciphering their biological behavior. In this short review, we summarize the main functions of Tspan8/Co-029 and its role in the biology of tumor cells. Based on data collected from recently reported studies, the possibilities of using antibodies to target Tspan8 in immunotherapy or radioimmunotherapy approaches are also discussed.

Keywords: tetraspanins; cancer; Tspan8; immunotherapy; radioimmunotherapy

1. Introduction

Tspan8 belongs to the tetraspanin molecular family of surface glycoproteins containing 33 members in humans, which are now referred to as Tspan1–33 (Figure 1). Tetraspanins are small membrane proteins (200–350 amino acids), which interact laterally with multiple partner proteins and with each other to form the so-called TEMs (tetraspanin-enriched microdomains). To qualify for membership in the tetraspanin family, a protein must have four transmembrane domains and several conserved amino acids, including an absolutely conserved CCG motif and two other cysteine residues that contribute to two crucial disulfide bonds within the second extracellular loop (EC2) (Figure 2). One or two additional disulfide bonds may also be found in EC2. The biological importance of tetraspanins is supported by functional consequences of genetic modifications that occur either spontaneously in humans or experimentally in mice. For instance, gene inactivation may affect fertility (CD9, CD81), and visual (RDS), kidney (CD151) or immunological functions (CD81, CD37) [1–4]. Since tetraspanins are not adhesion or signaling molecules, receptors or enzymes, the properties of these molecules are highly dependent on their ability to form TEMs with a hierarchical organization. Indeed, each tetraspanin has specific partners, including integrins, ADAM metalloproteases, growth factor receptors and histocompatibility antigens, that they are directly associated with through protein–protein interactions and form primary complexes with [5,6]. Coupled together, the latter can form second-order complexes through tetraspanin–tetraspanin interactions that may involve cholesterol and palmitoylation. In some cases, the function of these associated molecules has not yet been elucidated for the CD9P-1 and EWI2 (official protein names of PTGFRN and IGSF8) [7,8]. Some molecular experiments showed that tetraspanins may interfere with the properties (affinity of the integrin α6β1 for laminin-1 is modulated by the tetraspanin CD151) [9], the trafficking (CD81 controls the expression of CD19 at the B-lymphoid cell surface) [10] or membrane compartmentalization of associated molecules (such as ADAM10 by TspanC8) [11]. Detailed proteomic analysis of membrane molecules that are able to associate with CD9 and Tspan8 has been reported recently in colon carcinoma cell lines. Among other membrane proteins, E-cadherin and EGFR are associated with TM4 complexes. More specifically, the presence of Tspan8 in the membrane drives EGFR to tetraspanin complexes, which results in changes in motility behavior (see next paragraph) [12].

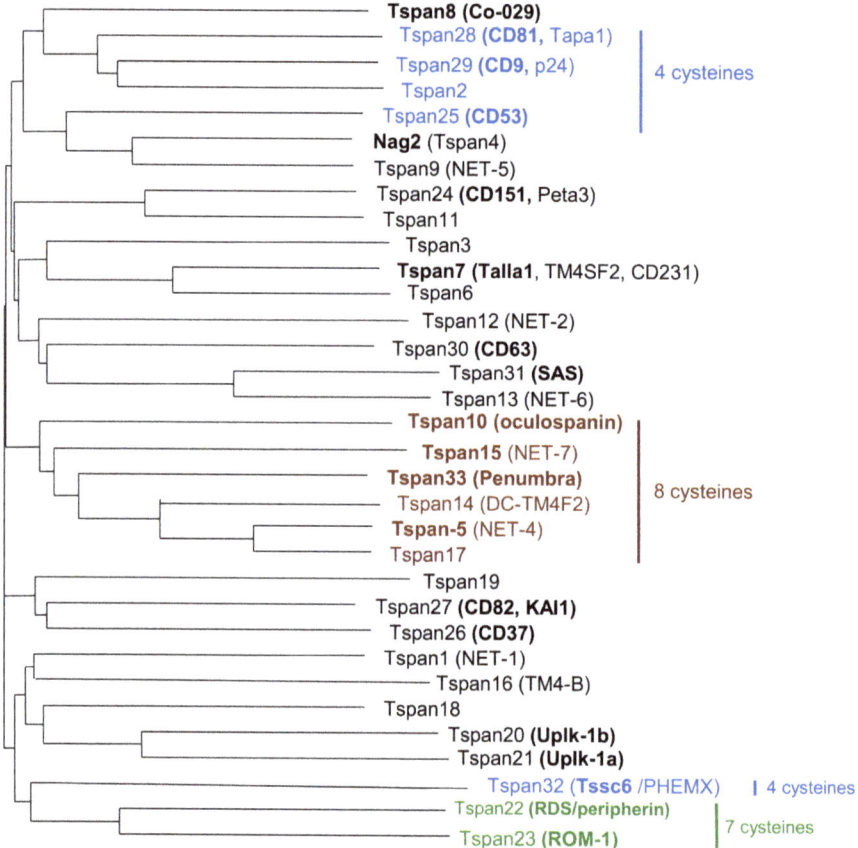

Figure 1. Homology tree between human tetraspanins. Protein sequences have been aligned to generate this distance tree. Bolded names correspond to commonly used ones. The number of cysteines in the extracellular loop EC2 is given when they are different from six cysteines.

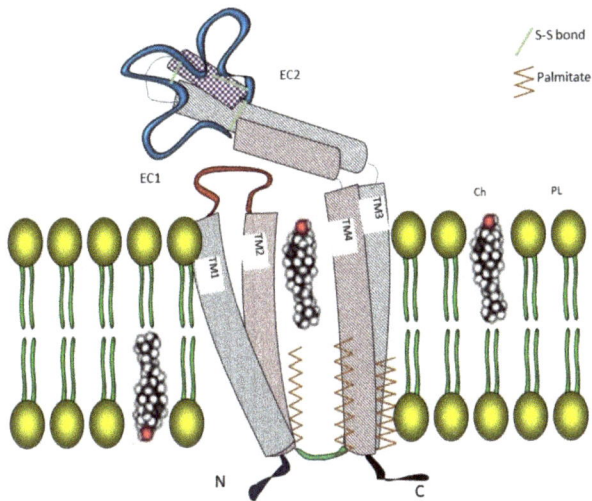

Figure 2. Schematic representation of Tspan8 in membrane. The transmembrane (TM) domains inserted in the phospholipid bilayer are palmitoylated with a cholesterol molecule in between these domains (by analogy with CD81 structure [13]). Among the two extracellular (EC) regions, the larger region contains six cysteines involved in disulfide bonds. EC1 and EC2 = extracellular domains 1 and 2; Ch = cholesterol; and PL = phospholipid.

Some tetraspanins are widely expressed (for example, CD81 and CD151) while others are more restricted (for example, CD37 and CD53 on lymphoid cells or RDS in retina). Several clinical observations and experimental data have correlated the expression of some tetraspanins with tumor metastatic potential. CD82 or CD9 expression is generally associated with favorable prognosis in different cancers [3]. On the contrary, CD151 and Tspan8 expression in tumor cells has been frequently associated with increased migration, proliferation and angiogenesis induction (Table 1). Mechanisms that could potentially explain the role of tetraspanins in tumors have been investigated experimentally using cellular models of overexpression in addition to knockdown or knockout animal models (reviewed in references [3,4,14–16]). The modulation of cellular properties, such as proliferation, cell migration and apoptosis, has been previously reported. Among other mechanisms, the knockout of CD37 leads to the occurrence of lymphomas that appear to be linked to the constitutive activation of the IL6 signaling pathway [17]. At a tissue level, an effect of Tspan8 on angiogenesis could be partially mediated by exosomes. More generally, the role of tetraspanins in tumor cell communication with their microenvironment through an effect on exosomal biogenesis is considered to be an important function of these molecules [18]. The changes in cell properties induced by the (over)expression of Tspan8 have been investigated in preclinical models. For example, the Isreco1 cell line derived from primary colorectal cancer (CRC) that does not express Tspan8 was compared with Is1-Co029, which was obtained by transduction to express Tspan8 at the same level as the two cell lines derived from metastases of the same patient. There was no difference in the motility of single cells plated on collagen, but RNAi targeting various surface molecules, such as E-cadherin, p120-catenin or EGFR, increased the motility of Is1-Co029, whereas no effect was observed on Isreco1 [12,19]. A possible link between Tspan8, E-cadherin and motility could be the signaling molecule p120-catenin, which is retained at the cell membrane through its affinity for E-cadherin. Furthermore, it has been reported to regulate Rho and Rac functions in cell adhesion and motility (reviewed in reference [19]). However, models using long-term established tumor cell lines in 2D settings could be misleading and it would be important to conduct experiments on cells derived from fresh tumors and cultured in 3D conditions as organoids that would better reflect the in-vivo conditions.

Table 1. Summary of studies dealing with biological consequences of Tspan8 targeting using specific antibodies.

Preclinical and clinical models	Effect of Tspan8 Expression and Modulation by Antibody or Tspan8-LEL Targeting on Migration/Invasion/Metastasis, Proliferation/Tumor Growth, Angiogenesis	References
Rat pancreatic adenocarcinoma cells (AS-Tspan8 vs. AS)	In vitro: similar proliferation of two AS cell lines Inhibition by anti-rat Tspan8 mAb D6.1 of AS-Tspan8 In vivo: increased metastasis formation of AS-Tspan8 (i.v., s.c. or i.f.p. injection)	[20]
Rat pancreatic adenocarcinoma cells (AS-Tspan8 vs. AS)	In vitro: increased endothelial cell branching blocked by mAb D6.1 In vivo: peritoneal carcinosis—increased vessel density (intravital microscopy) abolished by mAb D6	[21]
Highly metastatic rat pancreatic adenocarcinoma BSp73ASML (+/− Tspan8 knockdown)	In vitro: transwell migration and wound healing: reduced in BSp73ASML-Tspan8^{kd} and by mAb D6.1 in BSp73AMSL No effect of D6.1 on BSp73ASML single-cell motility In vivo: delayed metastasis and prolonged survival in BSp73ASML-Tspan8^{kd}	[22]
Human colorectal cancer cell lines: Isreco1 and Is-Co029(Tspan8) HT-29, SW480 and SW480-Tspan8	Patients: IHC: Tspan8 high expression correlated with worse prognosis In vitro: single cell-motility on collagen I increased by Ecad, p120ctn and EGFR RNAi when Tspan8 is expressed. This effect is reversed by anti-mouse Tspan8 mAb Ts29.1. No effect of mAb Ts29.1 or Ts29.2 on proliferation In vivo (nude mice): tumor growth reduced by i.p. injection of mAb Ts29.2 No effect on angiogenesis (IHC-CD34 labeling) Tumor growth inhibition by i.v. injection of [^{177}Lu]DOTA-Ts29.2	[12,19,23,24]
Human ovarian cell line—effect of Tspan8 RNAi, Tspan8-LEL-Fc, Tspan8-LEL IgG (human Ab selected by phage display)	In vitro: invasion in Matrigel-coated Transwell is inhibited by the 3 reagents In vivo: partial metastasis inhibition (SK-OV3-Luc) by i.v. injection of Tspan8-LEL IgG	[25]

i.v.: intravenous, i.p.: intraperitoneal, i.f.p: intrafootpad and s.c.: subcutaneous.

Experimental results and clinical trials using monoclonal antibodies (mAbs) suggest that some tetraspanins may be targeted in hematological malignancies and carcinomas [26]. In a similar way, Tspan8 appears to be an interesting candidate for the development of therapeutic antibodies, and different methods are discussed in the last part of this review.

2. Mechanisms and Requirements for the Use of Therapeutic Anti-Tetraspanin Antibodies

2.1. Molecular Mechanisms

Since antibodies are large proteins, their ability to reach their target may be limited by their diffusion inside different tissues and their components due to certain barriers, such as the hemato-encephalic barrier. However, since the permeability of tumor vessels is usually abnormal, diffusion appears to be increased in such tumor tissues [27,28]. Once located close to their biological target, the antibodies can enact different mechanisms of action.

2.1.1. Blocking Antibodies

According to current knowledge, the action of tetraspanins relies on their ability to regulate the function of their partner molecules. Even if the detailed molecular basis remains mostly unknown, the binding of mAbs on Tspan8 may result in the inhibition of cell migration, invasion, proliferation and angiogenesis in organized tissues (Table 1).

2.1.2. Cytotoxic Antibodies

Unconjugated antibodies mediate ADCC (antibody-dependent cell cytotoxicity) via the activation of accessory cytotoxic cells for killing target cells. Upon fixation on the cell surface, they recruit macrophages or NK cells through their Fc fragment, which can further destroy the target cell. The subclass and glycosylation of the Fc region are important parameters that determine the efficacy of ADCC. Furthermore, the ability of antibodies to mediate ADCC may be optimized through genetic modification of their Fc region.

On the contrary, radionuclide- or drug-conjugated antibodies have directly toxic effects in vivo.

Depending on the radionuclide used (nature of emissions, energy and so on), radionuclide-conjugated antibodies can efficiently treat the target cells and the neighboring cells, which can be of high value in the case of heterogeneous cell expression of the target molecule. In addition, radionuclide-conjugated antibodies can also allow for a combination of imaging and radiotoxicity. This will be detailed in the radionuclide-conjugated Tspan8 antibodies section.

When antibodies are conjugated with cytotoxic drugs, an internalization of the antigen/antibody complex is often necessary to allow drug delivery [29]. However, if the targeted protein is widely distributed, the use of these two main categories of antibody–drug conjugates may have deleterious effects on normal tissues. As a consequence, the careful evaluation of the pattern of expression of the target is a critical prerequisite for the development of a therapeutic antibody. However, recent progress in antibody-conjugated drugs has allowed one to target more specific released molecules in tumors. For instance, cleavage in acidic zones that occur in the highly proliferative zone or proteolytic cleavage by tumor enzymes, such as MMPs, increase specificity. Another stage was added with a pro-body approach, which consists of modifying the antibody with a small peptide that needs to be cleaved by a specific protease for antigen recognition [30].

2.2. Pattern of Expression

An ideal antigenic target should be expressed at a high intensity on the surface of tumor cells, especially tumor stem cells and not on normal cells. None of the molecules that are currently targeted by mAbs are able to fulfil these criteria and not surprisingly, tetraspanins do not escape this rule.

As mentioned above, the tissue distribution of tetraspanins is highly variable. A very restricted distribution of some tetraspanins has already been observed for peripherin/RDS found in the photoreceptors, UPk1a found on the urinary bladder epithelium or CD37 expressed mainly on B lymphoid cells. In contrast, other tetraspanins, such as CD9, CD63, CD81 or CD151, have a very large distribution and may be difficult to target in vivo. Tspan8 is expressed in a limited number of tissues and is mainly found on epithelial cells of the digestive tract. However, it is also located on the epithelial cells of the kidney, prostate and trachea [23]. The second aspect relates to the intensity ratio of Tspan8 in tumor compared to normal tissues, which is another crucial issue that needs to be addressed in order to avoid side effects. Increased Tspan8 expression in tumor tissues (colorectal and ovarian cancer, melanoma, hepatocellular and pancreatic carcinoma) is generally related to worse prognosis [19,25,31–33]. Therefore, Tspan8 appears to be an interesting target candidate for cancer treatment with mAbs.

2.3. Dodging Immune Neutralization

This important point has been widely studied and previously reviewed. Thus, this will not be detailed in this article. This is mainly realized through the humanization of the molecule but other methods have been previously reported [34].

3. Therapeutic Antibodies Directed toward the Tetraspanins CD9, CD151 and CD37 in Cancer

There are a few proofs of principle that have shown that targeting tetraspanins with antibodies might inhibit tumor growth or even induce partial or complete remission [35].

The effects of the anti-CD9 mAb ALB6 (IgG1) injected intravenously were investigated in a model of human gastric cancer (MKN-28) implanted subcutaneously in nude mice. A reduction of 60–70% in the size of the tumor in the treated group was observed compared to the control IgG-treated mice. At the same time, a significant reduction in cell proliferation and angiogenesis and an increase in apoptotic signals were observed [36]. Since this mAb is directed towards human CD9, damages to normal tissues were not evaluated. As CD9 is strongly expressed on many cellular types and particularly on platelets in humans, the use of this anti-CD9 antibody could lead to a loss of treatment efficiency and may trigger platelet activation or lysis depending on the nature of the Fc fragment [37]. However, Fc-mediated side effects could be avoided by genetic modifications of the antibody.

There have only been a few studies targeting tetraspanins in humans for therapeutic purposes. A cocktail of antibodies Ba1/2/3 directed respectively toward CD9, CD24 and CD10 to deplete the bone marrow of acute lymphoblastic leukemia patients for autologous bone marrow transplantation was investigated. Even if the specific role of each individual antibody was difficult to evaluate, an absence of toxicity against hematological stem cells was observed in these antibodies [38].

Due to its restricted specificity for differentiated cells of the B-cell lineage, CD37 was considered to be a potential target for the treatment for B-cell lymphoma using an anti-CD37 antibody radiolabeled with iodine-131 (β^-; $T_{1/2}$ = 8.02 d; 606 keV). Very encouraging results were obtained in comparison with an anti-CD20 antibody labelled with the same radionuclide [39]. However, since the use of unconjugated humanized anti-CD20 mAbs for B-cell lymphoma has been a very straightforward method for the improvement of treatment protocols, the use of anti-CD37 mAbs for the treatment of lymphoma and chronic lymphocytic leukemia was abandoned and only recently reintroduced. Several forms of therapeutic anti-CD37 antibodies, whether they are human or humanized, used in combination or alone (unconjugated antibodies (Bi 836826 and otlertuzumab) and drug conjugates (monomethyl auristatin E: AGS67E, maytansine: IMGN529)), or radiolabeled antibodies (^{177}Lu: belatutin) [40], have been developed and are currently undergoing clinical tests. Promising results have been obtained in the resistant forms of NHL (Non-Hodgkin Lymphomas) and CLL (Chronic Lymphocytic Leukemias).

Anti-CD151 antibodies inhibited metastasis spread and primary tumor growth in human tumor mouse models [41,42]. Despite their variable ability to disrupt the complex between CD151 and $\alpha3\beta1$ integrin, different anti-CD151 antibodies were reported to prevent metastasis formation in clinical models [35].

4. Treatment with Unconjugated Anti-Tspan8 Antibodies

Unconjugated mAbs may act through two different mechanisms, which are namely the mediation of ADCC or interference with molecular functions that are required for malignant cells to express their tumorigenicity. The functional activity of the anti-Tspan8 mAbs can be assessed to some extent in vitro but the link between tumor growth inhibition and either ADCC or functional inhibition could be difficult to determine in vivo.

Several studies were performed by Zöller's group with the rat pancreatic adenocarcinoma cells (AS-Tspan8 compared to AS). The anti-rat Tspan8 mAb D6.1 was found to inhibit cell proliferation in vitro [20]. Furthermore, in rat mesentery fragments cultured with tumor cells or their exosomes, increased endothelial cell branching linked to Tspan8 expression was blocked by mAb D6.1 [21]. These studies suggest that Tspan8 overexpression in rats promotes angiogenic activity and supports tumor growth while anti-rat Tspan8 mAbs can efficiently inhibit this process. In addition, increased vessel density observed by intravital microscopy was abolished after treatment with D6.1 in an in-vivo model of peritoneal carcinosis [21].

Anti-human Tspan8 mAbs (Ts29.1: IgG1 and Ts29.2: IgG2b) were produced by Boucheix's team. These antibodies had no effect on cell proliferation, migration or apoptosis for colorectal cancer (CRC) cell lines Isreco-1/Is1-Co029, SW480 (presenting spontaneously weak Tspan8 expression) and SW480-Co029 (overexpressing Tspan8 after gene transduction) in vitro. However, the 2D motility of Is1-Co029 was increased by RNAi targeting E-cadherin and p120-catenin while it only decreased after specific co-treatment with anti-Tspan8 mAbs [12,19]. EGFR blocking (mAb cetuximab or AG1478, a chemical EGFR inhibitor) in Is1-Co029 cells also induced an increase in cell motility, which was further blocked by treatment with anti-Tspan8 mAbs [12]. The observations in relation to EGFR inhibition were unexpected since Isreco-1 cell lines have a KRAS mutation, which should be associated with an inhibition of the EGFR function. Thus, this suggested that EGFR signaling may still be influenced when Tspan8 is expressed.

In a mouse model of CRC (SW480 vs. SW480-Co029), the growth of SW480-Co029 tumors was inhibited by up to 70% when treated in the early stages with the IgG2b anti-human Tspan8 mAbTs29.2 in vivo (initially 2 mg intraperitoneally, followed by 1 mg twice a week for 4 weeks). The same results were also observed in another CRC mouse model, which expressed spontaneously high levels of Tspan8 (HT29). The inhibition of the cell proliferation in vivo was demonstrated by a reduction of the mitotic index in HT29 tumor cells in Ts29.2-treated mice. These in-vivo data underlined the crucial role of Tspan8 in tumor growth and the therapeutic potential of anti-Tspan8 mAbs as a CRC treatment. The discrepancy between the in-vitro and in-vivo data on cell proliferation suggested that the binding of Ts29.2 to tumor cells may modify their response to signaling from the microenvironment. No significant differences between the treated and control mice were found when assessing the inflammatory infiltrate, angiogenesis (CD34) and apoptotic signal (Casp3). These findings did not support the hypothesis of ADCC.

In another approach targeting Tspan8, Park et al. [25] used phage display technology to produce a fully human mAb directed against Tspan8 LEL (large extra loop = EC2). For an in-vivo experiment, the mice that were intraperitoneally injected with SK-OV3-luc human ovarian cell line intravenously received either IgG or Tspan8–LEL IgG (10 mg/kg) twice a week until day 42 post inoculation. In the control IgG-treated group, a detectable luminescence signal in removed organs (ovary, pancreas, colon, heart, liver, spleen and kidney) was observed in 24 of 31 control mice whereas the incidence fell to 50% (15 of 30 mice) in the Tspan8–LEL IgG-treated group. This reduction of 35% was considered to be significant and the mice did not show any signs of severe toxicity.

5. Treatment with Radionuclide-Conjugated Anti-Tspan8 Antibodies

5.1. Radiolabeling of Antibodies

For radiotherapeutic purposes, antibodies are usually modified with grafted chelating moieties to allow radiolabeling with β^--emitter radionuclides like yttrium-90 (β^-; $T_{1/2}$ = 2.67 d; 2280 keV) or lutetium-177 (β^-; $T_{1/2}$ = 6.65 d; 498 keV) [43]. Advantageously, lutetium-177 can be used for both imaging and therapeutic purposes as β^- and γ radiations are generated during its decay. To date, the only radiolabeled mAb authorized for human treatment is the anti-CD20 [^{90}Y]ibritumomab tiuxetan (Zevalin®), which is administered as a second-line treatment to patients with non-Hodgkin lymphomas (NHLs) that are resistant to chemotherapy [44]. Although they were created several decades ago, radioimmunotherapy (RIT)sing β^--emitter—conjugated mAbs remains underused due to inherent issues concerning hematotoxicity, which is induced by the long biological half-life of mAbs in blood, and the low penetration of antibodies in solid tumors [43,45]. Thus, different strategies have been proposed to enhance RIT efficiency, including the use of α-particle emitters, pretargeting protocols and reduction/modification of the antibody size (nanobodies, affibodies and so on).

The use of α-particle emitters is of great interest for delivering high linear energy transfer (LET) in very small volumes (cell diameters of 50–100 µm) without affecting neighboring tissues. Among the increasing number of clinical studies using mAbs/peptides/ligands/radionuclides delivering α-particles [46], two mAbs radiolabeled with bismuth-213 (α; $T_{1/2}$ = 45.6 min; 5869 keV) (^{213}Bi-cDTPA-9.2.27 targeting MSCP in melanoma and ^{213}Bi-Hum195 mAb targeting CD33 in acute myeloid leukemia) have had positive results in terms of prognosis [47,48]. Moreover, challenging approaches using DOTA-mAbs radiolabeled with actinium-225 (α; $T_{1/2}$ = 10.0 d; 5580–5830 keV) are currently under investigation as this radionuclide decay generates francium-221 (α; $T_{1/2}$ = 4.79 min, 6300 keV), which has an interesting secondary radiotoxic effect [49]. This strategy should be applied for internalizing antibodies to concentrate α-particles in tumor cells.

To decrease hematotoxicity, different pretargeting strategies were developed to dissociate the mAb antibody and radionuclide injections [50]. One of the most interesting approaches involves the use of bio-orthogonal chemistry. In such strategies, the mAb and the delayed injected radioactive molecule are grafted with chemical entities that are highly reactive to each other but inert to chemical functions usually found on in-vivo molecules, such as proteins. This fast and specific reaction can advantageously take place in aqueous media, which is compatible with in-vivo applications. Another way of reducing side effects of RIT is to inject the radioactive molecule in a specific organ to avoid systemic irradiation. For example, this might involve intrahepatic metastases using arterial infusions [51].

Finally, different small protein forms (affibodies, nanobodies and so on) ranging from a few to 30 kDa with a shorter biological half-life in the blood circulation have been tested in preclinical RIT protocols [52] but mostly in nonradioactive applications. In clinical trials, one affibody is currently being investigated in Her2 breast cancer imaging [53].

5.2. Targeting Tspan8 with Radiolabeled Antibodies

Our team investigated the biodistribution of two monoclonal antibodies targeting human Tspan8, which were namely Ts29.1 and Ts29.2. These were grafted with DOTA and radiolabeled with indium-111 (γ; $T_{1/2}$ = 2.80 d; 171 keV; 245 keV). The measurement of the immunoreactive fraction revealed that the addition of DOTA-chelating moieties and radiolabeling did not modify the affinity of Ts29.2 for its target. The uptake of [^{111}In]DOTA-Ts29.2 in HT29 tumors was higher than that of [^{111}In]DOTA-Ts29.1 (Figure 3A,B). After this, further experiments were conducted on different models of xenografts [23]. Biodistribution studies on mice with both SW480-Co29/SW480 tumors demonstrated high specificity of [^{111}In]DOTA-Ts29.2 for Tspan8-expressing tumors. The same results were obtained using the Isreco-1 and Is1-Co029 models (Figure 4A,B). Further RIT experiments using this antibody were supported by the promising biodistribution and dosimetry results collected. During therapeutic studies, we observed that

[^{177}Lu]DOTA-Ts29.2 induced a significant reduction in HT29 xenograft growth, with molecular events sustaining the effects of the radiation in this model.

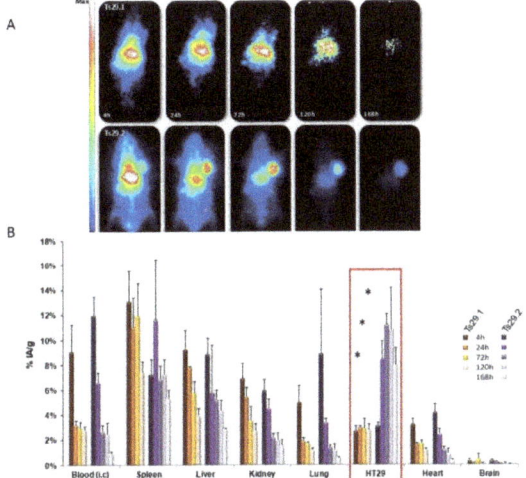

Figure 3. In-vivo selection of [^{111}In]DOTA-Ts29 antibodies for imaging and therapy in mice with HT29 colon carcinoma xenografts. Nude NMRI mice with HT-29 tumors were injected (i.v.) with 3.7 MBq of [^{111}In]DOTA-Ts29.1 (upper images) or [^{111}In]DOTA-Ts29.2 (lower images), which were imaged with a planar γ-camera at 4 h, 24 h, 72 h, 120 h and 168 h post injection (**A**). Biodistribution was performed after euthanasia and expressed as the percentage of activity injected per gram of tissue (%AI/g) of [^{111}In]DOTA-Ts29.1 (orange) or [^{111}In]DOTA-Ts29.2 (purple) (**B**). Radioactivity was measured using a γ-counter. Results are presented as the average percentage of injected dose/gram of tissue of three animals for each time point. The error bars represent the standard deviation. Biodistribution difference between the two mAbs: * $p < 0.05$ Fisher test.

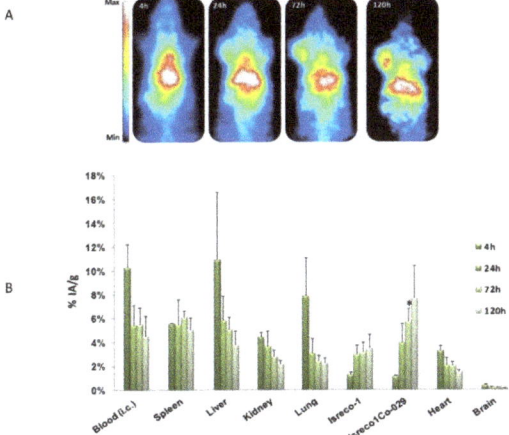

Figure 4. In-vivo specificity of [^{111}In]DOTA-Ts29.2 for Tspan8-expressing tumors. Nude NMRI mice with Isreco-1 (left shoulder) and Is1-Co29 (right shoulder) were injected (i.v.) with 3.7 MBq of [^{111}In]DOTA-Ts29.2 and imaged with a planar γ-camera at 4 h, 24 h, 72 h and 120 h post injection (**A**). Ex-vivo biodistribution study (%AI/g) of [^{111}In]DOTA-Ts29.2 (**B**) was determined on the same mice with the same protocol as Figure 3B. Biodistribution difference between the two tumors: * $p < 0.05$. Fisher test.

To initiate the pretargeting strategies, Ts29.2 was also modified by the addition of a transcyclooctene (TCO) to the lysine residues, which was evaluated in studies conducted in vitro and in vivo using a fluorescent tetrazine. We evaluated the best link size between TCO and TS29.2 and observed a higher fluorescent signal with Ts29.2-TCO without a PEG spacer, which can be explained by a higher isomerization rate of TCO to the inactive CCO form [54]. As tetrazin can be conjugated to a DOTA group, RIT with β^--emitters or α-particles will be considered. A recent preclinical study using such an approach had significant effects on mice xenografted with ovarian tumors and treated with an anti-CEA-TCO for 72 h before radionuclide injection [55].

5.3. Pros and Cons of RIT for Human Cancers: Focus on Targeting Tspan8

Stoichiometrically compared to its corresponding nonradiolabeled antibodies, [^{177}Lu]DOTA-Ts29.2 induced a greater slowing down of tumor growth. The main features in pretargeted radioimmunotherapy PRIT experiments were the reduction of proliferation and increase in apoptosis. As mentioned above, the treatment with nonradioactive antibodies (using 100-times more antibodies than in the [^{177}Lu]DOTA Ts29.2 experiments) also resulted in a slowing down of tumor growth with neither induction of apoptosis nor decrease in angiogenesis. In fact, the nonradioactive antibody should alter the interactions between tumor cells harboring Tspan8 and the microenvironment while its radiolabeled counterpart irradiates all surrounding cells after it attaches to its target antigen. This property should be interesting as it will decrease the number of so-called cancerous stem cells (CSCs) because Tspan8 has been identified on the surface of CSCs in pancreatic tumors [56]. RIT has been proven to be effective in stopping CSCs in melanomas using preclinical models, which utilized an IgM directed toward melanin and radiolabeled with rhenium-188 [57]. Conversely, Tspan8 is exposed on the surface of circulating exosomes [22], leading to potential blood radiotoxicity in RIT experiments. Apart from this potential disadvantage, one can imagine that targeting circulating exosomes will be of interest as these vesicles are implicated in metastatic spread [58]. As mentioned above, the hematotoxicity might be prevented by pretargeting strategies, which will be further reinforced by the use of blood clearing agents such as nonradiolabeled ligands conjugated to albumin [59]. As an example, this might allow their metabolism in the liver.

Tspan8 expression is restricted and this protein has been described as a significant contributor and potential therapeutic target in several cancer types. Even if secondary effects and immune system involvement cannot be evaluated on tumor-grafted mouse models used for these studies, targeting Tspan8 with radiolabeled antibodies seems to be an effective antitumoral therapy.

6. Conclusions

Tetraspanins may have a broad range of actions in cancers due to their intrinsic membrane localization (cell membrane or exosomes) and high numbers of their interacting molecules [3,26]. The aim of this article was to review recent preclinical attempts at targeting tetraspanins in cancer with a focus on Tspan8. Unconjugated antibodies and radionuclide-conjugated antibodies conceptually represent two different approaches for killing cancer cells through the expression of a surface molecule. Antibodies may have complex effects as they combine cell-mediated cytotoxicity and functional deleterious effects, such as apoptosis induction, or invasive growth and angiogenesis inhibition. This can occur directly or through microenvironment factors. For tetraspanins, it is still unknown how the targeting can alter the function of tumor cells in vivo, but their association with adhesion molecules, growth factor receptors or enzymes inside membrane molecular complexes leads to disturbance of the structure/composition of these complexes, which may result in modulation of migration and abnormal signaling into the cell and finally, inhibition of invasion/metastasis or even apoptosis. A better view and understanding of the behavior of tumor cells in real life would require improved models (such as 3D in-vitro setups with microenvironment reconstitution or syngeneic models in vivo). Although the mechanism of action of radionuclide antibodies is simple and straightforward, their manufacturing requires careful technical management and radioprotection protocols at all stages of their manipulation.

However, these offer interesting potential and should be pursued in the future. Innovative techniques have also been developed to reduce harmful effects that are linked to the antibodies binding to normal healthy tissue.

Funding: This research has been supported by INSERM-Transfert CoPOC program (MelCoMAb 2013–2016) and is now granted by the Ligue régionale contre le cancer du Puy de Dome (2019–2020).

Conflicts of Interest: The authors declare no conflict of interest.

References

1. Boucheix, C.; Rubinstein, E. Tetraspanins. *Cell. Mol. Life Sci.* **2001**, *58*, 1189–1205. [CrossRef] [PubMed]
2. Levy, S.; Shoham, T. The tetraspanin web modulates immune-signalling complexes. *Nat. Rev. Immunol.* **2005**, *5*, 136–148. [CrossRef] [PubMed]
3. Hemler, M.E. Tetraspanin proteins promote multiple cancer stages. *Nat. Rev. Cancer* **2014**, *14*, 49–60. [CrossRef] [PubMed]
4. Charrin, S.; Jouannet, S.; Boucheix, C.; Rubinstein, E. Tetraspanins at a glance. *J. Cell Sci.* **2014**, *127*, 3641–3648. [CrossRef]
5. Masse, I.; Agaësse, G.; Berthier-Vergnes, O. Tetraspanins in cutaneous physiopathology. *Med. Sci. (Paris)* **2016**, *32*, 267–273. (In French) [CrossRef] [PubMed]
6. Van Deventer, S.J.; Dunlock, V.-M.E.; van Spriel, A.B. Molecular interactions shaping the tetraspanin web. *Biochem. Soc. Trans.* **2017**, *45*, 741–750. [CrossRef] [PubMed]
7. Abache, T.; Le Naour, F.; Planchon, S.; Harper, F.; Boucheix, C.; Rubinstein, E. The transferrin receptor and the tetraspanin web molecules CD9, CD81 and CD9P-1 are differentially sorted into exosomes after TPA treatment of K562 cells. *J. Cell. Biochem.* **2007**, *102*, 650–664. [CrossRef]
8. Wang, H.-X.; Sharma, C.; Knoblich, K.; Granter, S.R.; Hemler, M.E. EWI-2 negatively regulates TGF-β signaling leading to altered melanoma growth and metastasis. *Cell Res.* **2015**, *25*, 370–385. [CrossRef]
9. Lammerding, J.; Kazarov, A.R.; Huang, H.; Lee, R.T.; Hemler, M.E. Tetraspanin CD151 regulates alpha6beta1 integrin adhesion strengthening. *Proc. Natl. Acad. Sci. USA* **2003**, *100*, 7616–7621. [CrossRef]
10. Shoham, T.; Rajapaksa, R.; Boucheix, C.; Rubinstein, E.; Poe, J.C.; Tedder, T.F.; Levy, S. The tetraspanin CD81 regulates the expression of CD19 during B cell development in a postendoplasmic reticulum compartment. *J. Immunol.* **2003**, *171*, 4062–4072. [CrossRef]
11. Saint-Pol, J.; Eschenbrenner, E.; Dornier, E.; Boucheix, C.; Charrin, S.; Rubinstein, E. Regulation of the trafficking and the function of the metalloprotease ADAM10 by tetraspanins. *Biochem. Soc. Trans.* **2017**, *45*, 937–944. [CrossRef] [PubMed]
12. Zhu, Y.; Ailane, N.; Sala-Valdés, M.; Haghighi-Rad, F.; Billard, M.; Nguyen, V.; Saffroy, R.; Lemoine, A.; Rubinstein, E.; Boucheix, C.; et al. Multi-factorial modulation of colorectal carcinoma cells motility—Partial coordination by the tetraspanin Co-029/Tspan8. *Oncotarget* **2017**, *8*, 27454–27470. [CrossRef] [PubMed]
13. Zimmerman, B.; Kelly, B.; McMillan, B.J.; Seegar, T.C.M.; Dror, R.O.; Kruse, A.C.; Blacklow, S.C. Crystal structure of a full-length human Tetraspanin reveals a cholesterol-binding pocket. *Cell* **2016**, *167*, 1041–1051. [CrossRef] [PubMed]
14. Zöller, M. Tetraspanins: Push and pull in suppressing and promoting metastasis. *Nat. Rev. Cancer* **2009**, *9*, 40–55. [CrossRef] [PubMed]
15. Charrin, S.; le Naour, F.; Silvie, O.; Milhiet, P.-E.; Boucheix, C.; Rubinstein, E. Lateral organization of membrane proteins: Tetraspanins spin their web. *Biochem. J.* **2009**, *420*, 133–154. [CrossRef] [PubMed]
16. Ashman, L.K.; Zoller, M. Tetraspanins in Cancer. In *Tetraspanins*; Berditchevski, F., Rubinstein, E., Eds.; Springer: Heidelberg, Germany, 2013; pp. 257–298.
17. De Winde, C.M.; Veenbergen, S.; Young, K.H.; Xu-Monette, Z.Y.; Wang, X.-X.; Xia, Y.; Jabbar, K.J.; van den Brand, M.; van der Schaaf, A.; Elfrink, S.; et al. Tetraspanin CD37 protects against the development of B cell lymphoma. *J. Clin. Investig.* **2016**, *126*, 653–666. [CrossRef] [PubMed]
18. Andreu, Z.; Yáñez-Mó, M. Tetraspanins in extracellular vesicle formation and function. *Front. Immunol.* **2014**, *5*, 442. [CrossRef] [PubMed]

19. Greco, C.; Bralet, M.-P.; Ailane, N.; Dubart-Kupperschmitt, A.; Rubinstein, E.; Le Naour, F.; Boucheix, C. E-cadherin/p120-catenin and tetraspanin Co-029 cooperate for cell motility control in human colon carcinoma. *Cancer Res.* **2010**, *70*, 7674–7683. [CrossRef]
20. Claas, C.; Seiter, S.; Claas, A.; Savelyeva, L.; Schwab, M.; Zöller, M. Association between the rat homologue of CO-029, a metastasis-associated tetraspanin molecule and consumption coagulopathy. *J. Cell Biol.* **1998**, *141*, 267–280. [CrossRef]
21. Gesierich, S.; Berezovskiy, I.; Ryschich, E.; Zöller, M. Systemic induction of the angiogenesis switch by the tetraspanin D6.1A/CO-029. *Cancer Res.* **2006**, *66*, 7083–7094. [CrossRef]
22. Yue, S.; Mu, W.; Erb, U.; Zöller, M. The tetraspanins CD151 and Tspan8 are essential exosome components for the crosstalk between cancer initiating cells and their surrounding. *Oncotarget* **2015**, *6*, 2366–2384. [CrossRef] [PubMed]
23. Maisonial-Besset, A.; Witkowski, T.; Navarro-Teulon, I.; Berthier-Vergnes, O.; Fois, G.; Zhu, Y.; Besse, S.; Bawa, O.; Briat, A.; Quintana, M.; et al. Tetraspanin 8 (TSPAN 8) as a potential target for radio-immunotherapy of colorectal cancer. *Oncotarget* **2017**, *8*, 22034–22047. [CrossRef] [PubMed]
24. Ailane, N.; Greco, C.; Zhu, Y.; Sala-Valdés, M.; Billard, M.; Casal, I.; Bawa, O.; Opolon, P.; Rubinstein, E.; Boucheix, C. Effect of an anti-human Co-029/Tspan8 mouse monoclonal antibody on tumor growth in a nude mouse model. *Front. Physiol.* **2014**, *5*. [CrossRef] [PubMed]
25. Park, C.S.; Kim, T.-K.; Kim, H.G.; Kim, Y.-J.; Jeoung, M.H.; Lee, W.R.; Go, N.K.; Heo, K.; Lee, S. Therapeutic targeting of tetraspanin8 in epithelial ovarian cancer invasion and metastasis. *Oncogene* **2016**, *35*, 4540–4548. [CrossRef] [PubMed]
26. Hemler, M.E. Targeting of tetraspanin proteins—Potential benefits and strategies. *Nat. Rev. Drug Discov.* **2008**, *7*, 747–758. [CrossRef] [PubMed]
27. Maeda, H.; Nakamura, H.; Fang, J. The EPR effect for macromolecular drug delivery to solid tumors: Improvement of tumor uptake, lowering of systemic toxicity and distinct tumor imaging in vivo. *Adv. Drug Deliv. Rev.* **2013**, *65*, 71–79. [CrossRef] [PubMed]
28. Matsumura, Y.; Maeda, H. A new concept for macromolecular therapeutics in cancer chemotherapy: Mechanism of tumoritropic accumulation of proteins and the antitumor agent smancs. *Cancer Res.* **1986**, *46*, 6387–6392.
29. Martin, C.; Kizlik-Masson, C.; Pèlegrin, A.; Watier, H.; Viaud-Massuard, M.-C.; Joubert, N. Antibody-drug conjugates: Design and development for therapy and imaging in and beyond cancer, LabEx MAbImprove industrial workshop, July 27–28, 2017, Tours, France. *MAbs* **2018**, *10*, 210–221. [CrossRef]
30. Lin, J.; Sagert, J. Targeting Drug Conjugates. In *Innovations for Next-Generation Antibody-Drug Conjugates*; Cancer Drug Discovery and Development; Humana Press: New York, NY, USA, 2018; pp. 281–298.
31. Berthier-Vergnes, O.; Kharbili, M.E.; de la Fouchardière, A.; Pointecouteau, T.; Verrando, P.; Wierinckx, A.; Lachuer, J.; Le Naour, F.; Lamartine, J. Gene expression profiles of human melanoma cells with different invasive potential reveal TSPAN8 as a novel mediator of invasion. *Br. J. Cancer* **2011**, *104*, 155–165. [CrossRef]
32. Kanetaka, K.; Sakamoto, M.; Yamamoto, Y.; Yamasaki, S.; Lanza, F.; Kanemitsu, T.; Hirohashi, S. Overexpression of tetraspanin CO-029 in hepatocellular carcinoma. *J. Hepatol.* **2001**, *35*, 637–642. [CrossRef]
33. Gesierich, S.; Paret, C.; Hildebrand, D.; Weitz, J.; Zgraggen, K.; Schmitz-Winnenthal, F.H.; Horejsi, V.; Yoshie, O.; Herlyn, D.; Ashman, L.K.; et al. Colocalization of the tetraspanins, CO-029 and CD151, with integrins in human pancreatic adenocarcinoma: Impact on cell motility. *Clin. Cancer Res.* **2005**, *11*, 2840–2852. [CrossRef] [PubMed]
34. Ahmadzadeh, V.; Farajnia, S.; Feizi, M.A.H.; Nejad, R.A.K. Antibody humanization methods for development of therapeutic applications. *Monoclon. Antib. Immunodiagn. Immunother.* **2014**, *33*, 67–73. [CrossRef] [PubMed]
35. Vences-Catalán, F.; Levy, S. Immune Targeting of Tetraspanins Involved in Cell Invasion and Metastasis. *Front. Immunol.* **2018**, *9*, 1277. [CrossRef] [PubMed]
36. Nakamoto, T.; Murayama, Y.; Oritani, K.; Boucheix, C.; Rubinstein, E.; Nishida, M.; Katsube, F.; Watabe, K.; Kiso, S.; Tsutsui, S.; et al. A novel therapeutic strategy with anti-CD9 antibody in gastric cancers. *J. Gastroenterol.* **2009**, *44*, 889–896. [CrossRef] [PubMed]
37. Worthington, R.E.; Carroll, R.C.; Boucheix, C. Platelet activation by CD9 monoclonal antibodies is mediated by the Fc gamma II receptor. *Br. J. Haematol.* **1990**, *74*, 216–222. [CrossRef] [PubMed]

38. Uckun, F.M.; Kersey, J.H.; Haake, R.; Weisdorf, D.; Ramsay, N.K. Autologous bone marrow transplantation in high-risk remission B-lineage acute lymphoblastic leukemia using a cocktail of three monoclonal antibodies (BA-1/CD24, BA-2/CD9 and BA-3/CD10) plus complement and 4-hydroperoxycyclophosphamide for ex vivo bone marrow purging. *Blood* **1992**, *79*, 1094–1104. [PubMed]
39. Press, O.W.; Eary, J.F.; Appelbaum, F.R.; Martin, P.J.; Badger, C.C.; Nelp, W.B.; Glenn, S.; Butchko, G.; Fisher, D.; Porter, B. Radiolabeled-antibody therapy of B-cell lymphoma with autologous bone marrow support. *N. Engl. J. Med.* **1993**, *329*, 1219–1224. [CrossRef]
40. Witkowska, M.; Smolewski, P.; Robak, T. Investigational therapies targeting CD37 for the treatment of B-cell lymphoid malignancies. *Expert Opin. Investig. Drugs* **2018**, *27*, 171–177. [CrossRef]
41. Palmer, T.D.; Martínez, C.H.; Vasquez, C.; Hebron, K.E.; Jones-Paris, C.; Arnold, S.A.; Chan, S.M.; Chalasani, V.; Gomez-Lemus, J.A.; Williams, A.K.; et al. Integrin-free tetraspanin CD151 can inhibit tumor cell motility upon clustering and is a clinical indicator of prostate cancer progression. *Cancer Res.* **2014**, *74*, 173–187. [CrossRef]
42. Haeuw, J.-F.; Goetsch, L.; Bailly, C.; Corvaia, N. Tetraspanin CD151 as a target for antibody-based cancer immunotherapy. *Biochem. Soc. Trans.* **2011**, *39*, 553–558. [CrossRef]
43. Larson, S.M.; Carrasquillo, J.A.; Cheung, N.-K.V.; Press, O.W. Radioimmunotherapy of human tumours. *Nat. Rev. Cancer* **2015**, *15*, 347–360. [CrossRef] [PubMed]
44. Ferrero, S.; Pastore, A.; Scholz, C.W.; Forstpointner, R.; Pezzutto, A.; Bergmann, L.; Trümper, L.; Finke, J.; Keller, U.; Ghione, P.; et al. Radioimmunotherapy in relapsed/refractory mantle cell lymphoma patients: Final results of a European MCL Network Phase II Trial. *Leukemia* **2016**, *30*, 984–987. [CrossRef] [PubMed]
45. Navarro-Teulon, I.; Lozza, C.; Pèlegrin, A.; Vivès, E.; Pouget, J.-P. General overview of radioimmunotherapy of solid tumors. *Immunotherapy* **2013**, *5*, 467–487. [CrossRef] [PubMed]
46. Makvandi, M.; Dupis, E.; Engle, J.W.; Nortier, F.M.; Fassbender, M.E.; Simon, S.; Birnbaum, E.R.; Atcher, R.W.; John, K.D.; Rixe, O.; et al. Alpha-Emitters and Targeted Alpha Therapy in Oncology: From Basic Science to Clinical Investigations. *Target Oncol.* **2018**, *13*, 189–203. [CrossRef] [PubMed]
47. Allen, B.J.; Singla, A.A.; Rizvi, S.M.A.; Graham, P.; Bruchertseifer, F.; Apostolidis, C.; Morgenstern, A. Analysis of patient survival in a Phase I trial of systemic targeted α-therapy for metastatic melanoma. *Immunotherapy* **2011**, *3*, 1041–1050. [CrossRef] [PubMed]
48. Rosenblat, T.L.; McDevitt, M.R.; Mulford, D.A.; Pandit-Taskar, N.; Divgi, C.R.; Panageas, K.S.; Heaney, M.L.; Chanel, S.; Morgenstern, A.; Sgouros, G.; et al. Sequential cytarabine and alpha-particle immunotherapy with bismuth-213-lintuzumab (HuM195) for acute myeloid leukemia. *Clin. Cancer Res.* **2010**, *16*, 5303–5311. [CrossRef] [PubMed]
49. Kraeber-Bodéré, F.; Rousseau, C.; Bodet-Milin, C.; Frampas, E.; Faivre-Chauvet, A.; Rauscher, A.; Sharkey, R.M.; Goldenberg, D.M.; Chatal, J.-F.; Barbet, J. A pretargeting system for tumor PET imaging and radioimmunotherapy. *Front. Pharmacol.* **2015**, *6*, 54.
50. Van de Watering, F.C.J.; Rijpkema, M.; Robillard, M.; Oyen, W.J.G.; Boerman, O.C. Pretargeted imaging and radioimmunotherapy of cancer using antibodies and bioorthogonal chemistry. *Front. Med. (Lausanne)* **2014**, *1*, 44. [CrossRef]
51. Venkatanarasimha, N.; Gogna, A.; Tong, K.T.A.; Damodharan, K.; Chow, P.K.H.; Lo, R.H.G.; Chandramohan, S. Radioembolisation of hepatocellular carcinoma: A primer. *Clin. Radiol.* **2017**, *72*, 1002–1013. [CrossRef]
52. Pruszynski, M.; D'Huyvetter, M.; Bruchertseifer, F.; Morgenstern, A.; Lahoutte, T. Evaluation of an Anti-HER2 Nanobody Labeled with 225Ac for Targeted α-Particle Therapy of Cancer. *Mol. Pharm.* **2018**, *15*, 1457–1466. [CrossRef]
53. Sörensen, J.; Sandberg, D.; Sandström, M.; Wennborg, A.; Feldwisch, J.; Tolmachev, V.; Åström, G.; Lubberink, M.; Garske-Román, U.; Carlsson, J.; et al. First-in-human molecular imaging of HER2 expression in breast cancer metastases using the 111In-ABY-025 affibody molecule. *J. Nucl. Med.* **2014**, *55*, 730–735. [CrossRef] [PubMed]
54. Rondon, A.; Ty, N.; Bequignat, J.-B.; Quintana, M.; Briat, A.; Witkowski, T.; Bouchon, B.; Boucheix, C.; Miot-Noirault, E.; Pouget, J.-P.; et al. Antibody PEGylation in bioorthogonal pretargeting with trans-cyclooctene/tetrazine cycloaddition: In vitro and in vivo evaluation in colorectal cancer models. *Sci. Rep.* **2017**, *7*, 14918. [CrossRef] [PubMed]

55. Houghton, J.L.; Membreno, R.; Abdel-Atti, D.; Cunanan, K.M.; Carlin, S.; Scholz, W.W.; Zanzonico, P.B.; Lewis, J.S.; Zeglis, B.M. Establishment of the In Vivo Efficacy of Pretargeted Radioimmunotherapy Utilizing Inverse Electron Demand Diels-Alder Click Chemistry. *Mol. Cancer Ther.* **2017**, *16*, 124–133. [CrossRef] [PubMed]
56. Heiler, S.; Wang, Z.; Zöller, M. Pancreatic cancer stem cell markers and exosomes—The incentive push. *World J. Gastroenterol.* **2016**, *22*, 5971–6007. [CrossRef] [PubMed]
57. Norain, A.; Dadachova, E. Targeted Radionuclide Therapy of Melanoma. *Semin. Nucl. Med.* **2016**, *46*, 250–259. [CrossRef]
58. Raposo, G.; Stoorvogel, W. Extracellular vesicles: Exosomes, microvesicles and friends. *J. Cell Biol.* **2013**, *200*, 373–383. [CrossRef] [PubMed]
59. Rossin, R.; Robillard, M.S. Pretargeted imaging using bioorthogonal chemistry in mice. *Curr. Opin. Chem. Biol.* **2014**, *21*, 161–169. [CrossRef]

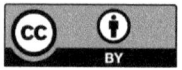

© 2019 by the authors. Licensee MDPI, Basel, Switzerland. This article is an open access article distributed under the terms and conditions of the Creative Commons Attribution (CC BY) license (http://creativecommons.org/licenses/by/4.0/).

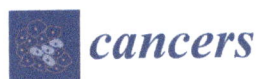

Review

The Changing Paradigm for the Treatment of HER2-Positive Breast Cancer

Aena Patel [1], Nisha Unni [1,*] and Yan Peng [2,*]

1. Department of Internal Medicine, Division of Hematology/Oncology, University of Texas Southwestern Medical Center, Dallas, TX 75390, USA; patel.aena@gmail.com
2. Department of Pathology, University of Texas Southwestern Medical Center, Dallas, TX 75390, USA
* Correspondence: nisha.unni@utsouthwestern.edu (N.U.); Yan.peng@UTSouthwestern.edu (Y.P.)

Received: 30 June 2020; Accepted: 22 July 2020; Published: 28 July 2020

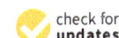

Abstract: For decades, HER2-positive breast cancer was associated with poor outcomes and higher mortality rates than other breast cancer subtypes. However, the advent of Trastuzumab (Herceptin) has significantly changed the treatment paradigm of patients afflicted with HER2-positive breast cancer. The discovery of newer HER2-targeted therapies, such as Pertuzumab (Perjeta), has further added to the armamentarium of treating HER2-positive breast cancers. This review highlights recent advancements in the treatment of HER2-positive diseases, including the newer HER2-targeted therapies and immunotherapies in clinical trials, which have paved (and will further update) the way for clinical practice, and become part of the standard of care in the neoadjuvant, adjuvant or metastatic setting.

Keywords: HER2-positive breast cancer; metastatic disease; neoadjuvant and adjuvant therapy; targeted therapy; immunotherapy

1. Introduction

Breast cancer is categorized into four different molecular subtypes: Hormone receptor (HR)-positive (+)/Human epidermal growth factor receptor 2 (HER2)-negative (−) (Luminal A); HR+/HER2+ (Luminal B); HR−/HER2+ (HER2-enriched); and HR−/HER2− (triple negative). The survival rate among patients differ based on the molecular subtype and stage. The survival rate at four years among women with HR+/HER2− is estimated to be 92.5%, followed by HR+/HER2+ at 90.3%, HR−/HER2+ at 82.7%, and HR−/HER2− at 77.0% [1]. The HER2 (human epidermal growth factor receptor 2) oncogene is positive in about 20% of primary invasive breast cancers [2]. It is well known that HER2 overexpression is associated with higher rates of disease recurrence and mortality. In addition, HER2+ breast cancers have a higher predilection to metastasize to the brain. However, during the last two decades, the treatments and outcomes for patients with HER2+ disease have shifted dramatically. Trastuzumab (Herceptin) was first approved in 1998 as the first anti-HER2 directed therapy in metastatic HER2+ invasive breast cancer. Prior to trastuzumab, historically, patients with metastatic HER2+ disease were treated with traditional chemotherapy regimens. A pivotal Phase III trial [3] of 469 women showed that adding trastuzumab to standard chemotherapy (paclitaxel or anthracycline/cyclophosphamide) resulted in improved response rates (50% versus 32%), extended time to progression (7.4 months versus 4.6 months), and improvement in median overall survival (25 versus 20 months) [3]. Relative risk of death was also reduced by 20% at a median follow up of 30 months. Since trastuzumab, multiple agents have been developed to treat patients with HER2+ disease.

The HER superfamily consists of four tyrosine kinase receptors: HER1 (epidermal growth factor receptor), HER2 (neu, c-erbB2), HER3 and HER4. When activated, these receptors cause epithelial cell growth and differentiation. The HER2 oncogene encodes for a glycoprotein receptor with intracellular tyrosine kinase activity, and has no known ligand [4]. On the other hand, the other three HER receptors have known ligands, and form homodimers or heterodimers upon ligand binding, with the HER2 receptor being the preferred dimerization partner. The HER2 receptor can heterodimerize with the other receptors, which results in autophosphorylation of the tyrosine residues. This autophosphorylation activates the MAPK (mitogen-activated protein kinase) pathway and the PI3K (phosphatidylinositol 3-kinase) pathways. The HER2, or epidermal growth factor receptor 2, is the target for many HER2-directed therapies.

Herceptin binds to subdomain IV of HER2 in order to disrupt HER2 signaling. HER2 testing is done via immunohistochemistry (IHC), which tests for the overexpression of the HER2 gene product, and fluorescence in situ hybridization (FISH) to test for HER2 gene amplification. The tumor is identified as HER2+ if IHC is 3+ (intense staining within >10% of the tumor cells), or if the ratio of HER2 and the chromosome 17 enumeration probe (HER2/CEP17) is ≥ 2 and the HER2 copy number signals/cell equals is ≥ 4. It is important to note that those with non-HER2-overexpressing breast cancers do not derive benefits from adjuvant trastuzumab. This was studied in a randomized trial of 3270 patients [5] with invasive breast cancer, with IHC scores of 1+ or 2+ and with FISH <2 (or if the ratio was not performed, HER2 gene copy number <4.0). The study found that adding trastuzumab to chemotherapy (either docetaxel plus cyclophosphamide, or doxorubicin and cyclophosphamide, followed by weekly paclitaxel for 12 weeks) did not improve disease-free survival, distant recurrence-free interval, or overall survival.

This is in line with the updated 2018 ASCO/CAP (American Society of Clinical Oncology/College of American Pathologists) guidelines. The 2018 ASCO/CAP guidelines [6] identify a testing algorithm to address the less commonly found clinical scenarios, in order to address the infrequent HER2 results that are of unclear significance. Another major revision in the 2018 guidelines includes the revision of the definition of IHC 2+. IHC2+ is now defined as invasive breast cancer with weak to moderate complete membrane staining observed in >10% of tumor cells.

Here, we will address the key trials that have led to a major change in how we treat HER2+ invasive breast cancer in the neoadjuvant, adjuvant and metastatic settings. In addition, we will also discuss newer therapies, such as bispecific antibodies, and trials that are ongoing.

2. Neoadjuvant Treatment

Neoadjuvant HER2-based therapy is typically used (as in other subtypes) in locally advanced breast cancer (Stage IIb with T3 disease, or Stage III), or in patients with an earlier stage HER2+ disease who desire breast conserving therapy, have limited axillary nodal involvement (N1) (which could potentially be converted to node-negative disease and therefore result in sentinel lymph node biopsy), or have had surgery postponed (due to a variety of reasons). Given that pathologic complete response is associated with improved event free survival (EFS) (HR (hazard ratio) of EFS 0.37, 95% CI (confidence interval) 0.32–0.43) and overall survival (HR OS 0.34, 95% CI 0.26–0.42) [7], neoadjuvant therapy can help us gauge which patients are at higher risk of relapse, and more aggressive therapy can be offered. HER2-directed therapy is typically added to a chemotherapy backbone.

Several studies have demonstrated the efficacy of trastuzumab in improving event free survival, pathologic complete response (pCR), and overall survival. Based on a 2012 meta-analysis, herceptin increased pathologic complete response rates from 23% to 40% when added to neoadjuvant chemotherapy [8]. In addition, in the Phase III NOAH (Neoadjuvant Herceptin) trial [9], the addition of herceptin increased pCR rates from 19% to 38%, and improved event free survival (EFS) from 43% to 58% (HR 0.64, 95% CI 0.544–0.930). Given the improvement of event free survival at a median follow up 5 years (from trastuzumab-containing neoadjuvant therapy followed by adjuvant trastuzumab, in patients with locally advanced or inflammatory breast cancer), this trial highlights the association between pathologic complete response and long-term outcomes of patients with HER2+ disease.

Despite the improvement in pathologic complete response and event free survival, 15% of patients will relapse after therapy with trastuzumab due to a resistance to herceptin. The proposed mechanisms have included structural defects within the HER2 receptor [10], the constitutive activation of downstream elements [11], the activation of the downstream pathways by other members of the HER family [10,11], or intracellular alterations that affect the PI3K pathway [10]. Therefore, additional therapeutic targets with different mechanisms of action have been extensively studied in combination with trastuzumab, in order to evaluate whether these combination therapies prolong time to resistance and treatment failure [4].

Pertuzumab (Perjeta) is another biological therapy that has been studied in patients with HER2+ breast cancer. Pertuzumab is a monoclonal antibody that binds to subdomain II of the HER2 receptor and thereby blocks the heterodimerization with HER3, subsequently inhibiting downstream signaling. Given that pertuzumab enhances locoregional responses, it was approved in 2013 for patients with locally advanced, inflammatory, or early stage HER2+ invasive breast cancer (with size >2 cm or node-positive disease). The addition of pertuzumab to herceptin in the neoadjuvant setting was assessed in the NEOSPHERE Trial [12]. In the NEOSPHERE trial, the percentage of patients who achieved pCR was significantly higher in the pertuzumab + herceptin + docetaxel arm (46%) versus the herceptin + docetaxel arm (29%). The addition of pertuzumab led to increased diarrhea, however rates of cardiotoxicity were not higher with the combination of herceptin and pertuzumab, as assessed in the TRYPHAENA Trial [13]. Criticisms of the NEOSPHERE trial include the small sample size, the lack of patients from the United States, the lack of a blinded pathology review and the chosen chemotherapy backbone (which is not typically used in the United States).

If comorbidities preclude the addition of chemotherapy to targeted HER2 therapy, the other options include herceptin + pertuzumab, based on one arm of the NEOSPHERE trial where pCR rates were 16.8% (95% CI: 10.3–25.3, $p = 0.0198$) with pertuzumab + herceptin, versus herceptin + docetaxel. Another option includes the addition of lapatinib + herceptin (given for 18 weeks) based on the PAMELA trial [14]. Lapatinib is a small-molecule inhibitor of the tyrosine kinase inhibitors of both HER1 and HER2. In this trial, pathologically complete response rates were seen in 30% of the patients with previously untreated HER2+, or Stage I–IIIA breast cancer. Although this is an option for patients not wanting chemotherapy, this approach has not been adapted into practice.

Several cytotoxic regimens have proved efficacious in the neoadjuvant/adjuvant setting, including TCH +/− P (docetaxel, carboplatin, herceptin, pertuzumab), PCH +/− P (paclitaxel, carboplatin, herceptin, pertuzumab) or an anthracycline-based regimen, such as AC-TH +/− P (doxorubicin, cyclophosphamide followed by a taxane such as paclitaxel or docetaxel with herceptin +/− pertuzumab) or FEC/EC-TH +/− P (fluoruracil, epirubicin, cyclophosphamide, herceptin, pertuzumab). It is important to note that the safety of pertuzumab has not been established when combined with a doxorubicin-containing regimen. In addition, the safety of pertuzumab for more than six cycles in early-stage breast cancer has also not been established.

For those with low-risk disease, or patients with comorbidities, alternatives include weekly paclitaxel with herceptin (+/− pertuzumab) or a combination of docetaxel with cyclophosphamide, in addition to herceptin, every 3 weeks for four cycles [15], based on the results in the adjuvant setting.

3. Adjuvant Treatment

Adjuvant chemotherapy is given to patients with HER2+ disease that is a node-positive, or a node-negative disease with tumors >1 cm in size. After completion of chemotherapy and herceptin (given concurrently), the standard of care is to continue herceptin for a total of 52 weeks. Studies have found an improvement in overall survival, with a hazard ratio of 0.67 (95% CI 0.57–0.80) [16], when herceptin is administered for 12 months in the adjuvant setting. Extension to 2 years did not improve the 10-year disease-free survival, as studied in the HERA trial [17]. There was no reported difference in 10-year disease-free survival when herceptin was given for 1 year versus 2 years (HR 1.02, 95% CI 0.89–1.17). In addition, the study found that the incidence of cardiotoxicity was higher in the group who received herceptin for 2 years (7.3% versus 4.4%).

In contrast, a duration of less than 1 year of anti-HER2-directed therapy was proven to be more detrimental in the PHARE trial [18], which showed that treating patients with herceptin for 6 months resulted in more deaths, shorter 2-year disease-free survival rates, and more distant recurrences.

However, there is some data to support the shorter duration of HER2-directed therapy if patients cannot tolerate 12 months. In the recently published PERSEPHONE trial [19], patients with early stage HER2+ breast cancer were randomized to receive either 12 months or 6 months of adjuvant herceptin. Patients who received herceptin for 6 months had 4-year DFS rates similar to those who received adjuvant herceptin for 12 months (89.4% versus 89.8%, HR 1.07, 95% CI 0.93–1.24). It is important to note that the absolute difference in the 4-year DFS was only 0.4%. The difference between the discordant results between the PHARE and PERSEPHONE trials, despite a near equivalence of hazard ratios in both studies, has been attributed to the chosen non-inferiority margin of each trial [20]. The PHARE trial had a non-inferiority margin of 1.15. The upper bound of the two-sided 95% confidence interval was less than 1.15 in the PHARE trial. However, in the PERSEPHONE trial, the non-inferiority margin was defined as an absolute decrease in the 4-year DFS rate of 3%, which resulted in a non-inferiority margin of 1.316. In addition, the two-sided confidence interval was 90% in the PERSEPHONE trial, which thereby increasing the chance of concluding non-inferiority. Pondé et al. [20] note that if the non-inferiority margin of 1.15 was used in the PERSEPHONE trial, then the non-inferiority goal would not have been reached. In terms of safety, the PERSEPHONE trial demonstrated that patients who received 6 months of adjuvant herceptin experienced less cardiotoxicity (3% versus 8%, $p < 0.0001$) and fewer severe adverse events (19% in the 6-month group versus 24% in the 12-month group, $p < 0.0002$). However, it is important to note that 90% of the patients in the PERSEPHONE trial received anthracycline-based treatments. In addition, given that more non-anthracycline-based regimens are used in the current climate, the benefit of shortening the duration of trastuzumab to 6 months, in terms of cardiac safety, is not clear.

The KATHERINE trial evaluated the safety and efficacy of kadcyla (ado-trastuzumab emtansine or T-DM1) for 14 cycles vs. herceptin in the adjuvant setting, in patients with residual disease after neoadjuvant HER2-directed therapy [21]. Kadcyla is an antibody–drug conjugate of herceptin linked to an antimicrotubule agent (DM1). Patients with HER2+ early breast cancer with residual disease who received T-DM1 had an improved 3-year DFS, compared to receiving trastuzumab (88% versus 77%; HR 0.50, 95% CI 0.39–0.64). Although the number of serious adverse events was higher in the T-DM1 group (13% versus 8%), switching to T-DM1 in the adjuvant setting is associated with a lower risk of distant recurrence (HR 0.60, 95% CI 0.45–0.79).

The seven-year update of the single-arm, Phase II APT (adjuvant paclitaxel and trastuzumab) trial continued to demonstrate excellent outcomes, with disease-free survival of 93% and a recurrence-free interval (RFI) of 97.5% in small, node-negative HER2+ breast cancers. Based on these encouraging results, herceptin and paclitaxel for 12 weeks, followed by herceptin alone to complete 1 year of treatment, has emerged as a very tolerable and effective treatment option in this subset of patients [22].

Dual anti-HER2-directed therapy is recommended and approved for high-risk disease (node-positive or node-negative, with tumor size >2cm) in the adjuvant setting. In the Phase III APHINITY trial [23], adding pertuzumab to herceptin and chemotherapy led to an improvement in 3-year disease-free survival (94.1 versus 93.2%; HR 0.81, 95% CI 0.66–1.00), with subgroup analysis showing improvement in the patients with node-positive disease (92 vs. 90.2%; HR 0.77, 95% CI 0.62–0.96) but no difference in those with node-negative disease.

Various options exist for the chemotherapy backbone in the adjuvant setting. If an anthracycline-based regimen is used, the recommendation is to administer HER2-directed therapy sequentially, given the increased risk of cardiotoxicity. For example, we administer dose-dense doxorubicin + cyclophosphamide, followed by a taxane + herceptin (+/− pertuzumab). If a nonanthracycline regimen is given, preference is given to chemotherapy and anti-HER2-directed therapy concurrently.

4. Extended Adjuvant Treatment

Another agent, neratinib (dual kinase inhibitor that irreversibly inhibits the pan-Her receptors), was shown to improve recurrence rates when given after completion of 1 year of herceptin [24]. In the Phase III ExTENET trial, women with early-stage HER2+ disease were randomly assigned to receive neratinib or a placebo after treatment with herceptin. There was an improvement in 5-year invasive disease-free survival (90.2% vs. 87.7%; HR 0.73, 95% CI 0.57–0.92), with a subgroup analysis showing a more pronounced benefit in patients with hormone receptor-positive disease. Diarrheal prophylaxis is recommended, given the high frequency of grade 3–4 diarrhea. The role of neratinib in the post-KATHERINE trial era is unknown.

5. Metastatic Disease

In patients with HER2+ metastatic breast cancer, four HER2-directed therapies are approved (herceptin, pertuzumab, kadcyla or lapatinib). For patients who want to avoid chemotherapy, single agent herceptin can be used, however with the caveat that with progression, chemotherapy should be considered. For patients with hormone receptor-positive and HER2+ cancers, a combination of endocrine therapy and HER2-directed therapy can be used. However, if the disease is rapidly progressive or if there is visceral involvement, HER2-directed therapy plus chemotherapy is typically recommended.

Patients are typically treated with herceptin and a taxane (docetaxel or paclitaxel) + pertuzumab. Addition of pertuzumab was shown to improve overall response rates (80% versus 69%), progression-free survival (median PFS 19 versus 12 months) and overall survival (medial OS 56.5 versus 40.8 months) in the CLEOPATRA trial [25]. However, the addition of pertuzumab to herceptin and docetaxel led to an increased incidence of diarrhea, neutropenia, rash and serious febrile neutropenia, without increasing the risk of cardiotoxicity.

Cytotoxic chemotherapy is usually discontinued after 6–12 months if patients achieve a response. If patients progress six months after receiving herceptin, triple therapy with herceptin, pertuzumab and a taxane can be re-introduced. However, if patients progress within six months of receiving herceptin, kadcyla (ado-trastuzumab emtansine) is recommended. In the Phase III EMILIA trial [26], patients who were previously treated with herceptin and a taxane were randomized to receive kadcyla or lapatinib + capecitabine. There was an improvement in progression-free survival (10 months vs. 6 months, HR 0.65, 95% CI 0.55–0.77), overall survival (median OS 31 months vs. 25 months; HR 0.68, 95% CI 0.55–0.85) and overall response rate (44% vs. 31%). Serious toxicities included thrombocytopenia (13% versus 0.2%) and a higher incidence of bleeding (30% versus 16% in the lapatinib + capecitabine arm). In the TH3RESA trial [27], for patients with unresectable, locally advanced, metastatic or recurrent HER2+ breast cancer, who had progressed while on two HER2-directed therapies (herceptin and lapatinib), kadcyla resulted in an improvement in progression-free survival (6.2 vs. 3.3 months; HR 0.53, 95% CI 0.42–0.66) and improvement in overall survival (22.7 vs. 15.8 months; HR 0.68, 95% 0.52–0.85). Given the data, kadcyla is usually considered in the second line setting. The Phase III MARIANNE trial [28] studied kadcyla in the first line setting. The study found that there was no significant difference between herceptin with a taxane versus kadcyla with a placebo versus kadcyla with pertuzumab. Upon progression while on kadcyla and trastuzumab-containing regimens, other options, such as lapatinib + capecitabine (given the improvement in time to progression compared to capecitabine alone), or a combination of anti-hormonal therapy along with anti HER2 therapy, can be considered. In the metastatic setting, HER2-directed therapy is often continued even with disease progression.

6. Brain Metastasis in HER2+ Disease

HER2-targeted therapies could be considered instead of locally directed therapies, such as radiation, in patients with brain metastasis from HER2+ breast cancer. After progression while on trastuzumab (with or without pertuzumab) with a taxane, trastuzumab-emtansine is typically utilized, based on the retrospective exploratory analysis from the EMILIA trial [29]. Among patients with CNS (central nervous system) metastasis, there was significant improvement in overall survival in the T-DM1 arm, compared to the lapatinib + capecitabine arm (hazard ratio of 0.38, $p = 0.008$, 26.8 months versus 12.9 months). The efficacy of capecitabine + lapatinib was studied in the LANDSCAPE trial [30]. In this trial, 66% of the patients (29 patients out of 44 patients) were found to have a partial response, with a median time to progression of 5.5 months. The 6-month overall survival was 90%. The combination of lapatinib and capecitabine is typically utilized as a later-line therapy.

The next line of therapy for patients with HER2+ CNS metastasis, after progression while on kadcyla, is typically a combination of tucatinib, capecitabine and trastuzumab [31]. Specifically in relation to brain metastases, 25% of the patients with brain metastases had a one-year PFS when treated with tucatinib with capecitabine and trastuzumab, compared to 0% in the trastuzumab + capecitabine arm (HR 0.48, 95% CI 0.34–0.69). The median PFS in the tucatinib arm was 7.6 months versus 5.4 months in the capecitabine + trastuzumab arm.

Another option for patients with HER2+ metastases is neratinib + capecitabine, based on the Phase II trial [32] that studied 49 patients with HER2+ brain metastasis. Among the lapatinib naïve patients, the objective response rate was 49%, with a median PFS of 5.5 months and overall survival 13.3 months. Among patients who received lapatinib previously, the objective response rate was 33%, with a median PFS of 3.1 months and overall survival of 15.1 months.

Bevacizumab, a monoclonal antibody against vascular endothelial growth factor A, is a systemic therapy option that has been studied in single-arm, Phase II studies [33], with reported response rates of >50% when added to a platinum-based regimen with cisplatin and etoposide.

7. Mechanism of Action of HER2-Directed Therapies and Resistance Mechanisms

As discussed above, the HER2 receptor is a transmembrane tyrosine kinase receptor that belongs to the human epidermal growth factor receptors (EGFR). It is expressed at a low level on the surface of epithelial cells, and is needed for development in several tissue types, such as the breast, ovary, central nervous system, lung, liver and kidney [10]. It is overexpressed in 25–30% of breast cancer cells. As shown in Figure 1, HER2 forms homodimers (binding of same receptor) or heterodimers (binding of different receptors) with other members of the human epidermal growth factor receptors. The HER2 protein can exist in an inactivated state, and dimerize independent of the binding of a ligand. The binding of a ligand induces phosphorylation of the receptors, which in turn activates the MAPK (mitogen-activated protein kinase) pathway and the PI3K (phosphatidylinositol 3-kinase) pathways.

The development of trastuzumab revolutionized the treatment of HER2+ breast cancer by introducing a monoclonal antibody that specifically targeted breast cancer cells that overexpressed aberrant HER2 receptors. Trastuzumab binds to the domain IV region of the extracellular site of the HER2 protein, thereby preventing dimerization, and subsequently signal transduction and cell survival. Pertuzumab is a monoclonal antibody that binds to domain II of the extracellular component of HER2, thereby preventing dimerization with Her1 and HER3. Ado-trastuzumab-DM1 (T-DM1, Kadcyla) combines the antibody (trastuzumab) with DM1 (anti-microtubule agent derived from maytansine), which then delivers the drug in the intracellular compartment [34]. Trastuzumab, pertuzumab and T-DM1 utilize antibody-dependent cellular cytotoxicity. Lapatinib is a dual tyrosine kinase inhibitor that reversibly binds to the tyrosine kinase receptors (EGFR or Erb1, and HER2 or ErbB2), thereby blocking the phosphorylation and activation of ERK (extracellular signal-regulated kinase) and AKT (protein kinase B). Neratinib, on the other hand, is an irreversible tyrosine kinase inhibitor of HER1, HER2 and HER4, thereby preventing the downstream signaling of the MAP kinase pathway and the AKT signaling pathways.

Although these HER2-targeted therapies have been proven to be efficacious in the various studies previously mentioned, studies have found that less than 35% of patients with HER2+ breast cancer initially respond to trastuzumab [10]. On the other hand, some patients acquire resistance after being on HER2-targeted therapies for several months after initial response. Several mechanisms of resistance to the trastuzumab-based therapy have been proposed [10]. Dr. Vu and colleagues [10] have shown that defects within the HER2 receptor, such as a truncated extracellular domain, prohibits the binding of trastuzumab to the receptor. For example, HER2 can mutate in a fashion that results in a truncated p95HER2 isoform, which inhibits the binding of trastuzumab due to the lack of the extracellular domain [35]. Studies have found that those who acquired the p95HER2 mutation were less likely to respond to trastuzumab as this mutated isoform results in constitutive kinase activity [36]. One way to overcome this form of resistance is to add lapatinib to trastuzumab, given that lapatinib acts intracellularly [37].

Another broad category in the different mechanisms of resistance includes elevations of other tyrosine kinase inhibitors. For example, studies have found that the cross-signaling between Insulin-like Growth factor-1 receptor (IGF-IR) and HER2 induces phosphorylation of HER2, and thereby activates signaling transduction [38]. Overexpression of c-met (tyrosine protein kinase met or hepatocyte growth factor receptor) has been found to confer resistance to trastuzumab [39].

Intracellular alterations can also cause resistance to HER2-targeted therapy. One such alteration involves the hyperactivation of the PI3K pathway by mutations or loss of PTEN (phosphatase and tensin homolog deleted on chromosome 10), which is a tumor suppressor gene that normally inhibits the PI3K pathway [35]. Patients with PTEN-deficient tumors had lower overall response rates to trastuzumab than patients with wild type PTEN [40]. Clinical trials, incorporating different drugs and combination strategies to overcome these mechanisms of resistance, are in progress.

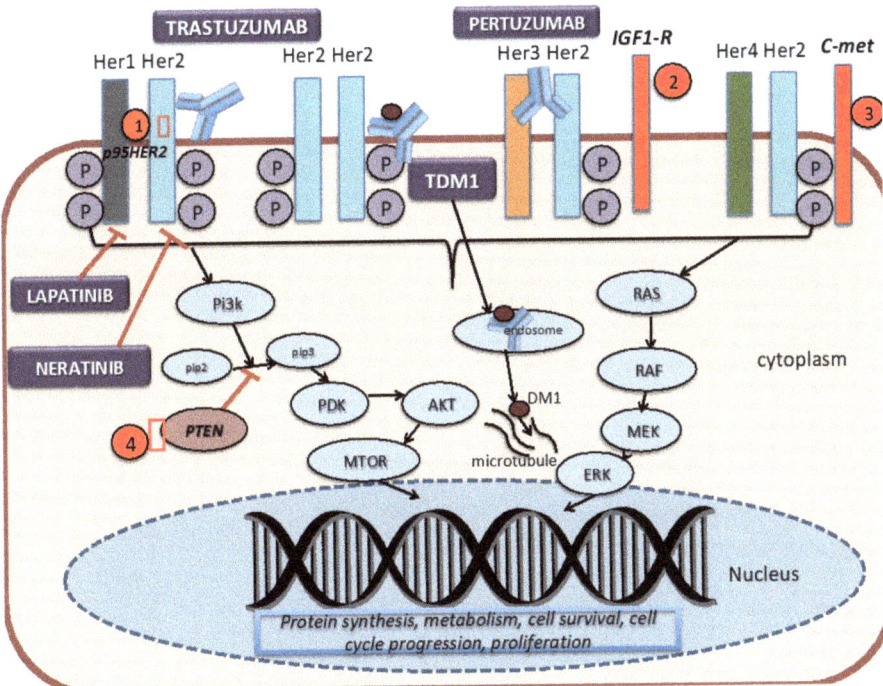

Figure 1. HER2 signaling pathway, mechanism of action of targeted therapies, and resistance mechanisms. 1. The truncated P95HER2 isoform results in the loss of the extracellular binding site for trastuzumab. 2.–3. Overexpression of other tyrosine kinase receptors, such as IGF1-R and C-met, can continue to trigger downstream signaling despite blockade by trastuzumab. 4. Mutations or loss of PTEN constitutively activates the PI3K signaling pathway.

Not much is known about the mechanisms of resistance to pertuzumab. However, one theory that has been proposed is the suppression of microRNA-150, which are small, noncoding, single-stranded RNAs, that negatively regulate the PI3K-AKT pathways. Studies in ovarian cancer [41,42] have found that the suppression of miRNA-150 resulted in decreased sensitivity to pertuzumab.

Given that combining trastuzumab with lapatinib targets both the intracellular and extracellular HER2 domains [37], combining these two drugs is an attractive strategy. However, acquired mechanisms of resistance to lapatinib often develop after chronic exposure to lapatinib. One theory is that lapatinib promotes the transcription of estrogen-positive genes, and therefore switches cell survival dependence from HER2 to estrogen receptors [43]. Another proposed mechanism involves the activation of AXL, a membrane-bound tyrosine kinase [44]. AXL has been associated with activation of the AKT/MTOR pathway [37].

The proposed theories concerning resistance to T-DM1 (kadcyla) include low tumor HER2 expression, poor internalization of the HER2-T-DM1 complexes, defective intracellular trafficking of the HER2-T-DM1 complex, and defective lysosomal degradation of T-DM1. These result in inadequate drug concentrations, and therefore cell death is halted [45]. Another proposed mechanism of resistance to T-DM1 is the presence of neuregulin b1 (NRG), which suppresses the cytotoxic activity of T-DM1 by triggering the formation of HER2-HER3 heterodimers. This heteromization activates the PI3K pathway, and thus leads to cell cycle proliferation independently of kadcyla [46,47]. SYD985, another HER2-targeting antibody-drug conjugate [48], is currently being studied in patients who develop resistance to T-DM1.

8. Newer HER2-targeted Therapies

Although trastuzumab (herceptin), pertuzumab (perjeta), Lapatinib (tykerb) and ado-trastuzumab emtansine (kadcyla) remain the most used HER2-targeted therapies in practice, other new HER2 therapies are being studied in clinical trials.

In the Phase III SOPHIA trial [49], margetuximab was compared to trastuzumab in patients with metastatic HER2+ breast cancer after progression while on the first, second or third line of therapy including kadcyla. In the study, the median age of the patients was 55 years. The backbone chemotherapy was of the investigator's choosing, between four systemic cytotoxic therapies (capecitabine—27% in each arm; eribulin—25% in each arm; gemcitabine—12% in each arm; vinorelbine—33% in each arm). Of note, more than 90% of the patients received kadcyla.

Margetuximab is a novel Fc-engineered monoclonal antibody that targets the HER2 oncoprotein. The Fc portion enhances the immune system in order to provide an added benefit. Of the patients in the study, 85% carried the CD16A 158F allele, which is shown to have a diminished response to trastuzumab. The patients who were homozygous for the CD16A-F allele appeared to attain longer progression-free survival with margetuximab compared to trastuzumab. Patients treated with margetuximab had a higher median PFS and higher overall response rates. The adverse reactions were similar between the two groups.

In the ALTERNATIVE trial [50], the addition of lapatinib to the trastuzumab and endocrine therapy (aromatase inhibitor) was studied in postmenopausal women with HER2+, hormone receptor-positive metastatic breast cancer. The addition of lapatinib to trastuzumab led to higher median progression-free survival (primary end point) and overall survival (see Table 1) rates.

Table 1. Trials of Newer HER2 Targeted Therapies.

Trial	Patients and Key Inclusion Criteria	Study Design	Results	Adverse Events
Phase III SOPHIA trial [49]	$n = 536$ Pre-treated (lines 1–3) HER2+ metastatic BC	MARG 15 mg/kg q3weeks vs. TRAS 8 mg/kg loading dose followed by 6 mg/kg q3w + investigator's choice (capecitabine, eribulin, gemcitabine or vinorelbine)	PFS: (HR 0.76, $p = 0.033$)–higher PFS if homozygous for CD16A-F allele Median PFS: 5.8 mo (MARG) vs. 4.9 months (TRAS) ORR: 22.1% (MARG) vs. 16.0% (TRAS); $p = 0.060$	Infusion reaction: 12.9% (MARG) vs. 3.8% (TRAS) Adverse events of any grade were similar between MARG and TRAS
Phase III ALTERNATIVE Trial, adding lapatinib to herceptin and aromatase inhibitor [50]	$n = 355$ Postmenopausal women with HER2+, HR+ MBC (had received prior ET and prior neoadjuvant or first line TRAS + chemo)	1:1 randomization LAP 1000 mg/d + TRAS ($n = 120$) + AI vs. LAP 1500 mg/d + AI ($n = 118$) vs. TRAS + AI ($n = 120$) AI: letrozole 2.5 mg/d, anastrozole 1 mg/d or exemestane 25 mg/d	Median PFS: 11.0 mo (LAP + TRAS + AI) vs. 5.7 mo (TRAS + AI) (HR = 0.62, $p = 0.0064$) vs. 8.3 mo (LAP + AI) (HR = 0.71, $p = 0.361$) ORR: 31.7% (LAP + TRAS + AI) vs. 13.7% (TRAS + AI) vs. 18.6% (LAP + AI)	
Phase IB HER2 CLIMB (TUC) trial [51]	$n = 60$ HER2+ metastatic BC, including patients with untreated or progressive brain metastasis	Not randomized TUC (300 mg bid) + CAP vs. TUC + TRAS vs. TUC + CAP + TRAS	RR: 42% (5/12) in patients with brain mets (TUC + CAP + TRAS) ORR: 61% (14/23) in the triple regimen Median duration of response: 11.0 (range, 2.9–18.6) in triplet regimen	Grade 1–2 in triplet regimen: diarrhea (33%), nausea (26%) and fatigue (15%) Dose-limiting toxicity: grade 4 cerebral edema in a patient with untreated brain metastasis who was not on steroids

BC, breast cancer; MARG, margetuximab; TRAS, trastuzumab; HR, hormone receptor; MBC, metastatic breast cancer; ET, endocrine therapy; LAP, lapatinib; AI, aromatase inhibitor; ORR, overall response rate; OS, overall survival; PFS, progressive free survival; TUC, tucatinib; CAP, capecitabine; RR, response rates.

The median progression-free survival associated with the combination of lapatinib with trastuzumab was 11 months, versus 5.7 months in the trastuzumab arm (HR 0.62, 95% CI 0.45–0.88). The data for overall survival was immature in the trial. The addition of lapatinib (and removal of pertuzumab) could be considered in patients who progressed after receiving trastuzumab, pertuzumab and an AI, if the disease is not rapidly progressive or if there is not a visceral crisis.

As of May 2020, there are two novel agents approved for the treatment of patients with advanced HER2+ breast cancer, and who have previously been treated.

In December 2019, the FDA approved trastuzumab deruxtecan-nxki (DS-8201a/Enhertu) in patients who have been previously treated with two or more prior anti-HER2 therapies in the metastatic setting. This approval was based on the results of an open-label, single group, phase 2 study with 184 patients who had previously received a median of six lines of therapy [52]. The primary end point of the DESTINY- Breast01 trial (Available online: https://clinicaltrials.gov/ct2/show/NCT03248492, identifier NCT03248492, last accessed 7/12/2020) was an overall response rate observed to be 60.9%, with patients achieving a disease control rate of 97.3%, median progression-free survival of 16.4 months and a median duration of response of 14.8 months. The median overall survival has not been reached. DS-8201 is an antibody–drug conjugate like kadcyla, but with a topoisomerase I inhibitor payload linked to a humanized monoclonal antibody, and to HER2, by a cleavable tetrapeptide linker. The most common adverse events noted were neutropenia, interstitial lung disease, anemia, nausea and alopecia. Death due to interstitial lung disease was reported in 2.2% of patients. Currently, ongoing trials are evaluating the effectiveness of DS-8201a against kadcyla in a randomized control trial (DESTINY-Breast03 trial; NCT03529110), as well as the effectiveness of capecitabine and herceptin or lapatinib (DESTINY-Breast02 trial; NCT03523585).

Based on the results of the HER2CLIMB trial [31], another novel HER2-targeted agent, tucatinib, was approved in April 2020 [31]. Tucatinib is an orally bioavailable, highly selective small-molecule HER2 tyrosine kinase inhibitor, which binds to the internal domain of the HER2 protein. Given the small size of the molecule, tucatinib is believed to cross the blood–brain barrier. It causes minimal EGFR inhibition, and hence is relatively well tolerated. Patients with previously treated, unresectable, locally advanced or metastatic HER2+ breast cancer were treated with either tucatinib + trastuzumab + capecitabine or with placebo + trastuzumab + capecitabine. The study allowed patients with untreated but asymptomatic brain metastasis to participate. Tucatinib combination therapy showed statistically significant improvements in progression-free survival at 1 year (primary end point), as well as in the overall survival at 2 years, in the overall population.

Given the high response rate, tucatinib combination is a promising therapy for previously treated HER2+ metastatic breast cancer patients, and could emerge as the go-to option, especially in patients with central nervous system involvement.

Neratinib is a pan-HER inhibitor, which has been recently approved in the metastatic setting, based on the NALA trial [53] and the TBCRC 022 [32]. In the Phase III NALA trial, neratinib plus capecitabine improved progression-free survival compared to lapatinib with capecitabine (12-month PFS was 29%, versus 15%). [53]. However, patients who received neratinib with capecitabine experienced more diarrhea. 25% of the patients in the neratinib plus capecitabine group experienced grade ≥ 3 diarrhea compared to 13% of the patients receiving lapatinib with capecitabine.

Pyrotinib and poziotinib are both irreversible pan-HER inhibitors. Pyrotinib has already received conditional approval in China, based on a Phase II trial which showed improved PFS in combination with capecitabine, with tolerable side effects [54]. A Phase III trial is currently ongoing (NCT03080895).

9. Novel Antibody Drug Conjugates (ADCs)

Following the success and FDA approval of two Antibody Drug Conjugates (ADCs), there are multiple other agents currently in clinical trials. Like DS-8201, these newer ADCs have a cleavable linker that accounts for what is called the "bystander effect". Bystander effect is responsible for the death of antigen-negative cells (both cancer cells and normal cells), hence it is important in both the efficacy and safety of the drug. Here we discuss a few ADCs with published clinical trial results.

These second-generation ADCs are thought to overcome the resistance of HER2+ cells to T-DM1. One of the ADCs currently in clinical trial, SYD985 (Trastuzumab Duocarmazine), was shown to be effective in T-DM1-resistant patient-derived tumor models [55]. Results of the dose-escalation/dose-expansion study with this agent demonstrated clinical activity in heavily pre-treated HER2+ patients, with a partial response of 33% and a median PFS of 7.6 months [55]. Currently, the Phase III randomized TULIP trial (NCT03262935) is evaluating the drug SYD985 against other standard of care options for previously treated HER2+ breast cancer patients.

Another ADC currently in Phase III trial is BAT8001 (Bio-Thera; NCT04185649), which uses a novel non-cleavable linker between trastuzumab and the maytansine payload. A phase I dose-escalation study (NCT04189211) revealed the drug to be safe, and it also showed efficacy in heavily pre-treated HER2+ patients. A randomized multi-center Phase III trial is ongoing in China [56].

RC48-ADC, or Distamab vedotin (RemeGen), is another antibody–drug conjugate with a cleavable cathepsin linker attached to the monomethyl auristatin E (MMAE) payload. In the Phase Ib/II trial, RC48 demonstrated good tolerability and efficacy. The disease control rate was seen to be 96.7%, with a 46.7% clinical benefit rate (CBR) [57]. A Phase II study is ongoing (NCT03500380).

DHES0815A (Genentech) is an engineered ADC, in which trastuzumab is conjugated with a stable linker to a highly toxic payload, pyrrolobenzodiazepine, and is the subject of an ongoing Phase I study (NCT03451162).

10. Bispecific Antibodies

These are molecules that recognize two different epitopes of the HER2 protein, and there are several of these currently in trials. In addition to these antibodies blocking tumor signaling pathways, they also engage immune cells and deliver payloads to destroy tumor cells [58].

ZW49 (Zymeworks) is a bispecific, biparatopic antibody, with an auristatin payload of an anti-HER2 biparatopic antibody, ZW25, which binds the same domains as trastuzumab (ECD2) and pertuzumab (ECD4). In pre-clinical breast cancer cell lines and PDX models, ZW49 has demonstrated anti-tumor activity [59]. A Phase I, dose-finding, multicenter, open-label trial is ongoing to assess the safety and tolerability of the drug (NCT03821233).

ZW25 increases tumor cell binding, improves receptor internalization and downregulates HER2 expression. A Phase I study showed a partial response rate of 33%, with a disease control rate of 50% [60].

BTRC4017A (Genentech) is currently being explored in a Phase Ia/b clinical trial (NCT03448042). It has a T-cell-dependent bispecific monoclonal antibody with two antigen recognition sites, one for HER2 and another one for the CD3 complex, which leads to the cross linking of HER2-expressing tumor cells and cytotoxic T lymphocytes.

TrasGex or Timigutuzumab is a glyco-optimized antibody, which has shown efficacy in a dose-escalation Phase I study by enhancing the antibody-dependent cell-mediated cytotoxicity [61]. However, it is unknown if the molecule is still being developed or not.

The experimental drug, NJH395 (Novartis), an immunoconjugate immune stimulator antibody conjugate (ISAC) consisting of a monoclonal anti-ErbB2 antibody conjugated to a TLR7 (Toll-like receptor 7) agonist, is another drug currently being studied in clinical trials (NCT0369771). No pre-clinical data is available yet.

11. Immunotherapy in HER2+ Disease

In addition to newer anti-HER2-targeted therapies, immunotherapy is being extensively studied given the ability of cancers to evade the immune system [62]. Different modalities are being utilized in immunotherapy to boost the patient's immune system so as to attack the cancerous cells. Immune checkpoint inhibitors, such as cytotoxic T-lymphocyte antigen-4 (CTLA-4) antibodies and programmed cell death-1 (PD-1)/programmed cell death-1 ligand (PD-L1) antibodies, are being studied in clinical trials. The expression of PDL-1 has been shown to be associated with unfavorable characteristics, such as HER2+ status in addition to large tumor sizes and high tumor grades [63]. Although PDL-1 therapy is approved for triple negative breast cancers [64], there is no approved PD-1/PDL-1 agent for the treatment of HER2+ breast cancers. In the Javelin Solid Tumor study (Phase Ib) [65], avelumab had an overall response rate of 3% (of the 168 patients in the study; 26 (15.5%) patients were HER2+), but a higher activity was seen if they exhibited PDL-1 expression. Most recently, in the single-arm, multicenter PANACEA trial [66], pembrolizumab was studied in patients with advanced HER2+ breast cancer, who progressed while on the trastuzumab or T-DM1 therapy in this Phase Ib/II trial. While six patients were enrolled in the phase Ib trial (all PDL-1-positive), 52 patients were enrolled in the phase II trial. Patients were tested for PDL-1 expression. Of the 52 patients in the phase II trial, 40 had PDL-1-positive tumors, and the remaining patients had PDL-1-negative tumors. Although no objective responses were seen in the PDL-1-negative patients, the disease control rate was 24% in PD-L1-positive patients, and the overall response rate was 39%. The most common adverse reaction that was noted was fatigue (21%).

12. Future Directions

Although patients do relatively well on the therapies previously mentioned, a subset of HER2+ breast cancer patients experienced relapse after neoadjuvant and adjuvant therapy, as well as resistance to existing therapies. A dual-targeted HER2 approach is typically used if there are no contraindications. However, what remains to be determined is whether adding a newer HER2-targeted therapy would increase progression-free survival, or whether immunotherapy would help in overcoming the resistance to HER2-targeted therapies. In addition, many trials did not utilize the updated 2018 ASCO (American Society of Clinical Oncology)/CAP (College of American Pathologists) guidelines on HER2 interpretation in breast cancer [6], which generated an increase in negative cases due to the more rigorous algorithm for identifying HER2+ patients. This algorithm helped to reclassify equivocal cases as either HER2+ or HER2−. Treatment of HER2 equivocal cases was not standardized, given the lack of data surrounding the clinical benefits of HER2-targeted therapies in this subset of patients. Since the 2018 guidelines reclassify these patients as either HER2+ or HER2−, the overtreatment of patients can be avoided, and costs can be saved.

There is still an unmet need for treatment of metastatic HER2+ breast cancer. Whether adding or utilizing immunotherapy upfront, like in other subtypes of breast cancer, can improve patient outcomes remains unknown. Different strategies are being employed to improve the efficacy of anti-HER2 therapy by combining existing approved therapies and exploring next-generation sequencing to target potential biomarkers, so as to overcome resistance and reduce side effects. There is much more to be studied in HER2+ breast cancer.

13. Conclusions

The discovery and implementation of new HER2-directed therapies in clinical practice has significantly changed how patients with HER2+ diseases are being treated. Although major strides have been made in treating patients with HER2+ diseases, studies are ongoing concerning the continued improvement of the outcomes for this subset of patients. Whether it is a combination of multiple HER2-directed therapies in the various settings, or the invention of immunotherapy, the treatment of HER2+ disease has resulted in better outcomes, including in progression-free survival and overall survival, compared to the outcomes of previous decades, and these will continue to evolve.

Funding: This research received no external funding.

Conflicts of Interest: Nisha Unni declares is serving on the advisory board of Eisai Inc. The other authors do not have a conflict of interest.

References

1. Howlader, N.; Cronin, K.A.; Kurian, A.W.; Andridge, R. Differences in Breast Cancer Survival by Molecular Subtypes in the United States. *Cancer Epidemiol. Biomark. Prev.* **2018**, *27*, 619–626. [CrossRef] [PubMed]
2. Slamon, D.J.; Clark, G.M.; Wong, S.G.; Levin, W.J.; Ullrich, A.; McGuire, W.L. Human breast cancer: Correlation of relapse and survival with amplification of the HER-2/neu oncogene. *Science* **1987**, *235*, 177–182. [CrossRef] [PubMed]
3. Slamon, D.J.; Leyland-Jones, B.; Shak, S.; Fuchs, H.; Paton, V.; Baiamonde, A.; Fleming, T.; Eiermann, W.; Wolter, J.; Pegram, M.; et al. Use of chemotherapy plus a monoclonal antibody against HER2 for metastatic breast cancer that overexpresses HER2. *N. Engl. J. Med.* **2001**, *344*, 783–792. [CrossRef] [PubMed]
4. Browne, B.C.; O'Brien, N.; Duffy, M.J.; Crown, J.; O'Donovan, N. Her-2 signaling and inhibition in breast cancer. *Curr. Cancer Drug Targets* **2009**, *9*, 419–438. [CrossRef] [PubMed]
5. Fehrenbacher, L.; Cecchini, R.S.; Geyer, C.E.; Rastogi, P.; Costantino, J.; Atkins, J.N.; Crown, J.P.; Polikoff, J.; Boileau, J.F.; Provencher, L.; et al. NSABP B-47/NRG Oncology Phase III Randomized Trial Comparing Adjuvant Chemotherapy With or Without Trastuzumab in High-Risk Invasive Breast Cancer Negative for HER2 by FISH and With IHC 1+ or 2. *J. Clin. Oncol.* **2020**, *38*, 444. [CrossRef]
6. Wolff, A.C.; Hammond, M.E.H.; Allison, K.H.; Harvey, B.E.; Mangu, P.B.; Bartlett, J.M.S.; Bilous, M.; Ellis, I.O.; Fitzgibbons, P.; Hanna, W.; et al. Human Epidermal Growth Factor Receptor 2 Testing in Breast Cancer: American Society of Clinical Oncology/College of American Pathologists Clinical Practice Guideline Focused Update. *J. Clin. Oncol.* **2018**, *36*, 2105–2122. [CrossRef]
7. Broglio, K.R.; Quintana, M.; Foster, M.; Olinger, M.; McGlothlin, A.; Berry, S.M.; Boileau, J.F.; Brezden-Masley, C.; Chia, S.; Dent, S.; et al. Association of Pathologic Complete Response to Neoadjuvant Therapy in HER2-Positive Breast Cancer With Long-Term Outcomes: A Meta-Analysis. *JAMA Oncol.* **2016**, *2*, 751–760. [CrossRef]
8. Cortazar, P.; Zhang, L.; Untch, M.; Mehta, K.; Costantino, J.P.; Wolmark, N.; Bonnefoi, H.; Cameron, D.; Gianni, L.; Valagussa, P.; et al. Pathological complete response and long-term clinical benefit in breast cancer: The CTNeoBC pooled analysis. *Lancet* **2014**, *384*, 164–172. [CrossRef]
9. Gianni, L.; Eiermann, W.; Semiglazov, V.; Lluch, A.; Tjulandin, S.; Zambetti, M.; Moliterni, A.; Vazquez, F.; Byakhov, M.J.; Lichinitser, M.; et al. Neoadjuvant and adjuvant trastuzumab in patients with HER2-positive locally advanced breast cancer (NOAH): Follow-up of a randomised controlled superiority trial with a parallel HER2-negative cohort. *Lancet Oncol.* **2014**, *15*, 640–647. [CrossRef]
10. Vu, T.; Claret, F.X. Trastuzumab: Updated mechanisms of action and resistance in breast cancer. *Front Oncol.* **2012**, *2*, 62. [CrossRef]
11. Nahta, R.; Esteva, F.J. Herceptin: Mechanisms of action and resistance. *Cancer Lett.* **2006**, *232*, 123–138. [CrossRef]
12. Gianni, L.; Pienkowski, T.; Im, Y.H.; Tseng, L.M.; Liu, M.C.; Lluch, A.; Starosławska, E.; de la Haba-Rodriguez, J.; Im, S.A.; Pedrini, J.L.; et al. 5-year analysis of neoadjuvant pertuzumab and trastuzumab in patients with locally advanced, inflammatory, or early-stage HER2-positive breast cancer (NEOSPHERE): A multicentre, open-label, phase 2 randomised trial. *Lancet Oncol.* **2016**, *17*, 791–800. [CrossRef]
13. Schneeweiss, A.; Chia, S.; Hickish, T.; Harvey, V.; Eniu, A.; Hegg, R.; Tausch, C.; Seo, J.H.; Tsai, Y.F.; Ratnayake, J.; et al. Pertuzumab plus trastuzumab in combination with standard neoadjuvant anthracycline-containing and anthracycline-free chemotherapy regimens in patients with HER2-positive early breast cancer: A randomized phase II cardiac safety study (TRYPHAENA). *Ann. Oncol.* **2013**, *24*, 2278–2284. [CrossRef]
14. Llombart-Cussac, A.; Cortés, J.; Paré, L.; Galván, P.; Bermejo, B.; Martínez, N.; Vidal, M.; Pernas, S.; López, R.; Muñoz, M.; et al. HER2-enriched subtype as a predictor of pathological complete response following trastuzumab and lapatinib without chemotherapy in early-stage HER2-positive breast cancer (PAMELA): An open-label, single-group, multicentre, phase 2 trial. *Lancet Oncol.* **2017**, *18*, 545. [CrossRef]
15. Jones, S.E.; Collea, R.; Paul, D.; Sedlacek, S.; Favret, A.M.; Gore, I., Jr.; Lindquist, D.L.; Holmes, F.A.; Allison, M.A.K.; Brooks, B.D.; et al. Adjuvant docetaxel and cyclophosphamide plus trastuzumab in patients with HER2-amplified early stage breast cancer: A single-group, open-label, phase 2 study. *Lancet Oncol.* **2013**, *14*, 1121–1128. [CrossRef]

16. Moja, L.; Tagliabue, L.; Balduzzi, S.; Balduzzi, S.; Parmelli, E.; Pistotti, V.; Guarneri, V.; D'Amico, R. Trastuzumab containing regimens for early breast cancer. *Cochrane Database Syst. Rev.* **2012**, *2012*. [CrossRef] [PubMed]
17. Cameron, D.; Piccart-Gebhart, M.J.; Gelber, R.D.; Procter, M.; Goldhirsch, A.; de Azambuja, E.; Castro, G., Jr.; Untch, M.; Smith, I.; Gianni, L.; et al. Herceptin Adjuvant (HERA) Trial Study Team. 11 years' follow-up of trastuzumab after adjuvant chemotherapy in HER2-positive early breast cancer: Final analysis of the HERceptin Adjuvant (HERA) trial. *Lancet* **2017**, *389*, 1195. [CrossRef]
18. Pivot, X.; Romieu, G.; Debled, M.; Pierga, J.Y.; Kerbrat, P.; Bachelot, T.; Lortholary, A.; Espié, M.; Fumoleau, P.; Serin, D.; et al. PHARE trial investigators. 6 months versus 12 months of adjuvant trastuzumab for patients with HER2-positive early breast cancer (PHARE): A randomised phase 3 trial. *Lancet Oncol.* **2013**, *14*, 741. [CrossRef]
19. Earl, H.M.; Hiller, L.; Vallier, A.L.; Loi, S.; McAdam, K.; Hughes-Davies, L.; Harnett, A.N.; Ah-See, M.L.; Simcock, R.; Rea, D.; et al. PERSEPHONE Steering Committee and Trial Investigators. 6 versus 12 months of adjuvant trastuzumab for HER2 positive (+) early breast cancer (PERSEPHONE): 4-year disease-free survival results of a randomised phase 3 non-inferiority trial. *Lancet* **2019**, *393*, 2599. [CrossRef]
20. Pondé, N.; Gelber, R.D.; Piccart, M. PERSEPHONE: Are we ready to de-escalate adjuvant trastuzumab for HER2-positive breast cancer? *NPJ Breast Cancer* **2019**, *5*, 1. [CrossRef] [PubMed]
21. Von Minckwitz, G.; Huang, C.S.; Mano, M.S.; Loibl, S.; Mamounas, E.P.; Untch, M.; Wolmark, N.; Rastogi, P.; Schneeweiss, A.; Redondo, A.; et al. KATHERINE Investigators. Trastuzumab Emtansine for Residual Invasive HER2-Positive Breast Cancer. *N. Engl. J. Med.* **2019**, *380*, 617. [CrossRef] [PubMed]
22. Tolaney, S.M.; Barry, W.T.; Dang, C.T.; Yardley, D.A.; Moy, B.; Marcom, P.K.; Albain, K.S.; Rugo, H.S.; Ellis, M.; Shapira, I.; et al. Adjuvant paclitaxel and trastuzumab for node-negative, HER2-positive breast cancer. *N. Engl. J. Med.* **2015**, *372*, 134. [CrossRef] [PubMed]
23. von Minckwitz, G.; Procter, M.; de Azambuja, E.; Zardavas, D.; Benyunes, M.; Viale, G.; Suter, T.; Arahmani, A.; Rouchet, N.; Clark, E.; et al. APHINITY Steering Committee and Investigators Adjuvant Pertuzumab and Trastuzumab in Early HER2-Positive Breast Cancer. *N. Engl. J. Med.* **2017**, *377*, 122. [CrossRef] [PubMed]
24. Martin, M.; Holmes, F.A.; Ejlertsen, B.; Delaloge, S.; Moy, B.; Iwata, H.; von Minckwitz, G.; Chia, S.K.L.; Mansi, J.; Barrios, C.H.; et al. ExteNET Study Group. Neratinib after trastuzumab-based adjuvant therapy in HER2-positive breast cancer (ExteNET): 5-year analysis of a randomised, double-blind, placebo-controlled, phase 3 trial. *Lancet Oncol.* **2017**, *18*, 1688. [CrossRef]
25. Swain, S.M.; Baselga, J.; Kim, S.B.; Ro, J.; Semiglazov, V.; Campone, M.; Ciruelos, E.; Ferrero, J.M.; Schneeweiss, A.; Heeson, S.; et al. CLEOPATRA Study Group. Pertuzumab, trastuzumab, and docetaxel in HER2-positive metastatic breast cancer. *N. Engl. J. Med.* **2015**, *372*, 724. [CrossRef]
26. Diéras, V.; Miles, D.; Verma, S.; Pegram, M.; Welslau, M.; Baselga, J.; Krop, I.E.; Blackwell, K.; Hoersch, S.; Xu, J.; et al. Trastuzumab emtansine versus capecitabine plus lapatinib in patients with previously treated HER2-positive advanced breast cancer (EMILIA): A descriptive analysis of final overall survival results from a randomised, open-label, phase 3 trial. *Lancet Oncol.* **2017**, *18*, 732. [CrossRef]
27. Krop, I.E.; Kim, S.B.; Martin, A.G.; LoRusso, P.M.; Ferrero, J.M.; Badovinac-Crnjevic, T.; Hoersch, S.; Smitt, M.; Wildiers, H. Trastuzumab emtansine versus treatment of physician's choice in patients with previously treated HER2-positive metastatic breast cancer (TH3RESA): Final overall survival results from a randomised open-label phase 3 trial. *Lancet Oncol* **2017**, *18*, 743. [CrossRef]
28. Perez, E.A.; Barrios, C.; Eiermann, W.; Toi, M.; Im, Y.H.; Conte, P.; Martin, M.; Pienkowski, T.; Pivot, X.; Burris, H.A.; et al. Trastuzumab Emtansine With or Without Pertuzumab Versus Trastuzumab Plus Taxane for Human Epidermal Growth Factor Receptor 2-Positive, Advanced Breast Cancer: Primary Results From the Phase III MARIANNE Study. *J. Clin. Oncol.* **2017**, *35*, 141. [CrossRef]
29. Krop, I.E.; Lin, N.U.; Blackwell, K.; Guardino, E.; Huober, J.; Lu, M.; Miles, D.; Samant, M.; Welslau, M.; Diéras, V. Trastuzumab emtansine (T-DM1) versus lapatinib plus capecitabine in patients with HER2-positive metastatic breast cancer and central nervous system metastases: A retrospective, exploratory analysis in EMILIA. *Ann. Oncol.* **2015**, *26*, 113–119. [CrossRef]
30. Bachelot, T.; Romieu, G.; Campone, M.; Diéras, V.; Cropet, C.; Dalenc, F.; Jimenez, M.; Rhun, E.L.; Pierga, J.Y.; Gonçalves, A.; et al. Lapatinib plus capecitabine in patients with previously untreated brain metastases from HER2-positive metastatic breast cancer (LANDSCAPE): A single-group phase 2 study. *Lancet Oncol.* **2013**, *14*, 64–71. [CrossRef]

31. Murthy, R.K.; Loi, S.; Okines, A.; Paplomata, E.; Hamilton, E.; Hurvitz, S.A.; Lin, N.U.; Borges, V.; Abramson, V.; Anders, C.; et al. Tucatinib, Trastuzumab, and Capecitabine for HER2-Positive Metastatic Breast Cancer. *N. Engl. J. Med.* **2020**, *382*, 597–609. [CrossRef] [PubMed]
32. Freedman, R.A.; Gelman, R.S.; Anders, C.K.; Melisko, M.E.; Parsons, H.A.; Cropp, A.M.; Silvestri, K.; Cotter, C.M.; Componeschi, K.P.; Marte, J.M.; et al. TBCRC 022: A Phase II Trial of Neratinib and Capecitabine for Patients With Human Epidermal Growth Factor Receptor 2-Positive Breast Cancer and Brain Metastases. *J. Clin. Oncol.* **2019**, *37*, 1081–1089. [CrossRef] [PubMed]
33. Lu, Y.S.; Chen, T.W.; Lin, C.H.; Yeh, D.C.; Tseng, L.M.; Wu, P.F.; Rau, K.M.; Chen, B.B.; Chao, T.C.; Huang, S.M.; et al. Taiwan Breast Cancer Consortium. Bevacizumab preconditioning followed by Etoposide and Cisplatin is highly effective in treating brain metastases of breast cancer progressing from whole-brain radiotherapy. *Clin. Cancer Res.* **2015**, *21*, 1851. [CrossRef] [PubMed]
34. Singh, J.C.; Jhaveri, K.; Esteva, F.J. HER2-positive advanced breast cancer: Optimizing patient outcomes and opportunities for drug development. *Br. J. Cancer* **2014**, *111*, 1888–1898. [CrossRef]
35. Scott, G.K.; Robles, R.; Park, J.W.; Montgomery, P.A.; Daniel, J.; Holmes, W.E.; Lee, J.; Keller, G.A.; Li, W.L.; Fendly, B.M. A truncated intracellular HER2/neu receptor produced by alternative RNA processing affects growth of human carcinoma cells. *Mol. Cell Biol.* **1993**, *13*, 2247–2257. [CrossRef]
36. Scaltriti, M.; Rojo, F.; Ocana, A.; Anido, J.; Guzman, M.; Cortes, J.; Di Cosimo, S.; Matias-Guiu, X.; Ramon y Cajal, S.; Arribas, J.; et al. Expression of p95HER2, a truncated form of the HER2 receptor, and response to anti-HER2 therapies in breast cancer. *J. Natl. Cancer Inst.* **2007**, *99*, 628–638. [CrossRef]
37. de Melo Gagliato, D.; Jardim, D.L.; Marchesi, M.S.; Hortobagyi, G.N. Mechanisms of resistance and sensitivity to anti-HER2 therapies in HER2+ breast cancer. *Oncotarget* **2016**, *7*, 64431–64446. [CrossRef]
38. Lu, Y.; Zi, X.; Zhao, Y.; Mascarenhas, D.; Pollak, M. Insulin-like growth factor-I receptor signaling and resistance to trastuzumab (Herceptin). *J. Natl. Cancer Inst.* **2001**, *93*, 1852–1857. [CrossRef]
39. Shattuck, D.L.; Miller, J.K.; Carraway, K.L. III.; Sweeney, C. Met receptor contributes to trastuzumab resistance of HER2-overexpressing breast cancer cells. *Cancer Res.* **2008**, *68*, 1471–1477. [CrossRef]
40. Nagata, Y.; Lan, K.H.; Zhou, X.; Tan, M.; Esteva, F.J.; Sahin, A.A.; Klos, K.S.; Li, P.; Monia, B.P.; Nguyen, N.T.; et al. PTEN activation contributes to tumor inhibition by trastuzumab, and loss of PTEN predicts trastuzumab resistance in patients. *Cancer Cell* **2004**, *6*, 1117–1127. [CrossRef]
41. Wuerkenbieke, D.; Wang, J.; Li, Y.; Ma, C. miRNA-150 downregulation promotes pertuzumab resistance in ovarian cancer cells via AKT activation. *Arch. Gynecol. Obstet.* **2015**. [CrossRef] [PubMed]
42. He, L.; Hannon, G.J. MicroRNAs: Small RNAs with a big role in gene regulation. *Nat. Rev. Genet.* **2004**, *5*, 522–531. [CrossRef] [PubMed]
43. Xia, W.; Bacus, S.; Hegde, P.; Husain, I.; Strum, J.; Liu, L.; Paulazzo, G.; Lyass, L.; Trusk, P.; Hill, J.; et al. A model of acquired autoresistance to a potent ErbB2 tyrosine kinase inhibitor and a therapeutic strategy to prevent its onset in breast cancer. *Proc. Natl. Acad. Sci. USA* **2006**, *103*, 7795–7800. [CrossRef] [PubMed]
44. Hafizi, S.; Dahlback, B. Signalling and functional diversity within the Axl subfamily of receptor tyrosine kinases. *Cytokine Growth Factor Rev.* **2006**, *17*, 295–304. [CrossRef]
45. Barok, M.; Joensuu, H.; Isola, J. Trastuzumab emtansine: Mechanisms of action and drug resistance. *Breast Cancer Res.* **2014**, *16*, 209. [CrossRef]
46. Holmes, W.E.; Sliwkowski, M.X.; Akita, R.W.; Henzel, W.J.; Lee, J.; Park, J.W.; Yansura, D.; Abadi, N.; Raab, H.; Lewis, G.D.; et al. Identification of heregulin, a specific activator of p185erbB2. *Science* **1992**, *256*, 1205–1210. [CrossRef]
47. Holbro, T.; Beerli, R.R.; Maurer, F.; Koziczak, M.; Barbas, C.F.; Hynes, N.E. The ErbB2/ErbB3 heterodimer functions as an oncogenic unit: ErbB2 requires ErbB3 to drive breast tumor cell proliferation. *Proc. Natl. Acad. Sci. USA* **2003**, *100*, 8933–8938. [CrossRef]
48. Nadal-Serrano, M.; Morancho, B.; Escrivá-de-Romaní, S.; Bernadó Morales, C.; Luque, A.; Escorihuela, M.; Espinosa Bravo, M.; Peg, V.; Dijcks, F.A.; Dokter, W.H.; et al. The Second Generation Antibody-Drug Conjugate SYD985 Overcomes Resistances to T-DM1. *Cancers* **2020**, *12*, 670. [CrossRef]
49. Rugo, H.S.; Im, S.-A.; Wright, G.L.S.; Escriva-de-Romani, S.; DeLaurentiis, M.; Cortes, J.; Bahadur, S.W.; Haley, B.B.; Oyola, R.H.; Riseberg, D.A.; et al. SOPHIA primary analysis: A phase 3 (P3) study of margetuximab (M) + chemotherapy (C) versus trastuzumab (T) + C in patients (pts) with HER2+ metastatic (met) breast cancer (MBC) after prior anti-HER2 therapies (Tx). *J. Clin. Oncol.* **2019**, *37*, 1000. [CrossRef]

50. Johnston, S.R.D.; Hegg, R.; Im, S.A.; Park, I.H.; Burdaeva, O.; Kurteva, G.; Press, M.F.; Tjulandin, S.; Iwata, H.; Simon, S.D.; et al. Phase III, randomized study of dual human epidermal growth factor receptor 2 (HER2) blockade with lapatinib plus trastuzumab in combination with an aromatase inhibitor in postmenopausal women with HER2-Positive, hormone receptor-positive metastatic breast cancer: ALTERNATIVE. *J. Clin. Oncol.* **2018**, *36*, 741.
51. Murthy, R.; Borges, V.F.; Conlin, A.; Chaves, J.; Chamberlain, M.; Gray, T.; Vo, A.; Hamilton, E. Tucatinib with capecitabine and trastuzumab in advanced HER2-positive metastatic breast cancer with and without brain metastases: A non-randomised, open-label, phase 1b study. *Lancet Oncol.* **2018**, *19*, 880–888. [CrossRef]
52. Modi, S.; Saura, C.; Yamshita, T.; Park, Y.H.; Kim, S.; Tamura, K.; Andre, F.; Iwata, H.; Ito, Y.; Tsurutani, J.; et al. Trastuzumab Deruxtecan in Previously Treated HER2-Positive Breast Cancer. *N. Engl. J. Med.* **2020**, *382*, 610–621. [CrossRef] [PubMed]
53. Saura, C.; Oliveira, M.; Feng, Y.H.; Dai, M.S.; Hurvitz, S.A.; Kim, S.B.; Moy, B.; Delaloge, S.; Gradishar, W.J.; Masuda, N.; et al. Neratinib plus Capecitabine versus lapatinib plus capecitabine in patients with HER2+ metastatic breast cancer previously treated with >2 HER-2 directed regimens: Findings from the multinational, randomized, Phase III NALA trial. *J. Clin. Oncol.* **2019**, *37*, 1002. [CrossRef]
54. Ma, F.; Ouyang, Q.; Li, W.; Jiang, Z.; Tong, Z.; Liu, Y.; Li, H.; Yu, S.; Feng, J.; Wang, S.; et al. Pyrotinib or Lapatinib Combined With Capecitabine in HER2-Positive Metastatic Breast Cancer With Prior Taxanes, Anthracyclines, and/or Trastuzumab: A Randomized, Phase II Study. *J. Clin. Oncol.* **2019**, *37*, 2610–2619. [CrossRef]
55. Banerji, U.; van Herpen, C.M.L.; Saura, C.; Thistlehwaite, S.; Moreno, V.; Macpherson, I.; Boni, V.; Rolfo, C.; Ede Vries, E.G.; Rottey, S.; et al. Trastuzumab duocarmazine in locally advanced and metastatic solid tumours and HER2-expressing breast cancer: A phase 1 dose-escalation and dose-expansion study. *Lancet Oncol.* **2019**, *20*, 1124–1135. [CrossRef]
56. Wang, S.; Xu, F.; Hong, R.; Xia, W.; Yu, J.C.; Tang, W.; Wei, J.; Song, S.; Wang, Z.; Zhang, L.; et al. Abstract CT053: BAT8001, a potent anti-HER2 antibody drug conjugate with a novel uncleavable linker to reduce toxicity for patients with HER2-positive tumor. *Cancer Res.* **2019**, *79*. [CrossRef]
57. Xu, B.; Wang, J.; Zhang, Q.; Liu, Y.; Ji, F.F.; Wang, W.; Fang, J. An open-label, multicenter, phase Ib study to evaluate RC48-ADC in patients with HER2-positive metastatic breast cancer. *J. Clin. Oncol.* **2018**, *36*, 1028. [CrossRef]
58. Suurs, F.; Lub-de Hooge, M.N.; deVries, E.; Groot, D. A review of bispecific antibodies and antibody constructs in oncology and clinical challenges. *Pharmacol. Ther.* **2019**, *201*, 103–119. [CrossRef]
59. Hamblett, K.J.; Barnscher, S.D.; Davies, R.H.; Hammond, P.W.; Hernandez, A.; Wickman, G.R.; Fung, V.K.; Ding, T.; Garnett, G.; Galey, A.S.; et al. Abstract P6-17-13: ZW49, a HER2 targeted biparatopic antibody drug conjugate for the treatment of HER2 expressing cancers. *Cancer Res.* **2019**, *79*. [CrossRef]
60. Meric-Bernstam, F.; Beeram, M.; Mayordomo, J.I.; Hanna, D.L.; Ajani, J.A.; Murphy, M.A.B.; Murthy, R.K.; Piha-Paul, S.A.; Bauer, T.M.; Bendell, J.C.; et al. Single agent activity of ZW25, a HER2-targeted bispecific antibody, in heavily pretreated HER2-expressing cancers. *J. Clin. Oncol.* **2018**, *36*, 2500. [CrossRef]
61. Forero-Torres, A.; Shah, J.; Wood, T.; Posey, J.; Carlisle, R.; Copigneaux, C.; Luo, F.R.; Wojtowicz-Praga, S.; Percent, I.; Saleh, M. Phase I trial of weekly tigatuzumab, an agonistic humanized monoclonal antibody targeting death receptor 5 (DR5). *Cancer Biother Radiopharm.* **2010**, *25*, 13–19. [CrossRef] [PubMed]
62. Ayoub, N.M.; Al-Shami, K.M.; Yaghan, R.J. Immunotherapy for HER2-positive breast cancer: Recent advances and combination therapeutic approaches. *Breast Cancer (Dove Med. Press)* **2019**, *11*, 53–69. [CrossRef] [PubMed]
63. Ghebeh, H.; Mohammed, S.; Al-Omair, A.; Qattan, A.; Lehe, C.; Al-Qudaihi, G.; Elkum, N.; Alshabanah, M.; Bin Amer, S.; Tulbah, A.; et al. The B7-H1 (PD-L1) T lymphocyte-inhibitory molecule is expressed in breast cancer patients with infiltrating ductal carcinoma: Correlation with important high-risk prognostic factors. *Neoplasia* **2006**, *8*, 190–198. [CrossRef] [PubMed]
64. Schmid, P.; Adams, S.; Rugo, H.S.; Schneeweiss, A.; Barrios, C.H.; Iwata, H.; Diéras, V.; Hegg, R.; Im, S.A.; Shaw Wright, G.; et al. Impassion130 Trial Investigators. Atezolizumab and Nab-Paclitaxel in Advanced Triple-Negative Breast Cancer. *N. Engl. J. Med.* **2018**, *379*, 2108–2121. [CrossRef]

65. Dirix, L.Y.; Takacs, I.; Jerusalem, G.; Nikolinakos, P.; Arkenau, H.T.; Forero-Torres, A.; Boccia, R.; Lippman, M.E.; Somer, R.; Smakal, M.; et al. Avelumab, an anti-PD-L1 antibody, in patients with locally advanced or metastatic breast cancer: A phase 1b JAVELIN solid tumor study. *Breast Cancer Res. Treat.* **2018**, *167*, 671–686. [CrossRef]
66. Loi, S.; Giobbie-Hurder, A.; Gombos, A.; Bachelot, T.; Hui, R.; Curigliano, G.; Campone, M.; Biganzoli, L.; Bonnefoi, H.; Jerusalem, G.; et al. International Breast Cancer Study Group and the Breast International Group. Pembrolizumab in trastuzumab-resistant, advanced, HER2-positive breast cancer (PANACEA): A single-arm, multicenter, phase 1b-2 trial. *Lancet* **2019**, *20*, 371–382. [CrossRef]

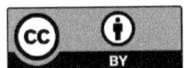

© 2020 by the authors. Licensee MDPI, Basel, Switzerland. This article is an open access article distributed under the terms and conditions of the Creative Commons Attribution (CC BY) license (http://creativecommons.org/licenses/by/4.0/).

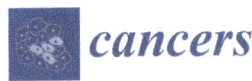

Review

Monoclonal Antibodies in Dermatooncology—State of the Art and Future Perspectives

Malgorzata Bobrowicz [1], Radoslaw Zagozdzon [2,3], Joanna Domagala [1,4], Roberta Vasconcelos-Berg [5], Emmanuella Guenova [6,7,*] and Magdalena Winiarska [1,*]

1. Department of Immunology, Medical University of Warsaw, 02-097 Warsaw, Poland; malgorzata.bobrowicz@wum.edu.pl (M.B.); j.b.stachura@gmail.com (J.D.)
2. Department of Clinical Immunology, Medical University of Warsaw, 02-006 Warsaw, Poland; Radoslaw.zagozdzon@wum.edu.pl
3. Department of Immunology, Transplantology and Internal Diseases, Medical University of Warsaw, 02-006 Warsaw, Poland
4. Postgraduate School of Molecular Medicine, 02-091 Warsaw, Poland
5. Department of Dermatology, University Hospital Basel, University of Basel, 4031 Basel, Switzerland; robertadermatousp@gmail.com
6. Department of Dermatology, University Hospital Zurich, University of Zurich, 8091 Zurich, Switzerland
7. Department of Dermatology, University of Lausanne, 1011 Lausanne, Switzerland
* Correspondence: magdalena.winiarska@wum.edu.pl (M.W.); emmanuella.guenova@unil.ch (E.G.)

Received: 30 July 2019; Accepted: 17 September 2019; Published: 24 September 2019

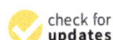

Abstract: Monoclonal antibodies (mAbs) targeting specific proteins are currently the most popular form of immunotherapy used in the treatment of cancer and other non-malignant diseases. Since the first approval of anti-CD20 mAb rituximab in 1997 for the treatment of B-cell malignancies, the market is continuously booming and the clinically used mAbs have undergone a remarkable evolution. Novel molecular targets are constantly emerging and the development of genetic engineering have facilitated the introduction of modified mAbs with improved safety and increased capabilities to activate the effector mechanisms of the immune system. Next to their remarkable success in hematooncology, mAbs have also an already established role in the treatment of solid malignancies. The recent development of mAbs targeting the immune checkpoints has opened new avenues for the use of this form of immunotherapy, also in the immune-rich milieu of the skin. In this review we aim at presenting a comprehensive view of mAbs' application in the modern treatment of skin cancer. We present the characteristics and efficacy of mAbs currently used in dermatooncology and summarize the recent clinical trials in the field. We discuss the side effects and strategies for their managing.

Keywords: dermatooncology; immune checkpoints; immunotherapy; monoclonal antibodies

1. Monoclonal Antibodies

Monoclonal antibodies (mAbs) targeting specific proteins are the most popular form of immunotherapy used in the treatment of cancer and non-malignant diseases. Since the first approval of anti-CD20 mAb rituximab in 1997 for the treatment of B-cell malignancies, the clinically used mAbs have undergone a remarkable evolution. Novel molecular targets are constantly emerging and the development of genetic engineering has facilitated the introduction of mAbs with modified structures. Recent advances in the field of monoclonal antibodies served to improve their safety, decrease immunogenicity and increase capabilities to activate the effector mechanisms of the immune system. Monoclonal antibodies are a booming market currently [1], making up a third of all new medicines introduced worldwide. The success of mAbs is remarkable in recent years with a record number of 12 novel antibodies registered in 2018 to treat a wide variety of diseases [2].

The concept of using antibodies to selectively target tumors has undergone a considerable evolution (excellently reviewed in [3]), since it has been proposed by Paul Ehrlich over a century ago. An update on the technological advances and novel registrations is published yearly by Hélène Kaplon and Janice Reichert in the mAbs journal [2].

The mechanisms of action of the currently used mAbs in dermatooncology can be generalized in five main directions: (1) The direct inhibition of oncogenic pathways with subsequent effects on cell growth and apoptosis e.g., targeting the epidermal growth factor receptor (EGFR), (2) the blockade of the formation of new blood vessels e.g., targeting vascular endothelial growth factor VEGF, (3) the opsonization of the target cells for its destruction utilizing the mechanisms of immune response e.g., targeting CD20, (4) the delivery of cytotoxic drugs to kill tumor cells e.g., mAb-cytotoxin conjugates such as anti-CD30 brentuximab vedotin and finally, (5) the activation of the impaired/exhausted immune response i.e., targeting negative immune regulators also known as immune checkpoints (ICs). Currently, particularly this last trend, awarded the 2018 Nobel Prize in Physiology or Medicine to Allison and Honjo, is of particular interest in the therapy of cancer.

Here we aim at presenting the established position, recent advances and perspectives in the treatment of cutaneous neoplasms with monoclonal antibodies.

Immune Checkpoints

The operational principle of the adoptive part of the immune system relies on two main functions: (1) Distinguishing self from non-self and (2) distinguishing safe from dangerous. This allows the immune effector cells to tolerate healthy cells of the organism, but also to ignore the non-self-commensals, such as the ones present in the intestine or on epidermis, as long as they do not induce tissue damage. However, once activated against a given antigen, the immune system shows a tendency of epitope spreading, which due to molecular mimicry could lead to cross-reactivity against bystander epitopes on healthy cells, especially under local proinflammatory conditions. Indeed, this phenomenon is thought to be responsible for a range of autoimmune disorders, including autoimmunity against skin antigens [4]. To prevent the bystander attack, the evolution has developed molecular mechanisms that tightly regulate the intracellular signal transduction following antigen recognition by T-cell receptor (TCR). These mechanisms have been commonly named "immune checkpoints". To properly discriminate the effector functions of lymphocytes, there are two main types of immune checkpoints: Negative (inhibitory) and positive (stimulatory). mAbs targeting negative ICs are commonly known as "immune checkpoint inhibitors" (ICIs).

The first molecule from the negative immune checkpoint family, cytotoxic T-lymphocyte-associated protein 4 (CTLA-4, CD152), was identified in 1987 [5] and its crucial role as a negative regulator of T cell activation was finally validated in 1995 [6,7]. CTLA-4 expression is dynamically upregulated in activated T cells and reaches the peak value between 24 and 48 hours following activation [8,9]. Once expressed, CTLA-4 potently competes with CD28 in binding to their cognate ligands, CD80 and CD86 [10], and thus strongly inhibits the priming phase of T cell activation [11]. CTLA-4 may also downregulate the intracellular signaling from the TCR complex via recruiting phosphatases [12], although the molecular events related to this phenomenon remain elusive. Subsequent studies by the 2018 Nobel Prize winner, Prof. James P. Allison, have demonstrated that, while indispensable for self-tolerance in the state of health, CTLA-4 is unfortunately also responsible for pathological tolerance towards malignant growth [13]. In consequence, monoclonal antibodies blocking CTLA-4 were shown to induce, in a "brake-off" mechanism, a potent antitumor response [13].

In parallel to studies on CTLA-4, the research group led by Prof. Tasuku Honjo, the second 2018 Nobel Prize awardee, has been focusing their studies on the Programmed Cell Death-1 (PD-1, CD279) receptor on immune cells [14]. PD-1 expression is also induced on activated T cells [15] and the cognate ligands for this molecule are PD-L1 and PD-L2, expressed on the target cells [16]. Therefore, the interaction between PD-L1/2 and PD-1 potently inhibits the effector phase of the cytotoxic immune response [17], which directly protects healthy tissues [18,19], but, when amplified in the tumor, also malignant cells [20]. Here again, monoclonal antibodies targeting either PD-1 or PD-L1 have been proved a powerful weapon against cancer [21], acting in the "brake-off" manner.

At present, mAbs targeting CTLA-4 and PD-1/PD-L1 axis have an established place in oncology. Their mechanism of action is summarized in the Figure 1. It should be noted that while the expression of CTLA-4 ligands—CD80 and CD86 is limited to antigen presenting cells (APC), PD-L1 and PD-L2 can be expressed both by APCs and tumor cells.

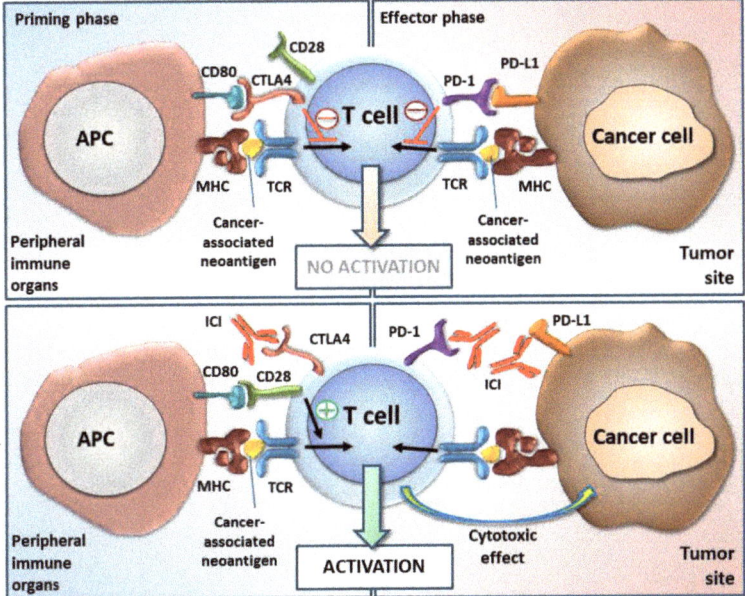

Figure 1. The mechanism of action of immune checkpoint inhibitors (ICIs).

Following the discoveries of the roles of CTLA4 and PD-L1/PD-1 in the malignant growth, targeting CTLA-4, PD-1 or PD-L1 with five agents (ipilimumab, cemiplimab, nivolumab, pembrolizumab and avelumab) has been established as registered therapies in the treatment of cutaneous neoplasms (Table 1). Additionally, two other checkpoint inhibitors (durvalumab and atezolizumab) are potential agents to be applied in dermatooncology (Table 1).

Following the success of targeting CTLA-4, PD-1 or PD-L1, a range of other molecules have been proposed to act as negative immune checkpoints protecting cancer tissue, and also proposed attractive targets for therapeutic antibodies (reviewed in [22]). The examples of such molecules are: Lymphocyte-activation gene-3 (LAG-3), T-cell immunoglobulin and mucin-domain containing-3 (TIM-3), T cell immunoreceptor with Ig and ITIM domains (TIGIT), V-domain Ig suppressor of T cell activation (VISTA) or B7/H3 (CD276), and more molecules are joining this list [23]. mAbs against these novel targets are still being investigated in Phase 1/2 clinical trials.

Table 1. Monoclonal antibodies (mAbs) targeting Cytotoxic T-Lymphocyte-Associated protein 4 (CTLA-4) and Programmed Cell Death-1 (PD-1)/PD-1 ligand-1 (PD-L1) currently in use in dermatooncology.

Name of the Agent	Molecular Target	Isotype	Source	Mechanism of Action	Trade Name	Registration Status in Dermatooncology	Most Relevant Clinical Trials
Ipilimumab	CTLA-4	IgG1	human	Triggers ADCC Blocks inhibitory APC—T cell interaction	Yervoy	2011—melanoma	NCT00636168 in MM, NCT01844505 in MM
Tremelimumab (CP-675206)	CTLA-4	IgG2	human	Reduced ADCC activity Blocks inhibitory APC—T cell interaction	NA	In clinical trials in melanoma	NCT00257205 in MM, NCT01704287 in MM
Cemiplimab REGN2810 (SAR439684)	PD-1	IgG4	human	Reduced ADCC activity Blocks inhibitory APC—T cell as well as tumor cell–T cell interaction	Libtayo	2018—CSCC	NCT03002376 in MM, NCT02383212 in BCC and CSCC, NCT02760498 in CSCC
Nivolumab	PD-1	IgG4	human	Reduced ADCC activity Blocks inhibitory APC—T cell as well as tumor cell–T cell interaction	Opdivo	2014—melanoma	NCT01844505 in MM, NCT01927419 in MM
Pembrolizumab (initially known as lambrolizumab)	PD-1	IgG4	humanized	Reduced ADCC activity Blocks inhibitory APC—T cell as well as tumor cell–T cell interaction	Keytruda	2014—melanoma	NCT02362594 in MM, NCT02243579 in CTLC
Atezolizumab	PD-L1	IgG1	humanized	Reduced ADCC activity Blocks inhibitory APC—T cell as well as tumor cell–T cell interaction	Tecentriq	In clinical trials in CTCL and melanoma	NCT03357224 in CTCL, NCT04020809 in MM, NCT01656642 in MM
Avelumab	PD-L1	IgG1	human	Triggers ADCC Blocks inhibitory APC—T cell interaction	Bavencio	2017—MCC	NCT01772004 in MM, NCT02155647 in MCC
Durvalumab (MEDI4736)	PD-L1	IgG1	human	Reduced ADCC activity Blocks inhibitory APC—T cell as well as tumor cell–T cell interaction	Imfinzi	In clinical trials in CTCL, melanoma and MCC	NCT02027961 in MM, NCT02643303 in CTCL

ADCC—antibody-dependent cell-mediated cytotoxicity, APC—antigen presenting cell, CSCC—cutaneous squamous cell carcinoma, CTCL—cutaneous T-cell lymphoma, NA—non-applicable, MCC—Merkel-cell carcinoma, MM—malignant melanoma.

2. Melanoma

Melanoma, the deadliest skin cancer, is responsible for the majority (approximately 75%) of deaths related to skin malignancies [24]. Melanoma formation is a result of a malignant transformation of melanocytes following the influence of both tumor-intrinsic and immune-related triggers [24,25]. The standard treatment for the localized disease consists of wide local excision with different safety margins [26]. Given a substantial recurrence risk after surgery, several attempts to develop adjuvant therapy have been made. Currently, the standard adjuvant therapy for recurrent locoregional disease includes anti-PD-1 nivolumab or pembrolizumab or dual BRAF-MEK inhibition by the combination of dabrafenib plus trametinib for *BRAF V600* mutated cases [24]. In metastatic disease, the combination of BRAF-MEK inhibitors is applied in *BRAF*-mutated patients, while the therapeutic options in unmutated patients have by now been scarce. In a small subset of patients with KIT kinase mutations, tyrosine kinase inhibitors have been tested with encouraging response rates characterized, however, by short duration [27]. Therefore, there was an urgent need for novel therapeutic option that is currently being fulfilled with the advent of checkpoint inhibitors.

2.1. Checkpoint Inhibitors in Melanoma Treatment

ICIs have an already established position in the treatment of melanoma. Melanoma is considered an immunogenic tumor due to a large number of somatic mutations mostly following ultraviolet damage from sun exposure. The subsequently produced tumor neoantigens are thus available for checkpoint inhibitor-reactivated immune cells [28]. The spontaneous regression of melanomas observed in some individuals is associated with functional T-cell activation [28]. Moreover, there is a body of evidence showing a link between impaired function of the immune system and melanoma proliferation [29]. Melanoma cells frequently evade the immune system by overexpressing negative immune checkpoints e.g. CTLA-4 [30]. PD-L1 can also be up-regulated following JAK-STAT activation [31]. Therefore, targeting ICs with mAbs have emerged as an attractive therapeutic option.

Initially, ICIs have been tested as adjuvants. The first trials concentrated on blocking CTLA-4 by ipilimumab. Encouraging results have been obtained in Phase III EORTC-18071 trial (NCT00636168) [32] on the adjuvant use of ipilimumab compared with placebo in patients with stage III melanoma, where a significant improvement in recurrence-free survival (RFS) has been achieved. Despite frequent adverse events (AEs), ipilimumab has been registered for patients with stage III melanoma at high risk of recurrence following complete resection in Oct 2015. The results of the EORTC 1325/Keynote-054 trial (NCT02362594) of pembrolizumab versus placebo in patients with stage III melanoma also demonstrated a significant improvement in RFS. Interestingly, a positive impact on RFS was noted in both PD-L1 positive and negative population and independently on the BRAF mutation status. [33]. Thus, pembrolizumab was approved as adjuvant therapy in stage III melanoma in Europe in Dec 2018 and by Food and Drug Administration (FDA) in Feb 2019. The superiority of checkpoint blockade with anti-CTLA-4 or anti-PD-1 mAbs to chemotherapy in the treatment of stage IV (metastatic) melanoma, has been proven in multiple randomized clinical trials (excellently reviewed in [24]).

The next step was the introduction of ICIs as a first-line therapy. Despite encouraging results of ipilimumab in terms of a marked increase in the percentage of long-term survival demonstrated in a pooled analysis from 12 clinical trials [34], due to its significant toxicity, anti-PD-1 nivolumab and pembrolizumab were further investigated. Given the positive impact on overall survival (OS) and low AE's rate when compared to ipilimumab [35,36], both agents were approved in 2014 and are now a standard treatment in advanced melanoma according to The National Comprehensive Cancer Network (NCCN) guidelines. Following the results of pivotal Phase I CheckMate-069 (NCT01927419) and Phase III Checkmate-067 study (NCT01844505) testing the efficacy of nivolumab vs. nivolumab + ipilimumab [37,38], the combination of these two agents have been approved for the treatment of unresectable or metastatic melanoma, firstly in BRAF unmutated cases in Oct 2015, which has been further expanded independently on the BRAF mutation status in Jan 2016. However, due to substantial toxicity of the combination, a more intense monitoring is recommended in case of the combinational treatment [39]. Tremelimumab, another anti-CTLA4 monoclonal antibody, is also being examined. Despite promising results from the phase I study (NCT00257205) [40], a Phase III clinical trial (NCT01704287) of tremelimumab in comparison to the standard of care—dacarbazine—showed no significant benefits [41].

Currently, also other agents targeting the PD-1/PD-L1 axis are being tested in advanced melanoma:

- Cemiplimab—a small exploratory tumor biopsy-driven study to understand the relationship between biomarkers and clinical response in melanoma patients (NCT03002376)—ongoing.
- Avelumab:
    - Combination immunotherapy with vaccine in subjects with melanoma who have progressed on or after chemotherapy and PD-1/PD-L1 therapy (NCT03167177)—not yet recruiting.
    - In metastatic or locally advanced solid tumors (NCT01772004)—preliminary results show durable responses, promising survival outcomes and an acceptable safety profile in patients with previously treated metastatic melanoma [42].
    - In combination with other cancer immunotherapies in advanced malignancies (NCT02554812)—currently recruiting.
- Durvalumab:
    - Phase 1 safety and tolerability in combination with dabrafenib and trametinib or with trametinib alone (NCT02027961)—awaiting results' publication.
- Atezolizumab—tested in numerous clinical trials.

2.2. Rituximab in Melanoma

Rituximab, a chimeric IgG1 kappa mAb targeting CD20 antigen, has an established use in the systemic treatment of B-cell malignancies. The interest in its use in melanoma is motivated by two different aspects of this disease. Firstly, CD20 has been identified as a marker of melanoma-initiating stem cells [43]. Regression of metastatic melanoma by targeting stem cells with rituximab has been described [44]. The second rationale for using rituximab is based on the concept of specific B-cell depletion [14]. Tumor-associated B-cells (TAB) have been identified in both primary and metastatic melanoma lesions [45–47] and the release of insulin-like growth factor by TABs leads to resistance to BRAF or MEK inhibitors [5]. By reducing the number of circulating B lymphocytes, rituximab might thus have a preventive effect on the development of drug resistance. However, the role of B cells in supporting the tumor growth and their possible use as a prognostic factor in melanoma patients are controversial [48–51], which is reflected by the conflicting results of rituximab's use in preclinical studies and clinical observations in melanoma patients. On one hand, B cells have been described as a pro-tumorigenic population that dampens immune responses through secretion of anti-inflammatory cytokines such as IL-4, IL-10 or TGFβ. On the other hand, B cells are vital elements in shaping an effective immune response by being efficient antigen-presenting cells (APCs) for the expansion of tumor-associated antigen-specific CD8+ and CD4+ T cells (reviewed in [52]).

In syngeneic mouse models depletion of mature CD20+ B cells was shown to promote melanoma growth [53,54]. Moreover, B-cell depletion has been shown to increase the efficacy of therapeutic anti-melanoma vaccines in a syngeneic murine model [55]. The results from a small trial testing the efficacy of anti-CD20 ofatumumab in stage IV metastatic melanoma resistant to BRAFV600E inhibitors also further support the benefit of the anti-CD20 approach in melanoma [56].

Moreover, a case series of seven patients with metastatic melanoma treated individually with rituximab, suggested that anti-CD20 therapy might be a therapeutic option for metastatic melanoma [57]. Reports suggesting that rituximab administration may lead to melanoma induction or worsening are also known [58,59]. A delayed growth of melanoma in B cell-deficient mice has been reported for D5 melanoma cell line [60]. However, data from a large cohort analysis established no increased risk of melanoma following rituximab treatment [61].

Recently, TABs have emerged as predictors of resistance to ICIs. [54]. The analysis of datasets from anti-PD1-treated melanoma patients revealed increased B-cell numbers in pre-therapy tumor samples in patients responding to immune checkpoints therapy.

2.3. Targeting LAG-3

Lymphocyte activation gene-3 (LAG-3, CD223) expressed on activated T, natural killer (NK) and B cells [62] is a negative regulatory protein for T cell function implicated in preventing tissue damage and autoimmunity [63,64]. In melanoma, LAG-3, frequently co-expressed with PD-1 was demonstrated on CD8+ tumor-infiltrating lymphocytes (TILs), leading to their clonal exhaustion and promotion of tumor growth [65]. An anti-LAG-3 mAb LAG525 is being tested in a phase 1/2 clinical trial in combination with an anti-PD-1 spartalizumab (NCT02460224). Another LAG-3 targeting mAb relatlimab (BMS-986016) alone and in combination with nivolumab is being tested in melanoma patients previously treated with anti-PD-1/PD-L1 therapy (NCT01968109). The preliminary results demonstrated encouraging initial efficacy with an objective response rate (ORR) of 16% and a disease control rate of 45% with benefit in some patients treated with anti-PD-1 [66].

2.4. Targeting TIGIT

TIGIT is a poliovirus receptor (PVR)-like protein containing Ig and ITIM domain with a well-established role in controlling immune suppression [67]. It is expressed on both T and NK cells, providing an opportunity to target the adaptive and innate arms of the immune system. TIGIT co-expression with PD-1 on CD8+ T cells was reported in melanoma [68,69] and its elevated expression correlates with poor prognosis. In in vitro studies, concomitant TIGIT and PD-1 blockade additively increased proliferation, cytokines production and degranulation of both tumor antigen-specific CD8+ T cells and CD8+ TILs from advanced melanoma patients [68]. Currently, three phase I clinical trials of different TIGIT-targeting molecules are opened in solid tumors, including melanoma, in combination with nivolumab—etiglimab (OMP-313M32)—NCT03119428, tiragolumab (MTIG7192A)—NCT02794571 and BMS-986207—NCT02913313.

2.5. Targeting TIM-3

T cell immunoglobulin-3 (TIM-3) detected on the surface of different types of immune cells is described as a direct negative regulator of T cells [70]. High TIM-3 levels on T cells are typical for exhaustion phenotype and correlate with poor prognosis in some tumors [64]. Interestingly, TIM-3 is also expressed by the melanoma cells themselves [71]. Data from the murine model showed promising results of TIM-3 targeting in combination with an anti-melanoma vaccine [72]. Since TIM-3 upregulation is associated with CD8+ T cells exhaustion in melanoma [73], clinical trials of two TIM-3 targeting mAbs—TSR-022 (NCT02817633) and MBG453 (as a single agent and in combination with PDR001—NCT02608268) are currently recruiting patients.

2.6. Targeting B7-H3

B7-H3 (CD276), a member of B7 family of immunoregulatory proteins expressed on dendritic cells, monocytes and macrophages is known to activate T-cells [74]. Its overexpression by melanoma cells and their microenvironment [75] results in immune escape and tumor proliferation [76,77]. Of note, B7-H3 shows limited expression in normal tissue, which may help to reduce the risk of adverse effects. Enoblituzumab (MGA271), a humanized anti-B7-H3 IgG1κ mAb, is being tested in combination with pembrolizumab in refractory cancer patients, including melanoma (NCT02475213). A phase I study of enoblituzumab in combination with ipilimumab in refractory melanoma (NCT02381314) has been completed and awaits the publication of the results.

2.7. Targeting VEGF

VEGF inhibition seems a rational approach in melanoma therapy, as the progression of this tumor from radial to the vertical growth phases has been associated with increased microvessel density [78]. Besides promoting angiogenesis, VEGF impairs dendritic cell maturation and modulates lymphocyte endothelial trafficking [79]. Bevacizumab, a humanized IgG1 anti-VEGF mAb registered in the management of diverse solid tumors e.g., colorectal, lung and ovarian cancer, showed encouraging results in phase II clinical trials in combination with the cytotoxic alkylating agents fotemustine (NCT01069627) [80] and temozolomide (NCT00568048) [81]. A large phase III study (ISRCTN 81261306) tested adjuvant bevacizumab vs. observation in melanoma patients at high risk of recurrence. Despite a significant improvement in the disease-free interval, no significant differences in the OS between treatment and observation groups have been reported [82]. Bevacizumab is being tested in advanced metastatic melanoma in combination with immune checkpoint inhibitors—atezolizumab (NCT03175432), pembrolizumab (NCT02681549), nivolumab/avelumab (NCT03167177), ipilimumab (NCT00790010, NCT01950390 and (NCT0215852). Incidence of the immune-mediated tumor vasculopathy induced by ipilimumab [83] led to a non-randomized clinical study assessing the efficacy of dual CTLA-4 plus VEGF inhibition [79] that reported a disease-control rate (DCR) of 67.4% and beneficial safety profile providing a basis for further investigation.

2.8. Targeting Chondroitin Sulfate Proteoglycan 4 (CSPG4)

CSPG4, a transmembrane proteoglycan, is a highly immunogenic tumor antigen associated with melanoma formation and poor prognosis [84]. Multiple studies showed its role in the survival, growth and motility of melanoma cells in vitro and tumor formation in vivo (reviewed in [85]). Although it has been suggested as a potentially attractive target, no clinical trials addressing CSPG4 targeting have been proposed yet.

3. Basal Cell Carcinoma and Cutaneous Squamous Cell Carcinoma

Basal cell carcinoma (BCC) and cutaneous squamous cell carcinoma (CSCC) are both linked to UV exposure, chemical carcinogens, ionizing radiation and immunosuppression [86]. BCC is the most common skin malignancy among the white population [87]. Although it rarely metastasizes, it can be locally destructive. BCC is most commonly cured by local resection and in case of metastatic disease some novel drug modalities i.e., hedgehog inhibitors have recently emerged. However, there is a lack of further therapeutic options for progressing patients [88]. CSCC is more aggressive than BCC and accounts for up to 20% of all deaths from skin cancer [86]. Here, the lack of effective therapeutic options for recurrent and metastatic patients also poses a considerable problem.

3.1. Checkpoint Inhibitors

In the treatment of metastatic BCC and CSCC there is also a large interest in ICIs supported by independent lines of evidence. First of all, early research in the murine models of UV-induced tumors showed immunosuppressive properties of the tumor microenvironment characterized by the onset of suppressor T cells [89]. High mutational burden present in BCC and CSCC, as a consequence of UV-exposure may elicit an effective immune response by inducing the expression of immunogenic tumor neoantigens [90]. This response can be further boosted by blocking the immunosuppressive checkpoint molecules. In fact, high mutation burden has been shown as a good response predictor to anti-PD-1 therapy in a panel of 12 different human tumors [91–93], where rapid expansion of neoantigen-specific T cell clones reactive to tumor neoantigens was observed. Data from the preclinical model of DMBA/PMA-induced carcinogenesis representing a multistage squamous cell carcinoma (SCC) development have also shown the efficacy of anti-PD-1 blockade in delaying the development of murine SCC [94].

There are several reports of response to the off-label treatment of BCC and CSCC with PD-1 targeting [95,96]. Other observations [97,98] have suggested that anti-PD-1 targeting may be a rational solution in BCC patients with acquired resistance to hedgehog pathway inhibition [97]. Substantial improvement in metastatic BCC with acquired resistance was noted after nivolumab [99] in five heavily pretreated patients with locally advanced and/or metastatic CSCC or baso-squamous carcinomas [100,101].

Pembrolizumab has been also tested in a small Phase II clinical trial (NCT02964559) in metastatic CSCC patients not curable by surgery or radiation. [102]. Data from a proof-of-principle, nonrandomized, open-label study of pembrolizumab with or without the hedgehog inhibitor vismodegib (NCT02690948) in patients with advanced BCCs showed no superiority of the combinational therapy vs. pembrolizumab alone and an acceptable safety profile [103].

A novel fully human anti-PD-1 monoclonal antibody—cemiplimab (formerly known as REGN2810)—is currently evaluated in BCC and CSCC (NCT02383212) [104]. The combined analysis of the phase 1 (NCT02383212) and phase 2 (NCT02760498) study in patients with locally advance or metastatic CSCC cemiplimab induced a response in approximately 50% of the patients [105]. The antibody received approval by US FDA in September 2018 for the treatment of patients with metastatic or locally advanced CSCC who are not candidates for curative surgery or curative radiation [106] and in April 2019 has been granted conditional marketing authorization in the EU for the same indication.

3.2. EGFR-Targeting

Before the advent of the era of ICIs, there has been a large interest in the targeting of epidermal growth factor receptor (EGFR). EGFR, a member of the family of transmembrane tyrosine kinases plays a pivotal role in signal transduction pathways regulating proliferation, invasion and metastasis [107]. mAbs targeting EGFR—cetuximab and panitumumab—are clinically used in solid tumors. There are several case reports showing their potential use with an acceptable safety profile in unresectable or recurrent CSCC [108–111]. It has also been suggested that anti-EGFR may improve response rates in CSCC when combined with other targeted therapies [112,113]. However, since other therapeutic options emerged i.e., hedgehog inhibitors in BCC and ICIs in CSCC, no further trials for cetuximab were undertaken.

4. Merkel-Cell Carcinoma

Merkel-cell carcinoma (MCC) is a rare and highly aggressive skin cancer in most cases caused by the Merkel cell polyomavirus (MCPyV or MCV) [114]. As the infection with MCV is common, additional cellular events together with loss of immunosurveillance are postulated to contribute to MCC development [115]. Indeed, an increased incidence of MCC has been reported for cancer patients [116,117], patients with immune deficiencies e.g., HIV infection [118], transplant recipients treated with immunosuppressive agents [119] as well as patients with autoimmune diseases on immunosuppression [120]. Until recently, chemotherapy has been offered to patients with advanced MCC. However, limited efficacy of regimens based on cyclophosphamide, doxorubicin and vincristine was reported leading to the introduction of platinum agents in combination with etoposide, that still offer only a short-term response [121]. Thus, preclinical and clinical studies testing targeted therapies in MCC including ICIs are currently underway (reviewed in [122]).

Checkpoint Inhibitors in MCC

Due to the immunogenicity of MCC [123] ICIs can be an effective approach in this malignancy. MCC-infiltrating CD8+ T cells, including MCPyV-specific T cells, have been shown to express high levels PD-1 and TIM-3, at far higher levels than T cells specific for other common human viruses [124]. Pembrolizumab was the first ICI to demonstrate objective tumor regressions in patients with MCC prompting its addition to the NCCN guidelines. A small single-arm, open-label Phase II clinical trial focused on treatment-naïve patients with stage IIIb or IV MCC (NCT02267603) showed a good tolerance [125]. Currently, the only registered ICI is avelumab that has been granted accelerated approval in Mar 2017 for the treatment of metastatic MCC, including chemotherapy-naïve individuals based on a multicenter Phase II clinical trial (NCT02155647) demonstrating a clinically meaningful and durable ORR [126]. The durability of responses to avelumab appears substantially superior comparing to historical trials of patients of chemotherapy [127–129]. The safety profiles of anti-PD-L1 antibodies administered to patients with MCC appear similar to those from previous trials involving patients with other tumor types. Combinational trials with avelumab are being considered e.g., with localized radiation or interferon-β (IFN-β) with or without adoptive immunotherapy of MCPyV T-antigen-specific T cells (NCT02584829) are currently ongoing.

Nivolumab's use has been investigated in the neoadjuvant setting for resectable MCC in a phase 1/2 trial (NCT02488759) [130]. Computed tomography scan results demonstrated tumor regression in 80% of patients.

Anti-CTLA-4 ipilimumab was also evaluated in an adjuvant trial following surgical resection of MCC (NCT02196961) [131]. However, after a median follow-up of 22.3 months, the enrollment to the study has been stopped due to the lack of efficacy of ipilimumab and a significantly increased incidence of adverse events. Another study aiming at assessing the combination of an anti-CTLA-4 tremelimumab with anti-PD-L1 durvalumab and polyinosinic-polycytidylic acid, and poly-L-lysine (polyICLC) (a TLR3 agonist; NCT02643303) is currently recruiting patients. [132]. Overall, these studies demonstrate the clear clinical benefit of immune checkpoint inhibition in MCC, which is superior to any form of therapy used hitherto.

5. Primary Cutaneous Lymphomas

Primary cutaneous lymphomas (PCTs) are a heterogeneous group composed of cutaneous T-cell lymphomas (CTCLs) accounting for 75–80% of all PCTs, and cutaneous B-cell lymphomas (CBCLs) representing 20–25% of PCTs [133]. According to the WHO EORTC classification, they are defined as non-Hodgkin lymphomas present in the skin without the evidence of extracutaneous disease at the time of diagnosis [134].

5.1. CTCL

CTCL arises from the malignant proliferation of skin-homing CD4+ T cells [135] and is typically a disease of elderly people [136,137]. The main two subtypes of CTCL include the most frequent mycosis fungoides (MF), accounting for approx. 60% of CTCL, and a rare leukemic variant—Sézary syndrome (SS)—representing around 5% of CTCL. The second most common group, representing approx. 25% of CTCL, is primary cutaneous CD30+ lymphoproliferative disorders (LPDs) including primary cutaneous anaplastic large lymphoma (C-ALCL) and lymphomatoid papulosis (LyP) [133].

In the majority of cases of CTCL, early-stage MF is diagnosed and the disease can be managed with active observation or topical therapy using corticosteroids, chemotherapy (mechlorethamine), immunomodulators (imiquimod), radiation or phototherapy [136]. The 5-year survival for these patients is around 90% compared with 30–50% for advanced disease [138]. Prognosis in SS is poor with an overall treatment response rates varying from 7.5 to 22.4 months [139]. Besides standard therapy (e.g., extracorporeal photopheresis (ECP), photochemotherapy, retinoids, radiation therapy, IFN-α, low dose methotrexate and polychemotherapy), small-molecule inhibitors and mAbs are currently being explored in this malignancy [140,141]. All those treatment modalities have, however, relatively low response rates ranging from 14% to 60% (mostly 20–30%) and median duration of response rarely exceeding 1 year [142]. Therefore, given the fact that allogeneic stem cell transplantation is the only curative option by now, there is a need for novel therapies in CTCL.

5.1.1. Alemtuzumab

Alemtuzumab, a humanized IgG1 kappa mAb targeting CD52 antigen expressed on both benign and malignant B and T cells, monocytes, macrophages, natural killer cells and a proportion of granulocytes [143] has originally been approved for the treatment of chronic lymphocytic leukemia (CLL). Given the expression of CD52 antigen on CD4+ T cells, there has been an increasing interest in applying alemtuzumab in CTCL. Alemtuzumab showed efficacy in managing erythroderma, plaque or skin tumors and importantly reduced pruritus. Results from a multicenter retrospective analysis carried among 39 patients with advanced CTCL (23 with SS and 16 with advanced MF) treated with alemtuzumab i.v. showed a 70% ORR in patients with SS and 25% ORR in patients with MF. The reason for its inefficacy in MF lies in the different origin of malignant T cells than in SS [144]. A presence of diffuse erythema has been suggested as a predictor of complete and durable response [145]. However, alemtuzumab increased the risk of infection due to depletion of B and T cells leading to cytomegalovirus (CMV) reactivation, fever of unknown origin and generalized herpes simplex infection. In the last years three clinical trials assessing alemtuzumab's efficacy in MF and SS have been completed (NCT00057967, NCT00047060 and NCT00057967), however their results have not been published so far.

5.1.2. Brentuximab Vedotin

Brentuximab vedotin (BV, formerly known as SGN-35) is an antibody-drug conjugate consisting of a CD30-directed monoclonal chimeric IgG1 antibody and monomethyl auristatin E (MMAE), a microtubule disrupting agent. CD30 is an excellent target for immunotherapies, both for mAb and chimeric receptor (CAR) lymphocytes due to its limited expression on non-malignant immune cells [146]. The mechanism of action of BV consists of the internalization of the drug-conjugate after binding to CD30-expressing cells, followed by the release of MMAE leading to cell cycle arrest and apoptosis [147,148]. BV, originally registered for the treatment of Hodgkin lymphoma and primary cutaneous large cell anaplastic T cell lymphoma (pcALCL), based on the results of phase III trial (NCT01578499) in Nov 2017 gained approval for CTCL patients who have received prior systemic therapy [149,150]. Another clinical trial of BV in CD30-positive ALCL, MF and LyP (NCT01352520) is ongoing with encouraging results in LyP and MF [151,152]. Due to the incidence of peripheral neuropathy, protocols with lower dosage have been suggested. The mAb also shows potential in the treatment of rare primary cutaneous natural killer/T-cell lymphoma with aberrant CD30 expression [153,154].

5.1.3. Mogamulizumab

Mogamulizumab, a humanized afucosylated IgG1 targeting CC chemokine receptor type 4 (CCR4) is the second mAb registered for the management of CTCL. CCR4, involved in cell trafficking of lymphocytes to the skin, is consistently expressed on the surface of tumor cells in T-cell malignancies [155,156]. Defucosylation of the mAb results in an increased affinity to FcγRIIIa (CD16), and enhanced antibody-dependent cell-mediated cytotoxicity (ADCC) [157]. It has been approved in Aug 2018 for the patients with relapsed or refractory CTCL after at least one prior systemic therapy. The registrations were based on the results of Phase III clinical trial (NCT01728805) including patients with relapsed MF or SS on either mogamulizumab or vorinostat. Median PFS for mogamulizumab reached 7.6 months and the ORR 28% compared to 3.1 months and 5% for vorinostat [158]. Moreover, in patients treated with mogamulizumab an improvement in some aspects of quality of life, including skin pain and fatigue were reported. Interestingly, the clinical response to mogamulizumab was not associated with skin CCR4 expression. [159]. Despite the relatively good safety profile of the antibody in clinical trials, some rare serious adverse events with potentially fatal outcome have been reported in clinical experience, mostly in patients with adult T-cell leukemia lymphoma (ATLL). [160,161]. By targeting CCR-4 mogamulizumab also eliminates nonmalignant regulatory T cells (Tregs) leading to autoimmune disorders [162] and predisposing to increased risk of graft-vs.-host disease (GVHD) after allogeneic bone marrow transplantation [163–166]. Therefore, in mogamulizumab-treated patients transplantation should be delayed for at least 50 days from the last dose and a Treg count prior to transplant has been suggested [167].

5.1.4. KIR3DL2 Targeting

KIR3DL2, also known as CD158k, a member of the killer cell immunoglobulin-like receptor (KIR) family, was initially identified as an inhibitory co-receptor on the surface of NK cells. In healthy individuals, KIR3DL2 is expressed by about 20% of NK cells and also by a small proportion of CD4$^+$ (5%) and CD8$^+$ (9%) T cells [168]. KIR3DL2 overexpression by MF and SS cells correlates with the disease stage and large cell transformation [169], as well as shorter survival [170]. Therefore, targeting KIR3DL2 raises hopes for developing the long-awaited CTCL-targeted therapy [171]. IPH4102, an anti-KIR2DL2 humanized IgG1 mAb effectively induces ADCC and immunophagocytosis [172], delays tumor growth and improves the overall survival in a xenograft mouse model. The results of a phase I study in MF and SS patients (NCT02593045) demonstrated a confirmed global overall response in 16 of 44 patients, and of those, 15 responses were observed in 35 patients with Sézary syndrome [173]. Moreover, a phase II trial of IPH4102 alone or in combination with chemotherapy in patients with advanced T cell lymphoma (NCT03902184) is currently recruiting patients.

5.1.5. Immune Checkpoint Inhibitors

Although the data on the expression pattern of PD-1 axis in CTCL are limited, they suggest a potential role of these negative immune regulators in the pathogenesis of CTCL and designate them as therapeutic targets. In general, these studies suggest a higher expression of PD-1 on CD4+ malignant cells in case of blood and skin of SS patients comparing to MF patients [174,175] and PD-1 has been proposed as a factor responsible for drug resistance in SS [176]. Our unpublished observations also indicate higher levels of PD-1 expression on CTLA + CD4 + cells in patients with a higher tumor burden. The particularity of CTCL in the context of the implementation of immune checkpoint inhibitors relies on the fact that the tumor itself arises from CD4+ T cells, a population of lymphocytes responsible for the priming of cytotoxic response. In CTCL both malignant and bystander T helper cells are characterized by Th2 bias, that results in skewed anti-tumor response [177]. A mounting body of evidence suggests that in CTCL both CD4+ and CD8+ cells have characteristics of immune exhaustion [178–180]. Therefore targeting immune checkpoints would have implications on the functionality of both helper and cytotoxic T cells. By now, the role of PD-1 axis has been much more investigated in CD8+ T cells [181]. It is not yet clear how targeting this pathway affects Th2 phenotype in CTCL. Studies in solid tumors suggest that blocking PD-1 may be effective in abrogating Th2 bias. PD-1 blockade was found to shift antigen-induced cellular reactivity toward a proinflammatory response, enhanced production of interferon-γ (IFN-γ), IL-2, TNF-α, IL-6 and reduced production of anti-inflammatory cytokines IL-5 and IL-13 [182]. In ex vivo studies, the inhibition of PD-1 downstream signaling increased IFN-γ secretion in a subset of patients, suggesting that PD-1 targeting may abolish suppressive phenotype of SS cells [174]. In CTCL by now promising results have been reported in phase II trial of pembrolizumab (NCT02243579) in heavily pretreated advanced-stage MF and SS patients [183,184]. Combination studies based on pembrolizumab are warranted in order to increase response rates.

Currently five open-label multicenter clinical studies of anti-PD-1 pembrolizumab in monotherapy and in combinations are ongoing and one trial for nivolumab is recruiting patients. However, as PD-1 has recently been demonstrated to act as a tumor suppressor in T-cell malignancies [185], it has been discussed that targeting PD-1 ligands may potentially offer a safer option in CTCL.

A study by Wilcox et al. demonstrated PD-L1 expression in peripheral blood CD4+ T cells in the majority of patients with leukemic CTCL, however only in 27% of patients' biopsies as evaluated with immunohistochemistry [186]. Its expression, was high in the tumor environment, particularly in the monocyte-derived compartment, where PD-L1 was expressed by 73% of cells. Currently, one trial of anti-PD-L1 atezolizumab (NCT03357224) in relapsed or refractory CTLC is active and another one for durvalumab (NCT03011814) is recruiting patients.

While the PD-1/PD-L1 has gained much interest in the therapy of CTCL, not much is known about CTLA-4 expression in this malignancy. Increased CTLA-4 expression has been reported on the surface of CD3+ T cells from MF patients, most prominently in patients with late-stage disease [187]. In an analysis of skin samples, Querfeld et al. observed higher expression of CTLA-4 on both CD4+ and CD8+ T cells. In our study, we observed no significant differences in CTLA-4 expression in CD4+ malignant vs. by-stander T cells in SS patients and healthy controls [188]. There is only a limited amount of data reports on the use of anti-CTLA-4 in CTCL. In a phase I clinical trial the combination of nivolumab and ipilimumab displayed a similar clinical safety and efficacy when compared with nivolumab monotherapy among pretreated patients with CTCL and peripheral T-cell lymphoma [189]. Currently, there are no active or recruiting clinical studies testing the efficacy of CTLA-4 targeting in CTCL.

5.1.6. CD47

CD47 is a principal ligand for signal regulatory protein alpha (SIRPα)—an immunoreceptor—expressed on all myeloid cells [190]. Binding to SIRPα results in a 'do not eat me' signal and suppresses phagocytosis by macrophages. Upregulation of CD47 by various types of cancer cells is one of the strategies of immunoevasion [191,192] contributing to poor prognosis for the patients [193,194]. CD47 is highly expressed on Sézary cells in the peripheral blood and skin and correlates with worse OS [195]. TTI-621, a recombinant fusion protein composed of human SIRPα N-terminal domain fused to the Fc receptor of IgG1 [196] not only blocks CD47's 'do not eat me' signal but also enhances phagocytosis of tumor cells by monocytes. By now, it is being tested in two Phase I trials. A single intratumoral injection resulted in a marked decrease in tumor size and in the number of circulating SS cells in MF and SS patients (NCT02890368). Moreover, upregulation of IFN-associated genes and alterations in innate immunity activation genes in peripheral blood and tumor tissue have been observed [197]. Due to these encouraging results, further trials of TTI-621 in the management of CTCL are warranted [198].

5.2. CBCL

According to the WHO EORTC joint classification B-cell-derived PCLs are classified into three major subtypes: The most common primary cutaneous follicle-center lymphoma (PCFCL), primary cutaneous marginal zone lymphoma (PCMZL) and the rarest but aggressive primary cutaneous diffuse large B-cell lymphoma, leg type (PCLBCL, LT) [199]. Both PCMZL and PCFCL types are characterized by an excellent prognosis, with 5-year survival rates higher than 90%, while for PCLBCL the 5-year survival rate is lower than 60% [200]. Due to the lack of randomized controlled trials in CBCL, the treatment recommendations of EORTC and International Society for Cutaneous Lymphoma (ISCL) are mostly based on small retrospective studies and institutional experience [201,202]. Patients with PCMZL and PCFCL are mostly treated with low-dose radiation therapy, while PCLBCL is managed with rituximab combined with chemotherapy with or without radiotherapy [200]. Anti-CD20 therapy is employed in PCFCL and PCMZL with more widespread skin involvement.

Rituximab

Rituximab applied intravenously is considered an alternative to the conventional treatment of PCFCL and PCMZL and is used in the treatment of PCLBCL, LT mainly in combination with cyclophosphamide, hydroxydaunorubicin [doxorubicin], Oncovin [vincristine], prednisone (CHOP) chemotherapy (R-CHOP). The treatment of PCDLBCL-LT is extrapolated from diffuse large B-cell lymphoma (DLBCL) due to morphologic, phenotypical and molecular genetic features as well as a clinical behavior they share [201,203]. However, it has to be noted that there is a lack of randomized clinical trials on this topic. Moreover, there are case reports on the use of rituximab as a monotherapy in PCLBCL, LT (reviewed in [204])

Data on the i.v. use of RTX in indolent CBCL are also case reports (reviewed in [204]). Intralesional application of RTX has been suggested as an alternative due to a better tolerance of treatment (the most common AE being injection-site pain) [205,206], lower dose and increased convenience for the patient with a slightly better outcome [201].

6. Problems with the Use of Checkpoint Inhibitors

In this part we will concentrate on discussing the problems concerning the clinical use of ICIs mainly in the context of melanoma.

6.1. Resistance to Immune Checkpoints

The application of ICIs encounters the problem of both primary (innate) as well as secondary (acquired) resistance. Three populations of patients—(1) responders, (2) patients with innate and (3) those with acquired resistance—have been identified by analyzing the results of the clinical trials [207–209].

In the case of anti-PD-1 targeting, the incidence of primary resistance has been reported in approximately 40% of untreated patients, 65% of the patients after progression on other therapies and in >70% of those treated with ipilimumab [209]. The primary insensitivity to immune checkpoints is related to insufficient T-cell and macrophage infiltration of the tumor, lack of PD-1 expression in the tissue, inadequate amount of neoantigens and low mutational burden. Moreover, immunosuppressive factors within the tumor microenvironment i.e., the presence of an innate anti-PD-1 resistance signature (IPRES) transcriptional signature (27), the absence of an interferon signature, increase in Tregs number, upregulation of PD-L1 molecule and the induction of indoleamine 2,3-dioxygenase (IDO) [209,210] also play an important role. Additionally, numerous studies aim at defining the role of the gut microbiome in the responsiveness to immunotherapy [211]. These studies are motivated by the fact that unmethylated CpG oligodeoxynucleotides abundantly present in the bacterial DNA enhance CD8+ T cell anti-tumor immunity by downregulating PD-1 expression via the IL-12 pathway. Moreover, the observations in germ-free animal models showed reduced numbers and impaired function of DCs and macrophages. Indeed, a higher diversity of the gut microbiome correlates to an increased response to anti-PD-1 monotherapy [212]. Overall, the results from preclinical in vivo studies of fecal transfer in a murine model of melanoma [213] and sequencing of the gut microbiota composition from 42 melanoma patients treated with anti-PD-1 [214] suggest a correlation between the presence of *Bifidobacterium* species and clinical response to this immunotherapy. In patients treated with ipilimumab specific bacteria genera i.e., *Faecalibacterium* and *Bacteroides* [215,216] were also associated with clinical response. Other studies (reviewed in [209,217]) suggest the influence of other bacterial species clearly indicating that further studies on this topic are warranted.

The secondary resistance concerns approximately 30% to 40% of patients showing an initial response to anti-PD-1. Although the mechanisms underlying the acquired resistance are not completely deciphered it seems that the upregulation of alternative immune checkpoints i.e., TIM-3 and LAG-3 [218], *JAK2* mutations resulting in disrupted IFN-γ [219] and decreased expression of human leukocyte antigen (HLA) molecules leading to decreased antigen presentation [220] play a role (reviewed in [209]).

Based on the finding from a retrospective study comparing the efficacy of ipilimumab monotherapy vs. ipilimumab + nivolumab in patients after progression on PD-1 inhibitors, ipilimumab seems an option for patients with acquired resistance [221]. Preclinical data from murine model suggest the efficacy of dual targeting of PD-1 together with the emerging immune checkpoints—LAG-3 [222] or TIM-3 [223].

6.2. Response Markers for Checkpoints Inhibitors

There is an unmet need for biomarkers that will identify patients more likely to respond to ICIs. The advances in the topic have been excellently reviewed in [224,225]. Here we aimed at accentuating the key aspects. As the blockage of PD-1/PD-L1 axis represents the most widely used ICI-based therapy, the majority of the cited studies concentrates on this aspect.

Data from clinical trials and cohort studies suggest that PD-L1 expression on tumor cells can be used as a predictor of response [226–231]. The expression of PD-L1 varies significantly depending on the melanoma subtype, which correlates with response to therapy [232]. However, its application as a single prediction marker of the therapy outcome has some limitation. Its expression undergoes dynamic changes in the course of treatment and as a result of inflammation [233,234] and there are reports on successful clinical outcome of anti-PD-1 treatment in PD-L1 negative cases [235]. Interestingly in Merkel cell carcinoma response has been observed independently on PD-L1 status [125]. PD-L1 expression in the tumor microenvironment has also been suggested to be more informative than its expression on the tumor cells [236,237]. Recently, soluble [238] and exosomal PD-L1 [239] have been presented as a possible predictor for anti-PD-1 therapy. High levels of circulating PD-L1 would suggest the exhaustion of T cells and the impossibility of their further reinvigoration following anti-PD-1 therapy. Interestingly, however, considerable changes in the levels of circulating PD-L1 prior to and during pembrolizumab [239] and ipilimumab [238] treatment have been observed and shown to correlate with clinical response. Some easily analyzable biochemical parameters have been suggested as potential response predictors e.g., lactate dehydrogenase (LDH) and S100, which are normally used as indicators of disease progression [240]. However, as all these markers do not correlate with the duration of response, they may identify patients with very high tumor burden that are unlikely to benefit from immunotherapies, but cannot be used as response predictors [225]. The same applies to the number of the organs involved by the tumor [241].

In terms of demographic factors it has been shown that although men are highly more susceptible to different types of tumors and have two-times higher risk of mortality from all cancers than women do [242], their relative survival benefit from ICI-based therapy is consistently higher than for women. Interestingly, the response to PD-1 blockage increases with age [243]. Paradoxically, despite the clear association between increased body-mass index (BMI) and the risk of developing and dying from various types of cancer [244], in a large retrospective study including a total of 2046 patients with metastatic melanoma obesity has been shown to increase response to all targeted therapies, including ICIs [245].

Features of the tumor microenvironment (TME) and the composition of the immune populations in the peripheral blood also associate with the response. Specifically, baseline levels of CD8+ TILs correlate with the likelihood of response. Moreover, the number of CD4+ TILs increases during therapy in responders [246], suggesting that the preexisting immunity is required for the ICI therapy efficacy. By analyzing the transcriptomes of 16,291 individual immune cells from 48 tumor samples of melanoma patients treated with ICI, two distinct states of CD8+ T cells associated with tumor regression or progression were defined by clustering [247]. The presence of the TCF7 transcription factor in CD8+ T cells that is crucial for their differentiation, self-renewal and reinvigoration has been presented to predict clinical response to checkpoint therapy. Since CD4+ T helper cells also play an important role in the tumor elimination e.g., by increasing the cytotoxic function of CD8+ cells and secretion of IL-2, several studies investigated them as a potential prognostic factor. An increase in central memory CD4+ T cells [248] and IL-9-producing CD4+ Th9 cells [249] has been reported exclusively in long-term responders to anti-PD-1 blockage. The recent advances in understanding the role of circulating myeloid-derived suppressor cells (MDSCs) in cancer progression also suggest that this population may play a role in defining survival and response to treatment [250]. Results from the studies in anti-PD-1-treated patients clearly show that a high percentage of MDSCs correlate with poor response to the therapy [251,252]. Further, the frequency of CD14+CD16-HLA-DRhi monocytes has been reported to predict progression-free and overall survival in response to anti-PD-1 immunotherapy [253].

Recently, it has been shown that antibodies specific for melanocyte differentiation antigens (MDAs) and cancer-testis antigens may be a response predictor for ICIs [254], suggesting also the importance of the interaction between B and T cells for the therapy outcome.

By now, it seems that tumor mutational burden together with T cell-inflamed gene expression profile exhibit the greatest predictive utility in identifying responders and nonresponders to anti PD-1 therapy, as shown in a large study in >300 patient samples with advanced solid tumors and melanoma (representing approx. 30% of the tested samples) from four KEYNOTE clinical trials [255]. Large-scale analyses in various cancers including patients with basal cell carcinoma and melanoma univocally reported that patients with intermediate to high mutational tumor burden assessed with next-generation sequencing (NGS) show a better clinical response to the PD-1/PD-L1 blockade [93,255,256]. The number of mutations undergoes a marked decrease in immunotherapy-responders, as reported by a study in 68 advanced melanoma patients treated with nivolumab. As demonstrated by a clonality analysis, the tumors in patients with Complete Response/Partial Response (CR/PR) undergo a substantial evolution in the course of the therapy, already after four weeks from the therapy start [228,234]. Upregulation of other immune checkpoints such as LAG-3 or TIM-3 was reported among others. Notably, these molecules remain candidates for co-targeting in combination treatment regimens in order to boost immunotherapy efficacy.

6.3. Managing Adverse Events

Since immune checkpoints under physiological conditions regulate the immune response to prevent autoimmunity bystander damage of the normal tissue, their inhibition leads to a plethora of immune-related AEs (irAEs). Moreover, exacerbation of already pre-existing conditions [257,258] is reported in ICIs-treated patients. The incidence of irAEs in patients treated with ICs and methods of management have been reviewed in [259,260]. The guidelines on the management of AEs have been prepared by several organizations [261,262].

Fortunately, fatal AEs, with their frequency of between 0.3% and 1.3% are less frequent than in case of other therapeutics [263]. However, they occur much earlier in the course of treatment than in the case of other therapies and evolve rapidly [264]. Data from metanalyses indicate that in case of ipilimumab-treatment the most frequent cause of death is colitis (approx. 70%), while targeting the PD-1/PD-L1 axis is most frequently associated with fatal pneumonitis (approx. 35%), hepatitis (approx. 20%) and neurotoxicity (approx. 15%).

In general the irAEs can affect every organ. However, some differences regarding the organ distribution can be identified in the populations of patients treated with anti-CTLA-4 or anti-PD-1/PD-L1. While both these populations suffer from colitis, endocrinopathies and cutaneous toxicity, pneumonitis and nephritis are typical for the group treated with anti-PD-1/PD-L1 [259]. Skin toxicities following immune checkpoint inhibition in melanoma have been thoroughly reviewed in [265] and are mostly observed in ipilimumab-treated patients. Skin-related side effects, experienced by around 60% of patients, are rarely severe and are mostly limited to rash and itching occurring at the beginning of the treatment, with its peak at the sixth week [266]. Targeting of PD-1 drugs induces less skin toxicity than ipilimumab with the incidence of some form of skin disorders around 40% [267,268]. Based on the by now the most comprehensive study by Hwang et al. the most frequent are rashes that can be divided into lichenoid reactions (17%) and eczema (17%) and the third most common adverse reaction, vitiligo (12%) [269]. A rash can be treated symptomatically with emollients, topical corticosteroids, oral antihistamines and oral corticosteroids in exacerbated cases. Vitiligo can be managed by the use of topical corticosteroids that induce repigmentation and the use of broad-spectrum photoprotection is highly required. Other forms of skin toxicities include severe pruritus, psoriasiform reactions, widespread erythema, DRESS syndrome, photosensitivity, sensitivity/skin toxicity in previously irradiated areas, ulcerations pyoderma gangrenosum-like, acneiform rash, eruptive keratoacanthomas, Sweet syndrome, Grover's disease, Stevens–Johnson syndrome/toxic epidermal necrolysis and erythema nodosum-like panniculitis.

Some authors suggest that cutaneous immune-related AEs of ICIs i.e., vitiligo and rash may be used as predictors of the clinical response. Indeed, analyses of nivolumab-treated melanoma patients indicate that the incidence of vitiligo and rash correlates with a significant OS improvement [270,271]. Other reports suggest that anti-PD-1-induced vitiligo associated with other toxicities, such as lichenoid reactions and eczema, can be a good prognosis marker [272].

7. Improving the Efficacy of ICIs

Beside strategies combining ICIs with other anti-tumor strategies i.e., conventional chemotherapy (reviewed in [273]), small-molecule inhibitors (reviewed in [274]), anti-angiogenic drugs and oncolytic viruses (both reviewed in [275]) and the already mentioned dual inhibition of immune checkpoints e.g., PD-1 and TIGIT, the efficacy of ICIs can also be improved by modulating the affinity of mAb to Fc receptors. Glyco-modification of the Fc portion of the antibody is routinely applied to eliminate ADCC induction in the case of two anti-PD-L1 IgG1 mAbs (atezolizumab and durvalumab) in order to avoid elimination of PD-1/PD-L1-expressing TILs [276]. Indeed, all anti-PD-1 directed mAbs belong to the IgG4 isotype with silenced ADCC activity. However, the utility of eliminating ADCC has been largely questioned by the efficacy of anti-PD-L1 avelumab [126] with non-suppressed ADCC activity. As the results of the studies in a murine tumor model strongly suggest that the activity of agents targeting PD-L1 relies on their binding to activating FcγR resulting in the altering myeloid subsets within the tumor microenvironment [277]. Recently, a defucosylated anti-PD-L1 mAb with increased affinity for FcγRIIIa has been engineered on the basis of atezolizumab and demonstrated encouraging in vitro results with increased CD8 T cell activation [278]. Therefore, glyco-optimization of the structures of ICIs may be of potential clinical benefit [279]. The anti-tumor efficacy dependent on the Fc-mediated effector functions has also been demonstrated for CTLA-4, TIGIT and VISTA (reviewed in [279]). However, this strategy is target-dependent, as the presence of FcγR-binding capacity compromises the anti-tumor activity of anti PD-1 mAbs [277]. In case of anti-PD-1 mAbs the attenuation of ADCC relies on the application of the IgG4 isotype. However, this isotype is considered anti-inflammatory and may result in a reduced anti-tumor efficacy, as it retains the binding to FcγRIIb [277]. Therefore, the efficacy of anti-PD-1 therapy may benefit from the development of agents with null FcγR-binding. It applies also to mAbs targeting co-inhibitory receptors i.e., TIM-3 and LAG-3 [279].

8. Conclusions and Perspectives

Skin is the human body's largest organ, and its easy accessibility offers an unprecedented gateway for early detection and diagnosis of diseases. Both, solid and hematological malignancies can arise in skin or secondarily affect it. The incidence of skin cancers has been increasing over the past decades up to 287,000 new cases for melanoma and 1.04 million new cases for non-melanoma in 2018 worldwide. This makes skin cancers a global health burden and a field of intense research contributing to the advancement of treatments in oncology overall. Increased knowledge about signaling and immune pathways led to the development of targeted therapies and immunotherapies representing recent breakthroughs in cancer therapy.

These therapies opened the way for personalized and precise treatment strategies, but they also confront physicians with novel adverse drug reactions, with the skin being again among the most commonly affected organs.

In light of the above, further research should aim to identify more antibody-targetable molecules, accumulate data on how to predict response to treatment and manage the adverse events. In particular, identifying novel molecular targets that may provide a solution to decreased efficacy of mAbs due to antigen loss as a result of selective pressure is of the utmost importance. While the intracellular molecules represent nearly half of the human proteome and provide an immense reservoir of potential novel targets, they have not yet been extensively explored in oncology [280]. Targeting intracellular molecules aims also at exploiting the products of their degradation by the proteasome that are subsequently presented in the context of MHC class I molecules and recognized by CD8+ T cells.

Antibodies targeting such MHC-peptide complexes, the so-called T-cell receptor-mimic (TCRm) antibodies expand the range of potential targets of immunotherapy without the problem with delivery, which is typical for intracellular antibodies [281]. Similar to conventional mAbs, TCRm antibodies activate various immune-dependent mechanisms i.e., ADCC and complement-dependent cytotoxicity (CDC). Such agents are being designed for melanoma treatment, however none of them has yet entered the clinic [280]. The use of bispecific mAbs also offers potential benefits in the context of the immune-rich skin microenvironment. An interesting example of the use of bispecific mAbs has been recently applied in in vitro studies, where a bispecific mAb targeting PD-L1xCSPG4 showed efficacy in the treatment of mixed cultures containing primary patient-derived CSPG4-expressing melanoma cells and autologous tumor-infiltrating lymphocytes [282]. Such bispecific mAbs may reduce the off-target binding to PD-L1-expressing normal cells that compromises on-target effect and is implicated in autoimmune-related (AEs).

Funding: This project was supported by the European Commission Horizon 2020 Program 692180-STREAMH2020-TWINN-2015 (MB, JD, MW), Polish National Science Centre 2015/18/E/NZ6/00702 (MB, JD, MW), 2015/19/B/NZ6/02862 (MW), EMBO (short-term fellowship nr. 7637 to MB), the Ministry of Science and Higher Education (2019/94/DIR/NN3 to MB), the Ministry of Science and Higher Education within "Regional Initiative of Excellence" Program in the years 2019-2022; Project number 013 / RID / 2018/19; Project budget PLN 12 million, the Promedica Stiftung (1406/M and 1412/M, both to EG), the Swiss Cancer Research Foundation (KFS-4243-08-2017 to EG). The funders had no role in study design, data collection and analysis, decision to publish, or preparation of the manuscript.

Conflicts of Interest: The authors declare no conflict of interest. The funders had no role in the design of the study; in the collection, analyses, or interpretation of data; in the writing of the manuscript, or in the decision to publish the results.

References

1. Sewell, F.; Chapman, K.; Couch, J.; Dempster, M.; Heidel, S.; Loberg, L.; Maier, C.; Maclachlan, T.K.; Todd, M.; van der Laan, J.W. Challenges and opportunities for the future of monoclonal antibody development: Improving safety assessment and reducing animal use. *MAbs* **2017**, *9*, 742–755. [CrossRef]
2. Kaplon, H.; Reichert, J.M. Antibodies to watch in 2019. *MAbs* **2019**, *11*, 219–238. [CrossRef]
3. Weiner, L.M.; Surana, R.; Wang, S. Monoclonal antibodies: versatile platforms for cancer immunotherapy. *Nat. Rev. Immunol.* **2010**, *10*, 317–327. [CrossRef]
4. Stevens, N.E.; Cowin, A.J.; Kopecki, Z. Skin barrier and autoimmunity-mechanisms and novel therapeutic Approaches for autoimmune Blistering diseases of the skin. *Front. Immunol.* **2019**, *10*, 1089. [CrossRef]
5. Brunet, J.F.; Denizot, F.; Luciani, M.F.; Roux-Dosseto, M.; Suzan, M.; Mattei, M.G.; Golstein, P. A new member of the immunoglobulin superfamily-CTLA-4. *Nature* **1987**, *328*, 267–270. [CrossRef]
6. Waterhouse, P.; Penninger, J.M.; Timms, E.; Wakeham, A.; Shahinian, A.; Lee, K.P.; Thompson, C.B.; Griesser, H.; Mak, T.W. Lymphoproliferative disorders with early lethality in mice deficient in Ctla-4. *Science* **1995**, *270*, 985–988. [CrossRef]
7. Tivol, E.A.; Borriello, F.; Schweitzer, A.N.; Lynch, W.P.; Bluestone, J.A.; Sharpe, A.H. Loss of CTLA-4 leads to massive lymphoproliferation and fatal multiorgan tissue destruction, revealing a critical negative regulatory role of CTLA-4. *Immunity* **1995**, *3*, 541–547. [CrossRef]
8. Linsley, P.S.; Greene, J.L.; Tan, P.; Bradshaw, J.; Ledbetter, J.A.; Anasetti, C.; Damle, N.K. Coexpression and functional cooperation of CTLA-4 and CD28 on activated T lymphocytes. *J. Exp. Med.* **1992**, *176*, 1595–1604. [CrossRef]
9. Lindsten, T.; Lee, K.P.; Harris, E.S.; Petryniak, B.; Craighead, N.; Reynolds, P.J.; Lombard, D.B.; Freeman, G.J.; Nadler, L.M.; Gray, G.S.; et al. Characterization of CTLA-4 structure and expression on human T cells. *J. Immunol.* **1993**, *151*, 3489–3499.
10. Qureshi, O.S.; Zheng, Y.; Nakamura, K.; Attridge, K.; Manzotti, C.; Schmidt, E.M.; Baker, J.; Jeffery, L.E.; Kaur, S.; Briggs, Z.; et al. Trans-endocytosis of CD80 and CD86: a molecular basis for the cell-extrinsic function of CTLA-4. *Science* **2011**, *332*, 600–603. [CrossRef]
11. Krummel, M.F.; Allison, J.P. CD28 and CTLA-4 have opposing effects on the response of T cells to stimulation. *J. Exp. Med.* **1995**, *182*, 459–465. [CrossRef]

12. Lee, K.M.; Chuang, E.; Griffin, M.; Khattri, R.; Hong, D.K.; Zhang, W.; Straus, D.; Samelson, L.E.; Thompson, C.B.; Bluestone, J.A. Molecular basis of T cell inactivation by CTLA-4. *Science* **1998**, *282*, 2263–2266. [CrossRef]
13. Leach, D.R.; Krummel, M.F.; Allison, J.P. Enhancement of antitumor immunity by CTLA-4 blockade. *Science* **1996**, *271*, 1734–1736. [CrossRef]
14. Ishida, Y.; Agata, Y.; Shibahara, K.; Honjo, T. Induced expression of PD-1, a novel member of the immunoglobulin gene superfamily, upon programmed cell death. *EMBO J.* **1992**, *11*, 3887–3895. [CrossRef]
15. Chikuma, S.; Terawaki, S.; Hayashi, T.; Nabeshima, R.; Yoshida, T.; Shibayama, S.; Okazaki, T.; Honjo, T. PD-1-mediated suppression of IL-2 production induces CD8+ T cell anergy in vivo. *J. Immunol.* **2009**, *182*, 6682–6689. [CrossRef]
16. Yokosuka, T.; Takamatsu, M.; Kobayashi-Imanishi, W.; Hashimoto-Tane, A.; Azuma, M.; Saito, T. Programmed cell death 1 forms negative costimulatory microclusters that directly inhibit T cell receptor signaling by recruiting phosphatase SHP2. *J. Exp. Med.* **2012**, *209*, 1201–1217. [CrossRef]
17. Freeman, G.J.; Long, A.J.; Iwai, Y.; Bourque, K.; Chernova, T.; Nishimura, H.; Fitz, L.J.; Malenkovich, N.; Okazaki, T.; Byrne, M.C.; et al. Engagement of the PD-1 immunoinhibitory receptor by a novel B7 family member leads to negative regulation of lymphocyte activation. *J. Exp. Med.* **2000**, *192*, 1027–1034. [CrossRef]
18. Guleria, I.; Khosroshahi, A.; Ansari, M.J.; Habicht, A.; Azuma, M.; Yagita, H.; Noelle, R.J.; Coyle, A.; Mellor, A.L.; Khoury, S.J.; et al. A critical role for the programmed death ligand 1 in fetomaternal tolerance. *J. Exp. Med.* **2005**, *202*, 231–237. [CrossRef]
19. Paluch, C.; Santos, A.M.; Anzilotti, C.; Cornall, R.J.; Davis, S.J. Immune Checkpoints as Therapeutic Targets in Autoimmunity. *Front Immunol.* **2018**, *9*, 2306. [CrossRef]
20. Iwai, Y.; Ishida, M.; Tanaka, Y.; Okazaki, T.; Honjo, T.; Minato, N. Involvement of PD-L1 on tumor cells in the escape from host immune system and tumor immunotherapy by PD-L1 blockade. *Proc. Natl. Acad. Sci. USA* **2002**, *99*, 12293–12297. [CrossRef]
21. Iwai, Y.; Terawaki, S.; Honjo, T. PD-1 blockade inhibits hematogenous spread of poorly immunogenic tumor cells by enhanced recruitment of effector T cells. *Int. Immunol.* **2005**, *17*, 133–144. [CrossRef]
22. Rotte, A.; Jin, J.Y.; Lemaire, V. Mechanistic overview of immune checkpoints to support the rational design of their combinations in cancer immunotherapy. *Ann. Oncol.* **2018**, *29*, 71–83. [CrossRef]
23. Mazzarella, L.; Duso, B.A.; Trapani, D.; Belli, C.; D'Amico, P.; Ferraro, E.; Viale, G.; Curigliano, G. The evolving landscape of 'next-generation' immune checkpoint inhibitors: A review. *Eur. J. Cancer* **2019**, *117*, 14–31. [CrossRef]
24. Schadendorf, D.; van Akkooi, A.C.J.; Berking, C.; Griewank, K.G.; Gutzmer, R.; Hauschild, A.; Stang, A.; Roesch, A.; Ugurel, S. Melanoma. *Lancet* **2018**, *392*, 971–984. [CrossRef]
25. Chin, L.; Garraway, L.A.; Fisher, D.E. Malignant melanoma: genetics and therapeutics in the genomic era. *Genes Dev.* **2006**, *20*, 2149–2182. [CrossRef]
26. Coit, D.G.; Thompson, J.A.; Albertini, M.R.; Barker, C.; Carson, W.E.; Contreras, C.; Daniels, G.A.; DiMaio, D.; Fields, R.C.; Fleming, M.D.; et al. Cutaneous melanoma; Version 2.2019; NCCN Clinical Practice Guidelines in Oncology. *J. Natl. Compr. Canc. Netw.* **2019**, *17*, 367–402. [CrossRef]
27. Guo, J.; Si, L.; Kong, Y.; Flaherty, K.T.; Xu, X.; Zhu, Y.; Corless, C.L.; Li, L.; Li, H.; Sheng, X.; et al. Phase II, open-label, single-arm trial of imatinib mesylate in patients with metastatic melanoma harboring c-Kit mutation or amplification. *J. Clin. Oncol.* **2011**, *29*, 2904–2909. [CrossRef]
28. Passarelli, A.; Mannavola, F.; Stucci, L.S.; Tucci, M.; Silvestris, F. Immune system and melanoma biology: A balance between immunosurveillance and immune escape. *Oncotarget* **2017**, *8*, 106132–106142. [CrossRef]
29. Mahmoud, F.; Shields, B.; Makhoul, I.; Avaritt, N.; Wong, H.K.; Hutchins, L.F.; Shalin, S.; Tackett, A.J. Immune surveillance in melanoma: From immune attack to melanoma escape and even counterattack. *Cancer Biol.* **2017**, *18*, 451–469. [CrossRef]
30. Weber, J. Overcoming immunologic tolerance to melanoma: targeting CTLA-4 with ipilimumab (MDX-010). *Oncologist* **2008**, *13* (Suppl. 4), 16–25. [CrossRef]
31. Garcia-Diaz, A.; Shin, D.S.; Moreno, B.H.; Saco, J.; Escuin-Ordinas, H.; Rodriguez, G.A.; Zaretsky, J.M.; Sun, L.; Hugo, W.; Wang, X.; et al. Interferon receptor signaling pathways regulating PD-L1 and PD-L2 expression. *Cell Rep.* **2017**, *19*, 1189–1201. [CrossRef]
32. Eggermont, A.M.; Chiarion-Sileni, V.; Grob, J.J.; Dummer, R.; Wolchok, J.D.; Schmidt, H.; Hamid, O.; Robert, C.; Ascierto, P.A.; Richards, J.M.; et al. Adjuvant ipilimumab versus placebo after complete resection

of high-risk stage III melanoma (EORTC 18071): a randomised, double-blind, phase 3 trial. *Lancet Oncol.* **2015**, *16*, 522–530. [CrossRef]
33. Eggermont, A.M.M.; Blank, C.U.; Mandala, M.; Long, G.V.; Atkinson, V.; Dalle, S.; Haydon, A.; Lichinitser, M.; Khattak, A.; Carlino, M.S.; et al. Adjuvant pembrolizumab versus placebo in resected stage III melanoma. *N. Engl. J. Med.* **2018**, *378*, 1789–1801. [CrossRef]
34. Schadendorf, D.; Hodi, F.S.; Robert, C.; Weber, J.S.; Margolin, K.; Hamid, O.; Patt, D.; Chen, T.T.; Berman, D.M.; Wolchok, J.D. Pooled analysis of long-term survival data from phase II and phase III trials of ipilimumab in unresectable or metastatic melanoma. *J. Clin. Oncol.* **2015**, *33*, 1889–1894. [CrossRef]
35. Wolchok, J.D.; Chiarion-Sileni, V.; Gonzalez, R.; Rutkowski, P.; Grob, J.J.; Cowey, C.L.; Lao, C.D.; Wagstaff, J.; Schadendorf, D.; Ferrucci, P.F.; et al. Overall survival with combined nivolumab and ipilimumab in advanced melanoma. *N. Engl. J. Med.* **2017**, *377*, 1345–1356. [CrossRef]
36. Robert, C.; Schachter, J.; Long, G.V.; Arance, A.; Grob, J.J.; Mortier, L.; Daud, A.; Carlino, M.S.; McNeil, C.; Lotem, M.; et al. Pembrolizumab versus ipilimumab in advanced melanoma. *N. Engl. J. Med.* **2015**, *372*, 2521–2532. [CrossRef]
37. Postow, M.A.; Chesney, J.; Pavlick, A.C.; Robert, C.; Grossmann, K.; McDermott, D.; Linette, G.P.; Meyer, N.; Giguere, J.K.; Agarwala, S.S.; et al. Nivolumab and ipilimumab versus ipilimumab in untreated melanoma. *N. Engl. J. Med.* **2015**, *372*, 2006–2017. [CrossRef]
38. Schadendorf, D.; Larkin, J.; Wolchok, J.; Hodi, F.S.; Chiarion-Sileni, V.; Gonzalez, R.; Rutkowski, P.; Grob, J.J.; Cowey, C.L.; Lao, C.; et al. Health-related quality of life results from the phase III CheckMate 067 study. *Eur. J. Cancer* **2017**, *82*, 80–91. [CrossRef]
39. Hassel, J.C.; Heinzerling, L.; Aberle, J.; Bahr, O.; Eigentler, T.K.; Grimm, M.O.; Grunwald, V.; Leipe, J.; Reinmuth, N.; Tietze, J.K.; et al. Combined immune checkpoint blockade (anti-PD-1/anti-CTLA-4): Evaluation and management of adverse drug reactions. *Cancer Treat Rev.* **2017**, *57*, 36–49. [CrossRef]
40. Ribas, A.; Camacho, L.H.; Lopez-Berestein, G.; Pavlov, D.; Bulanhagui, C.A.; Millham, R.; Comin-Anduix, B.; Reuben, J.M.; Seja, E.; Parker, C.A.; et al. Antitumor activity in melanoma and anti-self responses in a phase I trial with the anti-cytotoxic T lymphocyte–associated antigen 4 monoclonal antibody CP-675,206. *J. Clin. Oncol.* **2005**, *23*, 8968–8977. [CrossRef]
41. Ribas, A.; Kefford, R.; Marshall, M.A.; Punt, C.J.; Haanen, J.B.; Marmol, M.; Garbe, C.; Gogas, H.; Schachter, J.; Linette, G.; et al. Phase III randomized clinical trial comparing tremelimumab with standard-of-care chemotherapy in patients with advanced melanoma. *J. Clin. Oncol.* **2013**, *31*, 616–622. [CrossRef]
42. Keilholz, U.; Mehnert, J.M.; Bauer, S.; Bourgeois, H.; Patel, M.R.; Gravenor, D.; Nemunaitis, J.J.; Taylor, M.H.; Wyrwicz, L.; Lee, K.W.; et al. Avelumab in patients with previously treated metastatic melanoma: phase 1b results from the JAVELIN Solid Tumor trial. *J. Immunother. Cancer* **2019**, *7*, 12. [CrossRef]
43. Zabierowski, S.E.; Herlyn, M. Melanoma stem cells: the dark seed of melanoma. *J. Clin. Oncol.* **2008**, *26*, 2890–2894. [CrossRef]
44. Schlaak, M.; Schmidt, P.; Bangard, C.; Kurschat, P.; Mauch, C.; Abken, H. Regression of metastatic melanoma in a patient by antibody targeting of cancer stem cells. *Oncotarget* **2012**, *3*, 22–30. [CrossRef]
45. Hillen, F.; Baeten, C.I.; van de Winkel, A.; Creytens, D.; van der Schaft, D.W.; Winnepenninckx, V.; Griffioen, A.W. Leukocyte infiltration and tumor cell plasticity are parameters of aggressiveness in primary cutaneous melanoma. *Cancer Immunol. Immunother.* **2008**, *57*, 97–106. [CrossRef]
46. Erdag, G.; Schaefer, J.T.; Smolkin, M.E.; Deacon, D.H.; Shea, S.M.; Dengel, L.T.; Patterson, J.W.; Slingluff, C.L., Jr. Immunotype and immunohistologic characteristics of tumor-infiltrating immune cells are associated with clinical outcome in metastatic melanoma. *Cancer Res.* **2012**, *72*, 1070–1080. [CrossRef]
47. Hussein, M.R.; Elsers, D.A.; Fadel, S.A.; Omar, A.E. Immunohistological characterisation of tumour infiltrating lymphocytes in melanocytic skin lesions. *J. Clin. Pathol.* **2006**, *59*, 316–324. [CrossRef]
48. Ladanyi, A.; Kiss, J.; Mohos, A.; Somlai, B.; Liszkay, G.; Gilde, K.; Fejos, Z.; Gaudi, I.; Dobos, J.; Timar, J. Prognostic impact of B-cell density in cutaneous melanoma. *Cancer Immunol. Immunother.* **2011**, *60*, 1729–1738. [CrossRef]
49. Garg, K.; Maurer, M.; Griss, J.; Bruggen, M.C.; Wolf, I.H.; Wagner, C.; Willi, N.; Mertz, K.D.; Wagner, S.N. Tumor-associated B cells in cutaneous primary melanoma and improved clinical outcome. *Hum. Pathol.* **2016**, *54*, 157–164. [CrossRef]

50. Martinez-Rodriguez, M.; Thompson, A.K.; Monteagudo, C. A significant percentage of CD20-positive TILs correlates with poor prognosis in patients with primary cutaneous malignant melanoma. *Histopathology* **2014**, *65*, 726–728. [CrossRef]
51. Meyer, S.; Fuchs, T.J.; Bosserhoff, A.K.; Hofstadter, F.; Pauer, A.; Roth, V.; Buhmann, J.M.; Moll, I.; Anagnostou, N.; Brandner, J.M.; et al. A seven-marker signature and clinical outcome in malignant melanoma: a large-scale tissue-microarray study with two independent patient cohorts. *PLoS ONE* **2012**, *7*, e38222. [CrossRef]
52. Fremd, C.; Schuetz, F.; Sohn, C.; Beckhove, P.; Domschke, C. B cell-regulated immune responses in tumor models and cancer patients. *Oncoimmunology* **2013**, *2*, e25443. [CrossRef]
53. Shah, S.; Divekar, A.A.; Hilchey, S.P.; Cho, H.M.; Newman, C.L.; Shin, S.U.; Nechustan, H.; Challita-Eid, P.M.; Segal, B.M.; Yi, K.H.; et al. Increased rejection of primary tumors in mice lacking B cells: inhibition of anti-tumor CTL and TH1 cytokine responses by B cells. *Int. J. Cancer* **2005**, *117*, 574–586. [CrossRef]
54. DiLillo, D.J.; Yanaba, K.; Tedder, T.F. B cells are required for optimal CD4+ and CD8+ T cell tumor immunity: therapeutic B cell depletion enhances B16 melanoma growth in mice. *J. Immunol.* **2010**, *184*, 4006–4016. [CrossRef]
55. Perricone, M.A.; Smith, K.A.; Claussen, K.A.; Plog, M.S.; Hempel, D.M.; Roberts, B.L.; St George, J.A.; Kaplan, J.M. Enhanced efficacy of melanoma vaccines in the absence of B lymphocytes. *J. Immunother.* **2004**, *27*, 273–281. [CrossRef]
56. Somasundaram, R.; Zhang, G.; Fukunaga-Kalabis, M.; Perego, M.; Krepler, C.; Xu, X.; Wagner, C.; Hristova, D.; Zhang, J.; Tian, T.; et al. Tumor-associated B-cells induce tumor heterogeneity and therapy resistance. *Nat. Commun.* **2017**, *8*, 607. [CrossRef]
57. Winkler, J.K.; Schiller, M.; Bender, C.; Enk, A.H.; Hassel, J.C. Rituximab as a therapeutic option for patients with advanced melanoma. *Cancer Immunol. Immunother.* **2018**, *67*, 917–924. [CrossRef]
58. Peuvrel, L.; Chiffoleau, A.; Quereux, G.; Brocard, A.; Saint-Jean, M.; Batz, A.; Jolliet, P.; Dreno, B. Melanoma and rituximab: An incidental association? *Dermatology* **2013**, *226*, 274–278. [CrossRef]
59. Velter, C.; Pages, C.; Schneider, P.; Osio, A.; Brice, P.; Lebbe, C. Four cases of rituximab-associated melanoma. *Melanoma Res.* **2014**, *24*, 401–403. [CrossRef]
60. Inoue, S.; Leitner, W.W.; Golding, B.; Scott, D. Inhibitory effects of B cells on antitumor immunity. *Cancer Res.* **2006**, *66*, 7741–7747. [CrossRef]
61. van Vollenhoven, R.F.; Emery, P.; Bingham, C.O., 3rd; Keystone, E.C.; Fleischmann, R.; Furst, D.E.; Macey, K.; Sweetser, M.; Kelman, A.; Rao, R. Longterm safety of patients receiving rituximab in rheumatoid arthritis clinical trials. *J. Rheumatol.* **2010**, *37*, 558–567. [CrossRef]
62. Goldberg, M.V.; Drake, C.G. LAG-3 in Cancer Immunotherapy. *Curr. Top. Microbiol. Immunol.* **2011**, *344*, 269–278. [CrossRef]
63. Marin-Acevedo, J.A.; Dholaria, B.; Soyano, A.E.; Knutson, K.L.; Chumsri, S.; Lou, Y. Next generation of immune checkpoint therapy in cancer: new developments and challenges. *J. Hematol. Oncol.* **2018**, *11*, 39. [CrossRef]
64. Anderson, A.C.; Joller, N.; Kuchroo, V.K. Lag-3, Tim-3, and TIGIT: Co-inhibitory receptors with specialized functions in immune regulation. *Immunity* **2016**, *44*, 989–1004. [CrossRef]
65. Hemon, P.; Jean-Louis, F.; Ramgolam, K.; Brignone, C.; Viguier, M.; Bachelez, H.; Triebel, F.; Charron, D.; Aoudjit, F.; Al-Daccak, R.; et al. MHC class II engagement by its ligand LAG-3 (CD223) contributes to melanoma resistance to apoptosis. *J. Immunol.* **2011**, *186*, 5173–5183. [CrossRef]
66. Ascierto, P.A.; Melero, I.; Bhatia, S.; Bono, P.; Sanborn, R.E.; Lipson, E.J.; Callahan, M.K.; Gajewski, T.; Gomez-Roca, C.A.; Hodi, F.S.; et al. Initial efficacy of anti-lymphocyte activation gene-3 (anti–LAG-3; BMS-986016) in combination with nivolumab (nivo) in pts with melanoma (MEL) previously treated with anti-PD-1/PD-L1 therapy. *J. Clin. Oncol.* **2017**, *35*, 9520. [CrossRef]
67. Blake, S.J.; Dougall, W.C.; Miles, J.J.; Teng, M.W.; Smyth, M.J. Molecular Pathways: Targeting CD96 and TIGIT for Cancer Immunotherapy. *Clin. Cancer Res.* **2016**, *22*, 5183–5188. [CrossRef]
68. Chauvin, J.M.; Pagliano, O.; Fourcade, J.; Sun, Z.; Wang, H.; Sander, C.; Kirkwood, J.M.; Chen, T.H.; Maurer, M.; Korman, A.J.; et al. TIGIT and PD-1 impair tumor antigen-specific CD8(+) T cells in melanoma patients. *J. Clin. Investig.* **2015**, *125*, 2046–2058. [CrossRef]

69. Johnston, R.J.; Comps-Agrar, L.; Hackney, J.; Yu, X.; Huseni, M.; Yang, Y.; Park, S.; Javinal, V.; Chiu, H.; Irving, B.; et al. The immunoreceptor TIGIT regulates antitumor and antiviral CD8(+) T cell effector function. *Cancer Cell* **2014**, *26*, 923–937. [CrossRef]
70. He, Y.; Cao, J.; Zhao, C.; Li, X.; Zhou, C.; Hirsch, F.R. TIM-3, a promising target for cancer immunotherapy. *OncoTargets* **2018**, *11*, 7005–7009. [CrossRef]
71. Wiener, Z.; Kohalmi, B.; Pocza, P.; Jeager, J.; Tolgyesi, G.; Toth, S.; Gorbe, E.; Papp, Z.; Falus, A. TIM-3 is expressed in melanoma cells and is upregulated in TGF-beta stimulated mast cells. *J. Investig. Dermatol.* **2007**, *127*, 906–914. [CrossRef]
72. Baghdadi, M.; Nagao, H.; Yoshiyama, H.; Akiba, H.; Yagita, H.; Dosaka-Akita, H.; Jinushi, M. Combined blockade of TIM-3 and TIM-4 augments cancer vaccine efficacy against established melanomas. *Cancer Immunol. Immunother.* **2013**, *62*, 629–637. [CrossRef]
73. Fourcade, J.; Sun, Z.; Benallaoua, M.; Guillaume, P.; Luescher, I.F.; Sander, C.; Kirkwood, J.M.; Kuchroo, V.; Zarour, H.M. Upregulation of Tim-3 and PD-1 expression is associated with tumor antigen-specific CD8+ T cell dysfunction in melanoma patients. *J. Exp. Med.* **2010**, *207*, 2175–2186. [CrossRef]
74. Wang, J.; Chong, K.K.; Nakamura, Y.; Nguyen, L.; Huang, S.K.; Kuo, C.; Zhang, W.; Yu, H.; Morton, D.L.; Hoon, D.S. B7-H3 associated with tumor progression and epigenetic regulatory activity in cutaneous melanoma. *J. Investig. Dermatol.* **2013**, *133*, 2050–2058. [CrossRef]
75. Lee, Y.H.; Martin-Orozco, N.; Zheng, P.; Li, J.; Zhang, P.; Tan, H.; Park, H.J.; Jeong, M.; Chang, S.H.; Kim, B.S.; et al. Inhibition of the B7-H3 immune checkpoint limits tumor growth by enhancing cytotoxic lymphocyte function. *Cell Res.* **2017**, *27*, 1034–1045. [CrossRef]
76. Hofmeyer, K.A.; Ray, A.; Zang, X. The contrasting role of B7-H3. *Proc. Natl. Acad. Sci. USA* **2008**, *105*, 10277–10278. [CrossRef]
77. Flem-Karlsen, K.; Tekle, C.; Andersson, Y.; Flatmark, K.; Fodstad, O.; Nunes-Xavier, C.E. Immunoregulatory protein B7-H3 promotes growth and decreases sensitivity to therapy in metastatic melanoma cells. *Pigment Cell Melanoma Res.* **2017**, *30*, 467–476. [CrossRef]
78. Dewing, D.; Emmett, M.; Pritchard Jones, R. The roles of angiogenesis in malignant melanoma: Trends in basic science research over the last 100 years. *ISRN Oncol.* **2012**, *2012*, 546927. [CrossRef]
79. Hodi, F.S.; Lawrence, D.; Lezcano, C.; Wu, X.; Zhou, J.; Sasada, T.; Zeng, W.; Giobbie-Hurder, A.; Atkins, M.B.; Ibrahim, N.; et al. Bevacizumab plus ipilimumab in patients with metastatic melanoma. *Cancer Immunol. Res.* **2014**, *2*, 632–642. [CrossRef]
80. Del Vecchio, M.; Mortarini, R.; Canova, S.; Di Guardo, L.; Pimpinelli, N.; Sertoli, M.R.; Bedognetti, D.; Queirolo, P.; Morosini, P.; Perrone, T.; et al. Bevacizumab plus fotemustine as first-line treatment in metastatic melanoma patients: clinical activity and modulation of angiogenesis and lymphangiogenesis factors. *Clin. Cancer Res.* **2010**, *16*, 5862–5872. [CrossRef]
81. von Moos, R.; Seifert, B.; Simcock, M.; Goldinger, S.M.; Gillessen, S.; Ochsenbein, A.; Michielin, O.; Cathomas, R.; Schlappi, M.; Moch, H.; et al. First-line temozolomide combined with bevacizumab in metastatic melanoma: a multicentre phase II trial (SAKK 50/07). *Ann. Oncol.* **2012**, *23*, 531–536. [CrossRef]
82. Corrie, P.G.; Marshall, A.; Nathan, P.D.; Lorigan, P.; Gore, M.; Tahir, S.; Faust, G.; Kelly, C.G.; Marples, M.; Danson, S.J.; et al. Adjuvant bevacizumab for melanoma patients at high risk of recurrence: survival analysis of the AVAST-M trial. *Ann. Oncol.* **2018**, *29*, 1843–1852. [CrossRef]
83. Hodi, F.S.; Mihm, M.C.; Soiffer, R.J.; Haluska, F.G.; Butler, M.; Seiden, M.V.; Davis, T.; Henry-Spires, R.; MacRae, S.; Willman, A.; et al. Biologic activity of cytotoxic T lymphocyte-associated antigen 4 antibody blockade in previously vaccinated metastatic melanoma and ovarian carcinoma patients. *Proc. Natl. Acad. Sci. USA* **2003**, *100*, 4712–4717. [CrossRef]
84. Price, M.A.; Colvin Wanshura, L.E.; Yang, J.; Carlson, J.; Xiang, B.; Li, G.; Ferrone, S.; Dudek, A.Z.; Turley, E.A.; McCarthy, J.B. CSPG4, a potential therapeutic target, facilitates malignant progression of melanoma. *Pigment Cell Melanoma Res.* **2011**, *24*, 1148–1157. [CrossRef]
85. Ilieva, K.M.; Cheung, A.; Mele, S.; Chiaruttini, G.; Crescioli, S.; Griffin, M.; Nakamura, M.; Spicer, J.F.; Tsoka, S.; Lacy, K.E.; et al. Chondroitin sulfate proteoglycan 4 and its potential as an antibody immunotherapy target across different tumor types. *Front. Immunol.* **2017**, *8*, 1911. [CrossRef]
86. Bander, T.S.; Nehal, K.S.; Lee, E.H. Cutaneous Squamous Cell Carcinoma: Updates in Staging and Management. *Dermatol. Clin.* **2019**, *37*, 241–251. [CrossRef]

87. Gandhi, S.A.; Kampp, J. Skin cancer epidemiology, detection, and management. *Med. Clin. N. Am.* **2015**, *99*, 1323–1335. [CrossRef]
88. Sekulic, A.; Migden, M.R.; Basset-Seguin, N.; Garbe, C.; Gesierich, A.; Lao, C.D.; Miller, C.; Mortier, L.; Murrell, D.F.; Hamid, O.; et al. Long-term safety and efficacy of vismodegib in patients with advanced basal cell carcinoma: final update of the pivotal ERIVANCE BCC study. *BMC Cancer* **2017**, *17*, 332. [CrossRef]
89. Fisher, M.S.; Kripke, M.L. Suppressor T lymphocytes control the development of primary skin cancers in ultraviolet-irradiated mice. *Science* **1982**, *216*, 1133–1134. [CrossRef]
90. Chalmers, Z.R.; Connelly, C.F.; Fabrizio, D.; Gay, L.; Ali, S.M.; Ennis, R.; Schrock, A.; Campbell, B.; Shlien, A.; Chmielecki, J.; et al. Analysis of 100,000 human cancer genomes reveals the landscape of tumor mutational burden. *Genome Med.* **2017**, *9*, 34. [CrossRef]
91. Le, D.T.; Durham, J.N.; Smith, K.N.; Wang, H.; Bartlett, B.R.; Aulakh, L.K.; Lu, S.; Kemberling, H.; Wilt, C.; Luber, B.S.; et al. Mismatch repair deficiency predicts response of solid tumors to PD-1 blockade. *Science* **2017**, *357*, 409–413. [CrossRef]
92. Le, D.T.; Uram, J.N.; Wang, H.; Bartlett, B.R.; Kemberling, H.; Eyring, A.D.; Skora, A.D.; Luber, B.S.; Azad, N.S.; Laheru, D.; et al. PD-1 Blockade in tumors with mismatch-repair deficiency. *N. Engl. J. Med.* **2015**, *372*, 2509–2520. [CrossRef]
93. Goodman, A.M.; Kato, S.; Bazhenova, L.; Patel, S.P.; Frampton, G.M.; Miller, V.; Stephens, P.J.; Daniels, G.A.; Kurzrock, R. Tumor mutational burden as an independent predictor of response to Immunotherapy in diverse cancers. *Mol. Cancer* **2017**, *16*, 2598–2608. [CrossRef]
94. Belai, E.B.; de Oliveira, C.E.; Gasparoto, T.H.; Ramos, R.N.; Torres, S.A.; Garlet, G.P.; Cavassani, K.A.; Silva, J.S.; Campanelli, A.P. PD-1 blockage delays murine squamous cell carcinoma development. *Carcinogenesis* **2014**, *35*, 424–431. [CrossRef]
95. Lipson, E.J.; Bagnasco, S.M.; Moore, J., Jr.; Jang, S.; Patel, M.J.; Zachary, A.A.; Pardoll, D.M.; Taube, J.M.; Drake, C.G. Tumor regression and allograft rejection after administration of Anti-PD-1. *N. Engl. J. Med.* **2016**, *374*, 896–898. [CrossRef]
96. Winkler, J.K.; Schneiderbauer, R.; Bender, C.; Sedlaczek, O.; Frohling, S.; Penzel, R.; Enk, A.; Hassel, J.C. Anti-programmed cell death-1 therapy in nonmelanoma skin cancer. *Br. J. Dermatol.* **2017**, *176*, 498–502. [CrossRef]
97. Fischer, S.; Ali, O.H.; Jochum, W.; Kluckert, T.; Flatz, L.; Siano, M. Anti-PD-1 Therapy leads to near-complete remission in a patient with metastatic basal cell carcinoma. *Oncol. Res. Treat.* **2018**, *41*, 391–394. [CrossRef]
98. Lipson, E.J.; Lilo, M.T.; Ogurtsova, A.; Esandrio, J.; Xu, H.; Brothers, P.; Schollenberger, M.; Sharfman, W.H.; Taube, J.M. Basal cell carcinoma: PD-L1/PD-1 checkpoint expression and tumor regression after PD-1 blockade. *J. Immunother. Cancer* **2017**, *5*, 23. [CrossRef]
99. Ikeda, S.; Goodman, A.M.; Cohen, P.R.; Jensen, T.J.; Ellison, C.K.; Frampton, G.; Miller, V.; Patel, S.P.; Kurzrock, R. Metastatic basal cell carcinoma with amplification of PD-L1: exceptional response to anti-PD1 therapy. *NPJ Genom. Med.* **2016**, *1*. [CrossRef]
100. Borradori, L.; Sutton, B.; Shayesteh, P.; Daniels, G.A. Rescue therapy with anti-programmed cell death protein 1 inhibitors of advanced cutaneous squamous cell carcinoma and basosquamous carcinoma: preliminary experience in five cases. *Br. J. Dermatol.* **2016**, *175*, 1382–1386. [CrossRef]
101. Cannon, J.G.D.; Russell, J.S.; Kim, J.; Chang, A.L.S. A case of metastatic basal cell carcinoma treated with continuous PD-1 inhibitor exposure even after subsequent initiation of radiotherapy and surgery. *JAAD Case Rep.* **2018**, *4*, 248–250. [CrossRef]
102. Kudchadkar, R.R.; Yushak, M.L.; Lawson, D.H.; Delman, K.A.; Lowe, M.C.; Goings, M.; McBrien, S.; Mckellar, M.; Sieja, K.; Maynard, N.; et al. Phase II trial of pembrolizumab (MK-3475) in metastatic cutaneous squamous cell carcinoma (cSCC). *J. Clin. Oncol.* **2018**, *36*, 9543. [CrossRef]
103. Chang, A.L.S.; Tran, D.C.; Cannon, J.G.D.; Li, S.; Jeng, M.; Patel, R.; Van der Bokke, L.; Pague, A.; Brotherton, R.; Rieger, K.E.; et al. Pembrolizumab for advanced basal cell carcinoma: An investigator-initiated, proof-of-concept study. *J. Am. Acad. Dermatol.* **2019**, *80*, 564–566. [CrossRef]
104. Falchook, G.S.; Leidner, R.; Stankevich, E.; Piening, B.; Bifulco, C.; Lowy, I.; Fury, M.G. Responses of metastatic basal cell and cutaneous squamous cell carcinomas to anti-PD1 monoclonal antibody REGN2810. *J. Immunother. Cancer* **2016**, *4*, 70. [CrossRef]

105. Migden, M.R.; Rischin, D.; Schmults, C.D.; Guminski, A.; Hauschild, A.; Lewis, K.D.; Chung, C.H.; Hernandez-Aya, L.; Lim, A.M.; Chang, A.L.S.; et al. PD-1 Blockade with Cemiplimab in Advanced Cutaneous Squamous-Cell Carcinoma. *N. Engl. J. Med.* **2018**, *379*, 341–351. [CrossRef]
106. Markham, A.; Duggan, S. Cemiplimab: First Global Approval. *Drugs* **2018**, *78*, 1841–1846. [CrossRef]
107. Khan, M.H.; Alam, M.; Yoo, S. Epidermal growth factor receptor inhibitors in the treatment of nonmelanoma skin cancers. *Dermatol. Surg.* **2011**, *37*, 1199–1209. [CrossRef]
108. Eder, J.; Simonitsch-Klupp, I.; Trautinger, F. Treatment of unresectable squamous cell carcinoma of the skin with epidermal growth factor receptor antibodies—A case series. *Eur. J. Dermatol.* **2013**, *23*, 658–662. [CrossRef]
109. Bauman, J.E.; Eaton, K.D.; Martins, R.G. Treatment of recurrent squamous cell carcinoma of the skin with cetuximab. *Arch. Dermatol.* **2007**, *143*, 889–892. [CrossRef]
110. Seber, S.; Gonultas, A.; Ozturk, O.; Yetisyigit, T. Recurrent squamous cell carcinoma of the skin treated successfully with single agent cetuximab therapy. *OncoTargets* **2016**, *9*, 945–948. [CrossRef]
111. Maubec, E.; Petrow, P.; Scheer-Senyarich, I.; Duvillard, P.; Lacroix, L.; Gelly, J.; Certain, A.; Duval, X.; Crickx, B.; Buffard, V.; et al. Phase II study of cetuximab as first-line single-drug therapy in patients with unresectable squamous cell carcinoma of the skin. *J. Clin. Oncol.* **2011**, *29*, 3419–3426. [CrossRef] [PubMed]
112. Wollina, U. Update of cetuximab for non-melanoma skin cancer. *Expert Opin. Biol.* **2014**, *14*, 271–276. [CrossRef] [PubMed]
113. Kalapurakal, S.J.; Malone, J.; Robbins, K.T.; Buescher, L.; Godwin, J.; Rao, K. Cetuximab in refractory skin cancer treatment. *J. Cancer* **2012**, *3*, 257–261. [CrossRef] [PubMed]
114. Arora, R.; Chang, Y.; Moore, P.S. MCV and Merkel cell carcinoma: a molecular success story. *Curr. Opin. Virol.* **2012**, *2*, 489–498. [CrossRef] [PubMed]
115. Hughes, M.P.; Hardee, M.E.; Cornelius, L.A.; Hutchins, L.F.; Becker, J.C.; Gao, L. Merkel cell carcinoma: Epidemiology, target, and therapy. *Curr. Dermatol. Rep.* **2014**, *3*, 46–53. [CrossRef] [PubMed]
116. Youlden, D.R.; Youl, P.H.; Peter Soyer, H.; Fritschi, L.; Baade, P.D. Multiple primary cancers associated with Merkel cell carcinoma in Queensland, Australia, 1982–2011. *J. Investig. Dermatol.* **2014**, *134*, 2883–2889. [CrossRef] [PubMed]
117. Howard, R.A.; Dores, G.M.; Curtis, R.E.; Anderson, W.F.; Travis, L.B. Merkel cell carcinoma and multiple primary cancers. *Cancer Epidemiol. Biomark. Prev.* **2006**, *15*, 1545–1549. [CrossRef]
118. Engels, E.A.; Frisch, M.; Goedert, J.J.; Biggar, R.J.; Miller, R.W. Merkel cell carcinoma and HIV infection. *Lancet* **2002**, *359*, 497–498. [CrossRef]
119. Buell, J.F.; Trofe, J.; Hanaway, M.J.; Beebe, T.M.; Gross, T.G.; Alloway, R.R.; First, M.R.; Woodle, E.S. Immunosuppression and Merkel cell cancer. *Transpl. Proc.* **2002**, *34*, 1780–1781. [CrossRef]
120. Rotondo, J.C.; Bononi, I.; Puozzo, A.; Govoni, M.; Foschi, V.; Lanza, G.; Gafa, R.; Gaboriaud, P.; Touze, F.A.; Selvatici, R.; et al. Merkel cell carcinomas arising in autoimmune disease affected patients treated with biologic drugs, including Anti-TNF. *Clin. Cancer Res.* **2017**, *23*, 3929–3934. [CrossRef]
121. Iyer, J.G.; Blom, A.; Doumani, R.; Lewis, C.; Tarabadkar, E.S.; Anderson, A.; Ma, C.; Bestick, A.; Parvathaneni, U.; Bhatia, S.; et al. Response rates and durability of chemotherapy among 62 patients with metastatic Merkel cell carcinoma. *Cancer Med.* **2016**, *5*, 2294–2301. [CrossRef]
122. Harms, P.W.; Harms, K.L.; Moore, P.S.; DeCaprio, J.A.; Nghiem, P.; Wong, M.K.K.; Brownell, I.; International workshop on merkel cell carcinoma research working group. The biology and treatment of Merkel cell carcinoma: current understanding and research priorities. *Nat. Rev. Clin. Oncol.* **2018**, *15*, 763–776. [CrossRef]
123. Paulson, K.G.; Iyer, J.G.; Blom, A.; Warton, E.M.; Sokil, M.; Yelistratova, L.; Schuman, L.; Nagase, K.; Bhatia, S.; Asgari, M.M.; et al. Systemic immune suppression predicts diminished Merkel cell carcinoma-specific survival independent of stage. *J. Investig. Dermatol.* **2013**, *133*, 642–646. [CrossRef]
124. Afanasiev, O.K.; Yelistratova, L.; Miller, N.; Nagase, K.; Paulson, K.; Iyer, J.G.; Ibrani, D.; Koelle, D.M.; Nghiem, P. Merkel polyomavirus-specific T cells fluctuate with merkel cell carcinoma burden and express therapeutically targetable PD-1 and Tim-3 exhaustion markers. *Clin. Cancer Res.* **2013**, *19*, 5351–5360. [CrossRef]
125. Nghiem, P.T.; Bhatia, S.; Lipson, E.J.; Kudchadkar, R.R.; Miller, N.J.; Annamalai, L.; Berry, S.; Chartash, E.K.; Daud, A.; Fling, S.P.; et al. PD-1 Blockade with pembrolizumab in advanced merkel-cell carcinoma. *N. Engl. J. Med.* **2016**, *374*, 2542–2552. [CrossRef]

126. Kaufman, H.L.; Russell, J.; Hamid, O.; Bhatia, S.; Terheyden, P.; D'Angelo, S.P.; Shih, K.C.; Lebbe, C.; Linette, G.P.; Milella, M.; et al. Avelumab in patients with chemotherapy-refractory metastatic Merkel cell carcinoma: a multicentre, single-group, open-label, phase 2 trial. *Lancet Oncol.* **2016**, *17*, 1374–1385. [CrossRef]

127. Becker, J.C.; Lorenz, E.; Ugurel, S.; Eigentler, T.K.; Kiecker, F.; Pfohler, C.; Kellner, I.; Meier, F.; Kahler, K.; Mohr, P.; et al. Evaluation of real-world treatment outcomes in patients with distant metastatic Merkel cell carcinoma following second-line chemotherapy in Europe. *Oncotarget* **2017**, *8*, 79731–79741. [CrossRef]

128. Cowey, C.L.; Mahnke, L.; Espirito, J.; Helwig, C.; Oksen, D.; Bharmal, M. Real-world treatment outcomes in patients with metastatic Merkel cell carcinoma treated with chemotherapy in the USA. *Future Oncol.* **2017**, *13*, 1699–1710. [CrossRef]

129. D'Angelo, S.P.; Hunger, M.; Brohl, A.S.; Nghiem, P.; Bhatia, S.; Hamid, O.; Mehnert, J.M.; Terheyden, P.; Shih, K.C.; Brownell, I.; et al. Early objective response to avelumab treatment is associated with improved overall survival in patients with metastatic Merkel cell carcinoma. *Cancer Immunol. Immunother.* **2019**, *68*, 609–618. [CrossRef]

130. Topalian, S.L.; Bhatia, S.; Kudchadkar, R.R.; Amin, A.; Sharfman, W.H.; Lebbe, C.; Delord, J.-P.; Shinohara, M.M.; Baxi, S.S.; Chung, C.H.; et al. Nivolumab (Nivo) as neoadjuvant therapy in patients with resectable Merkel cell carcinoma (MCC) in CheckMate 358. *J. Clin. Oncol.* **2018**, *36*, 9505. [CrossRef]

131. Becker, J.C.; Hassel, J.C.; Menzer, C.; Kähler, K.C.; Eigentler, T.K.; Meier, F.E.; Berking, C.; Gutzmer, R.; Mohr, P.; Kiecker, F.; et al. Adjuvant ipilimumab compared with observation in completely resected Merkel cell carcinoma (ADMEC): A randomized, multicenter DeCOG/ADO study. *J. Clin. Oncol.* **2018**, *36*, 9527. [CrossRef]

132. Slingluff, C.L.; Dasilva, D.; Schwarzenberger, P.; Ricciardi, T.; Macri, M.J.; Ryan, A.; Venhaus, R.R.; Bhardwaj, N. Phase 1/2 study of in situ vaccination with tremelimumab + intravenous (IV) durvalumab + poly-ICLC in patients with select relapsed, advanced cancers with measurable, biopsy-accessible tumors. *J. Clin. Oncol.* **2017**, *35*, TPS3106. [CrossRef]

133. Willemze, R.; Jaffe, E.S.; Burg, G.; Cerroni, L.; Berti, E.; Swerdlow, S.H.; Ralfkiaer, E.; Chimenti, S.; Diaz-Perez, J.L.; Duncan, L.M.; et al. WHO-EORTC classification for cutaneous lymphomas. *Blood* **2005**, *105*, 3768–3785. [CrossRef]

134. Willemze, R.; Cerroni, L.; Kempf, W.; Berti, E.; Facchetti, F.; Swerdlow, S.H.; Jaffe, E.S. The 2018 update of the WHO-EORTC classification for primary cutaneous lymphomas. *Blood* **2019**, *133*, 1703–1714. [CrossRef]

135. Campbell, J.J.; Clark, R.A.; Watanabe, R.; Kupper, T.S. Sezary syndrome and mycosis fungoides arise from distinct T-cell subsets: a biologic rationale for their distinct clinical behaviors. *Blood* **2010**, *116*, 767–771. [CrossRef]

136. Wilcox, R.A. Cutaneous T-cell lymphoma: 2017 update on diagnosis, risk-stratification, and management. *Am. J. Hematol.* **2017**, *92*, 1085–1102. [CrossRef]

137. Scarisbrick, J.J.; Quaglino, P.; Prince, H.M.; Papadavid, E.; Hodak, E.; Bagot, M.; Servitje, O.; Berti, E.; Ortiz-Romero, P.; Stadler, R.; et al. The PROCLIPI international registry of early-stage mycosis fungoides identifies substantial diagnostic delay in most patients. *Br. J. Dermatol.* **2018**. [CrossRef]

138. Scarisbrick, J.J.; Prince, H.M.; Vermeer, M.H.; Quaglino, P.; Horwitz, S.; Porcu, P.; Stadler, R.; Wood, G.S.; Beylot-Barry, M.; Pham-Ledard, A.; et al. Cutaneous lymphoma international consortium study of outcome in advanced stages of mycosis fungoides and sezary syndrome: Effect of specific prognostic markers on survival and development of a prognostic model. *J. Clin. Oncol.* **2015**, *33*, 3766–3773. [CrossRef]

139. Janiga, J.; Kentley, J.; Nabhan, C.; Abdulla, F. Current systemic therapeutic options for advanced mycosis fungoides and Sezary syndrome. *Leuk. Lymphoma* **2018**, *59*, 562–577. [CrossRef]

140. Guenova, E.; Hoetzenecker, W.; Rozati, S.; Levesque, M.P.; Dummer, R.; Cozzio, A. Novel therapies for cutaneous T-cell lymphoma: what does the future hold? *Expert. Opin. Investig. Drugs* **2014**, *23*, 457–467. [CrossRef]

141. Saulite, I.; Hoetzenecker, W.; Weidinger, S.; Cozzio, A.; Guenova, E.; Wehkamp, U. Sezary syndrome and atopic dermatitis: Comparison of immunological aspects and targets. *Biomed. Res. Int.* **2016**, *2016*, 9717530. [CrossRef]

142. Photiou, L.; van der Weyden, C.; McCormack, C.; Miles Prince, H. Systemic treatment options for advanced-stage mycosis fungoides and sezary syndrome. *Curr. Oncol. Rep.* **2018**, *20*, 32. [CrossRef]

143. Buggins, A.G.; Mufti, G.J.; Salisbury, J.; Codd, J.; Westwood, N.; Arno, M.; Fishlock, K.; Pagliuca, A.; Devereux, S. Peripheral blood but not tissue dendritic cells express CD52 and are depleted by treatment with alemtuzumab. *Blood* **2002**, *100*, 1715–1720.
144. Clark, R.A.; Watanabe, R.; Teague, J.E.; Schlapbach, C.; Tawa, M.C.; Adams, N.; Dorosario, A.A.; Chaney, K.S.; Cutler, C.S.; Leboeuf, N.R.; et al. Skin effector memory T cells do not recirculate and provide immune protection in alemtuzumab-treated CTCL patients. *Sci. Transl. Med.* **2012**, *4*, 117ra117. [CrossRef]
145. Watanabe, R.; Teague, J.E.; Fisher, D.C.; Kupper, T.S.; Clark, R.A. Alemtuzumab therapy for leukemic cutaneous T-cell lymphoma: diffuse erythema as a positive predictor of complete remission. *JAMA Dermatol.* **2014**, *150*, 776–779. [CrossRef]
146. Grover, N.S.; Savoldo, B. Challenges of driving CD30-directed CAR-T cells to the clinic. *BMC Cancer* **2019**, *19*, 203. [CrossRef]
147. Ansell, S.M. Brentuximab vedotin. *Blood* **2014**, *124*, 3197–3200. [CrossRef]
148. Ansell, S.M. Brentuximab vedotin: delivering an antimitotic drug to activated lymphoma cells. *Expert. Opin. Investig. Drugs* **2011**, *20*, 99–105. [CrossRef]
149. Prince, H.M.; Gautam, A.; Kim, Y.H. Brentuximab vedotin: targeting CD30 as standard in CTCL. *Oncotarget* **2018**, *9*, 11887–11888. [CrossRef]
150. Prince, H.M.; Kim, Y.H.; Horwitz, S.M.; Dummer, R.; Scarisbrick, J.; Quaglino, P.; Zinzani, P.L.; Wolter, P.; Sanches, J.A.; Ortiz-Romero, P.L.; et al. Brentuximab vedotin or physician's choice in CD30-positive cutaneous T-cell lymphoma (ALCANZA): an international, open-label, randomised, phase 3, multicentre trial. *Lancet* **2017**, *390*, 555–566. [CrossRef]
151. Lewis, D.J.; Talpur, R.; Huen, A.O.; Tetzlaff, M.T.; Duvic, M. Brentuximab vedotin for patients with refractory lymphomatoid papulosis: An analysis of phase 2 results. *JAMA Dermatol.* **2017**, *153*, 1302–1306. [CrossRef]
152. Duvic, M.; Tetzlaff, M.T.; Gangar, P.; Clos, A.L.; Sui, D.; Talpur, R. Results of a phase II trial of brentuximab vedotin for CD30+ cutaneous T-cell lymphoma and lymphomatoid papulosis. *J. Clin. Oncol.* **2015**, *33*, 3759–3765. [CrossRef]
153. Poon, L.M.; Kwong, Y.L. Complete remission of refractory disseminated NK/T cell lymphoma with brentuximab vedotin and bendamustine. *Ann. Hematol.* **2016**, *95*, 847–849. [CrossRef]
154. Horwitz, S.M.; Advani, R.H.; Bartlett, N.L.; Jacobsen, E.D.; Sharman, J.P.; O'Connor, O.A.; Siddiqi, T.; Kennedy, D.A.; Oki, Y. Objective responses in relapsed T-cell lymphomas with single-agent brentuximab vedotin. *Blood* **2014**, *123*, 3095–3100. [CrossRef]
155. Ferenczi, K.; Fuhlbrigge, R.C.; Pinkus, J.; Pinkus, G.S.; Kupper, T.S. Increased CCR4 expression in cutaneous T cell lymphoma. *J. Investig. Dermatol.* **2002**, *119*, 1405–1410. [CrossRef]
156. Ishida, T.; Utsunomiya, A.; Iida, S.; Inagaki, H.; Takatsuka, Y.; Kusumoto, S.; Takeuchi, G.; Shimizu, S.; Ito, M.; Komatsu, H.; et al. Clinical significance of CCR4 expression in adult T-cell leukemia/lymphoma: its close association with skin involvement and unfavorable outcome. *Clin. Cancer Res.* **2003**, *9*, 3625–3634.
157. Shinkawa, T.; Nakamura, K.; Yamane, N.; Shoji-Hosaka, E.; Kanda, Y.; Sakurada, M.; Uchida, K.; Anazawa, H.; Satoh, M.; Yamasaki, M.; et al. The absence of fucose but not the presence of galactose or bisecting N-acetylglucosamine of human IgG1 complex-type oligosaccharides shows the critical role of enhancing antibody-dependent cellular cytotoxicity. *J. Biol. Chem.* **2003**, *278*, 3466–3473. [CrossRef]
158. Kim, Y.H.; Bagot, M.; Pinter-Brown, L.; Rook, A.H.; Porcu, P.; Horwitz, S.M.; Whittaker, S.; Tokura, Y.; Vermeer, M.; Zinzani, P.L.; et al. Mogamulizumab versus vorinostat in previously treated cutaneous T-cell lymphoma (MAVORIC): an international, open-label, randomised, controlled phase 3 trial. *Lancet Oncol.* **2018**, *19*, 1192–1204. [CrossRef]
159. Suzuki, Y.; Saito, M.; Ishii, T.; Urakawa, I.; Matsumoto, A.; Masaki, A.; Ito, A.; Kusumoto, S.; Suzuki, S.; Hiura, M.; et al. Mogamulizumab treatment elicits autoantibodies attacking the skin in patients with adult T cell leukemia-lymphoma. *Clin Cancer Res.* **2019**. [CrossRef]
160. Honda, T.; Hishizawa, M.; Kataoka, T.R.; Ohmori, K.; Takaori-Kondo, A.; Miyachi, Y.; Kabashima, K. Stevens-Johnson syndrome associated with mogamulizumab-induced deficiency of regulatory T cells in an adult T-cell leukaemia Patient. *Acta Dermatol. Venereol.* **2015**, *95*, 606–607. [CrossRef]
161. Ishida, T.; Ito, A.; Sato, F.; Kusumoto, S.; Iida, S.; Inagaki, H.; Morita, A.; Akinaga, S.; Ueda, R. Stevens-Johnson Syndrome associated with mogamulizumab treatment of adult T-cell leukemia/lymphoma. *Cancer Sci.* **2013**, *104*, 647–650. [CrossRef]

162. Bonnet, P.; Battistella, M.; Roelens, M.; Ram-Wolff, C.; Herms, F.; Frumholtz, L.; Bouaziz, J.D.; Brice, P.; Moins-Teisserenc, H.; Bagot, M.; et al. Association of autoimmunity and long-term complete remission in patients with Sezary syndrome treated with mogamulizumab. *Br. J. Dermatol.* **2019**, *180*, 419–420. [CrossRef]
163. Hosoi, H.; Mushino, T.; Nishikawa, A.; Hashimoto, H.; Murata, S.; Hatanaka, K.; Tamura, S.; Hanaoka, N.; Shimizu, N.; Sonoki, T. Severe graft-versus-host disease after allogeneic hematopoietic stem cell transplantation with residual mogamulizumab concentration. *Int. J. Hematol.* **2018**, *107*, 717–719. [CrossRef]
164. Fuji, S.; Inoue, Y.; Utsunomiya, A.; Moriuchi, Y.; Uchimaru, K.; Choi, I.; Otsuka, E.; Henzan, H.; Kato, K.; Tomoyose, T.; et al. Pretransplantation anti-CCR4 antibody mogamulizumab against adult T-cell leukemia/lymphoma is associated with significantly increased risks of severe and corticosteroid-refractory graft-versus-host disease, nonrelapse mortality, and overall mortality. *J. Clin. Oncol.* **2016**, *34*, 3426–3433. [CrossRef]
165. Ishida, T.; Jo, T.; Takemoto, S.; Suzushima, H.; Suehiro, Y.; Choi, I.; Yoshimitsu, M.; Saburi, Y.; Nosaka, K.; Utsunomiya, A.; et al. Follow-up of a randomised phase II study of chemotherapy alone or in combination with mogamulizumab in newly diagnosed aggressive adult T-cell leukaemia-lymphoma: impact on allogeneic haematopoietic stem cell transplantation. *Br. J. Haematol.* **2019**, *184*, 479–483. [CrossRef]
166. Dai, J.; Almazan, T.H.; Hong, E.K.; Khodadoust, M.S.; Arai, S.; Weng, W.K.; Kim, Y.H. Potential association of anti-CCR4 antibody mogamulizumab and graft-vs-host disease in patients with mycosis fungoides and sezary syndrome. *JAMA Dermatol.* **2018**, *154*, 728–730. [CrossRef]
167. Fuji, S.; Shindo, T. Friend or foe? Mogamulizumab in allogeneic hematopoietic stem cell transplantation for adult T-cell leukemia/lymphoma. *Stem Cell Investig.* **2016**, *3*, 70. [CrossRef]
168. Schmitt, C.; Marie-Cardine, A.; Bensussan, A. Therapeutic Antibodies to KIR3DL2 and Other Target Antigens on Cutaneous T-Cell Lymphomas. *Front. Immunol.* **2017**, *8*, 1010. [CrossRef]
169. Battistella, M.; Leboeuf, C.; Ram-Wolff, C.; Hurabielle, C.; Bonnafous, C.; Sicard, H.; Bensussan, A.; Bagot, M.; Janin, A. KIR3DL2 expression in cutaneous T-cell lymphomas: expanding the spectrum for KIR3DL2 targeting. *Blood* **2017**, *130*, 2900–2902. [CrossRef]
170. Hurabielle, C.; Thonnart, N.; Ram-Wolff, C.; Sicard, H.; Bensussan, A.; Bagot, M.; Marie-Cardine, A. Usefulness of KIR3DL2 to diagnose, follow-up, and manage the treatment of patients with Sezary syndrome. *Clin. Cancer Res.* **2017**, *23*, 3619–3627. [CrossRef]
171. Sicard, H.; Bonnafous, C.; Morel, A.; Bagot, M.; Bensussan, A.; Marie-Cardine, A. A novel targeted immunotherapy for CTCL is on its way: Anti-KIR3DL2 mAb IPH4102 is potent and safe in non-clinical studies. *Oncoimmunology* **2015**, *4*, e1022306. [CrossRef] [PubMed]
172. Marie-Cardine, A.; Viaud, N.; Thonnart, N.; Joly, R.; Chanteux, S.; Gauthier, L.; Bonnafous, C.; Rossi, B.; Blery, M.; Paturel, C.; et al. IPH4102, a humanized KIR3DL2 antibody with potent activity against cutaneous T-cell lymphoma. *Cancer Res.* **2014**, *74*, 6060–6070. [CrossRef] [PubMed]
173. Bagot, M.; Porcu, P.; Marie-Cardine, A.; Battistella, M.; William, B.M.; Whittaker, S.; Rotolo, F.; Ram-Wolff, C.; Khodadoust, M.S.; et al. IPH4102, a first-in-class anti-KIR3DL2 monoclonal antibody, in patients with relapsed or refractory cutaneous T-cell lymphoma: an international, first-in-human, open-label, phase 1 trial. *Lancet Oncol.* **2019**. [CrossRef]
174. Samimi, S.; Benoit, B.; Evans, K.; Wherry, E.J.; Showe, L.; Wysocka, M.; Rook, A.H. Increased programmed death-1 expression on CD4+ T cells in cutaneous T-cell lymphoma: implications for immune suppression. *Arch. Dermatol.* **2010**, *146*, 1382–1388. [CrossRef] [PubMed]
175. Cetinozman, F.; Jansen, P.M.; Vermeer, M.H.; Willemze, R. Differential expression of programmed death-1 (PD-1) in Sezary syndrome and mycosis fungoides. *Arch. Dermatol.* **2012**, *148*, 1379–1385. [CrossRef] [PubMed]
176. Wada, D.A.; Wilcox, R.A.; Harrington, S.M.; Kwon, E.D.; Ansell, S.M.; Comfere, N.I. Programmed death 1 is expressed in cutaneous infiltrates of mycosis fungoides and Sezary syndrome. *Am. J. Hematol.* **2011**, *86*, 325–327. [CrossRef] [PubMed]
177. Guenova, E.; Watanabe, R.; Teague, J.E.; Desimone, J.A.; Jiang, Y.; Dowlatshahi, M.; Schlapbach, C.; Schaekel, K.; Rook, A.H.; Tawa, M.; et al. TH2 cytokines from malignant cells suppress TH1 responses and enforce a global TH2 bias in leukemic cutaneous T-cell lymphoma. *Clin. Cancer Res.* **2013**, *19*, 3755–3763. [CrossRef]
178. Rubio Gonzalez, B.; Zain, J.; Rosen, S.T.; Querfeld, C. Tumor microenvironment in mycosis fungoides and Sezary syndrome. *Curr. Opin. Oncol.* **2016**, *28*, 88–96. [CrossRef]

179. Torrealba, M.P.; Manfrere, K.C.; Miyashiro, D.R.; Lima, J.F.; de, M.O.L.; Pereira, N.Z.; Cury-Martins, J.; Pereira, J.; Duarte, A.J.S.; Sato, M.N.; et al. Chronic activation profile of circulating CD8+ T cells in Sezary syndrome. *Oncotarget* **2018**, *9*, 3497–3506. [CrossRef]
180. Querfeld, C.; Leung, S.; Myskowski, P.L.; Curran, S.A.; Goldman, D.A.; Heller, G.; Wu, X.; Kil, S.H.; Sharma, S.; Finn, K.J.; et al. Primary T cells from cutaneous T-cell lymphoma skin explants display an exhausted immune checkpoint profile. *Cancer Immunol. Res.* **2018**, *6*, 900–909. [CrossRef]
181. Pauken, K.E.; Wherry, E.J. Overcoming T cell exhaustion in infection and cancer. *Trends Immunol.* **2015**, *36*, 265–276. [CrossRef]
182. Dulos, J.; Carven, G.J.; van Boxtel, S.J.; Evers, S.; Driessen-Engels, L.J.; Hobo, W.; Gorecka, M.A.; de Haan, A.F.; Mulders, P.; Punt, C.J.; et al. PD-1 blockade augments Th1 and Th17 and suppresses Th2 responses in peripheral blood from patients with prostate and advanced melanoma cancer. *J. Immunother.* **2012**, *35*, 169–178. [CrossRef] [PubMed]
183. Khodadoust, M.; Rook, A.H.; Porcu, P.; Foss, F.M.; Moskowitz, A.J.; Shustov, A.R.; Shanbhag, S.; Sokol, L.; Shine, R.; Fling, S.P.; et al. Pembrolizumab for treatment of relapsed/refractory mycosis fungoides and Sezary syndrome: Clinical efficacy in a Citn multicenter phase 2 study. *Blood* **2016**, *128*, 181.
184. Khodadoust, M.S.; Rook, A.; Porcu, P.; Foss, F.M.; Moskowitz, A.J.; Shustov, A.R.; Shanbhag, S.; Sokol, L.; Fling, S.P.; Li, S.; et al. Durable responses with pembrolizumab in relapsed/refractory mycosis fungoides and Sézary syndrome: Final results from a phase 2 multicenter study. *Blood* **2018**, *132*, 2896. [CrossRef]
185. Wartewig, T.; Kurgyis, Z.; Keppler, S.; Pechloff, K.; Hameister, E.; Ollinger, R.; Maresch, R.; Buch, T.; Steiger, K.; Winter, C.; et al. PD-1 is a haploinsufficient suppressor of T cell lymphomagenesis. *Nature* **2017**, *552*, 121–125. [CrossRef] [PubMed]
186. Wilcox, R.A.; Feldman, A.L.; Wada, D.A.; Yang, Z.Z.; Comfere, N.I.; Dong, H.; Kwon, E.D.; Novak, A.J.; Markovic, S.N.; Pittelkow, M.R.; et al. B7-H1 (PD-L1, CD274) suppresses host immunity in T-cell lymphoproliferative disorders. *Blood* **2009**, *114*, 2149–2158. [CrossRef] [PubMed]
187. Wong, H.K.; Wilson, A.J.; Gibson, H.M.; Hafner, M.S.; Hedgcock, C.J.; Berger, C.L.; Edelson, R.L.; Lim, H.W. Increased expression of CTLA-4 in malignant T-cells from patients with mycosis fungoides – cutaneous T cell lymphoma. *J. Investig. Dermatol.* **2006**, *126*, 212–219. [CrossRef] [PubMed]
188. Anzengruber, F.; Ignatova, D.; Schlaepfer, T.; Chang, Y.T.; French, L.E.; Pascolo, S.; Contassot, E.; Bobrowicz, M.; Hoetzenecker, W.; Guenova, E. Divergent LAG-3 versus BTLA, TIGIT, and FCRL3 expression in Sezary syndrome. *Leuk. Lymphoma* **2019**, 1–9. [CrossRef]
189. Ansell, S.; Gutierrez, M.E.; Shipp, M.A.; Gladstone, D.; Moskowitz, A.; Borello, I.; Popa-Mckiver, M.; Farsaci, B.; Zhu, L.; Lesokhin, A.M.; et al. A phase 1 study of nivolumab in combination with ipilimumab for relapsed or refractory hematologic malignancies (CheckMate 039). *Blood* **2016**, *128*, 183.
190. Matlung, H.L.; Szilagyi, K.; Barclay, N.A.; van den Berg, T.K. The CD47-SIRPalpha signaling axis as an innate immune checkpoint in cancer. *Immunol. Rev.* **2017**, *276*, 145–164. [CrossRef]
191. Huang, Y.; Ma, Y.; Gao, P.; Yao, Z. Targeting CD47: the achievements and concerns of current studies on cancer immunotherapy. *J. Thorac. Dis.* **2017**, *9*, E168–E174. [CrossRef] [PubMed]
192. Jaiswal, S.; Jamieson, C.H.; Pang, W.W.; Park, C.Y.; Chao, M.P.; Majeti, R.; Traver, D.; van Rooijen, N.; Weissman, I.L. CD47 is upregulated on circulating hematopoietic stem cells and leukemia cells to avoid phagocytosis. *Cell* **2009**, *138*, 271–285. [CrossRef]
193. Majeti, R.; Chao, M.P.; Alizadeh, A.A.; Pang, W.W.; Jaiswal, S.; Gibbs, K.D., Jr.; van Rooijen, N.; Weissman, I.L. CD47 is an adverse prognostic factor and therapeutic antibody target on human acute myeloid leukemia stem cells. *Cell* **2009**, *138*, 286–299. [CrossRef] [PubMed]
194. Willingham, S.B.; Volkmer, J.P.; Gentles, A.J.; Sahoo, D.; Dalerba, P.; Mitra, S.S.; Wang, J.; Contreras-Trujillo, H.; Martin, R.; Cohen, J.D.; et al. The CD47-signal regulatory protein alpha (SIRPa) interaction is a therapeutic target for human solid tumors. *Proc. Natl. Acad. Sci. USA* **2012**, *109*, 6662–6667. [CrossRef] [PubMed]
195. Johnson, L.D.S.; Banerjee, S.; Kruglov, O.; Viller, N.N.; Horwitz, S.M.; Lesokhin, A.; Zain, J.; Querfeld, C.; Chen, R.; Okada, C.; et al. Targeting CD47 in Sezary syndrome with SIRPalphaFc. *Blood Adv.* **2019**, *3*, 1145–1153. [CrossRef]
196. Weiskopf, K. Cancer immunotherapy targeting the CD47/SIRPalpha axis. *Eur. J. Cancer* **2017**, *76*, 100–109. [CrossRef] [PubMed]

197. Querfeld, C.; Thompson, J.; Taylor, M.; Pillai, R.; Johnson, L.D.; Catalano, T.; Petrova, P.S.; Uger, R.A.; Irwin, M.; Sievers, E.L.; et al. A single direct intratumoral injection of TTI-621 (SIRPαFc) induces antitumor activity in patients with relapsed/refractory mycosis fungoides and Sézary syndrome: Preliminary findings employing an immune checkpoint inhibitor blocking the CD47 "Do Not Eat" signal. *Blood* **2017**, *130*, 4076.
198. Folkes, A.S.; Feng, M.; Zain, J.M.; Abdulla, F.; Rosen, S.T.; Querfeld, C. Targeting CD47 as a cancer therapeutic strategy: the cutaneous T-cell lymphoma experience. *Curr. Opin. Oncol.* **2018**, *30*, 332–337. [CrossRef]
199. Varricchi, G.; Marone, G.; Mercurio, V.; Galdiero, M.R.; Bonaduce, D.; Tocchetti, C.G. Immune checkpoint inhibitors and cardiac toxicity: An emerging issue. *Curr. Med. Chem.* **2018**, *25*, 1327–1339. [CrossRef]
200. Wilcox, R.A. Cutaneous B-cell lymphomas: 2019 update on diagnosis, risk stratification, and management. *Am. J. Hematol.* **2018**, *93*, 1427–1430. [CrossRef]
201. Senff, N.J.; Noordijk, E.M.; Kim, Y.H.; Bagot, M.; Berti, E.; Cerroni, L.; Dummer, R.; Duvic, M.; Hoppe, R.T.; Pimpinelli, N.; et al. European Organization for Research and Treatment of Cancer and International Society for Cutaneous Lymphoma consensus recommendations for the management of cutaneous B-cell lymphomas. *Blood* **2008**, *112*, 1600–1609. [CrossRef] [PubMed]
202. Trautinger, F.; Eder, J.; Assaf, C.; Bagot, M.; Cozzio, A.; Dummer, R.; Gniadecki, R.; Klemke, C.D.; Ortiz-Romero, P.L.; Papadavid, E.; et al. European Organisation for Research and Treatment of Cancer consensus recommendations for the treatment of mycosis fungoides/Sezary syndrome—Update 2017. *Eur. J. Cancer* **2017**, *77*, 57–74. [CrossRef] [PubMed]
203. Willemze, R.; Hodak, E.; Zinzani, P.L.; Specht, L.; Ladetto, M.; Committee, E.G. Primary cutaneous lymphomas: ESMO Clinical Practice Guidelines for diagnosis, treatment and follow-up. *Ann. Oncol.* **2018**, *29*, iv30–iv40. [CrossRef] [PubMed]
204. Fernandez-Guarino, M.; Ortiz-Romero, P.L.; Fernandez-Misa, R.; Montalban, C. Rituximab in the treatment of primary cutaneous B-cell lymphoma: A review. *Actas Dermosifiliogr.* **2014**, *105*, 438–445. [CrossRef] [PubMed]
205. Penate, Y.; Hernandez-Machin, B.; Perez-Mendez, L.I.; Santiago, F.; Rosales, B.; Servitje, O.; Estrach, T.; Fernandez-Guarino, M.; Calzado, L.; Acebo, E.; et al. Intralesional rituximab in the treatment of indolent primary cutaneous B-cell lymphomas: an epidemiological observational multicentre study. The Spanish Working Group on Cutaneous Lymphoma. *Br. J. Dermatol.* **2012**, *167*, 174–179. [CrossRef] [PubMed]
206. Vakeva, L.; Ranki, A.; Malkonen, T. Intralesional rituximab treatment for primary cutaneous B-cell lymphoma: Nine finnish cases. *Acta Dermatol. Venereol.* **2016**, *96*, 396–397. [CrossRef] [PubMed]
207. Seto, T.; Sam, D.; Pan, M. Mechanisms of primary and secondary resistance to immune checkpoint inhibitors in cancer. *Med. Sci.* **2019**, *7*, 14. [CrossRef]
208. Jenkins, R.W.; Barbie, D.A.; Flaherty, K.T. Mechanisms of resistance to immune checkpoint inhibitors. *Br. J. Cancer* **2018**, *118*, 9–16. [CrossRef]
209. Gide, T.N.; Wilmott, J.S.; Scolyer, R.A.; Long, G.V. Primary and acquired resistance to immune checkpoint inhibitors in metastatic melanoma. *Clin. Cancer Res.* **2018**, *24*, 1260–1270. [CrossRef]
210. Hugo, W.; Zaretsky, J.M.; Sun, L.; Song, C.; Moreno, B.H.; Hu-Lieskovan, S.; Berent-Maoz, B.; Pang, J.; Chmielowski, B.; Cherry, G.; et al. Genomic and transcriptomic features of response to anti-PD-1 Therapy in metastatic melanoma. *Cell* **2017**, *168*, 542. [CrossRef]
211. Bhatt, A.P.; Redinbo, M.R.; Bultman, S.J. The role of the microbiome in cancer development and therapy. *CA Cancer J. Clin.* **2017**, *67*, 326–344. [CrossRef] [PubMed]
212. Wargo, J.A.; Gopalakrishnan, V.; Spencer, C.; Karpinets, T.; Reuben, A.; Andrews, M.C.; Tetzlaff, M.T.; Lazar, A.; Hwu, P.; Hwu, W.-J.; et al. Association of the diversity and composition of the gut microbiome with responses and survival (PFS) in metastatic melanoma (MM) patients (pts) on anti-PD-1 therapy. *J. Clin. Oncol.* **2017**, *35*, 3008. [CrossRef]
213. Sivan, A.; Corrales, L.; Hubert, N.; Williams, J.B.; Aquino-Michaels, K.; Earley, Z.M.; Benyamin, F.W.; Lei, Y.M.; Jabri, B.; Alegre, M.L.; et al. Commensal bifidobacterium promotes antitumor immunity and facilitates anti-PD-L1 efficacy. *Science* **2015**, *350*, 1084–1089. [CrossRef] [PubMed]
214. Matson, V.; Fessler, J.; Bao, R.; Chongsuwat, T.; Zha, Y.; Alegre, M.L.; Luke, J.J.; Gajewski, T.F. The commensal microbiome is associated with anti-PD-1 efficacy in metastatic melanoma patients. *Science* **2018**, *359*, 104–108. [CrossRef] [PubMed]

215. Chaput, N.; Lepage, P.; Coutzac, C.; Soularue, E.; Le Roux, K.; Monot, C.; Boselli, L.; Routier, E.; Cassard, L.; Collins, M.; et al. Baseline gut microbiota predicts clinical response and colitis in metastatic melanoma patients treated with ipilimumab. *Ann. Oncol.* **2017**, *28*, 1368–1379. [CrossRef] [PubMed]
216. Vetizou, M.; Pitt, J.M.; Daillere, R.; Lepage, P.; Waldschmitt, N.; Flament, C.; Rusakiewicz, S.; Routy, B.; Roberti, M.P.; Duong, C.P.; et al. Anticancer immunotherapy by CTLA-4 blockade relies on the gut microbiota. *Science* **2015**, *350*, 1079–1084. [CrossRef] [PubMed]
217. Wang, Y.; Ma, R.; Liu, F.; Lee, S.A.; Zhang, L. Modulation of gut microbiota: A novel paradigm of enhancing the efficacy of programmed death-1 and programmed death ligand-1 blockade therapy. *Front. Immunol.* **2018**, *9*, 374. [CrossRef]
218. Koyama, S.; Akbay, E.A.; Li, Y.Y.; Herter-Sprie, G.S.; Buczkowski, K.A.; Richards, W.G.; Gandhi, L.; Redig, A.J.; Rodig, S.J.; Asahina, H.; et al. Adaptive resistance to therapeutic PD-1 blockade is associated with upregulation of alternative immune checkpoints. *Nat. Commun.* **2016**, *7*, 10501. [CrossRef]
219. Zaretsky, J.M.; Garcia-Diaz, A.; Shin, D.S.; Escuin-Ordinas, H.; Hugo, W.; Hu-Lieskovan, S.; Torrejon, D.Y.; Abril-Rodriguez, G.; Sandoval, S.; Barthly, L.; et al. Mutations associated with acquired resistance to PD-1 blockade in melanoma. *N. Engl. J. Med.* **2016**, *375*, 819–829. [CrossRef]
220. Restifo, N.P.; Smyth, M.J.; Snyder, A. Acquired resistance to immunotherapy and future challenges. *Nat. Rev. Cancer* **2016**, *16*, 121–126. [CrossRef]
221. Zimmer, L.; Apuri, S.; Eroglu, Z.; Kottschade, L.A.; Forschner, A.; Gutzmer, R.; Schlaak, M.; Heinzerling, L.; Krackhardt, A.M.; Loquai, C.; et al. Ipilimumab alone or in combination with nivolumab after progression on anti-PD-1 therapy in advanced melanoma. *Eur. J. Cancer* **2017**, *75*, 47–55. [CrossRef] [PubMed]
222. Woo, S.R.; Turnis, M.E.; Goldberg, M.V.; Bankoti, J.; Selby, M.; Nirschl, C.J.; Bettini, M.L.; Gravano, D.M.; Vogel, P.; Liu, C.L.; et al. Immune inhibitory molecules LAG-3 and PD-1 synergistically regulate T-cell function to promote tumoral immune escape. *Cancer Res.* **2012**, *72*, 917–927. [CrossRef] [PubMed]
223. Sakuishi, K.; Apetoh, L.; Sullivan, J.M.; Blazar, B.R.; Kuchroo, V.K.; Anderson, A.C. Targeting Tim-3 and PD-1 pathways to reverse T cell exhaustion and restore anti-tumor immunity. *J. Exp. Med.* **2010**, *207*, 2187–2194. [CrossRef] [PubMed]
224. Kitano, S.; Nakayama, T.; Yamashita, M. Biomarkers for immune checkpoint inhibitors in melanoma. *Front. Oncol.* **2018**, *8*, 270. [CrossRef] [PubMed]
225. Hogan, S.A.; Levesque, M.P.; Cheng, P.F. Melanoma immunotherapy: Next-generation biomarkers. *Front. Oncol.* **2018**, *8*, 178. [CrossRef] [PubMed]
226. Topalian, S.L.; Hodi, F.S.; Brahmer, J.R.; Gettinger, S.N.; Smith, D.C.; McDermott, D.F.; Powderly, J.D.; Carvajal, R.D.; Sosman, J.A.; Atkins, M.B.; et al. Safety, activity, and immune correlates of anti-PD-1 antibody in cancer. *N. Engl. J. Med.* **2012**, *366*, 2443–2454. [CrossRef] [PubMed]
227. Ansell, S.M.; Lesokhin, A.M.; Borrello, I.; Halwani, A.; Scott, E.C.; Gutierrez, M.; Schuster, S.J.; Millenson, M.M.; Cattry, D.; Freeman, G.J.; et al. PD-1 blockade with nivolumab in relapsed or refractory Hodgkin's lymphoma. *N. Engl. J. Med.* **2015**, *372*, 311–319. [CrossRef] [PubMed]
228. Taube, J.M.; Young, G.D.; McMiller, T.L.; Chen, S.; Salas, J.T.; Pritchard, T.S.; Xu, H.; Meeker, A.K.; Fan, J.; Cheadle, C.; et al. Differential expression of immune-regulatory genes associated with PD-L1 display in melanoma: Implications for PD-1 pathway blockade. *Clin. Cancer Res.* **2015**, *21*, 3969–3976. [CrossRef] [PubMed]
229. Nguyen, L.T.; Ohashi, P.S. Clinical blockade of PD1 and LAG3–potential mechanisms of action. *Nat. Rev. Immunol.* **2015**, *15*, 45–56. [CrossRef]
230. Taube, J.M.; Klein, A.; Brahmer, J.R.; Xu, H.; Pan, X.; Kim, J.H.; Chen, L.; Pardoll, D.M.; Topalian, S.L.; Anders, R.A. Association of PD-1, PD-1 ligands, and other features of the tumor immune microenvironment with response to anti-PD-1 therapy. *Clin. Cancer Res.* **2014**, *20*, 5064–5074. [CrossRef]
231. Kollmann, D.; Ignatova, D.; Jedamzik, J.; Chang, Y.T.; Jomrich, G.; Baierl, A.; Kazakov, D.; Michal, M.; French, L.E.; Hoetzenecker, W.; et al. PD-L1 expression is an independent predictor of favorable outcome in patients with localized esophageal adenocarcinoma. *Oncoimmunology* **2018**, *7*, e1435226. [CrossRef] [PubMed]
232. Kaunitz, G.J.; Cottrell, T.R.; Lilo, M.; Muthappan, V.; Esandrio, J.; Berry, S.; Xu, H.; Ogurtsova, A.; Anders, R.A.; Fischer, A.H.; et al. Melanoma subtypes demonstrate distinct PD-L1 expression profiles. *Lab. Investig.* **2017**, *97*, 1063–1071. [CrossRef] [PubMed]

233. Vilain, R.E.; Menzies, A.M.; Wilmott, J.S.; Kakavand, H.; Madore, J.; Guminski, A.; Liniker, E.; Kong, B.Y.; Cooper, A.J.; Howle, J.R.; et al. Dynamic changes in PD-L1 expression and immune infiltrates early during treatment predict response to PD-1 blockade in melanoma. *Clin. Cancer Res.* **2017**, *23*, 5024–5033. [CrossRef] [PubMed]
234. Riaz, N.; Havel, J.J.; Makarov, V.; Desrichard, A.; Urba, W.J.; Sims, J.S.; Hodi, F.S.; Martin-Algarra, S.; Mandal, R.; Sharfman, W.H.; et al. Tumor and microenvironment evolution during immunotherapy with nivolumab. *Cell* **2017**, *171*, 934–949 e916. [CrossRef] [PubMed]
235. Grigg, C.; Rizvi, N.A. PD-L1 biomarker testing for non-small cell lung cancer: truth or fiction? *J. Immunother. Cancer* **2016**, *4*, 48. [CrossRef] [PubMed]
236. Herbst, R.S.; Soria, J.C.; Kowanetz, M.; Fine, G.D.; Hamid, O.; Gordon, M.S.; Sosman, J.A.; McDermott, D.F.; Powderly, J.D.; Gettinger, S.N.; et al. Predictive correlates of response to the anti-PD-L1 antibody MPDL3280A in cancer patients. *Nature* **2014**, *515*, 563–567. [CrossRef] [PubMed]
237. Khunger, M.; Jain, P.; Rakshit, S.; Pasupuleti, V.; Hernandez, A.V.; Stevenson, J.; Pennell, N.A.; Velcheti, V. Safety and efficacy of PD-1/PD-L1 inhibitors in treatment-naive and chemotherapy-refractory patients with non-small-cell lung cancer: A systematic review and meta-analysis. *Clin. Lung Cancer* **2018**, *19*, e335–e348. [CrossRef]
238. Zhou, J.; Mahoney, K.M.; Giobbie-Hurder, A.; Zhao, F.; Lee, S.; Liao, X.; Rodig, S.; Li, J.; Wu, X.; Butterfield, L.H.; et al. Soluble PD-L1 as a biomarker in malignant melanoma treated with checkpoint blockade. *Cancer Immunol. Res.* **2017**, *5*, 480–492. [CrossRef]
239. Chen, G.; Huang, A.C.; Zhang, W.; Zhang, G.; Wu, M.; Xu, W.; Yu, Z.; Yang, J.; Wang, B.; Sun, H.; et al. Exosomal PD-L1 contributes to immunosuppression and is associated with anti-PD-1 response. *Nature* **2018**, *560*, 382–386. [CrossRef]
240. Kaskel, P.; Berking, C.; Sander, S.; Volkenandt, M.; Peter, R.U.; Krahn, G. S-100 protein in peripheral blood: a marker for melanoma metastases: a prospective 2-center study of 570 patients with melanoma. *J. Am. Acad. Dermatol.* **1999**, *41*, 962–969. [CrossRef]
241. Diem, S.; Kasenda, B.; Martin-Liberal, J.; Lee, A.; Chauhan, D.; Gore, M.; Larkin, J. Prognostic score for patients with advanced melanoma treated with ipilimumab. *Eur. J. Cancer* **2015**, *51*, 2785–2791. [CrossRef] [PubMed]
242. Cook, M.B.; McGlynn, K.A.; Devesa, S.S.; Freedman, N.D.; Anderson, W.F. Sex disparities in cancer mortality and survival. *Cancer Epidemiol. Biomark. Prev.* **2011**, *20*, 1629–1637. [CrossRef] [PubMed]
243. Kugel, C.H., 3rd; Douglass, S.M.; Webster, M.R.; Kaur, A.; Liu, Q.; Yin, X.; Weiss, S.A.; Darvishian, F.; Al-Rohil, R.N.; Ndoye, A.; et al. Age correlates with response to Anti-PD1, reflecting age-related differences in intratumoral effector and regulatory T-cell populations. *Clin. Cancer Res.* **2018**, *24*, 5347–5356. [CrossRef] [PubMed]
244. Lauby-Secretan, B.; Scoccianti, C.; Loomis, D.; Grosse, Y.; Bianchini, F.; Straif, K.; International Agency for Research on Cancer Handbook Working Group. Body fatness and cancer—Viewpoint of the IARC working group. *N. Engl. J. Med.* **2016**, *375*, 794–798. [CrossRef] [PubMed]
245. McQuade, J.L.; Daniel, C.R.; Hess, K.R.; Mak, C.; Wang, D.Y.; Rai, R.R.; Park, J.J.; Haydu, L.E.; Spencer, C.; Wongchenko, M.; et al. Association of body-mass index and outcomes in patients with metastatic melanoma treated with targeted therapy, immunotherapy, or chemotherapy: a retrospective, multicohort analysis. *Lancet Oncol.* **2018**, *19*, 310–322. [CrossRef]
246. Tumeh, P.C.; Harview, C.L.; Yearley, J.H.; Shintaku, I.P.; Taylor, E.J.; Robert, L.; Chmielowski, B.; Spasic, M.; Henry, G.; Ciobanu, V.; et al. PD-1 blockade induces responses by inhibiting adaptive immune resistance. *Nature* **2014**, *515*, 568–571. [CrossRef] [PubMed]
247. Sade-Feldman, M.; Yizhak, K.; Bjorgaard, S.L.; Ray, J.P.; de Boer, C.G.; Jenkins, R.W.; Lieb, D.J.; Chen, J.H.; Frederick, D.T.; Barzily-Rokni, M.; et al. Defining T cell states associated with response to checkpoint immunotherapy in melanoma. *Cell* **2019**, *176*, 404. [CrossRef] [PubMed]
248. Takeuchi, Y.; Tanemura, A.; Tada, Y.; Katayama, I.; Kumanogoh, A.; Nishikawa, H. Clinical response to PD-1 blockade correlates with a sub-fraction of peripheral central memory CD4+ T cells in patients with malignant melanoma. *Int. Immunol.* **2018**, *30*, 13–22. [CrossRef] [PubMed]
249. Nonomura, Y.; Otsuka, A.; Nakashima, C.; Seidel, J.A.; Kitoh, A.; Dainichi, T.; Nakajima, S.; Sawada, Y.; Matsushita, S.; Aoki, M.; et al. Peripheral blood Th9 cells are a possible pharmacodynamic biomarker of nivolumab treatment efficacy in metastatic melanoma patients. *Oncoimmunology* **2016**, *5*, e1248327. [CrossRef]

250. Umansky, V.; Blattner, C.; Gebhardt, C.; Utikal, J. The Role of Myeloid-Derived Suppressor Cells (MDSC) in Cancer Progression. *Vaccines* **2016**, *4*, 36. [CrossRef]
251. Meyer, C.; Cagnon, L.; Costa-Nunes, C.M.; Baumgaertner, P.; Montandon, N.; Leyvraz, L.; Michielin, O.; Romano, E.; Speiser, D.E. Frequencies of circulating MDSC correlate with clinical outcome of melanoma patients treated with ipilimumab. *Cancer Immunol. Immunother.* **2014**, *63*, 247–257. [CrossRef] [PubMed]
252. Gebhardt, C.; Sevko, A.; Jiang, H.; Lichtenberger, R.; Reith, M.; Tarnanidis, K.; Holland-Letz, T.; Umansky, L.; Beckhove, P.; Sucker, A.; et al. Myeloid cells and related chronic inflammatory factors as novel predictive markers in melanoma treatment with ipilimumab. *Clin. Cancer Res.* **2015**, *21*, 5453–5459. [CrossRef] [PubMed]
253. Krieg, C.; Nowicka, M.; Guglietta, S.; Schindler, S.; Hartmann, F.J.; Weber, L.M.; Dummer, R.; Robinson, M.D.; Levesque, M.P.; Becher, B. High-dimensional single-cell analysis predicts response to anti-PD-1 immunotherapy. *Nat. Med.* **2018**, *24*, 144–153. [CrossRef] [PubMed]
254. Fassler, M.; Diem, S.; Mangana, J.; Hasan Ali, O.; Berner, F.; Bomze, D.; Ring, S.; Niederer, R.; Del Carmen Gil Cruz, C.; Perez Shibayama, C.I.; et al. Antibodies as biomarker candidates for response and survival to checkpoint inhibitors in melanoma patients. *J. Immunother. Cancer* **2019**, *7*, 50. [CrossRef] [PubMed]
255. Cristescu, R.; Mogg, R.; Ayers, M.; Albright, A.; Murphy, E.; Yearley, J.; Sher, X.; Liu, X.Q.; Lu, H.; Nebozhyn, M.; et al. Pan-tumor genomic biomarkers for PD-1 checkpoint blockade-based immunotherapy. *Science* **2018**, *362*. [CrossRef] [PubMed]
256. Johnson, D.B.; Frampton, G.M.; Rioth, M.J.; Yusko, E.; Xu, Y.; Guo, X.; Ennis, R.C.; Fabrizio, D.; Chalmers, Z.R.; Greenbowe, J.; et al. Targeted next generation sequencing identifies markers of response to PD-1 blockade. *Cancer Immunol. Res.* **2016**, *4*, 959–967. [CrossRef] [PubMed]
257. Johnson, D.B.; Sullivan, R.J.; Ott, P.A.; Carlino, M.S.; Khushalani, N.I.; Ye, F.; Guminski, A.; Puzanov, I.; Lawrence, D.P.; Buchbinder, E.I.; et al. Ipilimumab therapy in patients with advanced melanoma and preexisting autoimmune disorders. *JAMA Oncol.* **2016**, *2*, 234–240. [CrossRef]
258. Tocut, M.; Brenner, R.; Zandman-Goddard, G. Autoimmune phenomena and disease in cancer patients treated with immune checkpoint inhibitors. *Autoimmun. Rev.* **2018**, *17*, 610–616. [CrossRef]
259. Martins, F.; Sofiya, L.; Sykiotis, G.P.; Lamine, F.; Maillard, M.; Fraga, M.; Shabafrouz, K.; Ribi, C.; Cairoli, A.; Guex-Crosier, Y.; et al. Adverse effects of immune-checkpoint inhibitors: epidemiology, management and surveillance. *Nat. Rev. Clin. Oncol* **2019**. [CrossRef]
260. Wang, D.Y.; Johnson, D.B.; Davis, E.J. Toxicities Associated With PD-1/PD-L1 Blockade. *Cancer J.* **2018**, *24*, 36–40. [CrossRef]
261. Haanen, J.; Carbonnel, F.; Robert, C.; Kerr, K.M.; Peters, S.; Larkin, J.; Jordan, K.; Committee, E.G. Management of toxicities from immunotherapy: ESMO Clinical Practice Guidelines for diagnosis, treatment and follow-up. *Ann. Oncol.* **2018**, *29*, iv264–iv266. [CrossRef] [PubMed]
262. Puzanov, I.; Diab, A.; Abdallah, K.; Bingham, C.O., 3rd; Brogdon, C.; Dadu, R.; Hamad, L.; Kim, S.; Lacouture, M.E.; LeBoeuf, N.R.; et al. Managing toxicities associated with immune checkpoint inhibitors: consensus recommendations from the Society for Immunotherapy of Cancer (SITC) Toxicity Management Working Group. *J. Immunother. Cancer* **2017**, *5*, 95. [CrossRef] [PubMed]
263. Wang, D.Y.; Salem, J.E.; Cohen, J.V.; Chandra, S.; Menzer, C.; Ye, F.; Zhao, S.; Das, S.; Beckermann, K.E.; Ha, L.; et al. Fatal toxic effects associated with immune checkpoint inhibitors: A systematic review and meta-analysis. *JAMA Oncol.* **2018**, *4*, 1721–1728. [CrossRef] [PubMed]
264. Hellmann, M.D.; Ciuleanu, T.E.; Pluzanski, A.; Lee, J.S.; Otterson, G.A.; Audigier-Valette, C.; Minenza, E.; Linardou, H.; Burgers, S.; Salman, P.; et al. Nivolumab plus ipilimumab in lung cancer with a high Tumor mutational burden. *N. Engl. J. Med.* **2018**, *378*, 2093–2104. [CrossRef] [PubMed]
265. Boada, A.; Carrera, C.; Segura, S.; Collgros, H.; Pasquali, P.; Bodet, D.; Puig, S.; Malvehy, J. Cutaneous toxicities of new treatments for melanoma. *Clin. Transl. Oncol.* **2018**, *20*, 1373–1384. [CrossRef] [PubMed]
266. Macdonald, J.B.; Macdonald, B.; Golitz, L.E.; LoRusso, P.; Sekulic, A. Cutaneous adverse effects of targeted therapies: Part II: Inhibitors of intracellular molecular signaling pathways. *J. Am. Acad. Dermatol.* **2015**, *72*, 221–236, quiz 237-228. [CrossRef] [PubMed]
267. Minkis, K.; Garden, B.C.; Wu, S.; Pulitzer, M.P.; Lacouture, M.E. The risk of rash associated with ipilimumab in patients with cancer: a systematic review of the literature and meta-analysis. *J. Am. Acad Dermatol.* **2013**, *69*, e121–e128. [CrossRef]

268. Brahmer, J.R.; Tykodi, S.S.; Chow, L.Q.; Hwu, W.J.; Topalian, S.L.; Hwu, P.; Drake, C.G.; Camacho, L.H.; Kauh, J.; Odunsi, K.; et al. Safety and activity of anti-PD-L1 antibody in patients with advanced cancer. *N. Engl. J. Med.* **2012**, *366*, 2455–2465. [CrossRef]

269. Hwang, S.J.; Carlos, G.; Wakade, D.; Byth, K.; Kong, B.Y.; Chou, S.; Carlino, M.S.; Kefford, R.; Fernandez-Penas, P. Cutaneous adverse events (AEs) of anti-programmed cell death (PD)-1 therapy in patients with metastatic melanoma: A single-institution cohort. *J. Am. Acad. Dermatol.* **2016**, *74*, 455–461 e451. [CrossRef]

270. Freeman-Keller, M.; Kim, Y.; Cronin, H.; Richards, A.; Gibney, G.; Weber, J.S. Nivolumab in resected and unresectable metastatic melanoma: Characteristics of immune-related adverse events and association with outcomes. *Clin. Cancer Res.* **2016**, *22*, 886–894. [CrossRef]

271. Nakamura, Y.; Teramoto, Y.; Asami, Y.; Matsuya, T.; Adachi, J.I.; Nishikawa, R.; Yamamoto, A. Nivolumab therapy for treatment-related vitiligo in a patient with relapsed metastatic melanoma. *JAMA Dermatol.* **2017**, *153*, 942–944. [CrossRef] [PubMed]

272. Hua, C.; Boussemart, L.; Mateus, C.; Routier, E.; Boutros, C.; Cazenave, H.; Viollet, R.; Thomas, M.; Roy, S.; Benannoune, N.; et al. Association of vitiligo with tumor response in patients with metastatic melanoma treated with pembrolizumab. *JAMA Dermatol.* **2016**, *152*, 45–51. [CrossRef] [PubMed]

273. Yan, Y.; Kumar, A.B.; Finnes, H.; Markovic, S.N.; Park, S.; Dronca, R.S.; Dong, H. Combining immune checkpoint inhibitors with conventional cancer therapy. *Front. Immunol.* **2018**, *9*, 1739. [CrossRef] [PubMed]

274. Wang, M.; Liu, Y.; Cheng, Y.; Wei, Y.; Wei, X. Immune checkpoint blockade and its combination therapy with small-molecule inhibitors for cancer treatment. *Biochim. Biophys. Acta Rev. Cancer* **2019**, *1871*, 199–224. [CrossRef] [PubMed]

275. Longo, V.; Brunetti, O.; Azzariti, A.; Galetta, D.; Nardulli, P.; Leonetti, F.; Silvestris, N. Strategies to improve cancer immune checkpoint inhibitors efficacy, other than abscopal effect: A systematic review. *Cancers* **2019**, *11*, 539. [CrossRef] [PubMed]

276. Chen, D.S.; Irving, B.A.; Hodi, F.S. Molecular pathways: next-generation immunotherapy–inhibiting programmed death-ligand 1 and programmed death-1. *Clin. Cancer Res.* **2012**, *18*, 6580–6587. [CrossRef] [PubMed]

277. Dahan, R.; Sega, E.; Engelhardt, J.; Selby, M.; Korman, A.J.; Ravetch, J.V. FcgammaRs modulate the anti-tumor activity of antibodies targeting the PD-1/PD-L1 axis. *Cancer Cell* **2015**, *28*, 543. [CrossRef] [PubMed]

278. Goletz, C.; Lischke, T.; Harnack, U.; Schiele, P.; Danielczyk, A.; Ruhmann, J.; Goletz, S. Glyco-engineered anti-human programmed death-ligand 1 antibody mediates stronger CD8 T cell activation than its normal glycosylated and non-glycosylated counterparts. *Front. Immunol.* **2018**, *9*, 1614. [CrossRef]

279. Chen, X.; Song, X.; Li, K.; Zhang, T. FcgammaR-binding is an important functional attribute for immune checkpoint antibodies in cancer immunotherapy. *Front. Immunol.* **2019**, *10*, 292. [CrossRef]

280. Trenevska, I.; Li, D.; Banham, A.H. Therapeutic antibodies against intracellular tumor antigens. *Front. Immunol.* **2017**, *8*, 1001. [CrossRef]

281. Dubrovsky, L.; Dao, T.; Gejman, R.S.; Brea, E.J.; Chang, A.Y.; Oh, C.Y.; Casey, E.; Pankov, D.; Scheinberg, D.A. T cell receptor mimic antibodies for cancer therapy. *Oncoimmunology* **2016**, *5*, e1049803. [CrossRef] [PubMed]

282. Koopmans, I.; Hendriks, M.; van Ginkel, R.J.; Samplonius, D.F.; Bremer, E.; Helfrich, W. Bispecific antibody approach for improved melanoma-selective PD-L1 immune checkpoint blockade. *J. Investig. Dermatol.* **2019**. [CrossRef] [PubMed]

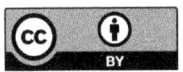

© 2019 by the authors. Licensee MDPI, Basel, Switzerland. This article is an open access article distributed under the terms and conditions of the Creative Commons Attribution (CC BY) license (http://creativecommons.org/licenses/by/4.0/).

MDPI
St. Alban-Anlage 66
4052 Basel
Switzerland
Tel. +41 61 683 77 34
Fax +41 61 302 89 18
www.mdpi.com

Cancers Editorial Office
E-mail: cancers@mdpi.com
www.mdpi.com/journal/cancers

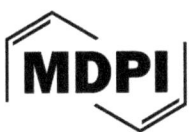

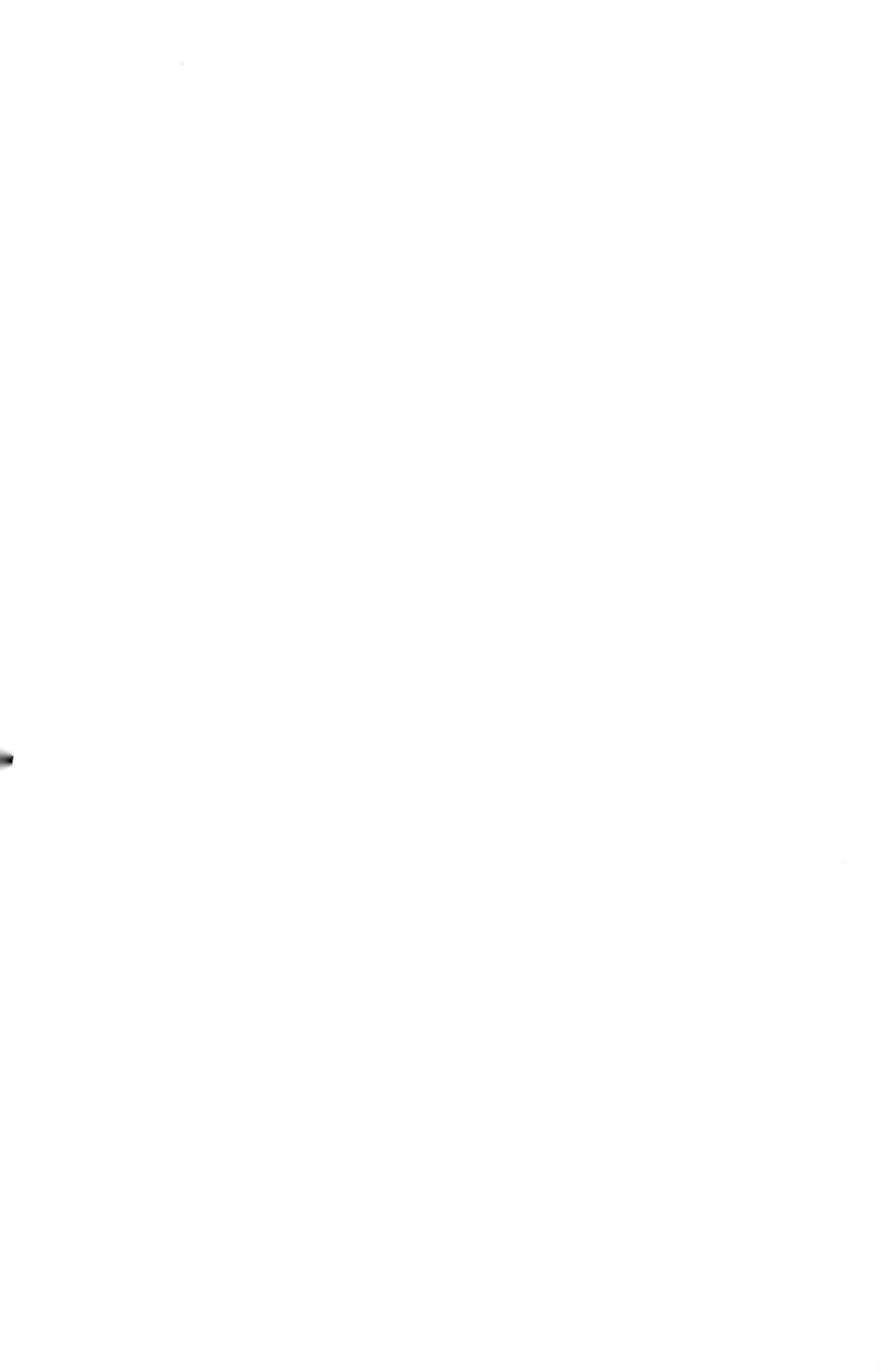

www.ingramcontent.com/pod-product-compliance
Lightning Source LLC
LaVergne TN
LVHW070152100526
838202LV00015B/1939